STUDY GUIDE
to
DSM-5-TR®

STUDY GUIDE
to
DSM-5-TR®

Edited by

Laura Weiss Roberts, M.D., M.A.
Alan K. Louie, M.D.
Matthew L. Edwards, M.D.

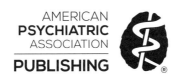

AMERICAN
PSYCHIATRIC
ASSOCIATION
PUBLISHING

Manufactured in the United States of America on acid-free paper
28 27 26 25 24   5 4 3 2 1

American Psychiatric Association Publishing
800 Maine Avenue SW, Suite 900
Washington, D.C. 20024-2812
www.appi.org

Library of Congress Cataloging-in-Publication Data

Names: Roberts, Laura Weiss, 1960- editor. | Louie, Alan K, 1955- editor. | Edwards, Matthew L., editor.
Title: Study guide to DSM-5-TR / edited by Laura Weiss Roberts, Alan K. Louie, Matthew L. Edwards.
Description: First edition. | Washington, D.C. : American Psychiatric Association Publishing, [2025] | Includes bibliographical references and index.
Identifiers: LCCN 2024029121 (print) | LCCN 2024029122 (ebook) | ISBN 9781615375554 (paperback ; alk. paper) | ISBN 9781615375561 (ebook)
Subjects: MESH: Diagnostic and statistical manual of mental disorders (Fifth edition, text revision) | Mental Disorders--diagnosis | Mental Disorders--classification | Diagnosis, Differential | Problems and Exercises | Case Reports
Classification: LCC R (print) | LCC R (ebook) | DDC 616.89001/2--dc23/eng/20240729
LC record available at https://lccn.loc.gov/2024029121
LC ebook record available at https://lccn.loc.gov/2024029122

British Library Cataloguing in Publication Data

A CIP record is available from the British Library.

To my wife and sons.

—Alan K. Louie

To Eric.

—Laura Weiss Roberts

In honor of Annie, and to Felicia, Ashley, and Silas,
with love and gratitude.

—Matthew L. Edwards

Contents

PART 1: Foundations

1 Diagnosis and DSM-5-TR 3

2 Arriving at a Diagnosis
APPLYING DSM-5-TR AND THE CLINICAL
INTERVIEW 17

3 Understanding Different Approaches to
Diagnostic Classification. 31

4 Beyond Diagnostic Classification
STRUCTURAL AND CULTURAL CONSIDERATIONS
AND DSM-5-TR 41

PART 2: DSM-5-TR Diagnostic Categories

5 Neurodevelopmental Disorders. 57

PART 3: Q&A

Contributors

Elias Aboujaoude, M.D., M.A.
Clinical Professor, Department of Psychiatry and Behavioral Sciences, Stanford University School of Medicine, Stanford, California

Bruce A. Arnow, Ph.D.
Professor, Department of Psychiatry and Behavioral Sciences, Stanford University School of Medicine, Stanford, California

Richard Balon, M.D.
Professor, Department of Psychiatry and Behavioral Neurosciences and Department of Anesthesiology, Wayne State University School of Medicine, Detroit, Michigan

Belinda S. Bandstra, M.D., M.A.
Health Sciences Associate Clinical Professor, Department of Psychiatry and Behavioral Sciences, University of California, Davis, School of Medicine, Davis, California

David Beckmann, M.D., M.P.H.
Program Director, Child and Adolescent Psychiatry Fellowship, and Assistant Professor, Department of Psychiatry and Human Behavior, Thomas Jefferson University, Philadelphia, Pennsylvania

Richa Bhatia, M.D.
Clinical Associate Professor, Department of Psychiatry and Behavioral Sciences, Stanford University School of Medicine, Stanford, California

Cara Bohon, Ph.D.
Clinical Associate Professor, Department of Psychiatry and Behavioral Sciences, Stanford University School of Medicine, Stanford, California

Kimberly L. Brodsky, Ph.D.
Staff Psychologist, Department of Psychiatry, Veterans Affairs Palo Alto Health Care System, Palo Alto; Clinical Associate Professor (Affiliated), Department of Psychiatry and Behavioral Sciences, Stanford University School of Medicine, Stanford, California

Christina F. Chick, Ph.D.
Instructor, Department of Psychiatry and Behavioral Sciences, Stanford University School of Medicine, Stanford, California

John H. Coverdale, M.D., M.Ed.
Professor, Department of Psychiatry and Behavioral Sciences, Center for Medical Ethics and Health Policy, Baylor College of Medicine, Houston, Texas

Whitney Daniels, M.D.
Clinical Associate Professor, Department of Psychiatry and Behavioral Sciences, Lucile Packard Children's Hospital, Stanford, California

Jennifer Derenne, M.D.
Clinical Professor, Department of Psychiatry and Behavioral Sciences, Stanford University School of Medicine, Stanford, California

Matthew L. Edwards, M.D.
Assistant Professor and Assistant Director of Residency Training, Department of Psychiatry and Behavioral Sciences, Stanford University School of Medicine, Stanford, California

Tobin J. Ehrlich, Ph.D.
Assistant Professor, Department of Neurology, University of Utah School of Medicine, Salt Lake City, Utah

Adrienne Gerken, M.D.
Director, Residency Program, and Assistant Professor, Department of Psychiatry and Human Behavior, Thomas Jefferson University, Philadelphia, Pennsylvania

Cheryl Gore-Felton, Ph.D.
Associate Dean for Academic Affairs, Stanford University School of Medicine; Walter E. Nichols, M.D. Professor and Senior Associate Chair, Department of Psychiatry and Behavioral Sciences, Stanford University School of Medicine, Stanford, California

Tamar Green, M.D.
Assistant Professor, Department of Psychiatry and Behavioral Sciences, Stanford University School of Medicine, Stanford, California

Thomas W. Heinrich, M.D.
Professor, Department of Psychiatry and Behavioral Medicine, Department of Family and Community Medicine, Department of Internal Medicine (Division of General Internal Medicine), Medical College of Wisconsin, Milwaukee, Wisconsin

Robert M. Holaway, Ph.D.
Assistant Professor, Palo Alto University, Palo Alto, California

David S. Hong, M.D.
Associate Professor, Department of Psychiatry and Behavioral Sciences, Stanford University School of Medicine, Stanford, California

Max Kasun, B.A.
Research Professional, Department of Psychiatry and Behavioral Sciences, Stanford University School of Medicine, Stanford, California

John Lauriello, M.D.
Daniel Lieberman Professor in Psychiatry and Human Behavior; Chair, Department of Psychiatry and Human Behavior; and Senior Vice President, Behavioral Health, Thomas Jefferson University, Philadelphia, Pennsylvania

Alan K. Louie, M.D.
Professor and Associate Chair—Education, Department of Psychiatry and Behavioral Sciences, Stanford University School of Medicine, Stanford, California

Brittany Matheson, Ph.D.
Clinical Assistant Professor, Department of Psychiatry and Behavioral Sciences, Stanford University School of Medicine, Stanford, California

Lucy Ogbu-Nwobodo, M.D., M.S., M.A.S.
Assistant Clinical Professor of Psychiatry, Associate Program Director of Psychiatry Residency Training, Associate Program Director of Public Psychiatry Fellowship, and Director of UCSF Post Baccalaureate and Outreach Programs, Department of Psychiatry and Behavioral Sciences, University of California, San Francisco, School of Medicine, San Francisco, California

Ruth O'Hara, Ph.D.
Senior Associate Dean for Research and Lowell W. and Josephine Q. Berry Professor, Department of Psychiatry and Behavioral Sciences, Stanford University School of Medicine, Stanford, California

Raquel Osorno, Psy.D.
Clinical Assistant Professor, Department of Psychiatry and Behavioral Sciences, Stanford University School of Medicine, Stanford, California

Michael J. Ostacher, M.D., M.P.H., M.M.Sc.
Staff Psychiatrist, Department of Psychiatry, Veterans Affairs Palo Alto Health Care System, Palo Alto; Professor, Department of Psychiatry and Behavioral Sciences, Stanford University School of Medicine, Stanford, California

Jodi Paik, M.F.A.
Editor, Department of Psychiatry and Behavioral Sciences, Stanford University School of Medicine, Stanford, California

Michelle Primeau, M.D.
Medical Director, Department of Sleep Medicine, Palo Alto Medical Foundation, San Carlos, California

Tahir Rahman, M.D.
Associate Professor, Department of Psychiatry, Washington University School of Medicine in St. Louis, St. Louis, Missouri

Daryn Reicherter, M.D.
Clinical Professor, Department of Psychiatry and Behavioral Sciences, Stanford University School of Medicine, Stanford, California

Laura Weiss Roberts, M.D., M.A.
Chairman and Katharine Dexter McCormick and Stanley McCormick Memorial Professor, Department of Psychiatry and Behavioral Sciences, Stanford University School of Medicine, Stanford, California

Willa Roberts, B.A.
Research Professional, Department of Psychiatry and Behavioral Sciences, Stanford University School of Medicine, Stanford, California

Allyson C. Rosen, Ph.D., ABPP-CN
Veterans Affairs Palo Alto Health Care System, Palo Alto, California

Ann C. Schwartz, M.D.
Professor, Department of Psychiatry and Behavioral Sciences, Emory University School of Medicine, Atlanta, Georgia

Daphne Simeon, M.D.
Adjunct Associate Clinical Professor, Department of Psychiatry, Mount Sinai School of Medicine, New York, New York

David Spiegel, M.D.
Willson Professor and Associate Chair of Psychiatry and Behavioral Sciences, Stanford University School of Medicine, Stanford, California

Mickey Trockel, M.D., Ph.D.
Professor, Department of Psychiatry and Behavioral Sciences, Stanford University School of Medicine, Stanford, California

Tonita E. Wroolie, Ph.D.
Clinical Professor, Department of Psychiatry and Behavioral Sciences, Stanford University School of Medicine, Stanford, California

Jerome Yesavage, M.D.
Veterans Affairs Palo Alto Health Care System, Palo Alto, California

Brian Yochim, Ph.D., ABPP-CN
San Francisco Veterans Affairs Medical Center, San Francisco, California

Maya Yutsis, Ph.D., ABPP-CN
Stanford University School of Medicine, Stanford, California

Sanno E. Zack, Ph.D.
Clinical Professor, Department of Psychiatry and Behavioral Sciences, Stanford University School of Medicine, Stanford, California

DISCLOSURES

The following contributors to this book have indicated a financial interest in or other affiliation with a commercial supporter, a manufacturer of a commercial product, a provider of a commercial service, a nongovernmental organization, and/or a government agency, as listed below:

Richa Bhatia, M.D.
Honorarium: Lippicott (section editor, *Current Opinion in Psychiatry*).

Jennifer Derenne, M.D.
Honoraria: Equip Health.

Adrienne Gerken, M.D.
Honorarium: WebMD.

David S. Hong, M.D.
Consultant/Stock: Little Otter, Inc.; ParentLab Inc.

John Lauriello, M.D.
Consultant: Bristol Meyers Squibb; *Employment:* Bristol Meyers Squibb; *Grant/Research Support:* Alkermes, Karuna Therapeutics, Teva.

Michael J. Ostacher, M.D., M.P.H., M.M.Sc.
Committee Chair: Neurocrine: Independent Data Monitoring.

The remaining authors have no competing interests to disclose.

Introduction

The *Diagnostic and Statistical Manual of Mental Disorders* (DSM) is the most widely used manual for assisting in the diagnosis of mental disorders. As such, it has tremendous influence over research, clinical care, education, and public policy relating to these disorders and to how clinicians, patients, families, and the public understand the disorders. Knowledge of and facility with DSM is a necessity for professionals who work with people living with or affected by mental disorders. DSM-5-TR, the text revision of the fifth full edition of this manual, is an essential resource for those training in all fields of physical and mental health. Of note, it is a valued clinical tool when applied in the context of whole people, keeping in mind an individual's ability to adapt, thrive, and engage, and in relation to genetic, biological, psychological, environmental, familial, and cultural considerations.

DSM-5-TR represents a decade of investigation and research since the publication of DSM-5 in 2013. Like its predecessor, DSM-5-TR embodies the tensions between what to keep of the old and what to change with the new—tensions that are natural and expected for all rapidly evolving fields such as psychiatry. Until the next edition, DSM-5-TR will be a key reference point in this evolution for further hypothesis testing and for comparison with other formal schemata with compatible but not identical aims, such as the National Institute of Mental Health's Research Domain Criteria (see www.nimh.nih.gov/research-priorities/rdoc/index.shtml) and the sequential iterations of the World Health Organization's *International Statistical Classification of Diseases and Related Health Problems* (ICD).

DSM-5-TR is the text revision of DSM-5. Revisions include changes to the text, references, diagnostic codes (several ICD-10-CM codes have been updated), and coding notes, as well as adjustments to diagnostic criteria, including some specifiers. Clarifications to diagnostic criteria or specifiers were made for more than 70 disorders. Three new disorders have been added: prolonged grief disorder, unspecified mood disorder, and stimulant-induced mild neurocognitive disorder. Additionally, symptom codes are provided for suicidal behavior and nonsuicidal self-injury in the chapter "Other Conditions That May Be a Focus of Clinical Attention." These codes can be used without any mental disorder diagnosis or can be coded along with a mental disorder diagnosis. Substantive changes to the coding of major and mild neurocognitive disorders went into effect on October 1, 2022. See the "Introduction" in DSM-5-TR for more details about the revisions.

DSM-5-TR includes a chapter for each diagnostic class. Each disorder is listed, and the authors have provided a careful analysis of key disorders within each diagnostic class, including updated epidemiological "statistical" information and evidence-informed criteria that must be met for a diagnosis of that disorder. Cultural consider-ations and associations with suicidality have also been added. The architecture of the text is essentially focused on psychopathology and is disorder-centered. Like DSM-5, the overarching structure of DSM-5-TR differs from previous DSM versions in that di-agnostic classes of disorders with overlapping or similar features have been placed, wherever possible, in an intentional sequence. Please note that, due to space consid-erations, the full diagnostic criteria for disorders have not been included in this *Study Guide*, and readers are referred to DSM-5-TR for this information. Our book serves as a resource for study and focuses on how to understand and apply DSM-5-TR.

We encourage our readers to consider DSM-5-TR as a resource for understanding the experiences of people living with mental disorders. The individual, personal expe-rience of having symptoms, signs, and disability associated with a condition—from the perspective of the affected individual and from that of the clinician—cannot be captured in mere criteria or reductionistic statistics. Clinicians may arrive at a diagno-sis that helps characterize, appreciate, and communicate the experience of a patient, but a person certainly cannot be reduced to a set of criteria, a diagnosis, or a list of di-agnoses. The biological, psychological, and sociological particulars of each individual, as a whole person, affect how an illness, a "diagnosis," is expressed. This *Study Guide to DSM-5-TR* aims to help translate the printed diagnostic criteria into the lived expe-riences of patients.

The *Study Guide* should be used side-by-side with the full text of DSM-5-TR. We take a patient-centered approach, complementing the more disorder-centered organi-zation of DSM-5-TR. A new chapter focusing on structural and cultural considerations in the diagnostic process has been added to Part 1 ("Foundations"). We also introduce consistent features in the diagnostic chapters to help make the concepts of DSM-5-TR come to life. For example, each of the chapters in Part 2 ("DSM-5-TR Diagnostic Cate-gories") offers case vignettes that illustrate patterns of illness, including expected and, at times, unexpected elements, and demonstrate how age, sex/gender, and several other cultural factors influence the cases. Other vignettes highlight patient-clinician in-teractions in the process of an interview and provide sample questions asked by the clinician to better appreciate the patient's unique experience of a disorder. The diagno-sis-oriented chapters in Part 2 provide "diagnostic pearls" and points of importance to daily clinical practice. Furthermore, the chapters in Part 2 include "Elements to Con-sider in the Cultural Formulation" sections and "Key Changes Between DSM-5 and DSM-5-TR" tables that bring attention to the changes that have been made in this text revision of DSM. The *Study Guide* provides a context for all of the diagnoses in DSM-5-TR, but instead of covering every diagnosis superficially, we chose to dive into greater detail ("in depth") for certain very interesting or very prevalent diagnoses that illustrate each diagnostic class.

Because this book is a study guide, we have tried to make it learner friendly to fa-cilitate the processes of registering new information from DSM-5-TR, recalling it, and then considering how it will apply in the reader's work. Part 1 puts DSM-5-TR in context in terms of explaining diagnostic frameworks and indicating how these might shape work with patients. Part 2 focuses on the diagnostic classes in DSM-5-TR. To stimulate learning about the disorders, each of these chapters has a self-assessment section, including "Key Concepts," "Questions to Discuss With Colleagues and Mentors," "Case-Based Questions" that describe complicated cases, and "Short-Answer Questions" with answers that are generally based on information in either the *Study Guide* or DSM-5-TR. Part 3 ("Q&A") is replete with more than 100 questions, including brief vignettes covering a wide range of diagnoses and patient circumstances to aid the application of DSM-5-TR to clinical work and training.

Some chapters of DSM-5-TR are not reviewed in this *Study Guide* due to space limitations. Examples include "Other Mental Disorders and Additional Codes," "Medication-Induced Movement Disorders and Other Adverse Effects of Medication," "Other Conditions That May Be a Focus of Clinical Attention," "Assessment Measures," "Culture and Psychiatric Diagnosis," "Alternative DSM-5 Model for Personality Disorders," and "Conditions for Further Study." The reader is encouraged to refer directly to DSM-5-TR to become familiar with these important elements. For instance, the DSM-5-TR chapter "Other Conditions That May Be a Focus of Clinical Attention" includes psychosocial stressors that may influence the presentation of a diagnosis. "Conditions for Further Study" describes conditions that are being studied to determine whether they should be considered as diagnoses in subsequent iterations of DSM. The learner will also find the chapters "Assessment Measures" and "Culture and Psychiatric Diagnosis" quite handy.

Because this *Study Guide* is a companion book to DSM-5-TR, its content intentionally parallels that of the latter. At times, the terminology and even phraseology here may be the same as in DSM-5-TR to provide a bridge between specific text in the *Study Guide* and DSM-5-TR. We have permission from the American Psychiatric Association to use material from DSM-5-TR.

The descriptions of people throughout this book—for example, in case vignettes and questions and answers—are hypothetical. Any resemblance to actual people is completely by chance, and names have been chosen randomly. Some of these descriptions of people include interactions with a clinician and questions that a clinician might ask. These described interactions are only meant to be illustrative, and the clinician questions are only sample questions. The descriptions are not of complete clinical interviews or analyses of cases, and many essential details have been omitted due to space limitations.

The authors of this *Study Guide* have attempted to ensure that all information is accurate at the time of writing and consistent with general psychiatric and medical standards. As medical research and practice continue to advance, however, information and standards may change. Specific situations may require a specific response not included in this *Study Guide*. The editors and authors cannot assume any legal liability for any mistakes of commission or omission in this book.

This is a study guide for a diagnostic and statistical manual. Therefore, it is not about therapies and interventions, and no information contained herein should be construed as providing treatment recommendations. For these reasons and because human and mechanical errors sometimes occur, we recommend that readers follow the advice of physicians directly involved in their care or the care of a member of their family.

The *Study Guide to DSM-5* was edited by two of us (L.W.R. and A.K.L.), and for this new *Study Guide to DSM-5-TR* we were joined by Dr. Matthew L. Edwards, who brought his expertise in general, forensic, and cultural psychiatry. We thank the many authors of the chapters and question-and-answer sections in both editions, who have been immensely generous with their expertise and responsiveness in preparing this book. We offer our unending appreciation to Gabriel Termuehlen, Max Kasun, and Jodi Paik at Stanford University School of Medicine, and to Ann M. Eng, DSM Managing Editor at American Psychiatric Association Publishing, for their outstanding support in preparing the *Study Guide*. We acknowledge with gratitude American Psychiatric Association Publishing; Simone Taylor, Publisher; Erika Parker, Acquisitions Editor; and Annie Birge, Acquisitions Coordinator, for making this project possible and advising us along the way. The editors thank their colleagues and families for their contributions and loving support.

We wish, most importantly, to thank *you*, dear reader—no matter what your discipline, profession, time of life, or walk of life—for your engagement with this *Study Guide*. We hope that our work will help in your learning and in your efforts to improve the lives of people who turn to you for understanding and for their care.

Laura Weiss Roberts, M.D., M.A.

Alan K. Louie, M.D.

Matthew L. Edwards, M.D.

PART 1

Foundations

CHAPTER 1

Diagnosis and DSM-5-TR

Laura Weiss Roberts, M.D., M.A.
Mickey Trockel, M.D., Ph.D.

Clinicians see patterns in the experiences, behaviors, and physical findings of their patients. They seek to understand the nature, timing, and sequence of their patients' experiences, findings, attributes, and behaviors—and in so doing, they diagnose.

The diagnosis is an interpretation or judgment made with more or less certainty regarding how the pattern recognized in one patient's life compares with that of others seen throughout clinical medicine. Through this comparative framework, a diagnosis may help guide the search for other distinguishing features of an illness process, reveal an underlying cause, inform the therapeutic approach to be undertaken, and suggest what the future holds for the patient and their loved ones. DSM-5-TR (American Psychiatric Association 2022) provides the current comparative framework for psychiatric illness.

DSM-5-TR is the revised version of the fifth edition of *Diagnostic and Statistical Manual of Mental Disorders*—a guidebook for characterizing significant mental health conditions that affect people throughout the world. DSM-5-TR has evolved to become more rigorous and comprehensive, as described in Chapter 3 of this *Study Guide*, "Understanding Different Approaches to Diagnostic Classification." It represents the current thinking of master clinicians and scientists in psychiatry, a specialty of medicine; in clinical psychology; and in related health professions. Its diagnoses are informed by evidence from the basic and clinical neurosciences and behavioral sciences. The diagnosis of mental health conditions, like that of physical health conditions, often relies on data that are descriptive or subjective in nature—at times with little empirical verification and often lacking clear biological explanation. (See Chapter 3 for greater detail on diagnostic classification systems and underlying questions of validity.) Because of these challenges, wherever possible DSM-5-TR includes the use of formal assessments or measures to bring greater consistency and precision to the diagnostic process. Taken together, the DSM-5-TR diagnoses represent a useful system for characterizing highly diverse phenomena across highly diverse settings.

Diagnostic hypotheses may guide additional data gathering, such as obtaining more detailed information about the patient's history or new laboratory results. The iterative process of hypothesis generation and empirical testing is paramount to arrive at a well-reasoned and carefully substantiated diagnosis, which supports the best outcome for the patient. Arriving at an accurate diagnosis is important to sound clinical care but brings burdens and risks to patients as well as benefits. The authority to render the diagnosis is the power to bring understanding and relief on one hand and the problem of labeling and possible stigmatization on the other. Lessening the weight of psychiatric disease burden while also seeking to "do no harm" can be a difficult balance to attain, especially given the prejudices and misunderstandings that exist throughout society related to neuropsychiatric diseases and related conditions. The hallmark of an excellent clinician is not simply the capacity to diagnose an illness correctly but also to appreciate the experience of the illness and the full meaning of having it "named" in the context of the patient's life.

Professional judgment is fostered by careful study of DSM-5-TR diagnostic criteria, coupled with clinical experience and informed by study of relevant basic and applied sciences. For both clinicians in training and experienced clinicians engaged in lifelong learning, the *Study Guide to DSM-5-TR* helps in this goal.

DSM-5-TR AND THE ROLES AND ATTRIBUTES OF DIAGNOSIS

There is a story about a man looking for his lost car keys on a dark evening. He searches only under the nearest lamppost, where he has enough light to see, although he likely dropped the keys a block away. Discerning the fundamental basis or underpinning of a patient's mental health complaint often requires looking where the light is dim at best. Despite increasing efforts to bridge the gap between neuroscience discovery and clinical practice, few findings have yet shed much light on the exact causes of psychiatric diseases (Insel 2009; Kendler 2016; Sullivan and Geschwind 2019). Although discouraging to some, the mystery of the functions and pathology of the human brain represents an extraordinary frontier. The many unanswered questions in neuroscience are a "call" to explore matters of importance to humankind.

Without definitive neuroscience to provide causal explanations of human health and disease, DSM-5-TR necessarily relies on descriptions—things patients experience and say about their experiences ("symptoms"), things observed by clinicians and others ("signs"), and, to a lesser extent, laboratory findings and neuroimaging results. DSM-5-TR, with its descriptive (phenomenological) rather than causal (etiological) approach, has a combination of scientific evidence and expert consensus opinion as its foundation. It is best understood as a systematic framework, informed by experience and evidence, that reflects maturation beyond prior diagnostic systems. Because DSM is a "living" document, it is certain to change with time.

DSM-5-TR has importance beyond clinical care, health science, and education in the health professions. It is used each day by teachers, attorneys, judges, policy makers, hospital administrators, insurers, and interested members of the public. For all who use the manual, it is important to remember that biomedical science is a human endeavor and that the history of medicine is rich with examples in which incremental, systematic, and evidence-driven approaches focusing on observable phenomena yielded remarkable improvements in health outcomes, even when underlying causes were unknown. Just as John Snow was able to identify that avoiding consumption of contaminated water prevented the spread of cholera *before* the identification of its bacterial cause, *Vibrio cholerae* (Paneth 2004), the use of empirically derived, descriptive, criteria-based diagnostic approaches can—and often does—yield relief of psychiatric morbidity. The causes of psychiatric morbidity involve many biological pathways and complicated environmental interactions that will be elucidated gradually in the coming decades (Sullivan and Geschwind 2019). While waiting for new and more clearly definitive scientific answers regarding the causes and prevention of mental illness, clinicians will use the increasingly rigorous and careful descriptive approach of DSM-5-TR in all settings, whether clinical, community, classroom, or courtroom.

For the clinician and the patient, the DSM-5-TR diagnosis serves many functions and has many attributes. It may be understood as a hypothesis, a way of communicating, a source of distress, a risk, and an experience of clarity. Each of these aspects is important and has bearing both on the clinician's approach and the patient's health.

Diagnosis as a Hypothesis

The DSM-5-TR diagnostic criteria allow clinicians to form hypotheses about their patients' mental health difficulties that imply commonality with other patients who present with similar symptom clusters and patterns. This process enables physicians to benefit from a knowledge base derived from the clinical history of other patients with the same diagnosis. This knowledge base serves as a foundation to build upon when evaluating clinical data and making treatment decisions.

Clinicians apply systematic reasoning to the clinical evaluation process by using clinical data to formulate and test diagnostic hypotheses. Researchers during the early conceptualization of diagnostic reasoning posited that establishing a clinical diagnosis involves hypothesis testing, in which a limited set of hypotheses formulated early in the process guides further data gathering (Elstein et al. 1978). Clinicians following health education methods often focus on this process and use initial presenting clinical data to create a *differential diagnosis*—a short list of plausible diagnosis hypotheses. Clinicians are taught to use the differential diagnosis to focus additional data gathering and to use evolving clinical information to narrow and refine the diagnostic possibilities. Application of evidence-based medicine adds precision to the process by employing decision theory, in which new data are used to adjust the estimated probability of diagnoses (Elstein and Schwartz 2002).

Experienced clinicians may use more efficient pattern recognition for routine medical cases and engage in deductive reasoning–driven hypothesis testing only when confronted with the most complex cases (Elstein and Schwartz 2002; Moayyeri et al. 2011). Nevertheless, careful hypothesis testing is uniquely useful during the process of psychiatric diagnosis, even for experienced clinicians. DSM-5-TR criteria are based almost entirely on latent (unobservable) variables, which reduces reliability and validity in any diagnostic process. Perhaps to a higher degree than in most other medical fields, the adage "knowing is the enemy of learning" is true in psychiatric diagnosis. Overreliance on pattern recognition to establish an efficient diagnosis dismisses the opportunity to discover an alternative and more accurate explanation of a patient's problem.

Consider a 30-year-old female with depressed mood, poor concentration, low energy, weight gain, and psychomotor slowing over the past 2 months. Her pattern "looks" like a major depressive episode. If the clinician looks no further, however, they may miss an underlying, and correctable, hypothyroid problem responsible for the patient's symptoms. The correct diagnosis would be readily discoverable through careful deductive reasoning to evaluate a limited set of plausible diagnoses. This example serves as a reminder of the importance of professional judgment in the use of DSM-5-TR criteria. The DSM-5-TR diagnostic system—which is oriented toward patterns of observations, findings, and symptoms rather than causal explanations—will give rise to superficial, premature, and incorrect diagnostic conclusions if applied carelessly. To fulfill professional responsibilities with patients, clinicians must engage in careful consideration of reasonable alternative diagnoses and must rigorously test diagnostic hypotheses against available data, even in apparently simple and straightforward cases.

Case Example: Importance of Refining a Diagnostic Hypothesis

Ms. Evans, age 27, was awaiting honorable discharge from her service with the U.S. Navy when her colleagues noticed she looked increasingly fearful and was talking about hearing voices telling her that the world was going to be destroyed in 2030. With Ms. Evans's permission, the evaluating psychiatrist interviewed one of her closest colleagues, who indicated that Ms. Evans had not been taking good care of her personal hygiene for several months. Ms. Evans admitted she was depressed. The psychiatrist also learned that Ms. Evans's performance of her military job duties had declined during this time and that her commanding officer had recommended she be evaluated by a psychiatrist approximately 2 weeks earlier for possible depression.

When interviewed, Ms. Evans endorsed believing that the world was going to end soon and indicated that several times she had heard an audible voice that repeated this information. She had a maternal uncle with schizophrenia, and her mother had a diagnosis of bipolar I disorder. Ms. Evans's toxicology screen was positive for tetrahydrocannabinol (THC). The evaluating psychiatrist informed Ms. Evans that they had made a tentative diagnosis of schizophrenia.

Questions to consider:

- What are your thoughts on this case regarding the tentative diagnosis of schizophrenia that the psychiatrist shared with Ms. Evans?
- Should the psychiatrist have made a tentative diagnosis?
- Should the psychiatrist have shared this information with Ms. Evans at this time?

- Will Ms. Evans's future situation, such as her clinical care, military status, employment, and family and personal life, be affected significantly by this diagnostic hypothesis?
- What substantiation may be possible with additional clinical data?
- What are the benefits and burdens that go with this diagnostic hypothesis?

An accurate psychiatric diagnosis opens the door to a growing body of evidence-based treatments and adaptive treatment algorithms (Lavori and Dawson 2008) that will help mental health clinicians tailor treatment to their individual patients. A hypothesized diagnosis also helps clinicians evaluate the observed treatment response against the expected treatment response as characterized in available literature describing other patients with the same diagnosis. This comparison may provide additional data that help them further refine their diagnostic hypothesis. At several points during the course of clinical care, open discussion of the working diagnostic hypothesis with the patient can facilitate collaborative, and ethically sound, treatment decision-making. When the clinician and the patient work together to make treatment decisions, the likelihood that treatment plans will be successfully implemented increases.

Diagnosis as a Way of Communicating

To the degree that the DSM-5-TR criteria are reliable, deriving a diagnosis facilitates precision and parsimony in clinical communication. A working diagnosis facilitates communication between individual patients and their clinicians, between members of a treatment team, between clinicians and researchers, and in conversations with families and stakeholders such as insurers, employers, and teachers. A diagnosis acts as a summary of descriptive information in all of these contexts.

Patients are increasingly aware of mental health diagnostic criteria because of internet-based health education. Although such information varies in accuracy, many patients now recognize symptoms of common diagnoses such as major depressive disorder. Some patients can and do present for mental health evaluation with an opening statement such as "I'm worried I have PTSD." Other patients accurately report a diagnosis they received previously from another clinician. Some patients may not present with a preconceived notion of their own diagnosis but will recognize some of the symptoms associated with their hypothesized diagnosis because of experience with a friend or family member who had the same diagnosis. In all of these scenarios, the diagnostic title conveys, to varying degrees, a large amount of shared understanding that facilitates communication.

Information sharing with a treatment team and in clinical consultation ideally will be efficient and accurate. A diagnosis rapidly identifies a wealth of information regarding clinical signs, symptoms, and probable course of illness that comes from volumes of relevant research and immense clinical experience. Consider the following beginning to a case presentation:

Mr. Samuels, a 25-year-old man, was brought to the emergency department by his father for assessment after he was found wandering in the park, muttering under his breath that he needed to get away from the FBI. He had left his house 2 days earlier after appearing increasingly anxious and withdrawn.

Now, consider the amount of additional information included in this initial case description by including a short statement regarding a clearly determined diagnosis:

> Mr. Samuels, a 25-year-old man *with a previously well-established diagnosis of schizophrenia*, was brought to the emergency department by his father for assessment after he was found wandering in the park, muttering under his breath that he needed to get away from the FBI. He had left his house 2 days earlier after appearing increasingly anxious and withdrawn.

The short description "a 25-year-old man with a previously well-established diagnosis of schizophrenia" immediately evokes a common understanding based on study of professional literature and experience with other patients with the same diagnosis. A careful listener will always be mindful of less likely possible explanations, but, when hearing the second presentation, they will likely be able to focus on a narrowed set of highly relevant concerns. An accurate diagnosis facilitates effective and efficient "dense" communication in clinical teaching, consultation, and all forms of treatment team collaboration.

Clinical diagnoses also convey salient information that, when coupled with associated epidemiology, helps guide public policy for funding of research and clinical services. Expert groups of clinicians determine diagnostic criteria. Epidemiologists then use those criteria to estimate incidence, prevalence, and other parameters that indicate the public health burden associated with the disease. One example is years lived with disability (YLD). Data from the Global Burden of Diseases, Injuries, and Risk Factors Study indicate that depressive disorders are the second largest contributor to worldwide YLDs, out of 371 diseases and injuries evaluated (Ferrari et al. 2024). Anxiety disorders, schizophrenia, autism spectrum disorder, alcohol use disorder, and other mental health disorders are also among the top 25 contributors to worldwide YLDs (Ferrari et al. 2024).

Diagnosis as a Source of Distress

Diagnoses with poor prognoses, such as schizophrenia, may bring more distress than hope. It is widely understood that among individuals who receive a diagnosis of schizophrenia, those with the greatest capacity to understand the nature of their illness are at greatest risk for subsequent depression and suicide (Crumlish et al. 2005; Kao and Liu 2011). In these cases, clinicians may appropriately wonder whether disclosing a diagnosis is likely to do more harm than good. The distress of living with severe symptoms that are only partially amenable to treatment is made even more severe by societal stigmatization. Patients experiencing mental illness may have more difficulty establishing and maintaining meaningful interpersonal relationships because of the intrinsic character of their diseases. People living with these conditions are likely to fear discrimination at work, in seeking housing, and in purchasing life and health insurance policies because of how mental disorders are viewed.

Although some psychiatric diagnoses may carry less burden of stigma now than in the past, data suggest that patients with psychotic illness were, in fact, more commonly stigmatized as violent and dangerous at the end of the twentieth century than they had been half a century earlier (Phelan et al. 2000). Subsequent data suggested that this stigmatizing perception stabilized but did not decrease (Pescosolido et al. 2010). A thought-provoking qualitative analysis of narrative interviews of 46 people with mental illness suggested that almost all people with mental illness worry about stigma (Dinos et al. 2004). Those with substance dependence or psychotic disorders are most affected by stigma, as poignantly illustrated in the remarks of an African Caribbean female with schizophrenia: "Schizophrenic is the worst diagnosis because I've heard it in the newspapers and on TV, that they are really mad schizophrenic people, they are very dangerous to society, they've got no control. So obviously I came under that category" (Dinos et al. 2004, p. 177). When speaking with people who have received psychiatric diagnoses, clinicians need to consider the distress of living with an illness process and the psychosocial impact of how the diagnosis is perceived.

In most clinical encounters, both significant benefits and detriments are associated with rendering a diagnosis. Diagnostic decisions are necessary to formulate treatment plans and to foster understanding and insight of the patient who must navigate the experience of illness and a system of care. Families and societal stakeholders (e.g., employers, insurers) may become involved, often introducing concerns and perhaps prejudices and greater sources of distress to the ill individual. In many cases, the understanding and legitimacy that a diagnosis offers patients are sources of hope. However, juxtaposed against these benefits are real risks of societal stigma and internal loss of self-esteem and self-efficacy (Corrigan and Watson 2002). Patients may benefit greatly from the clinician's willingness to weigh carefully the benefits and risks associated with rendering a diagnosis, the balance of which will vary across diagnostic categories and across individual patients within diagnostic categories.

Diagnosis as a Risk

In addition to their psychosocial benefits and risks, most psychiatric diagnoses lead to treatment plans that also convey probable benefits and risks. An appropriate view of benefits and risks inherent in the diagnostic process is further complicated by the reality that psychiatric diagnosis is not a process with perfect precision. Even when the brightest clinicians have the best training and the best intentions, their diagnostic conclusions will not be perfectly accurate. As summarized in Table 1–1, evaluation of the balance of benefits and risks associated with receiving a psychiatric diagnosis (and associated treatment where indicated) requires consideration of diagnoses that are accurate (true positive and true negative) and inaccurate (false positive and false negative).

TRUE-POSITIVE DIAGNOSES

Many individuals who present to a trained mental health clinician for evaluation will have a DSM-5-TR–defined diagnosis and will receive a diagnosis from their clinician that accurately categorizes the problem they present with. This true-positive diagno-

TABLE 1–1.   Summary considerations to keep in mind when rendering a psychiatric diagnosis

Diagnosed with the disorder

Has the disorder	**Does not have the disorder**
True-positive cases:	False-positive cases:
A. Most likely to benefit from research and clinical experience related to the diagnosis	A. Less likely to benefit from research and clinical experience related to the diagnosis
B. Likely to be subjected to typical side effect burden and economic cost of treatment, as well as psychosocial effects of the diagnostic label	B. Likely to be subjected to typical side effect burden and economic cost of treatment, as well as psychosocial effects of the diagnostic label
	More detrimental when side effect burden or economic cost of treatment is high, and when psychosocial effects of the diagnosis label are high

Diagnosed as not having the disorder

Has the disorder	**Does not have the disorder**
False-negative cases:	True-negative cases:
A. Subject to consequences of delayed treatment	A. Spared consequences and cost of unnecessary treatment
B. Potentially spared some exposure to typical side effect burden and cost of treatment, as well as psychosocial effects of the diagnostic label	B. Spared psychosocial effects of the diagnostic label
More detrimental when severity of illness is high and when benefit-to-risk ratio of treatment is high	

sis is what most readers probably thought of as we described the benefits and risks associated with psychiatric diagnoses. These are the patients most likely to benefit from the growing body of research defining effective treatment strategies for the problem they are experiencing. There are at least two reasons for this:

1. These patients are more likely than other patients to resemble individuals with the same diagnosis who participated in relevant clinical trials.
2. The clinician caring for these patients may be more effective in deriving treatment solutions on the basis of their own clinical experience of what has worked with other patients who had the same diagnosis.

A clinician who has derived a highly effective method for helping patients with bipolar I disorder stay on their medication will be of more benefit to a patient whom the clinician has accurately diagnosed with bipolar I disorder than they will be to a patient with major depressive disorder whom they have inaccurately diagnosed with bipolar I disorder.

FALSE-POSITIVE DIAGNOSES

Patients who are inaccurately labeled with a diagnosis experience all of the burdens associated with the hypothesized characterization, with significantly less benefit. They are less likely to benefit from a treatment plan built on an evidence-base for a diagnostic entity they do not actually have. This error is particularly unfortunate when the diagnosis indicates a lifetime of medication use that renders significant metabolic, cognitive, or other serious side effects. In some cases, the diagnostic error may not be the fault of the clinician. Consider the case of an adolescent who had a single manic episode while taking his friend's psychostimulant prescribed for ADHD. The clinician faces a difficult diagnostic puzzle if sufficient time has elapsed between the episode and a warranted toxicology screen, and the patient is denying use of substances because he fears being punished if his parents learn he illicitly used his friend's medication. The history of a single manic episode in this context may suggest a diagnosis of bipolar disorder to even the most careful and experienced clinician.

In many cases, however, an errant diagnosis can be avoided through appropriate assessment and understanding of diagnostic criteria. For example, consider the case of a young female who has a history of a manic episode while taking two antidepressant medications for treatment of a major depressive episode. An inappropriate diagnosis of bipolar disorder in this case can—and in similar actual cases does—lead to significant unnecessary exposure to the ill effects of mood-stabilizing or atypical antipsychotic medications, as well as the psychosocial burden associated with the errant diagnosis.

The likelihood of inappropriately receiving a psychiatric diagnosis may be increasing with each DSM version because of the rising number of officially canonized diagnoses. The original DSM (American Psychiatric Association 1952), published in the middle of the twentieth century, listed approximately 60 disorders, whereas DSM-5-TR lists more than 150. The iterations of the *International Classification of Diseases and Related Health Problems* (ICD) present an even greater concern in this respect because the ICD-11 has grown to include 55,000 codes. Clinicians who are socialized by their training to be wary of missing a diagnosis (i.e., those who are focused on preventing false-negative diagnoses) may be less cognizant of the potential harm associated with false-positive diagnoses. Nevertheless, the imperfect process of psychiatric diagnosis will also miss some diagnoses that should have been made.

FALSE-NEGATIVE DIAGNOSES

Failure to make a diagnosis that should have been made can also lead to unintended, unnecessary harm. A person who is looking for help for an underlying psychiatric illness that is not detected by a clinician will probably not receive optimal treatment—treatment that in some cases can be lifesaving. In the most extreme cases, this risk is alarmingly apparent. A substance-related disorder that leads to reckless driving and a traffic fatality could have been averted by timely diagnosis and treatment. A case of treatable postpartum depression inappropriately assumed to be a minor adjustment disorder may lead to detriments in parent-child interactions that are later associated with increased mental illness burden and decreased quality of life for years to come for the parent's newborn child.

Alternatively, some patients present with temporary anxiety, stress, or loss that is circumstantially bounded and may not warrant a psychiatric diagnosis. For these individuals the greatest diagnostic benefit a clinician may offer is reassurance that the experience does not convey a psychiatric diagnosis, along with appropriate support and assistance where warranted and desired.

TRUE-NEGATIVE DIAGNOSES

Although some individuals stand to lose benefits associated with a hoped-for diagnosis when seeking psychiatric evaluation, most will be relieved to know they do not have a significant mental health disorder. News that what ails them is not a suspected DSM diagnosis may indeed be reassuring to a bereaved patient, for example, and to others enduring difficult human experience. For a small minority of individuals, not receiving a certain diagnosis may mean failing to obtain insurance coverage for desired help or a lack of perceived legitimacy of their illness as sought from a clinical explanation. For example, a military veteran who experienced significant trauma during armed conflict but does not meet criteria for PTSD could interpret the accurate diagnostic message as meaning their experience is not thought to be as legitimate as that of others who do have PTSD. Still, for most patients, an accurate declaration of the absence of a significant mental health disorder will be welcome news.

In almost all circumstances, an accurate (true-positive or true-negative) diagnosis yields a more optimal benefit-to-risk ratio than an inaccurate (false-positive or false-negative) diagnosis. An accurate diagnosis maximizes the clinical benefit-to-risk ratio in spite of potential legal, economic, social, and other complicating variables.

Diagnosis as an Experience of Clarity

Most patients would like their clinicians' help with two things: 1) understanding the symptoms they are experiencing (Salmon et al. 2004), and 2) finding a solution to alleviate these symptoms. A diagnosis can help meet both of these needs.

An accurately rendered diagnosis clearly explored with a patient can help them feel that the clinician understands what they are going through and can draw from a clinical knowledge base that is derived from working with other patients who had the same problem and from the experience of colleagues who have worked with similar patients. Receiving a medical diagnosis can begin to give patients a sense of clarity, affirmation, or legitimacy in the experience of their condition. A clinical interview conducted with empathy and kindness—even by a novice or a learner in a clinical situation—is sufficient to help a patient feel that the clinician understands what they are experiencing. Hearing a professional diagnosis helps the patient feel that the clinician understands *why* they are feeling this way. This beneficial psychological effect may exist even though the DSM-based diagnoses are based much more on useful descriptive constructs than on validated biological models of pathology.

The experience of receiving a diagnosis may be particularly validating to psychiatric patients with emotional distress that is mostly unobservable or misunderstood by others. A diagnostic explanation can help a patient feel more understood and less harshly judged. Someone who experienced severe child abuse and has regular disturbing nightmares and a paralyzing fear of intimacy is likely to feel more understood and less judged after learning that many others exposed to similar traumatic experiences have reacted in the same way. The same patient may benefit from knowing that this reaction is officially termed *posttraumatic stress disorder* and is well recognized and studied. For this person, the diagnosis also extends hope for recovery and the restoration of a better life. For many individuals, a diagnosis may bring some, if somewhat paradoxical, comfort, such as the person with an eating disorder who has previously been told to "just *eat* something," someone with social anxiety disorder who has been told to "just get out of the house," or the profoundly depressed person who is unable to muster enough energy and motivation to get out of bed and has been told to "just snap out of it."

A good clinician will convey the clarity of a diagnosis wrapped in optimism and founded in a growing body of literature describing treatment strategies that have proven successful for patients with the same diagnosis. For example, a severely depressed patient and their clinician will have the option of selecting a best-fit treatment strategy that includes evidence-based psychotherapy, an antidepressant medication, or both. A patient with PTSD and their clinician can begin to map out an evidence-based treatment plan that—although challenging to implement when appropriately including a strategy such as cognitive processing therapy (Resick and Schnicke 1992) or prolonged exposure therapy (Foa et al. 1999)—offers evidence-based hope of significant, and even life-changing, recovery (Cusack et al. 2016). Patients with some anxiety disorders, including debilitating panic disorder, may be overjoyed to learn that their symptoms can be alleviated, in many cases, with 4–8 weeks of appropriate treatment (Gould et al. 1995). However, many patients present with dire need for relief from mental health problems for which decades of research have rendered less optimal solutions.

THE COMPASSIONATE DIAGNOSTICIAN

The task of the modern clinician is to use the wisdom and proven practices of the past while learning continuously about emerging evidence and working tirelessly to improve approaches to health care. Alleviating distress and enabling the greater well-being of patients should be goals that guide clinical practice in the DSM-5-TR era.

Diagnostic accuracy depends to a large extent on content mastery (Elstein and Schwartz 2002). Experts are more accurate than novices. Clinicians can accelerate their progress from novice to expert through study and clinical experience. Most training programs insist that budding clinicians study a significant amount of material before engaging in direct patient care. Although both study and clinical experience facilitate clinical content mastery, only one of these is accomplished without any burden to patients. This principle holds some truth for all clinicians. Study accelerates and supplements learning derived from clinical experience and helps clinicians optimize the benefit-to-risk ratio of care they provide to their patients. Careful study of DSM-defined diagnoses helps clinicians maximize diagnostic accuracy.

This *Study Guide* is designed to help clinicians at all levels of experience master the new DSM-5-TR diagnostic system. Happy studying!

SELF-ASSESSMENT

Questions to Discuss With Colleagues and Mentors

1. Have you ever made a diagnosis with unexpected results?
2. Have you ever delayed a diagnosis you wish you had made more rapidly?
3. When is rendering a psychiatric diagnosis most worrisome, in your experience? Why?
4. Are there clinical circumstances in which you have found it better to not share your diagnostic hypothesis with your patient? If yes, when?

Short-Answer Questions

1. To what degree is the DSM-5-TR diagnostic system based on neuroscientific discovery?
2. How do psychiatric diagnoses facilitate clinical communication?
3. What are some significant benefits to patients associated with an accurate psychiatric diagnosis?

Answers

1. The DSM-5-TR diagnostic system sought to incorporate recent best evidence and, where possible and appropriate, neuroscientific findings. DSM-5-TR is a phenomenologically oriented diagnostic system rather than an etiologically governed diagnostic approach.

2. In developing and refining a diagnostic hypothesis, the clinician must engage in a careful dialogue with the patient. The astute clinician seeks to clarify the patient's personal history, the symptoms experienced, the impact of living with an illness process, relevant background, and the patient's concerns. The dialogue may further allow the clinician to reconcile any incongruities among the patient's presentation and narrative, prior documentation, and collateral medical and psychosocial information.

3. Placing the patient's experience into a diagnostic framework can help them to understand features of the illness process and the anticipated outcomes. Receiving a diagnosis paradoxically can be reassuring and validating for patients who may believe that their symptoms are poorly understood by others.

RECOMMENDED READINGS

Corrigan PW (ed): On the Stigma of Mental Illness: Practical Strategies for Research and Social Change. Washington, DC, American Psychological Association, 2005

Frances AJ, Widiger T: Psychiatric diagnosis: lessons from the DSM-IV past and cautions for the DSM-5 future. Annu Rev Clin Psychol 8:109–130, 2012 22035240

Kraemer HC: Validity and psychiatric diagnoses. JAMA Psychiatry 70(2):138–139, 2013 23208663

Regier DA, Narrow WE, Clarke DE, et al: DSM-5 field trials in the United States and Canada, part II: test-retest reliability of selected categorical diagnoses. Am J Psychiatry 170(1):59–70, 2013 23111466

REFERENCES

American Psychiatric Association: Diagnostic and Statistical Manual: Mental Disorders. Washington, DC, American Psychiatric Association, 1952

American Psychiatric Association: Diagnostic and Statistical Manual of Mental Disorders, 5th Edition, Text Revision. Washington, DC, American Psychiatric Association, 2022

Corrigan PW, Watson AC: The paradox of self-stigma and mental illness. Clin Psychol 9:35–53, 2002

Crumlish N, Whitty P, Kamali M, et al: Early insight predicts depression and attempted suicide after 4 years in first-episode schizophrenia and schizophreniform disorder. Acta Psychiatr Scand 112(6):449–455, 2005 16279874

Cusack K, Jonas DE, Forneris CA, et al: Psychological treatments for adults with posttraumatic stress disorder: a systematic review and meta-analysis. Clin Psychol Rev 43:128–141, 2016 26574151

Dinos S, Stevens S, Serfaty M, et al: Stigma: the feelings and experiences of 46 people with mental illness. Qualitative study. Br J Psychiatry 184:176–181, 2004 14754832

Elstein AS, Schwartz A: Clinical problem solving and diagnostic decision making: selective review of the cognitive literature. BMJ 324(7339):729–732, 2002 11909793

Elstein AS, Shulman LS, Sprafka SA: Medical Problem Solving: An Analysis of Clinical Reasoning. Cambridge, MA, Harvard University Press, 1978

Ferrari AJ, Santomauro DF, Aali A, et al: Global incidence, prevalence, years lived with disability (YLDs), disability-adjusted life-years (DALYs), and healthy life expectancy (HALE) for 371 diseases and injuries in 204 countries and territories and 811 subnational locations, 1990–2021: a systematic analysis for the Global Burden of Disease Study 2021. Lancet 403(10440):2133–2161, 2024

Foa EB, Dancu CV, Hembree EA, et al: A comparison of exposure therapy, stress inoculation training, and their combination for reducing posttraumatic stress disorder in female assault victims. J Consult Clin Psychol 67(2):194–200, 1999 10224729

Gould RA, Ott MW, Pollack MH: A meta-analysis of treatment outcome for panic disorder. Clin Psychol Rev 15:819–844, 1995

Insel TR: Translating scientific opportunity into public health impact: a strategic plan for research on mental illness. Arch Gen Psychiatry 66(2):128–133, 2009 19188534

Kao YC, Liu YP: Suicidal behavior and insight into illness among patients with schizophrenia spectrum disorders. Psychiatr Q 82(3):207–220, 2011 20976555

Kendler KS: The nature of psychiatric disorders. World Psychiatry 15(1):5–12, 2016 26833596

Lavori PW, Dawson R: Adaptive treatment strategies in chronic disease. Annu Rev Med 59:443–453, 2008 17914924

Moayyeri A, Soltani A, Moosapour H, et al: Evidence-based history taking under "time constraint." J Res Med Sci 16(4):559–564, 2011 22091274

Paneth N: Assessing the contributions of John Snow to epidemiology: 150 years after removal of the broad street pump handle. Epidemiology 15(5):514–516, 2004 15308944

Pescosolido BA, Martin JK, Long JS, et al: "A disease like any other"? A decade of change in public reactions to schizophrenia, depression, and alcohol dependence. Am J Psychiatry 167(11):1321–1330, 2010 20843872

Phelan JC, Link BG, Stueve A, et al: Public conceptions of mental illness in 1950 and 1996: what is mental illness and is it to be feared? J Health Soc Behav 41:188–207, 2000

Resick PA, Schnicke MK: Cognitive processing therapy for sexual assault victims. J Consult Clin Psychol 60(5):748–756, 1992 1401390

Salmon P, Dowrick CF, Ring A, et al: Voiced but unheard agendas: qualitative analysis of the psychosocial cues that patients with unexplained symptoms present to general practitioners. Br J Gen Pract 54(500):171–176, 2004 15006121

Sullivan PF, Geschwind DH: Defining the genetic, genomic, cellular, and diagnostic architectures of psychiatric disorders. Cell 177(1):162–183, 2019 30901538

CHAPTER 2

Arriving at a Diagnosis

APPLYING DSM-5-TR AND THE CLINICAL INTERVIEW

Alan K. Louie, M.D.

John H. Coverdale, M.D., M.Ed.

Laura Weiss Roberts, M.D., M.A.

The clinical interview is a central process for arriving at a sound psychiatric diagnosis when using DSM-5-TR (American Psychiatric Association 2022). DSM-5-TR provides information, language, and formal criteria that together serve as tools that the diagnostician brings to the clinical interview to assist in ascertaining whether a psychiatric disorder is present. Making an accurate diagnosis requires construing and applying these tools in context—with real people, real situations, and real settings. For example, the DSM-5-TR criteria for panic attacks list the number, nature, and time course of symptoms that must be present, which may be relatively easy to assess with the patient. The criteria, however, do not detail how to determine whether the attacks occur in the setting of and are more related to the patient's obsessive-compulsive, substance use, or bipolar disorder. This determination is critical to making the appropriate diagnosis and is likely to rely on many contextual factors that are not interrogated by the DSM-5-TR criteria and are accessible only by asking questions, making observations, and performing examinations that constitute the whole clinical interview, beyond the criteria. Therefore, diagnosis will not be successful if it is based on using the DSM-5-TR criteria as a free-standing checklist; they must be paired with a complete clinical interview.

MAKING A DIAGNOSIS IN CONTEXT

A clinical interview is shaped by its context, which may be broken down by asking who, what, when, where, and why questions. Each of these questions should be considered explicitly for each clinical interview. For instance, who is the diagnostician conducting the interview, where is the interview situated, and when is the interview taking place? Is the person being interviewed a student being seen by a social worker in a college health center just before final exams, an individual meeting with a clinical psychologist to see if they meet the criteria to volunteer for a research protocol, or an incarcerated individual being evaluated by a forensic psychiatrist in a jail? The student, volunteer, and incarcerated person might all have the same diagnosis, but the context of each interview will influence the nature of the interaction and how each person looks, reacts to questions, and offers information. Taken one step further, people of different cultural and ethnic backgrounds, primary languages, sexes/genders, and ages will respond differently when seeking services for routine mental health needs in a familiar clinic versus seeking care in an unfamiliar emergency facility for acute and life-threatening needs. Many other scenarios may be imagined, covering people of varied intersectionalities, locations, and time frames, and each context will influence the presentation of a particular diagnosis. Attention to context matters because a formulaic or mechanical approach to making diagnoses in these highly diverse scenarios may lead to poorly executed interviews and possibly even incorrect diagnoses.

As a consequence, before starting the interview, the diagnostician should focus on the "why" and "what" questions. Why is the interview being conducted at this time? The answer to this question thus informs "what" type of interview should be performed, including the prioritization and framing of queries and topics to be covered in the interaction. Revisiting the three scenarios presented in the previous paragraph illustrates the salience of these questions and how their answers influence the effectiveness of the interview on a practical level:

- The first scenario involved a social worker meeting with a student at a college health center. This student was seeking help for psychological symptoms they were experiencing before their final exams. The social worker wanted the student to speak freely about these symptoms, and, to encourage this openness, they assured the student that their discussions would be confidential unless the student divulged information that the social worker was mandated to report (e.g., actively intending to harm another person). Notably, the social worker explained that they would not share information with the student's professors or dean, absent a reporting mandate. The interview questions clarified the student's mental health issues and led to development of a supportive treatment plan.
- In the second scenario, the volunteer was undergoing a screening interview to determine whether they met the inclusion and exclusion criteria set by a research protocol. The questions were not aimed at developing a treatment plan for the volunteer; indeed, the person had been informed that they should not expect the research study to benefit their mental health issues. This interview included an

informed consent procedure that described the protocol and key safeguards, such as approval and oversight by an institutional review board and a process for avoiding identification of the research volunteer in any subsequent publication.

- In the third scenario, the court set up the interview by the forensic psychiatrist. The forensic psychiatrist informed the incarcerated person at the beginning of the interview that they had been appointed by the court and could not serve in a clinical, caregiving role and that any responses would not remain confidential. In fact, any disclosures made by the incarcerated individual were likely to appear in a psychiatric report for the court. (The use of DSM-5-TR in a forensic setting is complicated, and readers should refer to the "Cautionary Statement for Forensic Use of DSM-5" in DSM-5-TR.)

These scenarios illustrate practical aspects of context that shape a clinical interview, but a more abstract notion of context also exists and has relevance when arriving at a diagnosis.

The Biopsychosocial Model

The biopsychosocial model is a view of context that appreciates, and is open-minded toward, the range of biological, psychological, and social factors that interact with and contribute to a patient's presentation and concerns. The biopsychosocial paradigm, proposed and developed by George Engel in 1977, posits that biological, psychological, and social domains together play a role in the development of disease or illness (Engel 1977). This model intends to encompass the full set of factors that pertain to human experience, including cultural and spiritual factors. The clinical interview guides patients in talking about what is important to them within each domain. The following text describes the model first in the social context and then in the psychological and biological contexts. The biopsychosocial model is antithetical to a reductionist approach.

SOCIAL CONTEXT

The practical questions of who, what, when, where, and why often address much of the social context. The social perspective is a natural starting place as the interview commences and as each party might wonder, "Why are we here and what are we doing here?" Usually, each party is taking on a role described in society—for example, as a therapist, researcher, patient, research volunteer, or incarcerated individual. Whether the parties agree about what these roles are and whether they accept their roles willingly is very important to the success of the interview. These issues are best understood, made transparent, and, if necessary, negotiated at the outset of the interview. This agreement is not only of ethical importance but also assists the interviewer in interpreting and assessing the patient's answers. For instance, when asking an adolescent patient about sexual behaviors, the degree to which the patient understands that the interviewer will not divulge the details to their parents is the social context influencing whether they are likely to be forthcoming. The social agreement is the foundation on which accurate, honest, and meaningful exchange rests during the clinical interview, including when checking if DSM criteria are met.

Going beyond the roles of interviewer and interviewee, social context also depends on the individuals' respective cultural and linguistic backgrounds. They may not fluently speak each other's language. Even with the assistance of a medical translator, the interviewer may not be sure that DSM criteria are truly met. For instance, the DSM-5-TR criteria for major depressive disorder in the English language inquire if "depressed mood" is present. Some languages do not have words that are clearly equivalent to these English words. Additionally, individuals raised in divergent cultures may actually experience and manifest a symptom, such as depressed mood, variably; in one culture, a person may experience depressed mood as a thought (e.g., "I think about depressing things"), whereas someone in another culture may experience it as a bodily sensation (e.g., "I am so fatigued"). The DSM-5-TR criteria were written mainly by people who have a Western view of the world, psychology, and psychiatry, and the diagnostician must judge how to weigh such factors when making a diagnosis.

Absent a significant linguistic difference, the interviewee and interviewer may well have some dissimilar cultural backgrounds, worldviews, or values. Even if both parties self-identify as members of the "mainstream" culture, differences in subcultures, intersectionalities, and families of origin should not be dismissed. For example, most DSM-5-TR criteria assess whether the patient reports being distressed or impaired by symptoms. This assessment, however, is mitigated by what level of distress or impairment the patient has accepted as a part of normal life or they are not embarrassed to disclose or what is an acceptable idiom of distress in their culture, subculture, and family.

PSYCHOLOGICAL CONTEXT

The psychological context involves the interviewee's characteristics and history as an individual. Each person brings to the clinical interview a unique mix of cognitive, emotional and temperamental, behavioral, and social attributes and competencies, products of both genetics and learning. The interviewer's awareness of these attributes and competencies assists in the application of DSM criteria. For instance, when assessing the criteria for major depressive disorder regarding "diminished ability to think or concentrate," knowing the interviewee's baseline cognitive function is valuable. Assessment of an adolescent's depressive complaint of decreased energy will differ depending on whether their usual behavior includes being a varsity athlete or an ardent video gamer. Individual characteristics may alternatively be described as personality traits. An interviewer may need to discern whether paranoid feelings are part of the interviewee's long-term personality style and approach to the world or a result of the repetitive use of amphetamines.

A more historical perspective is also valuable, in which the clinical interviewer gains some appreciation for the narrative of the interviewee and how they see the story of their life, with all its foreseen and unforeseen twists and turns. Patients experience symptoms, which sometimes meet DSM criteria, within the context of time and space in their lives. The interviewer seeks to understand where there are, or are not, correlations, or perhaps causality, between the symptoms and events in the patient's life narrative.

BIOLOGICAL CONTEXT

Now that we have touched on social and psychological contexts, the biological context remains. Psychiatry is a medical specialty concerned with human cognition, emotion, and behavior and how these are mediated, in health and pathology, by the brain. Although the "nurture" factors—that is, the social and psychological components—are strong determinants of a psychiatric diagnosis, the "nature" factors are also significant, especially for certain conditions. Indeed, a diagnosis may be understood to be a direct and inevitable result of an individual's fundamental biology (e.g., genetic and epigenetic makeup). With the historical disregard of psychiatric disorders by science, the challenges associated with advancing the scientific understanding of multidetermined complex genetic disorders, and the fact that the human genome was sequenced only very recently, this biological domain remains, for the most part, unexplored.

Currently, measures of biological markers that may correlate with or substantiate diagnoses are, for the most part, unavailable. Thus, we look to the future, when such markers, perhaps involving brain imaging or genetic findings, may be included in the DSM criteria. For now, weak proxies of these measures are elicited during an interview. For instance, an interviewer wants to know if an interviewee has a family history of a psychiatric disorder, especially if that disorder is thought to be highly heritable according to epidemiological data. Also, the interviewer searches for evidence of any medical disorder or the presence of substance or medication use that may be directly inducing symptoms of a given diagnosis on a biological level.

Summary

In sum, recognizing the social, psychological, and biological contexts in which symptoms in the DSM criteria occur is essential to accurate and appropriate psychiatric diagnosis. The biopsychosocial model reminds the interviewer of these three contexts, encouraging a multifaceted and holistic appreciation of the interviewee as a whole person. Viewing the person in multiple contexts sees them as more than the "sum of the parts," bringing a degree of humanism to the final diagnosis. Of note, the biopsychosocial model is only one proposed way to accomplish this. Another method deserving attention is the four perspectives (disease, dimensions, behaviors, and life stories) approach to psychiatry (McHugh and Slavney 1998).

The balance of this chapter addresses the details of "how" to conduct the interview and the psychiatric assessment in general. Interested readers may also wish to refer to the excellent resources on interviewing that informed this narrative, which are listed in the "Recommended Readings" section at the end of this chapter.

APPROACH TO THE PSYCHIATRIC INTERVIEW AND ASSESSMENT

The clinical interview and assessment in psychiatry are intended to identify whether a patient has a mental health problem, the nature of any problem(s), and the specific diagnoses. The assessment process is aimed at developing a comprehensive, valid, and reliable database for the purpose of ameliorating the problems with which the patient presented by identifying and treating specific medical and psychiatric diagnoses. The components of such a comprehensive approach include obtaining a history, conducting a mental status examination (MSE), investigating possible medical problems, pursuing collateral records and other informants (not covered in this chapter), administering relevant and validated assessment tools, and obtaining physical and laboratory examinations. The psychiatric interview serves to identify all of the factors (i.e., biological/medical, psychological, social/cultural) that influence the presenting problems and that pertain to the provision of safe and beneficial preventions and treatments.

Despite the clear objectives of the psychiatric interview and assessment, patients should be encouraged to talk about what is important to them during the assessment process, especially early in the interview. In patient-centered interviewing, the clinician helps the patient lead the conversation toward aspects of their life (i.e., psychosocial factors) that might be important for understanding the determinants of the problems and diagnoses. For example, homeless individuals who seek mental health care constitute a biopsychosocially vulnerable population with potential unmet needs. These needs could include undertreated medical, dietary, and psychiatric conditions complicated by victimization from crimes, violence, sexual exploitation, and alcohol and substance abuse. As noted earlier, a reductionist "checklist" approach to diagnosis alone is ineffective for identifying and managing the complex biopsychosocial problems with which these patients might present.

Before proceeding further, a note about professionalism in clinical interviewing. Each practitioner should sensitively acquire clinical data in accordance with their respective professional responsibilities and privileges. *Respect for persons* is the first and foremost principle in the clinical professions. Additionally, practitioners of all types of clinical licensure are urged to remember the professional virtues that are the ethical basis of clinical practice. The four fundamental professional virtues are integrity, compassion, self-effacement, and self-sacrifice. *Integrity* is the lifelong commitment to the practice of medicine in accordance with the standards of intellectual and moral excellence. *Compassion* in medicine is the deep regard for the experience of the patient and, as a corollary, the commitment to serve the well-being of the patient, including relief of the patient's pain and distress, through identification with the patient's distress. *Self-effacement* refers to the notion of humility. *Self-sacrifice* and *self-effacement* in medicine are apparent when the clinician sets aside personal concerns and interpersonal differences so that the patient's interests are best served. These virtues, introduced into the history of medical ethics by John Gregory (1724–1773), provide the basis for the fiduciary relationship and constitute the starting point for the clinical professional approach to psychiatric interviewing and assessment (McCullough 1998).

PSYCHIATRIC INTERVIEW

Psychiatric history taking necessitates a thoughtful, systematic, and disciplined inquiry. Although psychiatric interviews are dynamic and interactive processes, a general interview structure is required to promote efficiency and facilitate the recognition of diagnostic patterns and symptoms. This structure should be sufficiently flexible that the interviewer allows patients to talk about what is important to them, follows their cues and leads, and is sensitive to their mental state, comfort level, and personality style.

An interview with a new patient should begin with introductions, in which the interviewer makes a statement of purpose and notes the degree of confidentiality. The early phases of the interview are necessarily open-ended, with a focus on developing rapport and a therapeutic alliance. Allowing the patient to talk about what is important to them, listening and empathetically responding, deepening rapport, and seeking clarification should be priorities, especially for this beginning stage of the interview. Such an open-ended approach should be followed by screening for symptoms across diagnostic categories.

Some essential elements of the psychiatric interview include, but are not limited to, identifying information (e.g., age, sex/gender, marital status), the presenting problem, history of the presenting problem, past psychiatric history, suicidal or homicidal history, substance use history (including alcohol), medical history, family history, and personal and social histories. Part 2 of this *Study Guide* provides more details on how to obtain the psychiatric history in relation to specific diagnostic categories.

Interviewing Techniques

Eliciting accurate information from patients enriches clinical judgment, especially concerning clinical risks and consequences. Patients may be reluctant to reveal sensitive information for many reasons. Interviewers may also be reluctant to enter into areas that are uncomfortable for themselves, perhaps in anticipation of discomfort in the patient. Feelings of discomfort in the interviewer can unhinge judgment and impede further inquiry or, alternatively, might bias the patient toward a negative versus affirmative response. A key strategy for obtaining accurate information on sensitive issues is for the interviewer to recognize any feelings of discomfort or distress during the interview, in either the patient or the interviewer, and to prevent those feelings from becoming negatively influential.

Sensitive areas of inquiry include the patient's sexual history; legal and financial history; alcohol and drug use history; history of trauma, victimization, or violence; and suicidal or homicidal ideation. Inquiry into the possibility of a history of sexual abuse, for example, should be a routine part of interviewing.

A number of methods can be used for obtaining valid information (Shea 2016). One is to wait to ask questions of a potentially sensitive nature until later in the interview, after rapport is established. A second strategy is to provide the patient with a rationale for sensitive questions. For example, the interviewer might tell the patient that questions about sexual history are important for understanding risk for unwanted pregnancies and sexually transmitted infections. A third strategy is for the interviewer to follow up on leads that the patient provides and that open the gate into sensitive areas, while using language that facilitates and normalizes the expression of true responses.

In one approach to the last strategy, the interviewer asks questions that assume the patient has experienced a particular event or feeling. The patient's willingness to af-firm such an experience might become further enhanced by the interviewer telling the patient how such an experience or feeling is common, even expected, given certain circumstances. For example, when asking about suicidal feelings a depressed patient is experiencing, the interviewer might tell the patient that depression is commonly associated with suicidal feelings. Initial negative responses by the patient, especially when counterintuitive, should invite clarification and additional inquiry. Moreover, sometimes interviewers have to respectfully and compassionately explore difficult topics, including specific incidences and details of behaviors (e.g., sexual, abusive, suicidal, violent). For example, an interviewer may need to delve into whether arguing with a family member ever led to physical blows. As with the physical exam, the psychological exam may need to probe personal and sensitive areas that are usually avoided and considered too intrusive.

Interviewing Children and Older Adults

CHILDREN

When assessing children, clinicians should obtain information from a variety of sources, including family members, teachers, and school and medical records. Because children are sensitive to stress in families, family members are an especially important source of information. Furthermore, because very young children are less verbal and less able to sit still for a formal interview, their thoughts and feelings may need to be assessed by how they play and what they draw, as well as by what is attributed to objects such as dolls and stuffed animals. As in any vulnerable population, clinicians should be vigilant to identify possible neglect or abuse.

OLDER ADULT PATIENTS

Because new medical problems commonly arise in older age, along with unidentified or unmet medical needs, clinicians should thoroughly assess possible medical/biological contributions to a psychiatric presentation. Older age, rapidity of symptom onset, concomitant medical illnesses, and alcohol or substance abuse are examples of factors that should heighten suspicion of biological etiologies. Thus, the medical history, physical examination, laboratory tests, and ancillary investigations are routinely important in assessing all patients, but especially geriatric patients with psychiatric presentations. These patients are also vulnerable to adverse social circumstances, and a comprehensive assessment should determine their functional capacity and their ability to maintain safety in their home, as well as their risks for self-neglect and elder abuse. In addition, being careful to ensure that the older patient is physically comfortable and can hear the interviewer is essential for a successful interview.

Keeping Culture in Mind

Culture constitutes a wide developmental, social, and interpersonal matrix relevant to psychiatric diagnosis. It should be considered broadly and not be narrowly interpreted as a matter of ethnicity or race. Everyone has a distinctive personal culture that is determined by individual characteristics as diverse as their age, immigration history, religion, occupation, sexual orientation, school affiliation, club or sports membership, veteran status, linguistic capabilities, and so on. Given that people identify with a conglomerate of cultures and given the wide diversity of beliefs even within a respective culture, the clinician should approach each patient with humility and should respect cultural differences. They should learn about the cultural factors that can contribute to individual psychiatric presentations and integrate relevant protective or exacerbating factors into an understanding of why the patient presented. For example, immigrant or minority population status may be associated with challenges in accessing care, and any such barriers should be identified and addressed. Both clinicians and patients will be influenced by values related to their own cultures, and these may significantly affect the interaction between them as clinician and patient. For instance, cultures differ with regard to expectations about how authoritarian the clinician will be toward the patient and how questioning the patient will be toward the clinician.

DSM-5-TR provides a Cultural Formulation Interview in Section III, "Emerging Measures and Models." This interview is a structured approach to evaluating the interaction of culture and psychiatric and substance use disorders in a patient. Two versions are provided: one to administer to the patient and one for interviewing an informant about the patient. This structured interview guides clinicians through specific questions in a stepwise fashion, helping to define cultural factors and their possible influence on treatment. DSM-5-TR also discusses cultural concepts of distress in the "Culture and Psychiatric Diagnosis" chapter of Section III. For further discussion, see Chapter 4, "Beyond Diagnostic Classification: Structural and Cultural Considerations and DSM-5-TR" in this volume.

MENTAL STATUS EXAMINATION

The MSE assesses the specific details of the patient's appearance, responses, nonverbal communications, and other behaviors during the clinical interview. This structured assessment uses a relatively consistent terminology. The general components of the MSE often include appearance and behavior, motor activities, speech, affect and mood, form and content of thought, perception, and cognition. Table 2–1 lists some examples of details that might be found in each component of an MSE report. The table is not a universal or fully inclusive list; readers are directed to references on the MSE (e.g., Strub and Black 2000).

ASSESSMENT

The psychiatric interview and the MSE may be supplemented by any of the many validated and reliable assessment tools available, both self-administered and clinician-administered. These tools reduce subjectivity in assessments and enable a formal evaluation of outcomes of treatment. Some tools provide information across a range of diagnostic areas, whereas others focus on narrow areas, such as patients' emotional or cognitive abilities, or they may seek to determine the nature, severity, and duration of certain features of illness. Clinicians should learn about the strengths and weaknesses of diagnostic tools, including their validity, sensitivity, and specificity, and

TABLE 2–1.   Components of the mental status examination, with examples

Appearance and behavior: level of consciousness, attentiveness or distractibility, attitude toward the examiner, eye contact, clothing, grooming

Motor behavior: agitation or retardation, mannerisms, abnormal movements, gait

Speech: rate, volume, quantity, prosody

Affect and mood: *affect* is the feeling state of the patient as observed by the examiner (e.g., hostile, sad, happy, fearful, blunted, flat); *mood* is the patient's self-described feeling state (e.g., anxious, depressed, angry)

Form of thought (thought process): connectivity between ideas, perseveration, coherence, looseness of associations

Thought content: suicidal and/or homicidal ideas, intentions, or plans; delusions; obsessions

Perception: illusions, hallucinations, derealization, depersonalization

Cognition: orientation, attention, memory (different types), spatial abilities, abstract thinking, judgment, insight

Note.   Examples are not all-inclusive.

learn how to apply them for individual patients in conjunction with the psychiatric interview. DSM-5-TR includes the chapter "Assessment Measures" in Section III, "Emerging Measures and Models," that features the following measures:

- DSM-5 Self-Rated Level 1 Cross-Cutting Symptom Measure—Adult
- Parent/Guardian-Rated DSM-5 Level 1 Cross-Cutting Symptom Measure—Child Age 6–17
- Clinician-Rated Dimensions of Psychosis Symptom Severity
- World Health Organization Disability Assessment Schedule 2.0 (WHODAS 2.0)

Of note, each of these measures assesses symptoms in a dimensional manner— that is, the symptoms are rated according to points along a continuum (e.g., from mild to severe). This rating system is in contrast to systems that merely indicate in a categorical manner whether a symptom is present or absent. Most of the criteria in DSM-5-TR are categorical; in other words, the person is rated as either having a symptom or not having it. Dimensional ratings allow a more graduated and nuanced characterization of symptoms (see Chapter 3, "Understanding Different Approaches to Diagnostic Classification").

The DSM-5 Self-Rated Level 1 Cross-Cutting Symptom Measure, with separate versions for adults and children, is used to rate symptoms in a variety of domains along a continuum. Of note, the symptoms are not necessarily aligned with one diagnosis, and the endorsement of one symptom does not connote a specific diagnosis because several diagnoses may manifest the same symptom. For instance, the symptoms of sleep disturbance may apply to a number of possible diagnoses. Thus, the term *cross-cutting* is used because these symptoms cross diagnostic lines and provide a picture of the patient's presentation without assigning a diagnosis. This depiction of the patient's symptoms is holistic, and it complements and adds information to the categorical system of the DSM-5-TR diagnostic criteria.

In addition to the two cross-cutting measures, DSM-5-TR includes two other dimensional measures. The Clinician-Rated Dimensions of Psychosis Symptom Severity is a rating scale for the severity of eight symptoms of psychosis. The WHODAS 2.0 is used to measure the degree of disability, secondary to a health or mental health condition, experienced by the patient in everyday life during the past 30 days. It has a dimensional scale with a 5-point rating system ranging from having no problem doing a chore to not being able to do it at all. The 36 listed items include daily functions, such as moving about physically, grooming oneself, and interacting with people. This scale measures functioning without regard to diagnosis; disability may be secondary to any health or mental health condition, although knowledge of the specific condition(s) is not required.

The three types of scales in DSM-5-TR's "Assessment Measures" chapter may be considered along with the diagnostic interview. They are dimensional in construction and are not designed to make diagnoses. The diagnostic interview seeks to determine DSM-5-TR diagnoses; the assessment measures add value and nuance by attempting to quantify and track symptom severity and disabilities associated with the diagnoses made through the interview.

There is a potentially complex interplay between psychiatric and medical conditions. Medical conditions can cause psychiatric disorders, including mood, anxiety, psychotic, and cognitive disorders. Medical conditions can also adversely impact preexisting mental disorders. Also, patients with medical conditions might experience psychological problems, such as anxiety or depressive symptoms, that occur in connection with having been diagnosed with those conditions. In turn, preexisting psychiatric conditions can cause, underlie, or be associated with medical problems. Clinicians should be vigilant in identifying these interactions.

Physical exams and laboratory tests, in conjunction with the medical history and medical review of symptoms, serve to better identify salient medical issues. Identification of medical problems is an essential part of a comprehensive biopsychosocial prevention and treatment plan and may require collaborating with the patient's primary care and consultant physicians. The physical examination, when appropriate, should be thorough and adhere to examination standards. Laboratory and other diagnostic tests should be prudently ordered and justified in light of their relevance and costs.

SUMMARY

The clinical interview plays an essential role in arriving at an accurate diagnosis. How an interview is conducted is an expression of the interviewer's professionalism, and it serves as the cornerstone of the relationship between the clinician and patient. As described in this chapter, the clinical interview is grounded in a non-reductionist biopsychosocial model that gives importance to the whole person in context. Often, patients may be in distress or have significant impairments that become evident in a clinical interview, and sensitive information is—and should be—elicited in an indepth psychiatric interview. For these reasons, special care to address the comfort of and demonstrate respect toward the patient is warranted in psychiatry. The psychiatric interview, in particular, relies on a rigorous MSE and systematic inclusion of information from medical records and other informants, assessment (including formal measures), physical examination, and laboratory testing.

SELF-ASSESSMENT

Questions to Discuss With Colleagues and Mentors

1. How do you apply the biopsychosocial model for the practice of psychiatry and related fields?
2. How do the professional virtues of integrity, compassion, self-effacement, and self-sacrifice apply to the routine practice of psychiatry and related fields?
3. What methods, including wording of questions, do you use to facilitate patients' disclosure of sensitive information and to screen for selected disorders?
4. What areas of the comprehensive psychiatric interview do you find challenging or discomforting, and what steps do you take to increase your comfort and skills in those areas?
5. How do you incorporate a physical and laboratory examinations into your assessment of psychiatric patients?

Short-Answer Questions

1. What is the virtue of self-effacement, and what are the implications of it for managing patients from different cultures?
2. How should a clinician begin a psychiatric interview with a new patient?
3. What techniques can be used for eliciting accurate information from patients on sensitive topic areas?

Answers

1. **The virtue of self-effacement requires the clinician's humility. This virtue enables clinicians to put aside differences when these should not count as important in the clinical relationship. Clinicians should therefore strive to learn about the cultures of each of their patients and to respect their cultural differences.**

2. **A new interview should begin with a general introduction, a statement of purpose, and an explanation about the degree of confidentiality. Providing patients with an early opportunity to talk about what is important to them by using open-ended questions and by responding empathetically should help to develop rapport and a therapeutic alliance.**

3. **The interviewer should identify levels of discomfort in the interviewer or patient when asking questions that might impede sensitive and accurate**

inquiry. Factors that enhance patients' willingness to answer honestly include developing rapport before asking questions of a sensitive nature, explaining the rationale for the questions, gently following leads, using facilitative or normalizing language, getting behavioral details, and being flexible to patients' personality style.

RECOMMENDED READINGS

Jarvis GE, Kirmayer LJ, Gómez-Carrillo A, et al: Update on the Cultural Formulation Interview. Focus (Am Psychiatr Publ) 18(1):40–46, 2020 32047396

Poole R, Higgo R: Psychiatric Interviewing and Assessment. New York, Cambridge University Press, 2006

Shea SC: Psychiatric Interviewing: The Art of Understanding: A Practical Guide for Psychiatrists, Psychologists, Counselors, Social Workers, Nurses, and Other Mental Health Professionals, 3rd Edition. Philadelphia, PA, Elsevier, 2016

Sommers-Flanagan J, Sommers-Flanagan R: Clinical Interviewing, 7th Edition. New York, Wiley, 2023

Strub RL, Black FW: The Mental Status Examination in Neurology, 4th Edition. Philadelphia, PA, FA Davis, 2000

Trzepacz PT, Baker RW: The Psychiatric Mental Status Examination. New York, Oxford University Press, 1993

REFERENCES

American Psychiatric Association: Diagnostic and Statistical Manual of Mental Disorders, 5th Edition, Text Revision. Washington, DC, American Psychiatric Association, 2022

Engel GL: The need for a new medical model: a challenge for biomedicine. Science 196(4286):129–136, 1977 847460

McCullough LB: John Gregory and the Invention of Professional Medical Ethics and the Profession of Medicine. Dordrecht, The Netherlands, Kluwer Academic, 1998

McHugh PR, Slavney PR: The Perspectives of Psychiatry, 2nd Edition. Baltimore, MD, Johns Hopkins University Press, 1998

Shea SC: Psychiatric Interviewing: The Art of Understanding: A Practical Guide for Psychiatrists, Psychologists, Counselors, Social Workers, Nurses, and Other Mental Health Professionals, 3rd Edition. Philadelphia, PA, Elsevier, 2016

Strub RL, Black FW: The Mental Status Examination in Neurology, 4th Edition. Philadelphia, PA, FA Davis, 2000

CHAPTER 3

Understanding Different Approaches to Diagnostic Classification

Laura Weiss Roberts, M.D., M.A.

Giving a name, a diagnosis, to an illness or condition that is due to a specific and known cause is intuitively clear. Pneumococcal pneumonia, for example, is an illness in which the lung is infected with the bacterium *Streptococcus pneumoniae*. Typically affecting young children, older adults, or immunocompromised individuals, this infection may cause individuals to experience high fever, cough, shortness of breath, rapid breathing, and chest pain. Untreated, this infection can lead to death or enduring disability. And a person who has broken a leg in a bicycle accident will have, well, a broken leg, which might be characterized as being a compound, complete, comminuted, or compression bone fracture.

When the causes of an illness are not certain, the ways of sorting and classifying the dysfunction and disruption in health—assigning names or "diagnoses" to the problems—are less intuitive. In the context of mental illness, the origins of most psychiatric disorders are unknown, and definitive biomarkers for various disorders have yet to be discovered. Years ago, psychiatric diagnoses were based on assumptions—primarily untestable assertions of causality. Without clear etiology, pathogenesis, or discernible biomarkers, psychiatric diagnoses have thus become defined phenome-

Adapted from Ohayon MM, Roberts LW: "Understanding Different Approaches to Diagnostic Classification," in *Study Guide to DSM-5*. Edited by Roberts LW, Louie AK. Washington, DC, American Psychiatric Publishing, 2015, pp 33–46.

nologically—that is, by attaching the name of an illness to a specific set of symptoms and signs that together represent a psychiatric "syndrome."

The identification of clear boundaries between different syndromes is essential for the validity of diagnoses. Drawing such boundaries has proven difficult with major depression, anorexia nervosa, schizophrenia, PTSD, and alcohol dependence, among other illnesses. A clear diagnosis is useful to the extent that it provides information on possible etiology, treatment, and prognosis. Endeavoring to improve diagnostic classification is the intent of DSM-5-TR, which uses insights from clinical and epidemiological studies (American Psychiatric Association 2022). DSM-5-TR thus uses an approach that aligns with the manner in which a clinician reaches diagnostic conclusions: with each answer, the diagnosis becomes more refined.

Case Example: Refining a Diagnosis

Mr. Ramos, a 48-year-old man with a long-standing diagnosis of schizoaffective disorder, lost his daughter 1 year ago in an accident in which she was struck by a car. He is Hispanic, and throughout his life he has had very traditional religious values and beliefs. He tells his psychiatrist that he is "in despair" but feels comforted by "visits" from his daughter each night. He "sees" her in the flutter of his window curtain each night as he is falling asleep. Her visits started just a couple of months ago. He discussed his daughter's visits with his priest who, according to the patient, "at first" thought that the visits were "nice" but recently told the patient that he was "concerned" and thought the patient ought to "tell his doctor" about the visits.

Mr. Ramos has never used alcohol or other substances. He endorses feeling sad "nearly" every day, particularly in the mornings, and has lost 15 pounds. He says that the weight loss was unintended and that it is happening because his daughter is no longer there to cook his favorite dishes for him. He has adhered to his medication regimen, which includes medication for psychotic and mood symptoms. He has worked for more than 30 years on his family's ranch.

Questions to consider:

- What kinds of evidence does the psychiatrist have to help understand this clinical story?
- Mr. Ramos describes feeling "despair"—is this a symptom, and what is the differential diagnosis that goes with this finding?
- Mr. Ramos does not feel distressed by his daughter's "visits," yet they have become a cause for others' concern. How does this experience relate to the normative experience in the patient's religious community?
- What should be of greatest concern to the psychiatrist? For instance, what serious physical health problems occur as an individual falls asleep (e.g., hypnagogic hallucinations) at night?
- What additional clinical data are needed to refine the diagnostic picture?

When a diagnostic framework is created, clinical phenomena must be understood within, and may be organized into, different hierarchical levels and components. At a basic level, a clinician may assemble facts such as the results of laboratory tests, the scores on assessment scales, or the endorsement of symptoms or complaints on a checklist. In this context, a *fact* is a characteristic for which it is possible to define a normative value and its boundaries (e.g., a mean value with its standard deviation). For example, members of the general population sleep on average 6 hours and 35 minutes per night (Boulos et al. 2019). This amount—395 minutes—is a statistical norm. Different patterns of sleep represent variations or deviations from this norm and establish the range of variations in sleep behavior. Research may be performed to explore the extreme variations to this norm (e.g., two standard deviations from the norm, or the fifth and ninety-fifth percentiles) and can examine the health-related consequences for individuals whose sleep patterns are at the extremes. This process of identifying the norms and the extremes from normative values (in this case, sleep behavior) is an evidence-driven way of distinguishing highly specific clinical features that by definition signal the presence of specific diagnoses.

A list of facts does not assign relevance or importance to the individual items. Nevertheless, facts have value in that they can be used in research that may inform clinical care, such as in identifying norms in a given population. An example is the experience of hearing one's name spoken when no one is present. This "finding" could be seen as a symptom of a psychotic illness, but norm-based data reveal that this experience occurs commonly among individuals who are not in any sense "ill."

Complaints represent the clinician's second level of basic information. Diagnostic classification schemes also may be oriented toward categorizing patient *complaints*—that is, concerns reported by a patient. The complaint matters in that it reveals what the individual perceives as being a health problem. For health researchers, studying patient complaints can help in understanding what motivates individuals to seek help and how help seeking relates to symptom burden. Patient complaints, moreover, are reflective of the perceived need for care across larger groups and populations and may be used to evaluate the efficiency of health care providers in recognizing and meeting these perceived needs.

Symptoms are facts and patient complaints that relate to pathology and may be interpreted by the clinician. The clinician's medical knowledge and degree of specialization influence how well they discern and ascribe meaning to symptoms. Symptoms may then be the fundamental element in a diagnostic framework, although they may have a subjective component.

Diagnostic criteria are collections of symptoms and clinical observations that are grouped together to easily define clinical entities so that health care providers can reliably recognize them and communicate about them. These collections of symptoms and clinical observations can be assembled into syndromes, which allow for more refined efforts at validation of more specific diagnostic entities. Criterion-level investigation also presents the opportunity to explore the relationship between symptomatology and pathology or impairment, which affected individuals may ignore or not understand. Thus, a *syndrome* is a collection of criteria or symptoms necessary for a diagnosis. However, other possible diagnoses (the *differential diagnosis*) may not have been ruled out yet.

Disorders are based on the previous elements—facts, complaints, symptoms, criteria, and syndromes—and represent a well-defined collection of pathological elements grouped into a pattern recognized as necessary for a diagnosis to be made. Accuracy in defining diagnostic categories matters for precise communication among clinicians, researchers, and teachers. Diagnoses are valuable for people living with these conditions because appropriate interventions may be identified, introduced, and evaluated for their effectiveness.

INSIGHTS FROM EPIDEMIOLOGY

Traditionally, *binary models* are used to mark the existence of a diagnosis; that is, they indicate the presence or absence of symptoms and diagnoses. This approach is rather artificial in the sense that it allows little room for the perceptions and experiences of the individuals, which is particularly salient in psychiatry. Symptoms associated with mental illness are rarely black or white—they come in all shades of gray. For example, when a person endorses feeling "very" depressed or "somewhat" depressed, there is a sense that these reports are truly different for that individual. Using different and graduated ways of eliciting symptoms may improve the accuracy of diagnoses and reduce uncertainty at both the symptom and diagnosis levels.

In epidemiology, probabilistic and fuzzy models are two ways that clinicians can capture subtler, more nuanced findings regarding the presence of a disease process. The *probabilistic model* is shaped by Bayesian theory, and it attributes certainty degrees to the symptoms or the diagnosis. This approach allows for the creation of a natural framework that retains the characteristics of the diagnostic classification and can still be interpreted in the usual way in practice. The *fuzzy logic model* (Zadeh 1979) is based on the concept of reasoning in degrees and linguistic variables, as opposed to numerical or quantitative degrees. For example, one can feel "slightly" or "a lot" depressed during the day and experience feeling depressed "daily" or "nearly every day." The same can be said about continuous variables. For example, an individual may be considered obese when their BMI is 30 kg/m^2 or greater. What can be said about an individual whose BMI is 29.8 kg/m^2? Is the conclusion that this individual is not obese? A pure Boolean reasoning would conclude so, whereas a physician in real practice would not. In fuzzy logic, one can determine the degree of membership of "BMI" to the category "obese." Consequently, the fuzzy logic model has the advantage of accommodating the imprecision of the human language. Using fuzzy logic, diagnoses are given with different levels of certainty rather than absolute certainty (Ohayon 1999).

Thus, the models used to describe psychopathology are imperfect. Mainly, the validity of psychopathological models is verified through their ability to represent real phenomena via an identification mechanism between what is symbolic and what is real. Nevertheless, this mechanism is only and always a process of generalization because the model remains an unverified representation of the real phenomena.

Currently, categorical models are the most widely used in the world. The *International Classification of Diseases and Related Health Problems* (ICD) by the World Health Organization and DSM are two examples. With progress in the field of psychiatry, new classification entities are created; the objective is to achieve a better description of mental disorders while establishing a common language among researchers, clinicians, and mental health professionals. Nevertheless, these categorical models raise several concerns—mostly regarding their validity—because they are still anchored in phenomenology such as "facts" and "complaints." Some patients do not fit into any specific diagnostic category, whereas others fall into several. Despite the increased number of diagnoses, many disorders are not represented at all. The increased number of categories renders their use by clinicians more difficult. Furthermore, the strong co-occurrence between some diagnostic classes suggests an inadequacy in the newly created categories. Finally, the absence of correlations between proposed classification entities and the efficacy of the different pharmacological treatments raises further concerns about the classifications' validity.

DSM APPROACH

DSM was originally valued as a research tool to provide common guidelines for investigators rather than for its clinical utility. Over time, it has become firmly ingrained as the standard of psychiatric diagnosis among mental health professionals. Making a diagnosis is not a mathematical problem, however. The sum of diagnostic criteria does not necessarily provide the best answer. The concept of diagnosis implies the ability to sort uncertainties and to decide between equally plausible solutions. Progressively, the distinction between *concomitant diagnoses* (which are co-occurring and related) and *concurrent diagnoses* (which are co-occurring and separate) is vanishing. This distinction is crucial because it bears important consequences for epidemiology and clinical practice. Nonexclusive categorization essentially inflates the prevalence of some mental disorders. In the selection of treatment interventions, furthermore, the ambiguity and overlap of diagnostic categories increases the likelihood of nonresponse to treatment.

A classification system ideally works as a funnel, increasing the specificity in discerning or determining a given disease. For example, at the symptomatological level, 28.7% of the population endorses depressive symptoms. This prevalence progressively decreases to 5.2% of the population once the differential diagnosis is completed (Figure 3–1). Consequently, by itself, the presence of any depressive symptoms is helpful, but not in any way sufficient for planning treatment. Careful reflection on the differential diagnosis (i.e., engaging in the process of excluding other diagnoses) can help clinicians define a careful diagnosis and rule out other likely illness processes or diagnoses.

DSM-5 (American Psychiatric Association 2013) and DSM-5-TR preserve and advance the diagnostic classification scheme of DSM-IV (American Psychiatric Association 1994). DSM-5 developers sought to capture emerging scientific evidence to more clearly separate or at times align diagnostic categories and to provide a clearer rationale for elevating and refining specific diagnoses. The overarching metastructure of DSM-5 was very intentional, creating a spectrum in which similar diagnostic categories were placed nearer to one another where possible. DSM-5 included 157 separate disorders, compared with 172 separate disorders in DSM-IV. Interestingly, with the decrease in total disorders in DSM-5, 15 new disorders were introduced, 2 were eliminated (sexual aversion disorder and polysubstance-related disorder), and 22 were combined or consolidated with others. DSM-5-TR includes 3 new disorders (Table 3–1), as well as changes in the diagnostic criteria or specifiers for 70 disorders. Overall,

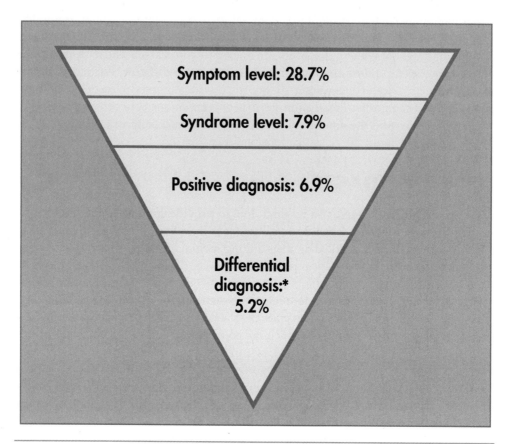

FIGURE 3–1. Prevalence of depressive symptoms and diagnosis in the general population.

Differential diagnosis refers to the positive diagnosis of a disorder, excluding alternative possible diagnoses.

Source. M.M. Ohayon, personal data, July 2013.

TABLE 3–1. Disorders newly introduced in DSM-5-TR

Prolonged grief disorder

Unspecified mood disorder

Stimulant-induced mild neurocognitive disorder

the classification of disorders emerging in childhood, sleep disorders, and substance-related disorders changed perhaps the most in DSM-5, whereas the personality disorders were preserved in their near-exact formulation from DSM-IV.

As discussed in detail throughout this *Study Guide*, DSM-5 and DSM-5-TR changed the diagnostic criteria in highly utilized, important, and long-standing disorders such as schizophrenia, bipolar disorder, major depression, PTSD, and ADHD. DSM-5 also moved away from "primary" and "secondary" attributions and eliminated the "not otherwise specified" language, instead employing "other specified" and "unspecified" conditions, bringing DSM-5 and DSM-5-TR closer to the language of the ICD system.

Diagnostic schemes are adaptive tools that evolve. Readers should seek to understand the value, application, and limitations of DSM-5-TR as well as other diagnostic classification approaches. For learners, DSM-5-TR will prove to be a helpful scaffolding for knowledge and will serve to inform clinical and scientific judgment, which is an expression of expertise and professionalism.

Case Example: The Difference Between the "Complaint" and the Diagnosis

Ms. Rush is a 26-year-old single woman completing her doctorate in biosciences. She is referred to a psychiatrist at the university mental health center because she has requested sleeping pills. "I just can't sleep," she says. Ms. Rush reports that she has had trouble sleeping since she was a teenager. She states that she wakes up several times each night and that this occurs three to four times per week ("it seems like every other night"). She sleeps, on average, 5 hours per night. She feels sleepy during the day and "has" to take a 1-hour nap almost every afternoon.

In the course of the initial visit, the psychiatrist learns that Ms. Rush has been experiencing difficulty with her doctoral studies and feels that her life has been "extremely stressful" for about 1 year. She has lost 14 pounds in the past year. ("I didn't try to lose the weight—it just happened from the stress.") Her BMI is 23 kg/m^2. Eight months ago, she and her boyfriend of 3 years broke up. Ms. Rush acknowledges that she wakes up every morning feeling extremely depressed and down; the feeling decreases during the day but is always present, every day. She says she cannot find any pleasure in her life. She feels that everything is taking an enormous effort. She is always tired and lacks energy even when she is not doing anything. Concentrating on her studies has become increasingly difficult. She feels like she is letting everybody down. She states that she does not think her decision to get the Ph.D. in biosciences was a good idea, that she will not get a job in her field in the future, but that now "there is no turning back." Ms. Rush says some days are so difficult that she thinks she should "finish it"—ending her life so that she will not be such a disappointment to her family and her mentor.

Ms. Rush denies previous psychiatric or medical history. She had "a difficult time" when she was in high school and says that this was about the same time that she started having difficulty sleeping. She does not drink coffee or caffeinated sodas, and she has never smoked cigarettes or used any drugs. She "almost never" drinks alcohol. She feels she should exercise more ("I try to take walks once or twice a week with my roommate"). She says that she has not had interest in sex for "more than a year."

On mental status examination, Ms. Rush is cooperative, looks thin, is dressed in athletic sweats and worn tennis shoes, and wears no jewelry or makeup. She sits very quietly, with little movement, and she answers most questions with few words, often by only a yes or no. Her speech is clear and normal in pitch, tone, and rhythm. She denies hallucinations but says that she sometimes hears someone calling to her as she falls asleep at night ("like someone is in my bedroom, but I call for my roommate and she isn't there"). She denies unusual thoughts or fears but "once in a while" she feels like she is being punished, as though there is a plan for everything to go wrong in her life.

Questions to consider:

- Difficulty sleeping is Ms. Rush's complaint and is the reason she is referred for psychiatric care at the university health center, but what are Ms. Rush's symptoms?

- How does the concept of a "funnel" apply to this case?
- How might the presenting complaint lead a clinician to give an incorrect diagnosis of a sleep disorder?

SELF-ASSESSMENT

Questions to Discuss With Colleagues and Mentors

1. What are the differences between a syndrome and a disorder? Why does this differentiation matter to a learner in the health professions?
2. What are the advantages to a diagnostic classification system that uses descriptive phenomenological criteria as opposed to etiological or causal-based criteria?
3. How do you handle overlapping diagnostic criteria for different disorders?
4. Why does ruling out other diagnoses matter in clinical practice? How does arriving at a differential diagnosis assist patient care?

Short-Answer Questions

1. Which of the following lists is correctly ordered in terms of greatest prevalence to least prevalence?

   A. Disorder, symptom, syndrome.
   B. Disorder, syndrome, symptom.
   C. Symptom, disorder, syndrome.
   D. Symptom, syndrome, disorder.
   E. Syndrome, symptom, disorder.

2. Weight loss can be considered which of the following?

   A. A fact.
   B. A complaint.
   C. A clinical sign.
   D. A diagnostic criterion.
   E. All of the above.

Answers

1. D.   Symptom, syndrome, disorder.

The list that is correctly ordered in terms of the greatest prevalence to least prevalence is symptom, syndrome, disorder. A diagnostic classification scheme narrows from widely experienced phenomena (such as a symptom of feeling sad or helpless) to a disorder (such as major depressive disorder).

2. E.   All of the above.

Weight loss may be a fact, a patient concern or complaint, a clinical sign, a diagnostic criterion, or all of the above depending on the clinical situation. For example, weight loss may be a fact, clinical sign, and diagnostic criterion in the circumstance of a patient with anorexia nervosa, but may not be a patient complaint.

RECOMMENDED READINGS

First MB, Yousif LH, Clarke DE, et al: DSM-5-TR: overview of what's new and what's changed. World Psychiatry 21(2):218–219, 2022 35524596

Regier DA, Narrow WE, Kuhl EA, et al (eds): The Conceptual Evolution of DSM-5. Washington, DC, American Psychiatric Publishing, 2011

REFERENCES

American Psychiatric Association: Diagnostic and Statistical Manual of Mental Disorders, 4th Edition. Washington, DC, American Psychiatric Association, 1994

American Psychiatric Association: Diagnostic and Statistical Manual of Mental Disorders, 5th Edition. Arlington, VA, American Psychiatric Association, 2013

American Psychiatric Association: Diagnostic and Statistical Manual of Mental Disorders, 5th Edition, Text Revision. Washington, DC, American Psychiatric Association, 2022

Boulos MI, Jairam T, Kendzerska T, et al: Normal polysomnography parameters in healthy adults: a systematic review and meta-analysis. Lancet Respir Med 7(6):533–543, 2019 31006560

Ohayon MM: Improving decision-making processes with the fuzzy logic approach in the epidemiology of sleep disorders. J Psychosom Res 47(4):297–311, 1999 10616225

Zadeh LA: A theory of approximate reasoning. Machine Intelligence 9:149–194, 1979

CHAPTER 4

Beyond Diagnostic Classification

STRUCTURAL AND CULTURAL CONSIDERATIONS AND DSM-5-TR

Matthew L. Edwards, M.D.

Lucy Ogbu-Nwobodo, M.D., M.S., M.A.S.

Belinda S. Bandstra, M.D., M.A.

The field of psychiatry recognizes that a diagnostic approach largely focused on pathology is only one lens to view the larger picture of mental health and well-being. Although DSM-5-TR (American Psychiatric Association 2022) is a shared language to communicate and describe mental disorders using a common set of symptoms, criteria, and considerations with a high degree of reliability, some factors that affect mental health and wellness do not neatly fall under diagnosable conditions but are nonetheless important to health outcomes and health care services. This chapter aims to outline social and cultural factors that influence health outcomes and access to health services and how these factors are represented in the DSM-5-TR framework.

We would like to acknowledge the contributions of Alyxian H.H. Guarneros Luna in the development of the case example for this chapter.

STRUCTURAL CONSIDERATIONS AND DSM-5-TR

Psychiatrists and public health experts have debated how and why mental health inequities persist. In a landmark paper titled "Social Conditions as Fundamental Causes of Disease," Link and Phelan (1995) argued that "social factors such as socioeconomic status and social support are likely 'fundamental causes' of disease" that create and maintain inequity. They acknowledged that these fundamental causes included factors such as race, income, gender, and social status, but even these considerations did not fully describe the impact of social influences on health. Their research led to extensive literature demonstrating that resource-poor and underrepresented racial groups have poorer health outcomes than their counterparts, regardless of socioeconomic status. These findings further support the observations that public policy, economics, and social systems all shape inequality, govern access to resources, and consequently may engender health inequity.

DSM-5-TR, like the *International Classification of Diseases* (ICD), acknowledges that there are nonpsychopathological factors that impact health, health services, and the larger health system. This addition to DSM-5-TR closes out the "Diagnostic Criteria and Codes" section with the chapter "Other Conditions That May Be a Focus of Clinical Attention," which includes such topics as abuse and neglect, relational and educational problems, occupational and housing problems, and economic problems. It also discusses issues related to the social environment; crime or interaction with the legal system; other psychosocial, personal, and environmental circumstances; access to medical and other health care; and circumstances of personal history. The factors, situations, and conditions included in this section may be assigned to a patient's treatment for a multitude of reasons, including if 1) it is the purpose of the encounter; 2) it may help explain the need for therapeutic intervention; 3) it may play a role in the initiation or exacerbation of a mental disorder; or 4) it should be considered in the overall management plan.

Most of these topics are connected to social determinants of health, which the World Health Organization (2008) defined as "the conditions in which people are born, grow, live, work, and age, and the systems put in place to deal with illness." Social conditions are influenced by the stratification of power and resources across all levels of society (World Health Organization 2008). Social determinants of health are known to play a role in psychiatric disorders and are often correlated with adverse health outcomes such as poor mental health, worsening mental illness, substance use disorders, increased morbidity, disability, and early mortality. Many social determinants of health are related to structural factors in our society and are shaped by the social, political, and economic institutions within our society.

DSM-5-TR recognizes descriptively that structural issues may be "a focus of clinical attention," and it provides a systematic list that may be useful to clinicians in documenting these issues. Structural competency would be a step further, to a point at which clinical practitioners recognize and intervene in the social, economic, and political conditions that produce health inequities. As clinicians move toward structural competence, they may begin to recognize how institutions, neighborhood contexts, economic forces, public policies, and health care delivery systems shape symptoms and disease. This framework provides a meaningful direction to expand the scope of interventions and responsibilities within health care systems, transcending the individual-level clinician-patient interactions toward larger systems-level factors that influence health.

Although DSM-5-TR mostly focuses on pathology-specific processes, most of the items in "Other Conditions That May Be a Focus of Clinical Attention" fall largely under social determinants of health and structural mental health issues—issues, therefore, that clinicians should recognize, document, and consider. By paying attention to these items, thought leaders in psychiatry also may develop a deeper understanding of social determinants so that access to therapeutic interventions and treatment can be less limiting and can more fully encompass the psychosocial needs of all individuals. There is a need for a broader awareness, understanding, and facility in describing these needs.

DSM-5-TR uses Z codes that are equivalent to previous V and Z codes from the ICD classification system. Z codes and V codes are also known as "factors influencing health status and contact with health services." In the past, V codes generally referred to areas of global functioning, such as interpersonal relationships, family cohesion, education, and work, that may bear on health and wellness. Meanwhile, Z codes referred to social determinants of health that may influence the experience of illness. Current Z codes are not specific to individuals with mental health conditions, nor do they necessarily imply that an individual may be at a greater risk of experiencing mental distress. Nevertheless, they describe situations and circumstances that may help explain an individual's health outcomes.

DSM-5-TR is one of several resources that list and classify disorders. Whereas DSM-5-TR and its related publications classify mental disorders and conditions, the ICD is a set of diagnostic conditions and codes that structure all medical conditions and diagnoses. It was developed by the World Health Organization in 1893, just as DSM was developed in 1952, with the intent of creating a standardized set of diagnostic criteria for medical conditions. The history of Z codes traces the medical field's recognition and acceptance of social, demographic, environmental, and emotional factors that shape health outcomes and access to health services. These codes are not medical conditions and do not appear in other classification systems within ICD or DSM. Rather, they reflect an extension of the thinking around factors that influence health and disease.

The first Z codes, including classifications for housing and economic instability, first appeared in ICD-9 in 1979. Over the past 40 years, these codes have grown to several thousand, including medication underdosing due to financial hardship (Z91.120), health impacts of underemployment or unemployment (Z56), other problems related to life management difficulty (Z73.89), and psychological trauma (Z91.4). These examples describe social determinants of health that are profoundly shaped by social, economic, and political factors that structure access to resources, such as education, money, and influence.

Individuals at greater risk for the detrimental effects of social determinants of health may be reluctant to discuss their social circumstances. Moreover, their clinicians may be reluctant to address these circumstances because of concerns regarding stigma, discrimination, and embarrassment of patients, who are often from marginalized backgrounds. However, not addressing social determinants of health such as education, financial well-being, housing, and food security will likely lead to worsened health outcomes and health and social inequities. Furthermore, addressing these issues in clinical settings leads to positive physical and mental health at the population level.

To be sure, Z codes are not the sole purview of DSM, but their inclusion reflects growing recognition of the social determinants of mental health—that is, the social determinants of health that specifically lead to mental health outcomes. Many of these outcomes and factors, from poverty and discrimination to structural racism, trauma, and proximity to interpersonal conflict, may be social determinants of both health and mental health; for example, discrimination may impact both, whereas stigma related to mental health conditions may have a greater impact on mental health.

Social determinants of physical and mental health are equally important because they often overlap and contribute to discrete and disproportionate effects on mental health. Moreover, there is a strong link between physical and mental health. Individuals with serious mental illness, for example, are more likely to die from preventable chronic illness than their counterparts without mental health conditions (Lawrence and Kisely 2010). A growing literature suggests that addressing social determinants of health can highlight inequities and inform treatments and interventions to mitigate them (Daniel et al. 2018; Shim and Compton 2018). Further research is needed to explore these relationships fully.

Although the research on the potential impact of Z codes is scant, there is a growing body of research on social causes as contributors to physical and mental diseases. Evidence indicates that socioeconomic status, demographic factors such as race and sex/gender, and other social characteristics are "fundamental causes of disease" because they structure access to health services and exposure to the adverse, deleterious, and detrimental social factors that influence disease (Link and Phelan 1995).

One example of a fundamental social cause of disease is limited education, which is associated not only with lower socioeconomic status but also with diabetes, heart disease, and cancer risk. The literature on social causes and social determinants of health show these associations. Although *social causes* may imply causation, these relationships are complex and shaped by many factors. Moreover, a given social cause can promote health while also serving as a risk factor for particular conditions or diseases. Racialization is one example of this type of factor; whereas race may be protective against some mental health conditions, such as suicidal ideation, it may worsen access to care and, in the process, worsen mental health outcomes. Suicidal ideation is another example of a social factor that may be a risk factor for some people and a protective factor for others (Stone et al. 2023). Recent trends have demonstrated a change in this relationship, however, which suggests increases in suicide rates among non-Hispanic American Indian or Alaska Native persons, non-Hispanic Black or African

American persons, and Hispanic persons. Recent research suggests that individuals with intersectional identities or multiple, marginalized identities may experience a higher prevalence of suicidal thoughts and behaviors (Forrest 2023).

Z codes may describe aspects of health and well-being that may not necessarily be addressed by biomedical interventions (e.g., food insecurity, homelessness, effects of involvement in the criminal legal system), but these aspects of health may nonetheless contribute to an individual's experience of illness. Thus, although the literature does not generally measure the direct impact of Z codes on health status, contact with the health system, or health outcomes, if systems can address some of the psychosocial stressors and other circumstances they capture, then these systems may more effectively address the social determinants of health.

Whereas a physician may document social determinants of health by listing a Z code or another description of adverse social circumstances, addressing these factors requires efforts outside typical professional medical activities. Some examples include physicians' efforts to expand supportive housing for individuals with severe and persistent mental illness in New York City; ensure equitable and adequate pay for entry-level or essential workers; and provide nutritional resources for individuals with food insecurity or promote access to nutritional foods among individuals who live in neighborhoods characterized as food deserts. There is no consistent approach to remunerating clinicians who include the social determinants of health in clinical documentation and assessment. Thus, the incentive to include these determinants is largely driven by individual factors, which may reflect cultural, social, institutional, or medical priorities.

CULTURAL CONSIDERATIONS AND DSM-5-TR

One of the primary goals of DSM-5-TR is to create a shared language for communicating and describing emotional, cognitive, and psychological experiences. DSM-5-TR plays an important role in providing the terms and grammar for understanding the different ways we experience emotional and mental distress. (Note that DSM has not always done this.) It serves as a tool to communicate and describe mental disorders using a common set of symptoms, criteria, and considerations with high reliability.

Shared language is culture, and clinicians should recognize that not every patient shares their language or culture. Different groups express psychological distress or define mental health differently (*cultural concepts of distress*). Different cultural groups may have different sources of vulnerability and resilience. Beliefs, behaviors, language, and modes of expression may differ across cultural groups, whether they are thought to explain an illness or to form a larger cultural syndrome. How (or whether) a patient expresses these to their clinician is also culturally determined.

DSM-5-TR recognizes that it communicates shared and different experiences across an increasingly diverse cultural landscape. The Cross-Cutting Review Committee on Cultural Issues focused on several considerations regarding how culture shapes the experience of mental illness. These considerations included

1. Cultural and social structural issues
2. Cultural norms and practices
3. Cultural concepts of distress
4. Influence of racism and discrimination on psychiatric diagnosis

The "Culture and Psychiatric Diagnosis" chapter in DSM-5-TR Section III highlights the Outline for Cultural Formulation. This framework for eliciting and considering information about culture is intended to support psychiatric diagnosis. The Cultural Formulation Interview (CFI) gives a structured example of addressing these issues with patients. Including the CFI underscores the large challenge of incorporating culture into the diagnostic process. Clinicians diagnose largely by gathering information, considering many possible explanations for an illness, and then gradually narrowing down diagnostic considerations as more information becomes available. In this way, psychiatric diagnosis begs for certainty, whereas understanding culture typically raises more questions than it answers. This practice of cultural humility is reflected in the types of questions discussed in the interview.

The CFI was developed as part of DSM-5. It contains 16 questions covering cultural background, identity, beliefs, and attitudes about mental health and treatment. It considers how individuals perceive their illness within the context of their culture, and it explores the factors that may encourage or discourage seeking mental health care. The questions that compose the CFI broadly map onto the cultural definition of presenting problems; perceptions of the cause, context, stressors, and supports; the role of cultural identity; and factors that shape disease experience, including means of coping, barriers, and help-seeking. These interview questions include

1. What brings you here today? People often understand their problems in their own way, which may be similar to or different from how doctors describe the problem. How would *you* describe your problem?
2. Sometimes people have different ways of describing their problem to their family, friends, or others in their community. How would you describe your problem to them?
3. What troubles you most about your problem?
4. Why do you think this is happening to you? What do you think are the causes of your problem? Some people may explain their problem as the result of bad things that happen in life, problems with others, a physical illness, a spiritual reason, or many other causes.
5. What do others in your family, your friends, or others in your community think is causing your problem?
6. Are there any kinds of support that make your problem better, such as support from family, friends, or others?
7. Are there any kinds of stresses that make your problem worse, such as difficulties with money, or family problems? Sometimes, aspects of people's background or identity can make their problem better or worse. By *background* or *identity*, I mean, for example, the communities you belong to, the languages you speak, where you or your family are from, your race or ethnic background, your gender or sexual orientation, or your faith or religion.

8. For you, what are the most important aspects of your background or identity?
9. Are there any aspects of your background or identity that make a difference to your problem?
10. Are there any aspects of your background or identity that are causing other concerns or difficulties for you?
11. Sometimes people have various ways of dealing with problems like yours. What have you done on your own to cope with your problem?
12. Often, people look for help from many different sources, including different kinds of doctors, helpers, or healers. In the past, what kinds of treatment, help, advice, or healing have you sought for your problem? What types of help or treatment were most useful? Not useful?
13. Has anything prevented you from getting the help you need—for example, money, work or family commitments, stigma or discrimination, or lack of services that understand your language or background?
14. Let's talk some more about the help you need. What kinds of help do you think would be most useful to you at this time for your problem?
15. Are there other kinds of help that your family, friends, or other people have suggested would be helpful for you now?
16. Sometimes doctors and patients misunderstand each other because they come from different backgrounds or have different expectations. Have you been concerned about this, and is there anything we can do to provide you with the care you need?

These questions help aid diagnosis. They enable clinicians to understand how culture alters the expression and experience of illness, whereas Z codes help a clinician understand other factors that influence a primary diagnosis. Thus, although the CFI may help a clinician arrive at a particular diagnosis in its cultural context, Z codes describe other factors that coexist with an illness in its social context. This emphasis on the differences between the two may belie that, when used together, the CFI and Z codes can comment on a wide range of sociocultural phenomena that impact illness.

Although cultural concepts of distress are well-intentioned and useful in some instances, they may have unintended consequences of "pathologizing nonwhite people on the basis of the assumption of static group practices and ways of being" (Shadravan and Barceló 2021, p. 37). It is crucial not to flatten the complexity of social groups and overlook the context in which systemic inequities persist and create unjust differences in social experience for many minoritized groups (Shadravan and Barceló 2021).

BARRIERS TO IMPLEMENTATION

DSM-5-TR and the CFI represent two useful tools to broaden social and cultural understanding when diagnosing and describing mental illness. Both tools are easily accessible, but implementing them may further increase documentation without the promise of available resources to address the problems they describe or to compensate or reimburse the clinician for either documenting Z codes or using the structured interview. As noted earlier, some clinicians may be reluctant to comment on sensitive social and cultural data for fear that such information may lead to discrimination, stigmatization, and additional barriers to care.

Clinicians may emphasize cultural and social explanations of mental illness differently. For instance, some clinicians may emphasize the social, political, and economic structures that shape health care access and outcomes. Structural competence has gained favor among a number of social scientists and clinicians, especially as a way to address the social determinants of health directly. Moreover, some clinicians may be reluctant to assign or attribute differences in health outcomes to values, beliefs, or characteristics of particular groups for fear that this may lead to typecasting particular cultures or pathologizing cultural beliefs and values.

UNDERSTANDING THE IMPACT OF CULTURE AND SOCIETY

Although similarities undoubtedly exist between social influences and cultural influences on health, discussing how culture and society structure health outcomes is helpful. Whereas *social conditions* refers to those aspects of society that influence how we live, *culture* refers to the values, norms, and practices that shape how we experience the world. Medical sociology and anthropology address many of the same questions but may focus on different attributes. Other scholars focus on the underlying social conditions influencing health and disease and on recognizing cultural factors at play.

The development of the CFI, much like the integration of the Z codes, reflected an effort to integrate cultural values, norms, and expressions of disease into the diagnostic framework of psychiatric practice. Both can be used to address social determinants of health and sociocultural factors that influence health outcomes, but the goals of the CFI differ significantly from those of the Z codes.

Whereas Z codes are actual diagnostic codes, the CFI provides a structure clinicians can utilize to help them gather, organize, understand, and integrate information about an individual's cultural background into their care. Z codes are a collection of diagnostic codes that convey information about non-medical factors that influence health outcomes; the CFI is a set of questions that identify cultural elements of an illness that complement the clinical interview. Neither fully addresses the impact of culture and society on an individual's life or illness, but they help convey and communicate information that the health system may use to improve health services and delivery.

Z codes provide a standardized way to track and measure particular data and social information about individuals across time and a variety of health settings. Cultural information gleaned from the CFI, however, is subject to more variability based on the individual patient and clinician and their understanding and interpretation of the information provided.

STRUCTURAL RACISM, STRUCTURAL CONSIDERATIONS, AND DSM-5-TR

Structural racism—defined by Camara Phyllis Jones (2000) as "differential access to the goods, services, and opportunities of society by race" (p. 1212)—has become more recently recognized as a fundamental cause of physical and mental health disparities, perpetuating inequities for historically excluded groups (Williams et al. 2019). For many, various elements of the conditions and factors described in DSM-5-TR's chapter "Other Conditions That May Be a Focus of Clinical Attention" can be intricately connected with a deeply entrenched societal system of structuring opportunities and values based on race. Thus, understanding racism can play a crucial role in then understanding the distribution of social determinants of health. In the United States, these "unequal distributions of health" disproportionately affect historically marginalized groups (World Health Organization 2008), particularly Black, Hispanic/Latino, and American Indian/Alaska Native people (Edwards et al. 2021; Williams and McAdams-Mahmoud 2019).

Structural racism inequitably limits opportunities for sociopolitical, economic, and financial advancement, contributing to poorer mental health. This complicated interplay has been illustrated by extensive research outlining differences in health outcomes among racially minoritized groups because of these structural factors (Paradies et al. 2015). This includes race-related inequities that lead to limited economic opportunities or poverty, food and housing insecurity, limited access to equitable health care, social exclusion or marginalization, limited educational opportunities, and excessive and unfair interactions with legal or carceral systems, among many others.

Exposure to racism is associated with poor mental health, including mood, anxiety, depression, and psychological distress. Social determinants of health are key drivers of mental health inequities within marginalized racial and ethnic communities and can be seen across multiple domains (Shim and Vinson 2021). Although not all-encompassing, this can be illustrated by some examples:

- Food insecurity in young adults has been associated with increased depression, suicidality, and substance misuse.
- Childhood family poverty has been shown to correlate with PTSD and depression diagnoses in adulthood, and countries with higher measures of inequality have increased incidences of schizophrenia.
- Poor access to educational opportunities has been shown to lead to a higher risk of poor mental health outcomes.
- Unemployment has been shown to contribute to mental health decline and poor life satisfaction.
- Interaction with criminal legal systems gives rise to reverberating factors that ultimately impair mental health.

Disadvantaged social contexts and status positions, such as racial or ethnic minoritized status, differentially expose individuals to social stressors and subsequent adverse mental health outcomes. Z codes do not explicitly reference race or ethnicity, but the circumstances underlying many of the conditions outlined within the codes can be connected to racism through various mechanisms. Thus, it is important to extend clinical approaches beyond the documentation of these psychosocial issues and to advance clinicians' understanding of the role racism can play in promoting some of these conditions. Mental health practitioners will require the necessary tools, training, and resources to identify and address the influence of racism and the structural causes of disease on health outcomes. Furthermore, rather than attributing disparities in mental health status to individual behavior or group-level differences in biology, a paradigm shift is needed to examine and consider the underlying systemic structural factors that lead to differences in mental health outcomes.

As discussed earlier, frameworks such as structural competency can allow for identifying, interrogating, and intervening in existing social structures and systems of racism that adversely affect the mental health of many minoritized communities. Some strategies to help address structural racism in mental health care include engaging in self-reflection, self-critiquing with a cultural and structural humility approach, educating oneself, and collaborating with patients and communities while maintaining an awareness of interpersonal privilege and power hierarchies in the health care system. Additionally, clinicians can apply a racial equity lens to change social norms and advocate for policy interventions that address the macro-level causes perpetuating inequities.

Case Example: Applying a Structural and Cultural Lens to DSM-5-TR

Ms. A is a 20-year-old woman who self-presents for initial evaluation and treatment. She has recently been discharged from the hospital for hitting herself enough to cause bruising, in the context of recurrent instances of being forcefully handled by a relative who is residing with her. Although she lives with her entire family and has brought up these instances with them, they have not validated her concerns and instead question her experience or tell her that she should stay out of his way.

In addition to assessing her primary psychiatric symptoms, how might DSM-5-TR conceptualize other conditions that may be a focus of clinical attention?

- Z91.52 Personal history of nonsuicidal self-harm
- Z69.81 Encounter for mental health services for victim of nonspousal or nonpartner adult abuse

Ms. A ends up leaving her home because of a recurrent experience of abuse and lives on the street, often sleeping on buses overnight. She remains employed as a food service worker and is able to obtain food only when she has shifts. She continues to try to see you on a regular basis but frequently cancels at the last minute or does not show up to appointments because of transportation challenges.

At this point, how might DSM-5-TR conceptualize other conditions that may be a focus of clinical attention?

- Z59.02 Unsheltered homelessness
- Z59.41 Food insecurity

What additional issues not represented in DSM-5-TR might affect her clinical care, and what might be structural interventions? Ms. A's challenges in obtaining consistent transportation are an additional structural issue impacting her health care access. Structural interventions might include recognizing that these difficulties are what contribute to her lack of regular attendance at appointments rather than "nonadherence to medical treatment" or other etiologies. Waiving fees or penalties for cancellation, adjusting appointment times to allow for easier transportation, and allowing for phone or virtual appointments rather than in-person appointments are all potential structural interventions.

> Ms. A identifies as queer Xicana and describes her estrangement from family as a major departure from the cultural and religious norms with which she grew up. As a child of immigrants who fled political hardship in their countries of origin, she is quick to minimize her own circumstance in comparison to her family's experience.

How might cultural issues contribute to her care? Understanding Ms. A's cultural identities will be helpful in identifying which pieces of her current situation are her primary stressors, and it will also help with understanding how her coping patterns and conceptualization of her distress may be related to intergenerational trauma. Recognizing her perspectives and experience is critical to aligning on shared goals of care. It may also be valuable to assess her exposure to racism, discrimination, and systemic institutional stigmatization in her current living situation, as well as her connection to cultural sources of support. Finally, it is important to understand how her cultural context shapes her view of medicine and health care and her relationship with you as her provider.

SELF-ASSESSMENT

Questions to Discuss With Colleagues and Mentors

1. How do structural issues affect clinician-patient interactions?
2. How do you use Z codes in your practice?
3. How can I address social norms and policies that perpetuate inequities in mental health?

Short-Answer Questions

1. When should criteria and codes from "Other Conditions That May Be a Focus of Clinical Attention" be assigned to a patient's treatment?
2. Which type of ICD code refers to social determinants of health that may influence the experience of illness?

Answers

1. There are many reasons why these codes should be assigned to a patient's treatment, such as 1) they identify the purpose of the encounter, 2) they help explain the need for therapeutic intervention, 3) they identify factors that play a role in the initiation or exacerbation of a mental disorder, or 4) they should be considered in the overall management plan.

2. Z codes refer to "factors influencing health status and contact with health services." They may account for non-psychopathological factors that influence health access, status, interaction with the health system, and outcomes. Many Z codes also correlate with social determinants of health that drive physical and mental health outcomes.

RECOMMENDED READING

Shim RS, Vinson SY (eds): Social (In)Justice and Mental Health. Washington, DC, American Psychiatric Association Publishing, 2021

REFERENCES

American Psychiatric Association: Diagnostic and Statistical Manual of Mental Disorders, 5th Edition, Text Revision. Washington, DC, American Psychiatric Association, 2022

Daniel H, Bornstein SS, Kane GC, et al: Addressing social determinants to improve patient care and promote health equity: an American College of Physicians position paper. Ann Intern Med 168(8):577–578, 2018 29677265

Edwards ML, Saenz SR, Collins R, et al: Social injustice and structural racism, in Social (In)Justice and Mental Health. Edited by Shim R, Vinson S. Washington, DC, American Psychiatric Association Publishing, 2021, pp. 47–61

Forrest LN, Beccia AL, Exten C, et al: Intersectional prevalence of suicide ideation, plan, and attempt based on gender, sexual orientation, race and ethnicity, and rurality. JAMA Psychiatry 80(10):1037–1046, 2023 37466933

Jones CP: Levels of racism: a theoretic framework and a gardener's tale. Am J Public Health 90(8):1212–1215, 2000 10936998

Lawrence D, Kisely S: Inequalities in healthcare provision for people with severe mental illness. J Psychopharmacol 24(4 Suppl):61–68, 2010 20923921

Link BG, Phelan J: Social conditions as fundamental causes of disease. J Health Soc Behav (Special Issue):80–94, 1995 7560851

Paradies Y, Ben J, Denson N, et al: Racism as a determinant of health: a systematic review and meta-analysis. PLoS One 10(9):e0138511, 2015 26398658

Shadravan SM, Barceló NE: Social injustice and mental health inequities, in Social (In)Justice and Mental Health. Edited by Shim RS, Vinson SY. Washington, DC, American Psychiatric Association Publishing, 2021

Shim RS, Compton MT: Addressing the social determinants of mental health: If not now, when? If not us, who? Psychiatr Serv 69(8):844–846, 2018 29852822

Shim RS, Vinson SY (eds): Social (In)Justice and Mental Health. Washington, DC, American Psychiatric Association Publishing, 2021

Stone DM, Mack KA, Qualters J: Notes from the field: recent changes in suicide rates, by race and ethnicity and age group—United States, 2021. MMWR Morb Mortal Wkly Rep 72(6):160–162, 2023 36757870

Williams DR, McAdams-Mahmoud A: Racism and mental health' pathways, evidence, and needed research, in Black Mental Health: Patients, Providers, and Systems. Edited by Griffith EEH, Jones BE, Stewart AJ. Washington, DC, American Psychiatric Association Publishing, 2019, pp. 269–281

Williams DR, Lawrence JA, Davis BA: Racism and health: evidence and needed research. Annu Rev Public Health 40:105–125, 2019 30601726

World Health Organization: International Statistical Classification of Diseases and Related Health Problems, 10th Revision. Geneva, World Health Organization, 1992

World Health Organization: Closing the Gap in a Generation: Health Equity Through Action on the Social Determinants of Health: Commission on Social Determinants of Health. Geneva, World Health Organization, 2008

PART 2

DSM-5-TR Diagnostic Categories

CHAPTER 5

Neurodevelopmental Disorders

Tamar Green, M.D.

David S. Hong, M.D.

"My son is too much to handle sometimes."

"I can tell my baby is different."

- Intellectual Developmental Disorders
  - Intellectual Developmental Disorder (Intellectual Disability)
  - Global Developmental Delay
  - Unspecified Intellectual Developmental Disorder (Intellectual Disability)
- Communication Disorders
  - Language Disorder
  - Speech Sound Disorder
  - Childhood-Onset Fluency Disorder (Stuttering)
  - Social (Pragmatic) Communication Disorder
  - Unspecified Communication Disorder
- Autism Spectrum Disorder
- Attention-Deficit/Hyperactivity Disorder
  - Attention-Deficit/Hyperactivity Disorder
  - Other Specified Attention-Deficit/Hyperactivity Disorder
  - Unspecified Attention-Deficit/Hyperactivity Disorder

- Specific Learning Disorder
- Motor Disorders
  - Developmental Coordination Disorder
  - Stereotypic Movement Disorder
  - Tic Disorders
  - Other Specified Tic Disorder
  - Unspecified Tic Disorder
- Other Neurodevelopmental Disorders
  - Other Specified Neurodevelopmental Disorder
  - Unspecified Neurodevelopmental Disorder

Development of the central nervous system is extremely intricate and complex. This has implications for the multitude of functions that it innervates. Thus, neurodevelopmental disorders encompass impairments across a broad range of functions. Although phenomenology and affected domains in this diagnostic category are heterogeneous, they are unified within a developmental framework—symptoms are acquired or inherited early in development and are characterized by a divergence from an expected trajectory for gaining skills. That is not to say that individuals can only be diagnosed with these disorders in childhood. Oftentimes, diagnoses may not be made until adulthood, or clinical history may reveal that symptoms that started in childhood continue to exist in an attenuated form later in life. However, as a general rule, symptoms in this diagnostic cluster demonstrate early onset, are highly influenced by genetic and familial risk factors, and have a fairly pervasive course across several stages of development. As with other diagnostic categories, impairments in this group of disorders must demonstrate a significant impact on adaptive functioning, typically manifesting in learning or work environments.

Included in this category is a broad range of disorders, but the diagnoses can be subgrouped generally according to the target cognitive or motor skill that demonstrates a disparity from typical development. Impairments in global domains such as intelligence fall under intellectual developmental disorders, and when specific speech and communication domains are affected, symptoms are characterized under communication disorders or specific learning disorders. Disordered social communication is categorized under autism spectrum disorder (ASD) or social communication disorder.

Some disorders show overlap and impairment across several domains, such as ADHD, in which executive function as well as motor inhibition are affected, whereas others may be restricted to motor dysfunction, such as developmental coordination disorder, stereotypic movement disorder, and chronic motor or vocal tic disorder. As a group, neurodevelopmental disorders are complex and heterogeneous both in etiology and clinical manifestations, while in other ways they share significant similarities in onset, course, and susceptibility to genetic and familial factors.

The approach to diagnosing a child with a neurodevelopmental disorder can be challenging in a number of ways. First, the nature of symptoms and the typical age at

TABLE 5–1. Key changes between DSM-5 and DSM-5-TR

Intellectual developmental disorder replaced the previous diagnosis of intellectual disability (with a continuous emphasis on using adaptive functioning rather than IQ scores to define the severity of intellectual developmental disorder).

When clinically relevant, specifiers for autism spectrum disorder now include associated conditions even when cause is not implied.

The role of bilingualism is now considered in the description of communication disorders.

Culture-related diagnostic issues have been updated to better address social determinants of health and sociocultural contexts.

Prevalence, associated features, and sex- and gender-related diagnostic issues have been updated in keeping with best evidence.

Association with suicidal thoughts or behavior has been added to all disorders in which data are available.

presentation (i.e., early development) often make it difficult to obtain all necessary information in a one-on-one clinical interview. As such, practitioners frequently need to be thoughtful and creative in acquiring information and may need to rely on other informants, such as family members, caretakers, and teachers, for additional clinical history. Standardized instruments designed to accommodate varying levels of developmental ability may also be of particular usefulness for this group. Furthermore, the early age at presentation often means that receiving a diagnosis of a neurodevelopmental disorder is the first interaction a family will have with the mental health system. As such, clinicians must be sensitive to the needs of the family throughout the process, especially because many disorders in this category are pervasive, and symptoms will impact functioning over several stages of development or in some cases will be lifelong. In a similar vein, practitioners can make a significant impact by helping families obtain an accurate diagnosis and navigate the challenges of acquiring comprehensive interventions. In fact, successful diagnosis and treatment planning often requires close interdisciplinary collaboration among mental health practitioners, medical specialists, educational staff, and agencies that provide specialized ancillary services.

Broad changes occurred in this diagnostic category between DSM-IV (American Psychiatric Association 1994) and DSM-5 (American Psychiatric Association 2013) (Table 5–1). Most notably, DSM-5 consolidated diagnoses around centralized domains of developmental delay and introduced diagnostic specifiers to characterize variations in symptom presentation. This change included consolidating social cognitive disorders under ASD and grouping impaired acquisition of academic skills under the specific learning disorder diagnosis. Likewise, DSM-5 broadened strict age criteria to accommodate clinical variability in diagnostic presentations during the developmental period for intellectual developmental disorder, ASD, and ADHD. DSM-5 also recategorized several diagnoses, including conduct disorder, oppositional defiant disorder, feeding and elimination disorders, social anxiety disorder, selective mutism, and reactive attachment disorder, and it introduced new diagnoses such as global developmental delay and social communication disorder.

IN-DEPTH DIAGNOSIS: INTELLECTUAL DEVELOPMENTAL DISORDER (INTELLECTUAL DISABILITY)

Parents have brought in a 6-year-old boy named Bryan to the clinic after being told by his school that Bryan is not ready to advance to first grade and will need to repeat a year. School reports indicate that he has not learned the alphabet and cannot count to 20 or recognize simple words by sight. He also has difficulty engaging with peers and teachers and has disruptive behaviors such as hand flapping and an inability to sit still or to pay attention during circle time. The school psychologist has just completed testing and found that Bryan has a full-scale IQ of 65 and scores below expected grade-level across several areas of academic achievement. Bryan was also noted to have "autistic traits" on a screening questionnaire.

Bryan's mother states that although she had difficulty getting pregnant, the pregnancy was otherwise uneventful, and Bryan was born full-term. She reports he was a "colicky" baby, had difficulty soothing and feeding, and was late to start walking and talking (almost age 2 years), but she disregarded these because she felt that "boys were usually late with this kind of thing." On examination, Bryan has prominent ears and a high forehead, appears anxious, avoids eye contact, and has poor speech enunciation. Although his mother has a history of anxiety, there is no family history of intellectual developmental disorder. Bryan is an only child.

In this case, Bryan's IQ falls just below two standard deviations from the mean (<70), and his behaviors demonstrate significant concerns in his adaptive functioning. Furthermore, Bryan presents with a constellation of symptoms that are consistent with fragile X syndrome, which is the most commonly inherited form of intellectual developmental disorder. Fragile X includes findings of characteristic facial features, stereotypic motor activity, possible autistic symptoms, and feeding problems during infancy. Although there is no clear evidence for family history of intellectual impairment, Bryan's mother has a history of anxiety and infertility problems, which may indicate that she carries a premutation. Fragile X syndrome is one of several genetic disorders that have a relatively high prevalence rate. Providers making an initial diagnosis of intellectual developmental disorder should be thoughtful about establishing an etiology when specific physical or medical features are present because that diagnosis may have significant impact on clinical management and family planning. Furthermore, Bryan likely presents with features of ADHD and possibly ASD. It is important to remember that no exclusion criteria exist for intellectual developmental disorder; therefore, the diagnosis should be given as long as criteria are met, even in the presence of other comorbid disorders.

Approach to the Diagnosis

Individuals with intellectual developmental disorder are typically diagnosed at an early age. In severe cases, evidence for delayed cognitive development will be seen in the first few years of life. With subtler presentations, referrals often occur after evidence of delays are detected in school settings. However, the diagnosis should reflect the presence of symptoms prior to adolescence (Criterion C). Given that clinical presentation and associated symptoms vary significantly with etiology, it is important to assess for signs of syndromic disorders even after establishing that criteria for diagnosis of intellectual developmental disorder are met. This entails conducting a thorough assessment of behavioral symptoms, developmental history, family history (three-generation family pedigree), and physical traits. Because most causes are linked to the period around birth, it is essential to obtain a thorough medical and developmental history for this period. Further acquisition of collateral information from school systems and referrals to genetic evaluation (e.g., karyotype or chromosomal microarray analysis and testing for specific genetic syndromes) and pediatric specialists (e.g., for metabolic screening or neuroimaging) may also be helpful for assessment and ongoing interdisciplinary management, if indicated.

Standardized intelligence testing establishes evidence of deficits in general mental abilities (Criterion A). Commonly, a score of two standard deviations from the mean is considered evidence of cognitive impairment—that is, a score less than or equal to 70±5 (when the mean score is 100 and standard deviation is 15). It is important to remember that full-scale IQ scores may not accurately represent intellectual ability; therefore, clinical judgment should be used to interpret whether attention, cultural or language biases, motivation, or uneven intellectual abilities are affecting overall testing performance.

Also, impaired cognition is necessary but not sufficient to make a diagnosis of intellectual developmental disorder. Patients should demonstrate evidence of impaired adaptive functioning, which indicates how well they are able to adapt to everyday life across academic or intellectual, social, and practical domains, and how well they demonstrate social norms of personal independence (Criterion B). Adaptive behavior will necessarily reflect factors of age and sociocultural influences; therefore, these aspects should always be considered carefully when making a diagnosis. Particularly for individuals with more severe impairments, it is helpful to obtain information regarding adaptive functioning from other reliable informants or from evaluations or standardized testing specifically geared toward assessing adaptive behavior. It is important to note that DSM-5-TR (American Psychiatric Association 2022) categorizes the severity of intellectual developmental disorders based on an individual's level of functioning relative to unaffected peers, rather than using IQ scores. Lastly, no exclusion criteria exist for this disorder, so if the criteria are met, a diagnosis should be made regardless of any comorbid disorder.

Getting the History

A family brings in their young daughter because of her cognitive delays. The interviewer determines whether the child lags behind expected age-appropriate development in general mental abilities, including assessing her overall acquisition of intellectual milestones and academic achievement. The interviewer also asks, "When did you first notice that your daughter might be having delays in her development?" and establishes that the onset of deficits was prior to adolescence. Evaluation of impairments should assess reasoning, problem-solving, abstract thinking, judgment, and learning. The interviewer asks, "Has your daughter ever had psychological testing or an IQ test?" and determines whether any standardized assessment on adaptive scales has been done. If results are available, the interviewer should interpret them with careful clinical judgment to establish whether global mental performance deviates significantly from the population mean and whether other conditions may not better explain performance deficits. The interviewer then asks the parents and the patient to review the child's physical, medical, and family history as well as any environmental exposures, maintaining a high degree of suspicion for any factors that may explain the underlying cause of intellectual impairment. The interviewer then asks the child and her parents, "How do these symptoms present challenges for day-to-day function? School or work performance? Relationships with others?" and further determines the severity of function in academic, social, and practical domains.

As is typical with intellectual developmental disorder, this child is referred because of concerns by caregivers that she is having problems with cognitive development. The interviewer characterizes the nature of these deficits through the clinical interview and neuropsychological testing and ascertains that they represent global difficulties with general mental abilities. The interviewer determines whether any factors may indicate a specific etiology or cause by conducting a thorough clinical history, and they also will want to conduct a physical examination, paying particular attention to neurological signs or dysmorphic features. They may also consider the usefulness of referring this child to colleagues in other specialties if they have a high index of suspicion for a specific cluster of diagnoses. The interviewer will also want to ascertain how intellectual impairments are affecting specific domains of function. Collateral information from other providers, colleagues, and caretakers would be useful to determine the patient's adaptive function across various contexts.

Tips for Clarifying the Diagnosis

- Establish level of general cognitive abilities: what are the individual's scores on standardized testing?
- Are there mitigating factors regarding the individual's performance on intelligence testing? Are cognitive abilities affected across domains?
- Obtain collateral information on how intellectual impairments are affecting function in academic, social, and practical domains.
- When were problems with intellectual function first diagnosed? Prior to adolescence?
- Is intellectual impairment accompanied by other developmental or physical impairments or by medical or family history that would suggest a specific etiology?

Consider the Case

Mr. Mendez, a 26-year-old man, is currently hospitalized for alcohol intoxication and withdrawal symptoms on the medical unit. Referral is made to the consultation-liaison psychiatry service to assess the patient and provide input on his alcohol dependence and psychosocial issues. The internal medicine service is frustrated that the patient is a "frequent flyer" with numerous similar hospitalizations over the past several years. He lives with his mother and has had significant difficulty independently managing activities of daily living since being hit by a car while riding his bike when he was 11 years old. Mr.

Mendez sustained significant head trauma at that time and has since had sustained cognitive deficits without progressive decline. His mother and close-knit family have since cared for him; however, they have had an increasingly difficult time managing him over the past several years. Maladaptive behaviors consist of poor insight; impaired cognitive abilities to reason, organize, and attend to basic self-care; and extreme impulsivity (they note that despite his small stature and some physical limitations, he often gets into fights in the neighborhood). Mr. Mendez receives disability assistance for moderate intellectual developmental disorder and works part-time for his brother stocking shelves; however, his family reports that after receiving any pay, Mr. Mendez immediately spends it on alcohol, leading to frequent inebriation and increased use of emergency services.

The patient in this case has an acquired etiology for intellectual developmental disorder, evidenced by a dramatically altered trajectory of cognitive development after sustaining serious head trauma during the developmental period. Because his condition likely results from traumatic brain injury, it would be appropriate to additionally give a diagnosis of major neurocognitive disorder characterized by a loss of cognitive functioning. Further information regarding psychological testing is needed; however, clinical assessment suggests that he falls within the moderate range of impairment in the conceptual domain, given that he retains some verbal ability and apparently has skills that allow him to work for his brother. The degree of impairment in the practical domain—impulsivity, excessive alcohol intake, inability to demonstrate progress toward independence—suggests an overall level of adaptive functioning that falls under the severe subtype. Providers should also consider to what extent Mr. Mendez's cultural identification may influence his family's perceptions of, or expectations for, his overall adaptive functioning. It is also clear in Mr. Mendez's case that his intellectual developmental disorder is a lifelong pervasive condition and demonstrates some of the challenges that occur during transition from childhood to adulthood for individuals with these impairments. Although services are in place for children with intellectual developmental disorder through the school system and federal and state agencies, available services for adults with this condition are often more variable. In conjunction with varying levels in independence and insight in decision-making, the ability for adults with intellectual developmental disorders to navigate the medical system can be challenging. In the case of Mr. Mendez, it has resulted in high use of emergency medical services and difficulty establishing appropriate care for comorbid disorders, such as likely alcohol dependence in this instance.

Differential Diagnosis

The differential diagnosis of intellectual developmental disorder is relatively limited because there are no exclusion criteria for this disorder. The diagnosis should be made when criteria are met, regardless of whether other diagnostic criteria are also fulfilled. Nevertheless, other psychiatric diagnoses should certainly be ruled out, including childhood-onset dementia, a neurodegenerative condition characterized by an ongoing decline from higher levels of cognitive function rather than the generally stable course of intellectual developmental disorder. Furthermore, it should be established that the patient's intelligence is globally affected; if his deficits are narrowly limited to specific cognitive domains, diagnoses of specific learning disorder or communication disorder may be preferred. It is also important to consider that impairments in these domains may make it difficult to assess global intellectual function, whether because of inability to participate in psychological testing or to variable engagement or motivation in the assessment environment. This consideration also applies to the domain of social communication in ASD, in which limited social engagement may influence an individual's ability to participate in assessment and testing, although intellectual developmental disorder is also quite commonly comorbid with ASD.

Given that the diagnosis of intellectual developmental disorder does not have exclusion criteria, mastery of diagnostic criteria is relatively straightforward. The primary points regarding diagnosis are to assess whether impairments in general mental ability are not better explained by deficits in specific, restricted domains that may be falsely skewing testing of general mental abilities. A number of other diagnoses will also significantly influence aspects of cognitive function, including ADHD, mood disturbances, psychosis, and certain medical conditions. However, attention to the time of onset; determination of an episodic versus pervasive, steady course; and clear establishment of the developmental trajectory may help in establishing the diagnosis. As discussed in DSM-5-TR, emphasis should also be placed on determining an underlying etiology, especially because the clinical manifestation of symptoms may vary significantly within this heterogeneous diagnostic group.

Unsurprisingly, more severe forms of intellectual developmental disorder tend to be diagnosed earlier in development and may be associated with identifiable syndromes, whereas individuals with milder impairment may not be detected until school age. Historically, intellectual developmental disorder was overdiagnosed in marginalized racial and ethnic groups, but the disorder occurs in all races and ethnicities.

Individuals with a diagnosis of intellectual developmental disorder with co-occurring mental disorders are at risk for suicide but might manifest atypically. They may think about suicide, make suicide attempts, and die from suicide. Thus, screening for suicidal thoughts is essential. Because of a lack of awareness of risk and danger, accidental injury rates may also be increased.

Summary

- Intellectual developmental disorder represents global impairment of mental ability across cognitive domains.
- Psychological testing can confirm Criterion A deficits in general mental abilities but may not reflect severity of functioning.
- Diagnosis of intellectual developmental disorder must always reflect impairment in adaptive functioning (Criterion B); cognitive impairment alone is not sufficient for diagnosis.
- Clinical approach to children with intellectual developmental disorder should include thorough developmental, family, and clinical histories to increase sensitivity for detecting syndromic manifestations.
- There are no exclusion criteria for diagnosis of intellectual developmental disorder, and it should be diagnosed whenever the criteria are met, regardless of its occurrence with other comorbid diagnoses.

IN-DEPTH DIAGNOSIS: AUTISM SPECTRUM DISORDER

The parents of a 2.5-year-old boy named Adam brought him to the outpatient child and adolescent psychiatry clinic with concerns that he speaks only three words ("mama," "dada," and "baby") and has not established a relationship with his parents or with his 5-year-old sister. They report that, in retrospect, Adam did not seem "responsive" as an infant. They recall he did less cooing and had decreased eye contact and copying of facial expressions compared with his older sister's behavior at the same age. However, they became most concerned when he still had not acquired words by age 2. They noted that over the past year, he has made only minimal gains in language skills—he speaks three words and appears to follow some simple commands, although neither of these behaviors is generally consistent or in context. He does not point or use gestures effectively; if he wants something, he will take them by the hand to an area and grunt, often becoming frustrated and having a temper tantrum if they are not able to figure out what he wants. Adam also does not engage with peers and will completely ignore his sister, at times crawling over her to get where he wants to be. He primarily plays alone and obsessively with toys, lining up blocks by color or spinning wheels on trucks rather than rolling trucks on the floor. Adam is also somewhat clumsy for his age and frequently makes odd stretching postures with his fingers, but his medical history is otherwise unremarkable, and his hearing has tested within normal limits. Family history is significant only for a paternal uncle who is "a bit odd" and "the black sheep of the family."

Adam's case demonstrates significant impairments in social reciprocity, structural language, and interactive play. These signs were evident early in childhood, although initial signs were likely already detectable in infancy. The solitary and restricted nature of Adam's play significantly diverges from what would be expected from age-matched peers. Similarly, his odd finger posturing likely demonstrates restricted and stereotyped motor behaviors, which is also consistent with ASD. Adam's expressive and receptive language is significantly delayed; however, more notably in this case, he does not demonstrate other means of social communication, whether through nonverbal means, coordinated gestures, or expressions. It would be important to assess Adam's intellectual ability, although it will likely be challenging to obtain an accurate portrayal given that his social deficits may interfere with engagement in psychological testing and thereby affect performance. Although not presented here, it would also be important to screen for mood and anxiety symptoms as well as problems with inattention to assess whether other neuropsychiatric syndromes are contributing to his social deficits or are comorbid with an ASD diagnosis. Furthermore, additional clarity on the initial age of parental concern, whether Adam had demonstrated any sustained period of a typical developmental trajectory, and assessment for signs of any genetic predisposition or associated syndrome would be warranted. In this particular case, given a presumptive diagnosis of ASD, Adam likely exhibits impairments in social communication of level 3 severity—further information regarding rigidity (including whether he demonstrates self-injurious behaviors) would be helpful in determining the degree of severity for restricted behaviors; however, his symptoms likely fall at least within a level 2 severity.

Approach to the Diagnosis

The ASD diagnostic category encompasses impairments in social cognitive abilities. In DSM-IV, distinct deficits in social interaction and social communication were required for the diagnosis; in DSM-5 and DSM-5-TR, the Criterion A impairments fall under three required categories: 1) social-emotional reciprocity, 2) nonverbal communicative behaviors, and 3) social interaction. In order to meet Criterion A, an individual must demonstrate persistent deficits in all three domains. Although a number of psychiatric disorders of childhood adversely impact social functioning, either generally or in specific contexts, the core features of Criterion A indicate pervasive impairment across social cognitive abilities that are integral for appropriate interpersonal relatedness. As an example, rather than impairment in language ability causing problems with social communication, the hallmark of ASD is the inability to effectively understand or use the social aspects of language. The same holds true for nonverbal communication or the maintenance of relationships. At times, discriminating the exact nature of these symptoms may be challenging, in which case structured social cognitive assessments may be useful in providing additional information.

Patients must also demonstrate at least two characteristics of restricted or repetitive behaviors (Criterion B), which can encompass repetitive speech, motor mannerisms, and the use of objects, specific interests, rituals, or rigidity around routines. In DSM-5, restrictive or repetitive sensory behaviors also fall within this category, including sensitivity to textures, excessive touching or smelling of objects, and obsession with specific sights or sounds. Symptoms consistent with ASD must also be diagnosed in early childhood (Criterion C) and cause significant impairment in adaptive functioning (Criterion D).

Previously, several additional subtypes were also used to describe social impairments, including Asperger's disorder, childhood disintegrative disorder, and pervasive developmental disorder not otherwise specified. DSM-5-TR continues to largely consolidate these diagnoses within the ASD diagnostic category under the rubric of shared social cognitive deficits representing the core feature of impairment, using specifiers to denote the severity levels. DSM-5-TR defines the severity level for symptoms falling under social communication and restricted behaviors and lists specifiers for additional deficits in intelligence or language ability; for association with a genetic, medical, or environmental condition; and for neurodevelopmental, mental, or behavioral problems if they contribute to the functional impairments or to the treatment plan. Nevertheless, co-occurring diagnosed mental disorders should be listed separately.

Getting the History

A pediatrician refers a 4-year-old boy to the child psychiatry clinic because of concerns around the boy's delayed language and limited interaction with family members. The parents report their concerns that the child's development has differed significantly from that of his siblings. The interviewer asks them, "Can you tell me about his interactions with you and other family members?" The child's mother becomes tearful, stating that she always knew something was "wrong" and should have come to the doctor earlier, but she appears to have difficulty describing her child's symptoms in detail. The interviewer asks, "How does he respond when you play with him?" and the parents respond that he has never engaged in games such as peek-a-boo, appears relatively uninterested in looking at their faces or eyes, and is generally oblivious to the presence of others. The interviewer determines whether the child has circumscribed stereotyped behaviors or interests that include at least two of the four symptom clusters for restricted and repetitive behaviors. The parents report prominent sensory reactivity and cognitive rigidity. The interviewer inquires about verbal and motor development, with specific attention to the child's delays in language. The interviewer also asks, "When did you first notice problems with language and social behaviors?" and establishes whether the child had acquired skills during the first years of life that were subsequently lost. The interviewer then asks, "How are his symptoms affecting his day-to-day functioning at home and at preschool?" and determines whether any formal testing, including intelligence assessments, or any medical or genetic workup has been completed.

The symptoms in this case likely meet criteria for ASD. The child demonstrates pervasive developmental deficits in social-emotional reciprocity, nonverbal communication, and maintenance of relationships. It may be challenging to evaluate children with ASD, particularly when structural language impairments are present. Therefore, it is often important to obtain their history from the family and other collateral sources to develop a comprehensive picture of the child's skills in various contexts. Additionally, social cognitive abilities may be difficult for individuals or family members to characterize. Here, the psychiatrist is able to prompt the family by asking broad questions, which may be followed by more specific inquiries to establish that symptoms meet criteria for the condition. They also screen for other psychiatric disorders; however, a further assessment of the child's general mental abilities is needed to determine whether his social deficits are in line with or exceed his other mental abilities. This would help in determining if the child meets criteria for the diagnosis. After establishing that social cognitive impairments exist, the psychiatrist also carefully ascertains how the symptoms fall under specifiers defined in DSM-5-TR.

Tips for Clarifying the Diagnosis

- Does the child have difficulty understanding the perspective of others? How does this difficulty manifest in the child's use of language, gestures, or play?
- Would their problems with social interaction be better explained by anxiety or specific social contexts, or are their symptoms fairly pervasive across contexts and individuals?
- Are the child's interests and activities narrower than would be expected given their age and cultural or socioeconomic background?
- What is the developmental history regarding the onset of their symptoms? Do they have accompanying deficits in language or general intelligence?
- Do their social impairments exceed what would be expected, given their level of intelligence?
- What is the effect on the child's functioning for social communication and restrictive or repetitive behaviors?

Consider the Case

A 17-year-old man named Jon is self-referred to the clinic for "having trouble getting along with people." Jon has traditionally done well academically, particularly in his stated interests of math and history, and when prompted he can expound at length on dates and events of colonial American history. He describes himself as being "socially awkward" and initially asked to come to the clinic because of his increasing feelings of isolation. Jon has a supportive family and has one or two friends at school who share his interest in computers and video games. He watches public programming on television but never watches sitcoms because he does not understand "why people find them funny." Jon has never had a romantic partner and rarely socializes with peers after school or on the weekend, although he admits that he would like to do so. He is not able to recollect details from his childhood clearly but states that he always felt different from other kids and never had "best friends" growing up. He states that his parents never told him he was behind developmentally and otherwise reports no notable psychiatric or medical history. During the interview, Jon presents as fairly robotic, with a flattened tone and stilted, adult-like language, which almost sounds like he is quoting text. When spoken to, Jon appears uncomfortable, avoiding eye contact and instead appearing to stare intently at the interviewer's mouth. During the review of depressive symptoms, Jon states that "maybe" he feels down at times and goes on to express that people who commit suicide are "stupid" because there is always a logical reason to stay alive.

Jon demonstrates pervasive social deficits across contexts that are affecting his adaptive functioning, particularly in contrast to his desired level of social interaction. His impairments are largely isolated to social functioning rather than general developmental delays; in fact, a cursory overview may suggest he is generally functioning at a high level, particularly given the apparent absence of intellectual impairment or language deficits. This may also explain why he is presenting for assessment at a much later age than is typical for ASD. However, despite his relative strengths, Jon has significant social difficulties engaging with others, and certain aspects of his clinical history such as his limited peer interactions and narrow interests may represent characteristic features of the disorder. It would be important for the interviewer to get an understanding of the depth of Jon's interactions with his friends and his ability to develop and maintain those relationships, as well as to consider whether cultural differences affect the nature of his social interactions. Jon's stated inability to reciprocally understand others' perspectives may also be reflected in his lack of enjoyment or understanding of sitcoms, as well as observed signs of nonverbal communication such as impaired eye contact during the interview. He also demonstrates stereotyped speech and restricted interests in specific areas, although the extent to which these interests are excessively perseverative or circumscribed should be further assessed.

Determining the onset of symptoms is more challenging for individuals who present in late adolescence or adulthood. In Jon's case, it would be useful to obtain collateral information from his family or friends to establish the developmental course of his symptoms. Also, how his symptoms affect his functioning should be carefully assessed, especially because Jon's older age at diagnosis suggests he may have already developed compensatory strategies for any social deficits. In previous categorizations, his symptoms may have fallen under the diagnosis of Asperger's disorder or high-functioning autism; however, using DSM-5-TR schema, a diagnosis with specifiers denoting the absence of accompanying intellectual or language impairments would be indicated. Furthermore, other comorbid disorders should be screened for, particularly depressive symptoms in Jon's case, because mood, anxiety, and attention disorders may either contribute to or result from core deficits in social functioning, and these disorders are associated with increased risk for suicide and suicide attempts in adolescents with ASD, even after adjustment for demographic factors.

Differential Diagnosis

Many psychiatric disorders have accompanying impairments in social functioning, but ASD is distinguished by social cognitive deficits representing the primary reason for symptoms. As an example, intellectual developmental disorder may be difficult to differentiate from ASD because global impairments in mental functioning generally affect all cognitive domains, including social processing. However, a diagnosis of ASD should be made in the case of an individual with intellectual developmental disorder when impairments in social communication and interaction exceed what would be expected for the individual's developmental level. Similarly, impairments in language, particularly receptive language, may also lead to secondary impairments in social functioning, requiring careful sensitivity on the part of an interviewer in defining the nature of core symptoms. In other instances, core social deficits may be present but not be accompanied by restricted or repetitive behaviors, as is the case in selective mutism and social communication disorder. In contrast, the presence of unusual motor stereotypies or repetitive behaviors without the core deficits in social communication would be better categorized under stereotypic movement disorder, OCD, or obsessive-compulsive personality disorder. The ubiquitous nature of social deficits and restrictive behaviors means there is a high degree of symptom overlap with other psychiatric disorders. It is also quite common for ASD to coexist with other conditions, if and when criteria are specifically met for comorbid disorders.

Evaluation of ASD may be complicated by the impairment in communication that is a primary feature of this condition, which may lead to misinformation during the diagnostic process. As an example, screening questions for psychotic symptoms may be interpreted literally; a positive response to whether the person "hears voices when alone" may mean that the patient is listening to the radio rather than experiencing primary psychotic symptoms. Therefore, communication with individuals affected by ASD requires thoughtfulness about how they perceive and understand information. If further diagnostic clarification is needed because of limited history or communication difficulties, standardized social cognitive assessments should also be considered. In clinical samples, females with ASD were more likely to demonstrate better reciprocal conversation and integration of verbal and nonverbal behavior and fewer repetitive behaviors, although variance in degree of symptoms is also generally higher among females than among males with the disorder.

Lastly, it should be noted that DSM-5 centralized diagnoses characterized by impaired social communication and restrictive behavior with the goal of consolidating shared features across these diagnoses. Therefore, practitioners should pay particular attention to clarifying aspects of the diagnosis that may help distinguish variations in clinical presentation by carefully screening for specifiers included under this diagnosis. DSM-5-TR's ASD diagnostic category does not include subtypes, per se, but instead relies on specifiers to indicate 1) severity of social communication deficits and repetitive behaviors, 2) recognized regression from established skills, 3) age at first concern, and 4) accompanying intellectual, structural language, or other medical, genetic, or acquired conditions.

Summary

- Criteria for ASD define core features of social dysfunction; additional specifiers may be used to establish modifying factors, including age at onset, severity, accompanying language or intellectual impairment, and presence of other related conditions.
- Specific attention should be focused on social impairments and whether these rise from problems innately resulting from social cognitive abilities rather than problems in other domains affecting social functioning.
- Restrictive and repetitive criteria may encompass a range of motor, interest, or behavioral aspects.
- Impairments will be pervasive and sustained, although manifestations will vary according to intellectual and language ability, as well as factors such as age.
- Compensatory strategies may influence presentation and time of diagnosis.

IN-DEPTH DIAGNOSIS: ATTENTION-DEFICIT/ HYPERACTIVITY DISORDER

The mother of a 7-year-old boy named Shawn comes to the clinic because he is experiencing problems in school, and she is concerned that "he never sits still for a second." She reports that she has had multiple complaints over the past 2 years from Shawn's teachers, who state that his behavior is extremely disruptive—he is often getting out of his seat, talking with other classmates, and getting into arguments with peers during recess. His mother also has concerns about his behavior at home, although to a lesser degree than the concerns from school staff. She notes that he has always been an active child, in contrast to when he seems to focus intently on an activity for hours at a time, such as playing video games. However, she notes that he frequently gets out of his chair during meals, can never sit through a whole service at church, and tends to be more oppositional with boundaries than his siblings. He frequently loses his jackets and gloves and often forgets to complete or turn in homework assignments. Shawn's mother also describes him as being very impulsive ("he is always saying the first thing on his mind"), which has caused problems with friends and family members on several occasions. Furthermore, when his attention is captured by a particular idea, he acts on it immediately, to the extent that he has walked out of a store or restaurant into the street by himself, causing his family to be extremely concerned about his personal safety. During the interview, Shawn demonstrates a high degree of motor activity, jitters his legs constantly for the 5 minutes he is sitting in his chair, and wanders around the room, handling objects on the clinician's desk and frequently interrupting the conversation between the clinician and parent.

This case demonstrates a typical presentation of ADHD during an initial evaluation. Shawn has difficulty with symptoms on both the inattention domain and the hyperactivity-impulsivity spectrum and likely would fall under the descriptive specifier for the combined presentation. Although this constellation of symptoms is fairly common, care should also be taken to ensure that his level of activity exceeds high normal motor activity for male children of his age. Given that identification rates and symptom ratings of ADHD vary between cultural groups, his mother's interpretation of his behaviors should also be considered using a culturally competent approach. The variability of Shawn's symptoms should also be considered—although he appears able to maintain attention on activities that he finds interesting, his predominant symptoms over the past several months indicate significant difficulty engaging in tasks that require sustained mental effort, resulting in impaired functioning at school and at home. Additional collateral information, including parent and teacher rating scales, teacher interviews, or classroom observation, may be helpful in providing a more comprehensive picture of Shawn's symptoms across contexts. On the basis of the clinical interview, the severity of his symptoms likely would fall within the moderate to severe range. It also should be clarified whether his difficulties in school are solely related to ADHD, because these symptoms may mask specific learning disorders or other neurocognitive impairment. A thorough screening for other psychiatric conditions frequently comorbid with ADHD would be helpful, including an assessment of mood and anxiety symptoms and an evaluation of disruptive or oppositional behavior.

Approach to the Diagnosis

Diagnosis of ADHD is challenging given the heterogeneous clinical nature of the disorder. Because ADHD symptoms may vary significantly over time and context, a high degree of suspicion and careful screening and assessment practices are required. The core features for ADHD in DSM-5-TR fall along two axes: inattention and hyperactivity-impulsivity. Impairments in either of these domains can present with a relatively broad range of symptoms; therefore, care should be taken to ensure that individuals meet required criteria before a diagnosis. This includes taking a thorough history to identify time of onset and placing symptoms in the context of where the individual is in their development. Furthermore, it is important to obtain family and medical history because risk factors such as low birth weight; toxin exposure; in utero exposure to smoking, substances, or alcohol; first-degree relatives with ADHD; or environmental stressors such as abuse and neglect may provide additional clues about the diagnosis. As listed in the differential diagnosis, a number of psychiatric and medical etiologies may also affect an individual's overall ability to maintain attention, motor activity, or impulse control; therefore, careful screening is needed to rule out alternative etiologies. However, because individuals often will also meet criteria for other comorbid diagnoses, particularly disruptive behaviors, criteria for these diagnoses should be carefully reviewed. Collateral information is also particularly useful in this diagnostic category for establishing both the diagnosis and the degree of functional impairment due to symptoms. This information may include standardized assessments from family members and teachers and neuropsychological testing.

Because the clinical presentation for ADHD is temporally and contextually variable, care should be taken with DSM-5-TR specifiers in defining presentations. Coding specifiers should include the patient's predominant symptom presentation for the previous 6 months and characterizations of severity from mild to severe. Classifications include combined, predominantly inattentive, and predominantly hyperactive/impulsive, in addition to a course specifier indicating partial remission of symptoms.

Getting the History

A 6-year-old boy is brought into the pediatrician's office for a well-child check. Upon review of symptoms, his parents reveal that he has been having difficulty at school because of disruptive behaviors. The clinician asks the family, "What reports have you been receiving from school that have caused you to be concerned?" The parents respond that at a recent teacher conference, they were told that their son had difficulty paying attention, sitting still during class, and following instructions, but they feel that this may be due largely to teacher-student fit because his teacher in the previous year seemed better equipped to deal with these issues. The clinician follows up by asking the parents, "Can you tell me more about your son's development?" and asking for specific landmarks in cognitive and motor milestones and other environmental, academic, or social factors that they feel might be influencing their son's current behavior in the classroom. The clinician asks, "Have you noticed similar behaviors at home?" and pays careful attention to determine if more than six symptoms are met under criteria for either inattention or hyperactivity-impulsivity. The parents describe symptoms of increased motor activity, although they feel that this activity may be normative because "all boys are active." They also report significant disorganization, impulsivity, and intrusiveness when he plays with siblings. The clinician then gently asks, "Do you feel these issues might be affecting your son's ability to thrive at school or in his relationships with his peers?" The clinician also asks the child how he feels things are going in school and at home, providing specific prompts as needed, such as whether he forgets what his teacher is saying in class, feels as if he cannot sit still, or often forgets his things at school or home. They also review his medical, developmental, and family history to screen for risk factors that may provide additional diagnostic clues and assess carefully for other medical or psychiatric conditions that may be contributing to the diagnosis. With the parents' consent, they provide standardized assessment forms for the parents and their son's teachers to fill out prior to the next appointment.

The pediatrician uses open-ended questions to contextualize the child's difficulties in school, carefully reviewing whether his symptoms are consistent with an atypical developmental trajectory in the core features of inattention and hyperactivity-impulsivity. They also systematically assess whether other disorders might better explain the diagnosis or be comorbid with the patient's ADHD symptoms. Further investigation of mood and anxiety symptoms, as well as learning disorders, would be useful. The pediatrician is also sensitive to the parents' apparent concern about pathologizing the patient's behavior by assessing whether they feel that symptoms exceed normative variation and are significantly affecting the patient's adaptive functioning. Additionally, the pediatrician makes sure to obtain history from the patient regarding symptom presentation and effect on day-to-day function, while arranging to gather further information from collateral sources through the use of standardized screening measures that may help establish a diagnosis.

Tips for Clarifying the Diagnosis

- When did symptoms first present? Do symptoms exceed behavior that would be appropriate for the individual's stage of development?
- How do symptoms present in different contexts, and what are others' impressions of the individual's behavior in those environments?
- Have other diagnoses been ruled out, including medical etiologies that may better explain the clinical presentation?
- Which symptom clusters have been predominant over the past 6 months along the dimensions of inattention-distractibility and hyperactivity-impulsivity?

Consider the Case

Ms. Jain, a 36-year-old woman, presents to the clinic for an "ADD evaluation." She reports lifelong problems with attention and organization, stating that she remembers always "daydreaming" in class. Although she managed to do fairly well in school, getting mostly high grades, she really started to struggle after beginning college. Ms. Jain remembers having significant problems managing her time, forgetting to turn in assignments, and often being described as forgetful and "dreamy" by her parents and teachers. Although she was able to manage a full course load, she always felt she had to work "three times as hard" as her peers to achieve the same results. After college, these problems crossed over into her professional work, where she is currently having significant difficulty organizing her office ("my desk is a chaotic mess"), has been missing important meetings, and has been receiving negative feedback from managers regarding her organizational style. At home, she frequently misplaces her keys and mobile phone around the house, and her lack of organization and impulsivity have been a source of frustration for her and her spouse. Ms. Jain particularly feels that symptoms have worsened since she gave birth to her two children; she needed to cut back from work after feeling overwhelmed with balancing full-time work and raising a family. Her 6-year-old son recently received a diagnosis of ADHD, which prompted her to consider whether she also had the diagnosis. Medical history is otherwise significant for a remote history of an eating disorder during adolescence and weekly migraines for which the patient takes opiate pain medications.

As seen in this case, diagnosis of ADHD in adults may be challenging, particularly when determining whether the person demonstrated symptoms prior to age 12. Obtaining historical records and collateral information from family and school sources may be of use in establishing this diagnostic criterion. However, with regard to her current symptoms, it is likely that Ms. Jain meets criteria of having at least five symptoms of ADHD, with particularly prominent symptoms in the inattention cluster. This symptom presentation is more likely for females with ADHD and is also more common in adults because symptoms in the hyperactivity domain are more likely to attenuate over the course of development. This difference in symptom presentation may partly explain why Ms. Jain's impairments were not diagnosed earlier in life (even though symptoms appear to have been evident at that time), which is important because childhood symptoms are required for the diagnosis. As an adult, Ms. Jain may face some additional challenges in obtaining an appropriate diagnosis for

ADHD. This challenge may be in part because of the difficulty in assessing the pervasiveness of symptoms over development but may additionally reflect her clinician's concerns that comorbid diagnoses are influencing her attention and cognitive function, as well as reservations about the high potential for misuse or abuse of first-line ADHD medications. However, careful clinical assessment should still allow an appropriate diagnosis to be established. In Ms. Jain's case, this assessment should include comprehensive screening for anxiety and depression symptoms, assessment of interpersonal issues and adaptive functioning at home and at work, screening for abuse or misuse of pain medications, and a general medical workup.

ADHD symptoms may vary over the developmental span, with motor hyperactivity tending to attenuate toward adulthood. However, many individuals may continue to exhibit the full syndrome, or symptoms within domains of inattention, poor planning, or impulsivity, well into adulthood. It should be noted that in older adolescents (i.e., older than 17 years) and adults, only five symptoms are required within a cluster to meet criteria. Diagnosis of ADHD may be challenging because the clinical expression of symptoms may vary significantly depending on age, context, and environment. Similarly, risk and prognostic factors for ADHD are fairly heterogeneous and include a range of temperamental, environmental, genetic, and medical associations. Given the unstable presentation of symptoms over time and context, specifiers characterizing the most prominent symptoms in the preceding 6 months are used to define level of severity and presentation, which encompass variations of severity between the core symptom clusters of inattention and hyperactivity-impulsivity. ADHD is also associated with impairments in sociobehavioral domains and increased rates of comorbidity with other psychiatric disorders. Cultural factors also appear to influence rates of diagnoses: Black and Latinx children are diagnosed less frequently than non-Latinx White children. Sex differences are also evident in rates of diagnosis, with young males being diagnosed twice as often as young females in the general population. In contrast, adult males are only 1.6 times more likely to be diagnosed than adult females.

Differential Diagnosis

A number of psychiatric disorders affect higher cognitive functions of attention, motor, and impulse control. Similarly, symptoms of ADHD may be particularly difficult to discriminate from normative behaviors in early childhood. Oppositional defiant disorder and intermittent explosive disorder are also characterized by impaired impulse control, but specific features of hostility, aggression, and negativity are absent in individuals with ADHD alone, although emotion dysregulation is frequently observed. Hyperactivity is also seen in children with normative, high motor activity in the absence of other symptoms but should be distinguished from stereotypic movement disorder, ASD, and Tourette's disorder, in which motor behaviors are usually fixed and repetitive rather than generalized. Overall difficulties with attention, particularly in the school environment, may also be affected by mild intellectual developmental disorder and specific learning disorders, which can lead to frustration or disinterest in academic activities, although comorbid diagnoses can also be made when inattention persists in nonacademic tasks. Similarly, depressive, bipolar, anxiety, and psychotic disorders will affect attention or hyperactivity-impulsivity, although such effects are often clearly tied to specific mood or anxiety states and are more episodic in nature. External etiologies such as substance use disorders, sleep disorders, and side effects from prescribed medications (e.g., bronchodilators, thyroid hormones) may also closely mimic symptoms of ADHD and require a thorough history and workup during assessment. Lastly, reactive attachment disorder and personality disorders share several nonspecific traits regarding emotional dysregulation and disorganization problems with inattention that require ongoing observation and assessment to distinguish these disorders from ADHD. ADHD is associated with an increased risk of suicide attempts when comorbid with mood, conduct, or substance use disorders.

Summary

- Symptoms in the ADHD diagnostic category may vary significantly across contexts and developmental stages.
- Obtaining collateral information may be very helpful for establishing a comprehensive picture of the patient's symptoms and adaptive functioning in different environments.
- Impairments will broadly span clusters of inattention and hyperactivity-impulsivity, and predominant symptoms in these domains over the most recent 6 months will assist in establishing subtype.
- Difficulties with attention and hyperactivity can either mimic or be comorbid with a broad range of other etiologies, necessitating a thorough diagnostic evaluation and workup.

SUMMARY: NEURODEVELOPMENTAL DISORDERS

Neurodevelopment is a dynamic process by which individuals acquire capacities in cognitive, physical, language, and socioemotional domains. This process is influenced by many factors, and the general framework and timeline by which these skills are acquired share many characteristics. Divergence from the expected sequence of events may reflect a derailment of the developmental process, and attention should be paid to how biological, psychological, or environmental factors may be affecting an individual's progress. The neurodevelopmental disorders diagnostic category is designed to capture the presence of abnormal developmental processes and to identify clinical symptoms that indicate an underlying pathological process. The domains affected may be heterogeneous, but the pervasive nature of symptoms over early developmental stages is shared in this group of disorders. Furthermore, symptoms for these groups may have significant effect on an individual's functioning, with potentially severe consequences.

ELEMENTS TO CONSIDER IN THE CULTURAL FORMULATION

- Neurodevelopmental disorders occur across all ethnic and racial groups.
- Sociocultural factors play a central role in how neurodevelopmental conditions are ascertained, diagnosed, and treated, requiring thoughtful approaches in formulation and treatment planning.
- Expectations regarding developmental course and variation from longitudinal trajectories are often influenced by social norms and cultural contexts.
- Sometimes clinicians and patients misunderstand each other because they come from different backgrounds or have different expectations.
- In some instances, sociocultural elements may interface directly with core features of a condition, such as in specific learning disorder, where differences in linguistic systems may result in different manifestations of reading difficulties.
- Perception of symptoms by informants (e.g., parents, teachers) may be influenced by sociocultural frameworks, leading to over- or underdiagnosis or even misdiagnosis in some instances, such as in ASD and ADHD, in which symptoms may be mislabeled as disruptive behavior.
- Furthermore, these sociocultural factors also interact with mental health care delivery and access, as well as other complex social determinants of health. In many cases this results in delayed diagnosis for children in marginalized racial or ethnic groups across a number of neurodevelopmental conditions.
- Treatment planning should incorporate patient and family cultural frameworks when considering treatment selection, as well as culturally informed psychoeducation around associated stigma, understanding of etiologies and causes, and anticipated outcomes.

DIAGNOSTIC PEARLS

- A concrete knowledge of developmental milestones is important for making accurate diagnoses.
- Comprehensive family histories may provide significant information in establishing a diagnosis because many of these disorders are believed to have a strong genetic predisposition.
- Thorough medical histories will be useful in defining syndromes associated with neurodevelopmental disorders—physical examination findings and neurological signs may be particularly helpful.
- Increased access and affordability of comprehensive genetic testing may make such testing a useful clinical modality for disorders in this category, particularly intellectual developmental disorder and autism spectrum disorder.
- Collateral sources of information and standardized assessments are useful for diagnosis, particularly for individuals who are not able to participate fully in the diagnostic process.

- *Stereotypies* are abnormally frequent, non-goal-directed repetitive movements that are seemingly driven and nonfunctional motor behaviors (e.g., hand shaking or waving, body rocking, head banging, self-biting).
- *Distractibility* refers to difficulties concentrating and focusing on tasks and difficulty maintaining goal-focused behavior, including both planning and completing tasks. Attention is easily diverted by extraneous stimuli.

SELF-ASSESSMENT

Key Concepts: Double-Check Your Knowledge

What is the relevance of the following concepts to the various neurodevelopmental disorders?

- Developmental milestones
- General intelligence
- Cognitive subdomains
- Social cognition
- Attention
- Hyperactivity
- Motor ability

Questions to Discuss With Colleagues and Mentors

1. What distinguishes normative from atypical development? What defines early stages of development? How is adolescence defined?
2. What defines ability—how does ability differ among social, cognitive, executive functioning, or motor control domains?
3. How do impairments in neuropsychological domains interact with temperament, motivation, mood, or environment to define diagnoses?
4. What is the best way to screen for alternative etiologies for presenting symptoms? At what point is it best to make a referral or involve other team members? How much workup is appropriate for less commonly seen etiologies?
5. How much does making the appropriate diagnoses affect treatment and clinical outcome?
6. How do you approach the treatment of patients with more than one disorder in this diagnostic category?

Case-Based Questions

PART A

Gregory is a 13-year-old male who was diagnosed prenatally with Down syndrome. His parents report a history of mild to moderate developmental delays—Gregory's first words were at age 1.5 years, and he started walking at age 2 years. Medical history is significant for surgical repair of a septal defect in infancy, short stature, vision impairment requiring glasses, and mild hearing loss bilaterally. His parents have brought him in for evaluation because of a recent increase in maladaptive behaviors at his middle school. Reports indicate that he is increasingly distracted and has trouble maintaining attention in his special day classroom. They also state that he is more irritable and aggressive with his peers and staff.

What might be some contributing factors to Gregory's difficulties at school?   Several issues are relevant in this case, most of which revolve around Gregory's diagnosis of Down syndrome. It would be important to determine the extent of his cognitive abilities and to assess for other conditions such as specific learning disorder, ADHD, mood disorders, or difficulties arising from related medical conditions.

PART B

Gregory's parents have brought his individualized education program report, which includes results for psychological testing over the past several years. His full-scale IQ is in the 60–65 range, and academic achievement testing reveals lower scores across all domains. Teacher feedback suggests that Gregory has appeared withdrawn and less interested in class over the past several months, despite the absence of significant changes in his curriculum or classroom environment. He has also had a recent medical evaluation, including a hearing assessment, which showed no changes from his previous exam a year ago.

How do you determine whether symptoms represent natural variation in the course of intellectual developmental disorder or emergence of a distinct disorder?   Psychological testing suggests that Gregory has general cognitive deficits, which is common for individuals with Down syndrome. However, intellectual impairments in this condition follow a relatively steady course. Although increasing cognitive demands may make existing deficits more pronounced as individuals progress through school, this change does not fully explain the relatively recent difficulties that Gregory has been experiencing. Similarly, sensory impairments may also result in academic and behavioral changes, but Gregory's medical issues appear to be addressed in the current case. Taken together, further evaluation for evidence of other psychiatric diagnoses would be warranted.

PART C

More detailed history reveals that Gregory had problems with sustaining attention with difficult tasks when he was younger, although his parents did not feel it significantly affected his adaptive functioning at the time, particularly because he had a very supportive home and school environment. They also do not recollect that he was particularly fidgety or impulsive. When asked, Gregory focuses less on problems with attention or distractibility and instead endorses symptoms of depressed mood. He states that he increasingly feels alone and "different" from his peers and has many days when he feels too "sad" to go to school.

Does Gregory have ADHD and/or a depressive disorder?   Comorbid disorders are commonly seen with intellectual developmental disorder, which is not surprising given that impairments in general intellectual functioning may also contribute to difficulties in other cognitive domains, such as attention. Gregory's history suggests that he may have had at least some symptoms of ADHD in childhood, although his symptoms likely did not meet full criteria at that time. Furthermore, as seen here, it is also evident that he experiences depressive symptoms. Depressive disorders are not uncommon in Down syndrome and can be seen in intellectual developmental disorder at large. Cognitive impairments often contribute to significant difficulties in navigating school and home environments, thereby creating stressors that may exacerbate or contribute to depressive symptoms. In turn, severe depressive symptoms may affect domains of attention and concentration. Gregory's case illustrates the interrelatedness of cognitive and socioemotional functions, as well as the means by which cognitive difficulties can also affect behavior and adaptive functioning. Further evaluation is warranted in his case because he may in fact have symptoms consistent with both ADHD and a depressive disorder.

Short-Answer Questions

1. Rank in order the age at onset for intellectual developmental disorder, global developmental delay, unspecified intellectual developmental disorder, autism spectrum disorder, ADHD, and Tourette's disorder.
2. List three causes for intellectual developmental disorder.
3. Name at least three cognitive functions subserving general mental ability.
4. What psychological testing must be conducted for intellectual developmental disorder?
5. What constitutes a "severe" level of severity for intellectual developmental disorder?
6. Which of the following symptoms fall under the diagnostic criteria of autism spectrum disorder: limited facial expressions, echolalia, inaccurate word reading, clumsiness, lack of interest in peers, decreased sensitivity to temperature, self-injurious behavior?
7. Describe sex differences in the presentation of autism spectrum disorder.
8. How might one differentiate between the symptoms of bipolar disorder and ADHD?
9. List four medical conditions that may mimic symptoms of ADHD.
10. Are individuals with ADHD at risk for increased substance abuse?
11. Circumlocution is a hallmark of which neurodevelopmental disorder?
12. What is a difference in presentation for adults with ADHD in comparison with that for children with ADHD?
13. How might intellectual developmental disorder be differentiated from specific learning disorder? Can these diagnoses coexist?
14. Which motor skills are affected in developmental coordination disorder?
15. Name at least two conditions to screen for when evaluating an individual for stereotypic movement disorder.
16. What is the distinguishing characteristic of Tourette's disorder from other tic disorders?

Answers

1. Global developmental delay (younger than 5 years), unspecified intellectual developmental disorder (older than 5 years), ADHD (younger than 12 years), and Tourette's disorder (younger than 18 years). Autism spectrum disorder no longer has a specific age cutoff of 3 years; instead, it is defined as symptoms being present in early childhood. Onset of intellectual developmental disorder is by adolescence.

2. Three causes: 1) Down syndrome (trisomy 21) is the most common cause of intellectual developmental disorder; 2) fragile X syndrome represents the most common *inherited* cause; and 3) phenylketonuria is a metabolic disorder that leads to impairments in intellectual ability if left untreated.

3. General mental ability is a comprehensive concept that broadly defines how individuals understand and process information. For the purpose of DSM-5-TR, this ability includes functions of reasoning, problem-solving, planning, abstract thinking, judgment, academic learning, and practical learning.

4. Commonly used tests to assess general mental ability include the Wechsler Intelligence Scale for Children, Stanford-Binet Intelligence Scales, and the Differential Ability Scales. All of these instruments generate an overall age-normed standard score with a mean of 100, and impairment is considered as scores falling two standard deviations below the mean. Standardized assessments such as the Vineland Adaptive Behavioral Scales and the American Association on Mental Retardation Adaptive Behavior Scale may be used to characterize adaptive functioning.

5. "Severe" impairment within social, conceptual, and practical domains entails the following items: social—limited to nonverbal communication to initiate and respond to social interactions and impaired understanding of social contexts; conceptual—relatively simple use of objects and limited grasp of numerical or functional concepts (e.g., time, money); practical—requires assistance for all activities of daily living and needs ongoing supervision in decisions for personal well-being. If degree of severity differs between domains, the overall level of severity that best describes the individual's functioning should be selected.

6. Limited facial expressions and lack of interest in peers are characteristic deficits in social communication and interaction in autism spectrum disorder, while echolalia and decreased sensitivity to temperature represent typical restricted and repetitive behaviors associated with the diagnosis. Although subtle motor deficits may be observed in children with the disorder, clumsiness is not a specific diagnostic feature. Likewise, self-injurious behavior may be observed in autistic children with severe features but is not part of the diagnostic criteria. Inaccurate word reading may suggest a diagnosis of language disorder or specific learning disorder.

7. Males are three to four times more likely to be diagnosed with autism spectrum disorder than females, and there is some evidence to suggest that females are more likely to have accompanying intellectual impairment. Symptoms vary more in females with autism spectrum disorder, and, as a group, they may have better reciprocal conversation, shared interests, and integration of verbal and nonverbal behavior.

8. Young children with bipolar disorder may also present with increased motor activity, impulsivity, and problems with attention and irritability, particularly during hypomanic and manic episodes. However, these symptom presentations tend to be more episodic in nature and correlate with changes in mood state. The nature of motor activity is also usually more goal-directed.

9. A wide range of conditions may also lead to problems with attention, hyperactivity, and impulsivity. Some medical etiologies include side effects from medications (e.g., bronchodilators, neuroleptics, thyroid medications), thyroid disease, lead poisoning, obstructive sleep apnea, substance abuse, and sensory impairments such as hearing loss.

10. Evidence suggests that individuals with ADHD have increased risk for alcohol and other drug abuse, particularly for those whose symptoms persist into adolescence and adulthood. Development of comorbid characteristics such as conduct disorder or antisocial personality disorder may also identify individuals at risk.

11. Circumlocution represents the use of word substitution or unnecessarily roundabout language in order to avoid saying problematic words. It is a diagnostic feature seen in childhood-onset fluency disorder (stuttering).

12. Adults with ADHD may be less likely to have overt symptoms of increased motor activity, but they may still experience an increased internal sense of restlessness or have difficulty participating in sedentary activities. Also, for older adolescents (older than 17 years) and adults with the disorder, only five symptoms from the inattention and/or hyperactivity-impulsivity domains are required for diagnosis.

13. Intellectual developmental disorder characterizes general mental ability, whereas specific learning disorder defines an individual's ability to acquire skills in one or more academic domains, including reading, writing, or arithmetic. General intelligence affects performance in specific academic skills, and individuals with specific learning disorder should also be evaluated for intellectual developmental disorder. Both diagnoses may be appropriate if difficulties in an academic skill exceed what would be expected given an individual's general intelligence.

14. Developmental coordination disorder covers a broad range of fine and gross motor skills, including general clumsiness, catching objects, handwriting, and riding a bike.

15. Trichotillomania and OCD should be considered when evaluating an individual for stereotypic movement disorder because in some instances they will be the more appropriate diagnosis.

16. Tourette's disorder can be distinguished from persistent motor or vocal tic disorder by virtue of having *both* motor and vocal features; it differs from provisional tic disorder in terms of duration of symptoms (longer than 1 year).

REFERENCES

American Psychiatric Association: Diagnostic and Statistical Manual of Mental Disorders, 4th Edition. Washington, DC, American Psychiatric Association, 1994

American Psychiatric Association: Diagnostic and Statistical Manual of Mental Disorders, 5th Edition. Arlington, VA, American Psychiatric Association, 2013

American Psychiatric Association: Diagnostic and Statistical Manual of Mental Disorders, 5th Edition, Text Revision. Washington, DC, American Psychiatric Association, 2022

CHAPTER 6

Schizophrenia Spectrum and Other Psychotic Disorders

David Beckmann, M.D., M.P.H.

Adrienne Gerken, M.D.

Tahir Rahman, M.D.

John Lauriello, M.D.

"My neighbors are saying terrible things about me. I can hear them through the vents."

"I need to have a brain scan to find the transmitter and get it out of there."

- Delusional Disorder
- Brief Psychotic Disorder
- Schizophreniform Disorder
- Schizophrenia
- Schizoaffective Disorder
- Substance/Medication-Induced Psychotic Disorder
- Psychotic Disorder Due to Another Medical Condition

Schizophrenia and the other psychotic disorders in this category all feature prominent psychosis. Psychosis is a symptom, not a diagnosis in and of itself, and can be a presenting symptom of other disorders not in this category. It can be defined as a break in reality testing, such as experiencing perceptions without a corresponding stimulus (i.e., hallucinations) or holding a fixed belief or set of beliefs that is not culturally accepted by most people (i.e., delusions). Schizophrenia can also affect thinking, communication, and behavior. Ever-growing research supports genetic, biochemical, and anatomical markers of schizophrenia, as well as clues to how these and environmental factors (e.g., trauma) may contribute to its pathogenesis. Less research has been conducted on the other psychotic disorders.

Psychosis is a critical element of the schizophrenia diagnosis because hallucinations and delusions make up two of the five possible symptoms in Criterion A. The other three symptoms are disorganized speech, grossly abnormal psychomotor activity (including catatonia), and negative symptoms. Individuals must exhibit at least two of these symptoms, one of which must be a hallucination, a delusion, or disorganized speech lasting at least 1 month. There must also be significant disturbances in functioning secondary to the symptoms, with a wide range of functional domains possibly affected (e.g., school, work, interpersonal relationships). To receive a diagnosis of schizophrenia, the symptoms and disturbance of functioning must total at least 6 months in duration. If the duration of illness is greater than 1 month but less than 6 months, the diagnosis of schizophreniform disorder should be used. If the symptoms are present for at least 1 day but less than 1 month, the diagnosis of brief psychotic disorder should be considered. Brief psychotic disorder can be further characterized depending on whether it occurs with or without a marked stressor or within 4 weeks postpartum. It should be noted that because these diagnoses depend on duration of illness, the diagnosis may evolve with ongoing symptoms.

An important exclusion for the diagnosis of schizophrenia occurs if the symptoms of Criterion A are caused by a mood disorder. Thus, major depressive disorder or bipolar disorder must be ruled out. If the psychosis is present only when there is an identifiable mood episode, then the psychosis is part of a mood disorder. A useful analogy is that the mood disorder is the fuel for the psychosis. Remove the fuel (i.e., resolve the mood disturbance), and the psychosis is snuffed out. However, in some situations, a person's symptoms can meet the diagnosis of a mood disorder, but when the mood disorder is not clinically present, the symptoms of a psychotic disorder remain—the fuel for the psychosis is independent of the mood disorder. In this situation, the diagnosis of schizoaffective disorder should be considered if the duration of independent psychosis is at least 2 weeks. In DSM-5-TR, the mood disorder, even if treated, must be present for most (>50%) of the lifelong illness (American Psychiatric Association 2022). Substance/medication-induced psychotic disorder and psychotic disorder due to another medical condition must also be ruled out before a diagnosis of a primary psychotic disorder is appropriate.

If Criterion A is not met, several other diagnoses in this category may be considered. For example, if an individual manifests delusions alone for at least 1 month, and the delusions do not markedly affect functioning, a delusional disorder should be considered. Subtypes of delusional disorder include erotomanic, grandiose, jealous,

TABLE 6–1. Key changes from DSM-5 to DSM-5-TR

Diagnostic criteria have been changed to clarify that the onset of substance/medication-induced psychotic disorder occurs after substance/medication usage.

Under diagnostic criteria for other specified schizophrenia spectrum and other psychotic disorder, the name of one entry has been changed from "delusional symptoms in partner" to "delusional symptoms in the context of relationship," with some further clarification.

For schizophrenia, even the changes from DSM-IV-TR (American Psychiatric Association 2000) to DSM-5 were evolutionary, rather than revolutionary, but recent research has further supported that these changes were appropriate.

Outside of the diagnostic criteria, cultural considerations were added and robustly updated for the assessment of psychotic symptoms and for each specific diagnosis.

Smaller updates were made to many of the specific diagnoses' diagnostic features, development and course, risk and prognostic factors, or differential diagnosis to reflect the most recent evidence.

persecutory, somatic, and mixed. Some individuals manifest pervasive social and interpersonal difficulties that are "psychosis-like" but do not meet the full symptom picture. Such individuals are often odd or eccentric and detached from others by an apparent lack of empathy or intimacy. In these cases, the diagnosis of schizotypal (personality) disorder may apply. In other cases, subclinical forms of delusions, hallucinations, and disorganized speech come to attention. In some instances, the only disturbance is a pattern of abnormal movements and behavior identified as part of catatonia (which is no longer its own diagnosis but can occur in various disorders). Additionally, the "Other Specified Schizophrenia Spectrum and Other Psychotic Disorder" section provides diagnoses of further research interest, such as persistent auditory hallucinations and attenuated psychosis syndrome. Finally, psychosis that cannot be definitively placed in a specific disorder should be diagnosed as unspecified schizophrenia spectrum and other psychotic disorder, which is intended primarily to serve as a temporary diagnosis when limited information is available.

Other than very minor wording changes made for clarity (specifically in the "Other Specified Schizophrenia Spectrum and Other Psychotic Disorder" and "Substance/Medication-Induced Psychotic Disorder" sections), the diagnostic criteria of the psychotic disorders did not change from DSM-5 (American Psychiatric Association 2013) to DSM-5-TR. Changes outside of diagnostic criteria (e.g., prevalence, risk and prognostic factors) are highlighted throughout this chapter. See Table 6–1 for a summary of the minor changes made to diagnostic criteria.

Diagnosing and treating persons with schizophrenia and the other psychotic disorders pose unique challenges. Many clinicians and family members have personal experiences with the symptoms of other mental illnesses. For example, feeling sad, anxious, or overly preoccupied are common experiences; even if they do not progress to a diagnosis of a mental illness, individuals may be able to extrapolate to what more extreme symptoms might resemble. In contrast, hallucinations and delusions are singular experiences. A clinician may merely be able to say, "I can only imagine what you are going through." If clinicians do not have a personal frame of reference for understanding the psychotic illnesses, they can only wonder how hard this illness is for the person manifesting these symptoms, both initially and then chronically. Although the clinician may not be able to truly understand what the person is experiencing (and thus should avoid phrases such as "I understand what you're going through"), they can understand and empathize with the distress and feelings of alienation resulting from these illnesses.

Experiencing psychosis can be frightening for patients and their loved ones alike, and it will often lead to many questions about prognosis. If the symptoms are less than 6 months in duration and either schizophreniform disorder or brief psychotic disorder is diagnosed, the clinician should communicate a wait-and-see perspective. If the diagnostic criteria exceed the 6-month mark, then a discussion about managing and living with a potentially chronic disorder must ensue. In either case, the clinician's experience with the psychotic disorders is critical. An experienced clinician who has worked with many patients with psychosis is usually aware of the highly variable outcomes, which depend on patients' insight into their illness, premorbid level of functioning, availability of psychosocial resources, and family and social supports. Clinicians should align themselves with their patients' goals and emphasize their patients' strengths and resilience.

IN-DEPTH DIAGNOSIS: SCHIZOPHRENIA

Mr. Kennedy is a 19-year-old sophomore in college who was brought in by his parents because of concerns that his grades were worsening and that he seemed "distant and distracted" on the rare occasions when he interacted with them. He had done well in his freshman year but has had significant worsening of his grades over the past semester. His parents noted that they started to see changes when he came home after his first year; he was working at a fantasy card store and often came home smelling of cannabis. He reluctantly agreed to see a psychiatrist, and during the initial evaluation he was withdrawn and reluctant to talk. The psychiatrist asked to see him alone and tried to build an alliance with him by asking about the games he liked to play. He seemed to brighten at this question and described a particular video game he had been playing recently. Although he said most people think of it as just a game, he knew better. He explained that he hears the voice of the "Grand Sorcerer," who told him that people around him are pawns in a larger game of good versus evil, and that he can unlock the secrets of this larger game through specific actions within the video game. The psychiatrist asked questions to clarify a timeline, and Mr. Kennedy said he had been hearing the Grand Sorcerer since the previous summer (7 months before this evaluation). With further questioning, Mr. Kennedy said that these communications initially occurred while using cannabis. However, because of an agreement with his parents, he has not used cannabis or other substances for 3 months. A urine toxicology screen performed that day was negative for Δ^9-tetrahydrocannabinol (Δ^9-THC) and other substances.

This case highlights several hallmark characteristics of a person with presumed schizophrenia. First, Mr. Kennedy is a late-adolescent male who has demonstrated a disturbance in his expected level of functioning—a good student who is now failing his classes. The change in his behavior has alarmed his family, and they are seeking some explanation from the psychiatrist. As in many cases, Mr. Kennedy's use of cannabis clouds the picture. In this case, ongoing symptoms months after ceasing use argues against a purely substance-induced disorder, although substance use can precipitate the onset of psychotic symptoms. The psychiatrist is able to engage Mr. Kennedy in an open conversation about fantasy games, which allows the patient to discuss his hallucinations and beliefs in an informal dialogue. He hears the "Grand Sorcerer's" voice, talks to that voice, and has an elaborate belief system centered on the game. The psychiatrist formulates a preliminary diagnosis of schizophrenia based on the presence of psychosis, disturbance of functioning, and duration of symptoms greater than 6 months. A substance/medication-induced psychotic disorder may still be possible, but at this point that diagnosis is less likely because Mr. Kennedy has not used substances for a length of time.

Approach to the Diagnosis

Although the identification of hallucinations and delusions would seem to be the starting point for diagnosing schizophrenia, a change in level of functioning is most often the beginning of the diagnostic journey. The teenager whose grades are plummeting or the new army recruit who is not doing well in boot camp either seeks help or raises enough concern that others facilitate an evaluation. Clear indications of delusions and hallucinations direct the clinician toward schizophrenia and the related psychotic disorders. However, the presenting symptoms are often not clear-cut and may include misrepresentations, misattributions, and misperceptions, not frank delusions or hallucinations. The clinician begins to explore the symptoms, eliciting specific examples of each one. Understanding, in detail, a person's individual experiences is critical. Are the voices coming from within their head, or do they attribute the voices to an external source? Is it their own voice or someone else's? Is the individual's avoidance of others a product of a delusion, a result of extreme shyness, or simply a way to deal with living in a well-documented dangerous neighborhood?

Listening to how the individual speaks and puts together their thoughts is also a useful window into the patient's information processing. Factors such as level of education and primary language should be considered but rarely explain frank disorganization or poverty of speech. Talk to the person's family and friends: What do they say about the person's thought process, especially whether it has changed?

Understanding the role of mood in diagnosing schizophrenia is also important: although not part of the diagnostic criteria, persons with schizophrenia often experience symptoms of depression and, rarely, mania. It is critical to understand the relationship between mood and psychotic symptoms—if they occur only during mood episodes, this likely represents affective psychosis (i.e., bipolar disorder or major depressive disorder with psychotic features). Clear symptoms of psychosis that remain during periods of euthymia (when mood episode remits or is adequately treated) lead the clinician's diagnostic algorithm to either schizophrenia or schizoaffective disorder. Distinguishing these two diagnoses relies on a careful timeline of the temporal relationship between these types of symptoms over months and years. If the mood episodes are present for most (≥50%) of the illness history, the diagnosis of schizoaffective disorder is more appropriate.

Clinicians should not jump to a diagnosis of schizophrenia without conducting a comprehensive review of all other causations. Substances (prescribed or otherwise) are a common cause of psychosis, and substance-induced psychosis is likely becoming more common as the legal landscape of cannabis use becomes more permissive. Atypical features of psychosis, or co-occurring medical/neurological symptoms, also warrant a more robust workup for medical causes. Attentive psychiatrists have discovered many nonpsychiatric diagnoses, including autoimmune disorders, infections, heavy metal poisoning, and malignancies.

On the other hand, clinicians should not shy away from the diagnosis of schizophrenia if all evidence points to it. The reluctance to tell patients and their families that the diagnosis is schizophrenia may be understandable but is counterproductive. Sometimes the diagnosis feels premature, despite the patient clearly meeting the minimum 6 months (often 1–2 years); sometimes the diagnosis can be too demoralizing for a clinician who recalls other chronic and disabled patients with schizophrenia. Patients and families also often have a skewed view of the illness because years of stigma have painted (inaccurately) a one-dimensional picture of schizophrenia. The large number of patients diagnosed under DSM-IV's psychosis not otherwise specified (American Psychiatric Association 1994) belied the original intent of that diagnosis; making such a diagnosis may be an attempt to avoid or forestall a difficult conversation. It is hoped that DSM-5-TR's unspecified schizophrenia spectrum and other psychotic disorder diagnosis is not similarly used.

Getting the History

> Mr. Rivera presents to the clinic after a referral from his primary care doctor. His doctor is concerned that Mr. Rivera is overly occupied with a cough that does not appear to have an "organic cause." In the doctor's office, Mr. Rivera seems distant and appears at times to look away and talk to himself.

The psychiatrist should initially approach such a situation with an open mind and a wide differential diagnosis; it is possible that these symptoms may be psychiatric, or they may be from another medical cause that has not yet been found (patients with diagnosed mental illness are particularly likely to experience "diagnostic overshadowing," in which providers anchor to psychiatric causes and do not perform an adequate medical workup). Such interviews are usually best started with very open-ended questions about how the clinician can be helpful and the patient's understanding from their referring provider. A common response to such questions is a variation on "I'm here because the doctor says it's all in my head." One response to such a statement is: "It is possible for physical symptoms to come from what happens in your mind, but I don't know if that's the case for you. Can you begin by telling me a bit about the cough?" The psychiatrist goes beyond eliciting the symptoms of the cough (e.g., frequency, productive or not, other physical symptoms) and asks about Mr. Rivera's concerns about the cough. "What do you think is causing the cough? Is there something specific you're worried about?"

> In the interview, Mr. Rivera seems to look away and talk to himself. The psychiatrist asks, "I can't help noticing that you seem to be talking to someone besides me in the room. Are you comfortable telling me about that?" Mr. Rivera responds that he is hear-

ing his mother talk to him, even though she died 3 years previously. The psychiatrist asks what he and his mother talk about, and although he is initially guarded, eventually he explains that his mother warns him to be afraid of the germs that are everywhere. The psychiatrist asks how long he has been able to communicate with his mother and how he feels about it. If the patient is not providing the desired type of answer, more closed-ended follow-up questions may be useful, such as, "Do you find it helpful? Or frightening? Or something else entirely?" Mr. Rivera says he has spoken with his mother for the past year, and he feels it is a great help to talk to her. As he speaks, he talks with little emotion, so to delve further, the psychiatrist asks Mr. Rivera about his feelings when she died. He expresses very little emotion when responding that at first he was upset but that now he understands that she is still able to talk to him as if she were alive. The psychiatrist asks if his cough has affected his work and learns that Mr. Rivera no longer works because there are "too many germs out there." When asked if he takes any prescribed medicine, traditional remedies, or other substances to help with the cough and germs, Mr. Rivera states that he took prescribed antibiotics for a while but no longer does. He has consulted a healer in his neighborhood with a shared cultural background who told him to breathe the steam from boiling water infused with garlic, which he does about once per week. He denies using alcohol, cannabis, or other substances.

One of the most interesting aspects of working with patients with psychotic disorders can be summarized by the adage "Once a clinician sees one case of schizophrenia, the clinician has seen one case of schizophrenia." Psychosis always comes in the context of the patient's life, family, stressors, and past events. Mr. Rivera presents with a physical symptom, which is a common entry into treatment. The facts about the physical symptom and its meaning to him are critical. Other patients might present after an identifiable breakdown in their functioning, a failed semester, or a new job they could not handle. Still others have had psychological difficulties from childhood and are diagnosed with various other illnesses that either coexisted with or were harbingers of a fully manifested psychosis. The psychiatrist needs to be open-minded about the individual details but understand that central themes tend to emerge after working with many patients. These themes include preoccupations with beliefs that negatively affect functioning and unusual thinking and behaviors that point to schizophrenia. Certain ways of expressing thoughts, often disconnected from the full range of emotions, are indicators of schizophrenia. The experienced clinician understands that schizophrenia is not a "one visit" diagnosis but requires multiple assessments over time to confirm.

Tips for Clarifying the Diagnosis

- First, determine if psychosis is present. Ask the person about hearing voices or seeing things that others do not; delve into the details of these experiences. Many people, including those with trauma-related and autism spectrum disorders, will use terms such as "hearing voices" to describe ego-dystonic intrusive thoughts. Although these cannot be distinguished perfectly, it can be useful to ask questions such as "Does the voice sound like it's coming from inside your head, or are you hearing it with your ears the same way you're hearing my voice?" Observing that a patient is "responding to internal stimuli" (i.e., attending to their hallucinations) may also suggest that someone is experiencing psychosis. This is not a necessary feature, however, and many persons with schizophrenia have learned to ignore or avoid reacting to hallucinations they experience.

• The timeline of symptoms is essential. Consider epidemiological clues such as age at onset and whether symptoms of psychosis were preceded by a prodromal period. The temporal relationship between psychosis and any mood symptoms, substance use, or changes in physical health, will help distinguish schizophrenia from schizoaffective disorder and primary psychotic disorders from psychosis secondary to a mood disorder, substance use, or medical condition.

• Understand the person's cultural beliefs. A potentially helpful tip is to ask the patient's family members how they feel about the issues the patient has reported. For example, if the family believes that dead relatives can speak to them, this experience may not be a delusion.

• People often understand their problems in their own way, which may be similar to or different from how doctors describe the problem.

• Understanding an individual's overall level of functioning is important for diagnosis, as well as for prognosis and management. Understanding their educational or career trajectory prior to experiencing symptoms can help clarify the significance of recent changes.

• Sometimes substances cause or exacerbate symptoms of psychosis, but individuals may ascribe more to substance use than is accurate.

• A deeper understanding of a person's beliefs may provide valuable information. When a patient describes persecutory delusions, for example, questions about who they believe is after them and why might reveal more about the patient's level of insight or uncover significant grandiosity.

Consider the Case

Ms. Smythe is a 42-year-old recent immigrant to the United States. She cites political and economic reasons for leaving her home, parents, and extended family. She has been unable to find work in her previous field as a hospital administrator, so she supports herself by working as a cleaner in a hotel. She has made some acquaintances at work and at church but misses her old life, especially her parents, whom she hopes to bring to the United States. In church, she enrolled in a vocational program that helps members find higher-paying work. While Ms. Smythe was in the program, the minister noticed that she was becoming increasingly disheveled and distracted. When asked about this, she became tearful and upset. She said everything was going so well until a man began to follow her home from work. At first, she thought nothing of it, but now she was sure that he was a member of the secret police from her country of origin. Somehow, he has been able to put listening devices in her apartment and has slipped tracking devices into her food, which she can taste when she eats. When asked why anyone would go to such lengths to follow her, she whispers that she is the rightful president of her country and that the man is attempting to stop her from taking power. The minister suggests she speak to someone at the community clinic and arranges for an appointment with a psychiatrist. On interview, the psychiatrist notes that Ms. Smythe seems preoccupied and repeatedly looks out the window. When the psychiatrist asks what she is looking at, she states nonchalantly that city buses with a certain advertisement are sending her codes from loyalists in her homeland. The psychiatrist notes that she is speaking slowly and calmly and does not appear markedly distressed or agitated. She reports sleeping well and going to work as scheduled. She denies any history of substance use, including alcohol, nicotine, and cannabis. She was diagnosed 5 years ago with hyperthyroidism, which is under good control.

Ms. Smythe presents with both typical and atypical features of schizophrenia. At 42 years old, she seems a bit "old" for the diagnosis, but there is a second, much smaller, peak of onset during middle age, particularly for females. Her move to the United States is a significant stressor, compounded by having to leave her family. It is also not known whether she might have had previous or subclinical episodes in her native country. The minister noticed a change in her, but she is still able to work and take care of herself. Her belief that she is being followed, the messages from the city buses (delusions of reference), and the possible gustatory hallucinations point to a psychotic manifestation. However, it is important to determine whether some of her experiences may be related to the culture and political climate of her native country. It is possible, for example, that she may have to be much more independent in the United States than she had previously been accustomed. This could lead to a sense of insecurity that might present as paranoia. She might also have had traumatic events in her past that make her wary of others, so her psychotic symptoms may be intertwined with posttraumatic symptoms. As with all diagnoses, collecting information from family and friends may shed some light on many of these issues.

Determining whether Ms. Smythe's psychotic symptoms are secondary to a mood disorder is critical to making an accurate diagnosis. She believes herself to be a political leader—an apparently grandiose belief—but she has no symptoms or external observations of mania (e.g., pressured speech). Thyroid abnormalities can lead to psychosis, and although no evidence of that has been seen, a full thyroid panel should be obtained, as well as toxicology and metabolic screenings, despite her report of not using substances. Other medical workup is not routinely necessary to diagnose schizophrenia, but any other clues should be followed to rule out secondary psychoses (e.g., brain MRI if neurological abnormalities are present). Depending on how long these symptoms have been occurring and how much they have affected her functioning, the presumptive diagnosis of schizophrenia could be confirmed.

Studies have found that first- and particularly second-generation immigrants are at increased risk for developing schizophrenia. The adversities of migration include racial discrimination, poverty, and disrupted families. The fact that the risk is even higher in persons whose parents immigrated ("second-generation immigrants") may suggest that some risk stems from challenges related to one's identity and belonging within a social group. Similarly, members of marginalized groups in general have higher rates of schizophrenia when living in areas with low proportions of members of that group.

People who are Black, Indigenous, and persons of color (BIPOC) do not appear to be at marked increased risk of schizophrenia, but disparities in access to and quality of care mean that BIPOC patients are more likely to be misdiagnosed, receive less or lower-quality treatment, and experience less favorable outcomes. The field of psychiatry must acknowledge its own history in generating some of these disparities. In particular, changes that were made to the diagnostic criteria for schizophrenia in DSM-II (American Psychiatric Association 1968) highlighted hostility and aggression as prominent features; these changes exacerbated structural racism, regardless of whether this was intended. Physicians were more likely to describe BIPOC patients with these terms and diagnosed Black Americans with schizophrenia much more commonly, resulting in negative consequences including prolonged or indefinite hospitalization.

These and other historical factors (e.g., racist policies that have resulted in marginalized communities having reduced access to resources) are largely beyond the control of individual providers. However, interpersonal issues are also at play. For example, persons from BIPOC communities are more likely to have experienced mistreatment in medical settings and thus may present with guardedness or suspicion. This might be interpreted as paranoia or negative symptoms and lead to an inaccurate diagnosis of schizophrenia. Even when presented with a standardized case vignette, psychiatrists are more likely to assign a diagnosis of schizophrenia if the patient is described as Black and to assign bipolar disorder if the patient is described as White, demonstrating that provider bias remains a significant factor in diagnosis. This includes implicit biases associating BIPOC patients with schizophrenia, which might cause providers to "anchor" to this diagnosis and fail to ask appropriate questions to elicit the presence of a mood episode. Similarly, White patients are more likely to be offered the most effective treatments, such as electroconvulsive therapy and clozapine, compared with BIPOC patients. Being aware of one's own implicit biases, as well as those of medical systems and society in general, is an essential step in compensating for these disparities. When a large first-episode psychosis program created interventions that were specifically tailored to marginalized populations using the program, most differences by race or ethnicity were eliminated.

In addition to the impact of historical and ongoing racism and other biases, cultural factors may affect how patients present. For example, it may be culturally normative for a person to hear the voice of God or to believe that demons or spirits are responsible for causing distress. Discordance between the patient's and the clinician's spoken languages (and culturally relevant nonverbal communications) might also be misinterpreted as disorganization, alogia, or simply abnormal. This risk can be mitigated by using a trained medical interpreter whenever possible and asking the interpreter for their impressions of thought process and word usage after the interview. Again, collateral sources of information about what is culturally normative (e.g., from family members, religious leaders) can be enormously helpful.

The relationship between exposure to substances—particularly cannabis—and the development of schizophrenia has also long been of interest to researchers. Individuals with schizophrenia are more likely to use cannabis and more likely to have used cannabis heavily prior to developing symptoms of psychosis when compared with their peers; causality, however, has historically been difficult to demonstrate. As cannabis becomes more widely accepted and available, however, its role as a risk factor is becoming clearer. In Europe, youth who used high-potency (THC >10%) cannabis at least daily were twice as likely to develop schizophrenia compared with peers who did not use cannabis. Like other risk factors discussed here, most people who use cannabis heavily in youth will not develop schizophrenia; therefore, an underlying (presumably genetic) risk is likely also necessary.

Persons with schizophrenia also have increased morbidity and mortality related to higher rates of obesity and use of substances, particularly cigarettes. The reasons for this are complex and include overlapping genetic risk. Medications used to treat schizophrenia also play a role because most antipsychotics can cause weight gain, and many atypical antipsychotics risk other metabolic problems (including decreased insulin sensitivity).

Persons with schizophrenia use medical services less often, and they may distrust the medical system, lack insurance, or be wary of clinician stigma. The mortality risk for schizophrenia is a growing concern. Individuals with schizophrenia have a two- or threefold increase in risk of early mortality, and life expectancy is reduced by nearly a quarter of a century, to just under 60 years. It is incumbent on the treating psychiatrist to recognize and address some of these issues as part of the larger illness (e.g., addressing smoking cessation and weight management).

Differential Diagnosis

The differential diagnosis of schizophrenia is a process of eliciting the cardinal symptoms represented in Criterion A and then determining whether these symptoms might be represented by another disorder. Functional impairment frequently brings people to the attention of health care providers. The degree of functional impairment might help differentiate between more circumscribed disorders such as delusional disorder or mood disorders, although the degree of functional impairment in schizophrenia is highly variable. If the person has a noticeable presentation of depression or mania, mood disorders and schizoaffective disorder should be immediately considered. The number of episodes and the recovery from psychosis with resolution of mood symptoms help differentiate mood disorders from schizophrenia. The continued manifestation of psychosis when mood symptoms are absent or adequately treated for at least 2 weeks directs the differential to either schizoaffective disorder or schizophrenia. Distinguishing these two can be difficult and requires a careful retrospective bookkeeping of the percentage of mood disorder versus the overall length of the psychotic illness.

Other important differentiators include length of illness and plausible alternative explanations for the symptoms. Along a time continuum, brief psychotic disorder lasts less than 1 month; schizophreniform disorder, less than 6 months; and schizophrenia and schizoaffective disorder, longer than 6 months. If either an underlying medical condition or use of illicit substances is a possible source of the psychotic symptoms, it must be eliminated as the potential cause. The treatment of underlying medical conditions and the assurance that there is no ongoing substance use, when applicable, may lead to complete resolution of the symptoms and confirm a diagnosis of psychotic disorder due to another medical condition or substance/medication-induced psychotic disorder. Personality disorders must also be considered (e.g., schizotypal personality disorder) and usually include a long-standing pattern of behavior without the full-blown presentation of psychosis seen in schizophrenia. In addition to the overlap in symptoms seen in Cluster A personality disorders, people with significant trauma histories or borderline personality disorder may experience psychotic or psychotic-like symptoms at times of high stress. Persons with autism spectrum disorder (ASD) may also experience psychotic-like symptoms and may describe experiences very differently compared with their neurotypical peers. Teenagers and young adults with ASD often present diagnostic challenges when describing psychotic-like symptoms: this tends to be a stressful time for all youth, particularly those with ASD, but this is also the time when we would expect the initial manifestations of schizophrenia to emerge.

Approximately 5%–6% of individuals with schizophrenia die from suicide, about 20% attempt suicide on one or more occasions, and many more have significant suicidal ideation. Those most at risk are persons with command hallucinations (i.e., voices telling the person to engage in suicide) as well as younger males with co-occurring substance use (one meta-analysis found each of these features—youth, male sex, and substance use—to be independent risk factors). Other risk factors include having depressive symptoms or feelings of hopelessness, unemployment (or underemployment), a greater number of hospital admissions, and proximity to a hospitalization or episode of psychosis. Although earlier age at onset tends to result in more severe symptoms, persons who develop schizophrenia later in life are at higher risk of suicide. This, like higher IQ, may suggest that the role of insight in this potentially devastating illness is two-sided. Despite the frequency with which it is portrayed in the media, the association between schizophrenia and violence is small; persons with schizophrenia often face enormous stigma and are much more likely to be victims of violence rather than perpetrators.

Summary

- Schizophrenia and the other psychotic disorders under this category all share the common manifestation of psychosis. Psychotic thinking is a symptom, not a diagnosis by itself, and can be a presenting symptom of other disorders not in this category.
- Schizophrenia is a serious mental disorder affecting thinking, communication, and behavior. Psychosis is a critical element of this diagnosis; hallucinations and delusions make up two of the five symptoms in Criterion A. The other three symptoms are disorganized speech, grossly abnormal psychomotor activity, and negative symptoms.
- Persons must meet at least two of these symptoms, and one must be a hallucination, delusion, or disorganized speech lasting at least 1 month.
- There must be significant disturbances in functioning secondary to the symptoms, with a wide range of functional domains possibly affected (e.g., school, work, interpersonal relationships) for at least 6 months.
- Meta-analyses have found an estimated lifetime prevalence of schizophrenia to be between 3 and 7 per 1,000. However, the results of prevalence studies vary widely, and this may be an underestimate.
- Depending on the criteria, sex differences may not exist; however, estimates emphasizing negative symptoms tend to suggest higher rates in males.
- Immigration conveys a higher rate of schizophrenia, which could be because of the stress of a new culture and the effects of displacement.

- Age at onset is typically in the late teens and early twenties and is slightly younger in males than in females.
- Risk factors proposed for schizophrenia include family history, winter birth, older paternal age, dose-dependent cannabis use, and obstetrical complications, but no single risk factor has been clinically predictive. Candidate genes have been identified, but they alone are not yet a definitive "test" for schizophrenia.
- Morbidity data for persons with schizophrenia are often difficult to capture, but it is widely accepted that those with schizophrenia are more likely to experience obesity (often worsened by antipsychotic medication) and substance use, particularly cigarette use. These co-occurring concerns warrant attention from the psychiatrist or a closely collaborating primary care provider.
- Cultural differences may have a substantial impact on how symptoms of psychosis present. Separately, systemic racism, xenophobia, and other biases lead to high rates of misdiagnosis when patients present with psychosis. It is essential for providers to recognize their own implicit biases and to ensure that symptoms are interpreted in an appropriate context.
- Clinicians should take extra care when interpreting symptoms of psychosis in patients from BIPOC and other marginalized communities. Specifically, suspicion or guardedness may represent paranoia, or it may be an understandable response to historical or personal mistreatment. If the presence of psychosis is established, beware of unconsciously jumping to conclusions about the appropriate diagnosis and ensure that alternate diagnoses—including bipolar disorder and major depressive disorder with psychotic features—have been adequately considered.
- Individuals with schizophrenia have two to three times the risk of early mortality, and their life expectancy is reduced by nearly a quarter of a century.

IN-DEPTH DIAGNOSIS:
SCHIZOAFFECTIVE DISORDER

Ms. Hill is a 30-year-old woman who presents to the psychiatric clinic because she has been hearing a disparaging voice during the past month. After learning a little bit about her life, the psychiatrist asks questions about her history, and she confirms that this is not the first time she has heard the voice and that a previous psychiatrist diagnosed and treated her for major depressive disorder with psychotic features. Further questioning reveals that her first depressive episode was near the end of high school; she was prescribed medication at that time with good results. She had no significant symptoms for several years, during which time she graduated from college, married, and had her first child. She had a second depressive episode when she was 27 during the postpartum period after her second child was born. This episode was severe enough that she became isolated, had poor sleep and appetite, and began to hear the voice of a former high school teacher, who said negative things about her. She believed that the teacher was going to report her to the authorities and that she would lose custody of her children. This led to her first hospitalization, during which she responded well to a regimen of both antidepressant and antipsychotic medications. After a year of euthymia without psychosis, she was gradually tapered off of her medications and stopped seeing her psychiatrist. She continued to feel well for about a month, but then 1 month ago began to hear whispers of the voice of her former teacher and those of other people from her past. She denies any current problems with her mood, energy, sleep, or appetite, and the evaluating psychiatrist does not appreciate any signs of mania or depression. For a while Ms. Hill thought that the voices would pass quickly because she was not feeling depressed this time, but they have been getting louder. The psychiatrist shares their diagnostic thoughts, and together they arrive at a treatment plan that involves restarting both antidepressant and antipsychotic medications.

This case illustrates some of the classic features of schizoaffective disorder. Ms. Hill started with depressive symptoms earlier in life, and only during a subsequent depressive episode did she begin to have symptoms consistent with Criterion A for schizophrenia. In her case, she experienced both hallucinations (the teacher's voice) and a delusion (that the teacher would report her to child custody authorities). When she first began to exhibit psychotic symptoms, she was in a full depressive episode. At that point in her history, Ms. Hill's symptoms were most consistent with major depressive disorder with psychotic features. The psychiatrist prudently kept her on both the antidepressant (for her recurrent depression) and the antipsychotic (for a suitably conservative period). After a year, an attempt to wean the antipsychotic medication seems reasonable. In this case, however, Ms. Hill's psychotic symptoms returned while her mood was euthymic. Because she reports hearing the voices for more than 2 weeks, she has established a period of psychosis independent from her mood disorder. She has also had depression for more than 50% of the time since she first experienced psychosis (most of that time with successful treatment), thus fulfilling the criterion of having mood symptoms for the majority of her illness.

Approach to the Diagnosis

Schizoaffective disorder is a diagnosis that must be made with the patient's clinical timeline in mind. Because it is an amalgam of periods of disordered mood or psychosis, determining the relative components of each is critical. Clinicians should first determine the mood component, and then determine whether the patient has had a period of normal mood during which they have demonstrated the cardinal symptoms of schizophrenia delineated in Criterion A. Alternatively, clinicians may start with the Criterion A symptoms of schizophrenia and subject that diagnosis to the possibility of a concurrent mood disorder. Symptoms of depression are more common than symptoms of mania, and mood symptoms typically precede psychosis, but illness course is variable. Only when the patient's mood is stable and psychotic symptoms remain is the possibility of schizoaffective disorder or schizophrenia entertained. Differentiating the latter two diagnoses requires determining the cumulative time the patient has spent in mood episodes.

It is often difficult to explain the diagnosis of schizoaffective disorder to patients and families, who tend to categorize illnesses into either a mood or a psychotic disorder. Indeed, prior to DSM-5, this diagnosis was likely applied too liberally (e.g., to persons with schizophrenia and mood symptoms or with mood disorders and symptoms of psychosis). The diagnosis has also been historically misapplied as something of a catchall when a patient has some features of psychosis and some of mood symptoms but there is not enough information to definitively clarify the diagnosis. However, schizoaffective disorder requires that criteria for these two disorders be met separately and suggests two distinct mechanisms of action. Providing "fuel" for these symptoms may be a useful analogy: different fuels (e.g., neuroreceptors, aberrant neuronal connections) may independently ignite the symptoms of the mood disorder and the symptoms of Criterion A of schizophrenia.

Notice the distinction between psychosis and the Criterion A symptoms of schizophrenia: the diagnosis of schizoaffective disorder requires at least two symptoms in Criterion A, including at least one of the first three:

1. Delusions
2. Hallucinations
3. Disorganized speech
4. Grossly abnormal psychomotor behavior, including catatonia
5. Negative symptoms, such as diminished emotional expression or avolition

Although meeting Criterion A is necessary for the overall diagnosis, hallucinations or delusions are sufficient to satisfy the need for 2 weeks of psychotic symptoms in the absence of a mood episode.

Getting the History

A 32-year-old man presents to the clinician's office with a chief complaint of depression that began when he lost his job 6 months ago. In the interview, he reports that he has been a victim of "unknown forces" since graduating from high school. These forces are malevolent and keep him from succeeding at work and with personal relationships. He purchased heavyweight "blackout" blinds for his bedroom so that the forces cannot spy on him. He recently visited his primary care doctor for a yearly checkup and, aside from elevated cholesterol, has no active medical problems. He lives with his parents, who accompany him to the appointment. With the patient's permission, the psychiatrist asks the parents about these symptoms. They were aware that he had been depressed but are surprised about "the forces." They had assumed he put the heavy blinds on his windows to help him sleep. In discussing family history, his father explains that the family was not in touch with the patient's biological mother, but that she had experienced a "nervous breakdown."

This patient presents a diagnostic challenge to the clinician. The information provided is insufficient to diagnose a specific mood or psychotic disorder, and questions about both the nature and timing of his symptoms are essential to discriminate between these diagnoses. The clinician should start with the patient's presenting complaint, which in this case is depression. We often ask people to describe their depression: "Depression may mean different things to different people. Can you describe your depression to me?" A person may give a classic description of major depression; however, depression may also mean feeling flat or unemotional. In the latter case, a stronger suspicion of negative symptoms of schizophrenia should be entertained. Assuming the case example patient does describe many of the symptoms of major depression, it would be very helpful to elicit the length of time each episode lasts and the total number of episodes. If he is unsure, the clinician could ask whether he can remember the worst episode or one that was particularly memorable (e.g., because he had suicidal thoughts or was hospitalized). The clinician needs to sketch in their mind (or even record on paper) the approximate length of time the patient has had a mood problem, which is essential for making the final diagnosis.

The patient in this case has no overt history of a manic episode. Sometimes this history can be elicited by referring to the person's suspicions: "Is there something special about you that may explain why someone would want to spy on you and keep you from being successful?" This question may bring out symptoms of grandiosity, which can be explored more deeply for periods of mania. A further evaluation of the possible symptoms of Criterion A of schizophrenia is then necessary. This patient described paranoia and persecutory thinking, so a next question might be whether he ever hears or sees evidence of these forces. His speech seems organized, but allowing him to talk freely may draw out some disorganization. Close observation of his movements may show some abnormalities, and a discussion with him and his family may bring out negative symptoms. Finally, confirming that his hallucinations or delusions occur in the absence of a mood episode is critical. Asking him, "Do the forces bother you, even when you think your mood is in a pretty even state?" may help to define a period of psychosis without the co-occurring mood disorder. The path for making this diagnosis may be summarized as an uninterrupted period of illness, more than half of which meets criteria for a mood disorder, with overlapping Criterion A symptoms and at least 2 weeks of delusions or hallucinations without mood symptoms, leading to the diagnosis of schizoaffective disorder.

Tips for Clarifying the Diagnosis

- Start by establishing the presence of a major depressive or manic episode. Note that many psychiatric disorders feature some mood symptoms; full criteria should be applied rigorously.
- Determine whether the patient satisfies Criterion A for schizophrenia (noting that one symptom must be hallucinations, delusions, or disorganized speech).
- Determine if any hallucinations or delusions have occurred for at least 2 weeks while the mood disorder is not present (or is treated to remission).
- Last, calculate how much of the patient's treatment history has occurred either during a mood episode or while the patient was taking medication. If that time is greater than 50% of the total, then schizoaffective disorder should be considered the most likely diagnosis.

Consider the Case

Mr. Williams is an 18-year-old man who is seen by a psychiatrist at the local jail after being arrested for shoplifting. At the time of his arrest, he was agitated, talking rapidly, and saying that the "voices" were screaming in his head. He argued that he was not shoplifting because he owned the store but that no one believed him because he is Black. He further described that he owned many stores in the area and that the world depended on his collecting and combining objects from the stores correctly. He had been walking around the city, in and out of stores, for 3 days to find these "relics," not even stopping to sleep for more than a few hours.

The jail physician initially suspects a substance-induced condition, but a few days later Mr. Williams's symptoms have not improved, and his urine toxicology result is negative. He is diagnosed with bipolar disorder, current episode manic, and he is prescribed an antipsychotic and mood stabilizer with good effect. He is ultimately sentenced to probation that includes ongoing psychiatric care and living with his parents, and he is discharged with only the mood stabilizer.

The psychiatrist working with Mr. Williams in the community learns that his only psychiatric history was being diagnosed with oppositional defiant disorder when he was 14 years old after a series of behavioral concerns at school. He has never been hospitalized but has spent time in juvenile justice facilities. Initially, Mr. Williams seems to be doing well: he is not having mood symptoms and has enrolled in a local community college. However, a month into classes, he tells his mother that he is hearing voices again—whispers at first, then full conversations. He believes that the voices are being beamed into his head by satellite as part of a government experiment. Despite the severity of his psychosis, his mood remains normal, and he does not manifest any signs or symptoms of mania or depression. The psychiatrist recommends antipsychotic therapy, which markedly improves his symptoms.

Mr. Williams is another example of how schizoaffective disorder may present, although his case is less typical. Mr. Williams is relatively young, without an established diagnosis of mood disorder or history of Criterion A schizophrenia symptoms. This scenario also highlights, however, some of the biases that can further interfere with arriving at the correct diagnosis. BIPOC youth, particularly Black male children, are more likely to have psychiatric symptoms be interpreted as opposition and to receive a diagnosis of oppositional defiant disorder or receive punishment with no diagnosis at all. Persons of marginalized racial and ethnic groups are also more likely to have these behaviors addressed through the criminal justice, rather than mental health, system. It is possible that Mr. Williams showed symptoms of mania or psychosis previously that were met with disciplinary rather than treatment measures. Once incarcerated, adequate diagnosis and treatment were delayed based on an assumption that his symptoms were substance induced, an assumption that may not have been made in a different treatment setting.

Based on the information provided, the jail psychiatrist's ultimate presumptive diagnosis of bipolar disorder—and their approach to treating this—were reasonable. However, these diagnoses should never be seen as immutable, and with additional information, the recurrence of psychosis in the absence of a mood episode made schizoaffective disorder the most appropriate diagnosis.

Differential Diagnosis

Identifying schizoaffective disorder is an exercise in differential diagnosis. Embedded in the diagnosis are elements of both schizophrenia and a major mood disorder. By definition, one must distinguish this diagnosis from three other diagnoses: schizophrenia, major depression with psychotic features, and bipolar disorder. Uncoupling the psychotic symptoms from the mood disorder and having a mood disorder for more than half the time are essential. Of note, if the patient is experiencing psychosis for the first time, the same differential for schizophrenia must be considered: those with psychotic symptoms lasting less than 1 month may have a brief psychotic disorder, whereas those with psychotic symptoms lasting less than 6 months may have schizophreniform disorder. The presence of an established mood disorder does not preclude the possibility of these diagnoses.

As with other psychotic disorders, substance-induced and medical causes must be ruled out. Cluster A personality disorders may have psychotic-like symptoms, and diagnoses that feature affective instability (e.g., intermittent explosive disorder) can have overlap with features of mania. Borderline personality disorder can feature both labile affect and, at times of stress, psychotic-like features. Rapid changes in mood (minutes to hours) can be a useful clue to differentiate this from episodes of mania (which typically last days to months).

Because of the overlap between mood and psychotic disorders, it is relatively common for a diagnosis to change to schizoaffective disorder (e.g., in a person diagnosed with schizophrenia after the course of mood symptoms becomes more apparent) or for a diagnosis of schizoaffective disorder to evolve into a different mood or psychotic disorder. In the latter case, it is much more common for the diagnosis to change to schizophrenia than to bipolar disorder or major depressive disorder.

Schizoaffective disorder appears to be at most one-third as common as schizophrenia, with one Finnish study finding a lifetime prevalence estimate of 0.3% using DSM-IV criteria (the more stringent diagnostic criteria of DSM-5-TR suggest a similar study conducted today would find an even lower prevalence). The typical age at onset of schizoaffective disorder is during early adulthood, usually older than that of schizophrenia. The prognosis for schizoaffective disorder is highly variable, with some prognostic value in the relative severity of the psychotic symptoms. Although the overall prognosis is highly heterogeneous, individuals with schizoaffective disorder achieve, on average, better functional outcomes than those with schizophrenia, and not as good functional outcomes as those with bipolar disorder. The incidence of schizoaffective disorder is at least slightly higher among females than among males—a difference that is mostly accounted for by increased incidence among females with depression. The lifetime risk of suicide for schizophrenia and schizoaffective disorder is 5%, and the presence of depressive symptoms is correlated with a higher risk for suicide.

Summary

- Schizoaffective disorder is an admixture of mood and schizophrenia-like disorder during an uninterrupted period. Both diagnostic groups have to be confirmed during the lifetime course of the disorder.
- Establishing an independent period of at least 2 weeks (i.e., in the absence of a mood episode) with delusions or hallucinations is necessary.
- A careful calculation of how much of the person's treatment history has been either during an overt mood episode or while successfully being treated with medication is critical. If that time is greater than 50% of the total, then schizoaffective disorder should be strongly considered.
- The prevalence of schizoaffective disorder is estimated to be less than one-third of that of schizophrenia, assuming careful adherence to the criteria. It is slightly more common in females.

IN-DEPTH DIAGNOSIS: DELUSIONAL DISORDER

Ms. Gordon is a 39-year-old woman brought to the emergency department by police for reportedly harassing a local celebrity. She presents as calm, appears to have good hygiene, makes good eye contact, and communicates clearly in a linear and logical fashion with health care staff. When she is asked about the harassment complaints involving the celebrity, however, she becomes upset and explains that the two of them have a special connection and are destined to marry. Ms. Gordon has been writing the celebrity love letters and trying to call him for 2 years; tonight she tried to approach him near his home. When asked further questions about this "relationship," she explains in elaborate detail how they met online and how they are destined to be married tonight.

Her mental status examination is unremarkable beyond the belief that she is supposed to marry this celebrity, and further questions on this topic begin to cause her significant distress. She is eventually given a low dose of an antipsychotic to keep her calm and help her sleep. Her sister arrives later and provides more details: at first the family believed that Ms. Gordon genuinely had a relationship with this man, but they quickly realized this was not true. Her sister confirms that aside from her preoccupation with the celebrity, she appears to have normal mood, sleep, energy, and activity levels.

This case highlights the important aspects of delusional disorder, erotomanic type. Ms. Gordon had a fixed, false belief that she was to marry the celebrity. The belief is rigidly held and cannot be reasoned away by others. She does not meet criteria for schizophrenia because she does not have any other symptoms from Criterion A. Her speech is logical and goal-directed, and she has no disorganized thoughts or behavior. Her level of functioning appears remarkably intact except for the ramifications of this circumscribed belief. Note that the criteria for delusional disorder do allow for the presence of hallucinations as long as they are not prominent and are related to the delusional theme (e.g., if Ms. Gordon occasionally hears the celebrity calling her name when she passes his house).

Ms. Gordon does not meet criteria for a mood disorder. She is upset that she cannot be with the celebrity but otherwise shows no indication of either depression or manic symptoms. The term "erotomanic" should not be confused with bipolar mania. A person with mania could have such a delusion, but they would also have other classic manic symptoms, such as decreased need for sleep and elevated activity level.

Other possible causes of psychosis (e.g., substances, delirium, or major neurocognitive disorders) were carefully ruled out. Although less applicable to this case, delusions may also be about one's own body, in which case body dysmorphic disorder should be considered, or about one's need to engage in certain behaviors, which should raise suspicion for obsessive-compulsive and related disorders.

Approach to the Diagnosis

Directly confronting patients and explicitly stating that their delusions are not true is rarely fruitful, particularly if the clinician is not well known to them. It is unlikely to change their beliefs and may compromise the treatment alliance. Expressing agreement with delusional beliefs is dishonest and may also be counterproductive. A nonjudgmental, curious, and comforting approach that validates the patient's distress (rather than delusional beliefs) is best. Focusing on other topics to build alliance prior to discussing areas directly related to the delusions may be advantageous, as might early involvement of the patient's family.

In delusional disorder specifically, delusions are typically not "bizarre." Plausible scenarios with themes such as jealousy, persecution, erotomania, or having a special relationship with an important person are much more common than beliefs about imminently invading extraterrestrials or having one's mind controlled by means of an implanted chip. These less plausible beliefs may point the clinician more in the direction of schizophrenia or a mood disorder with psychotic features.

The diagnosis of delusional disorder is made after conducting a careful history and examination. External informants and collateral data are often needed from family members, friends, and old records. The person may not discuss their delusions with the examiner openly, so the symptoms may go undetected without external information. The person's history should be examined carefully for mood symptoms such as manic episodes with psychosis or depression with psychosis. Mania, for example, often features delusions of grandeur and may inflate one's importance in society, families, or peer groups. However, people experiencing mania also exhibit other symptoms, such as decreased need for sleep, elevated activity and energy levels, agitation, and mood cycling. People with psychotic depression often exhibit nihilistic delusions and may also have ego-syntonic hallucinations, as well as mood symptoms such as diminished interest in activities, crying spells, hopelessness, and lethargy. A complete family and social history, as well as a medical history, should be obtained to help determine genetic and psychosocial issues in the person's life.

Getting the History

A 27-year-old woman presents to the emergency department with her mother for evaluation of distress related to her belief that her husband is having an extramarital affair. Her mother describes that the family was initially shocked that her son-in-law would do that, but further conversations quickly clarified that her daughter's concerns were not based in reality. The psychiatrist tries to understand the patient's concerns and her thought process in reaching this conclusion. The psychiatrist validates the patient's distress, noting that it must be very upsetting to feel betrayed, and asks nonconfrontational questions, such as "When did you get suspicious about your husband's affair? How did you find out? Is there any particular evidence that led you to believe this? Do you believe he is still having an affair? Can you explain more?"

The psychiatrist keeps an open mind—including for the possibility that the patient's concerns are not a delusion—but the patient is unable to explain her concerns with evidence or logic. She agrees it is likely a delusion, so the psychiatrist looks for the presence of other symptoms of psychosis, asking questions such as "Do you hear voices when you are alone? Or see things that other people do not see? Do you ever feel like you are being watched or followed? Do you ever notice messages meant just for you, like from the television or radio?" In addition to symptoms of psychosis, the psychiatrist carefully screens for substance use, mood symptoms, and trauma history.

Psychiatrists must often rely on collateral sources of data for making the proper diagnosis. Sometimes this information becomes necessary in emergencies when a person cannot communicate well or is unable to establish a discourse with the clinician. In other situations, gathering these data requires patience and written permission from the person. In either type of situation, it is helpful for the clinician to gather relevant clinical information from third parties, such as close relatives or friends. Persons with psychosis often have disorganized thoughts, delusions, or active hallucinations, which can make it difficult to gather enough information to make a proper assessment. Collateral information can be essential even when evaluating patients who present with clearly described symptoms and substantial insight. For example, many of the diagnostic criteria for psychiatric conditions require time durations for symptoms to be present. Relying on the person's report alone can be misleading, as any patient may get confused about details of their own history, particularly if the illness is causing impairment to cognition or memory.

Tips for Clarifying the Diagnosis

- Obtain collateral sources of information, such as interviews with family members, past psychiatric records, and a comprehensive evaluation of the person's psychosocial and medical history.
- Carefully rule out common causes of psychosis, such as mania or depression with psychosis.
- Relying on only the patient interview can be misleading. Detecting delusions often requires external interviews.
- Confronting delusions directly is rarely fruitful and can make people guarded and distrustful. Early interviews should focus on developing a trusting relationship and rapport.
- Toxicology screening and other medical and neuroimaging testing may be indicated to rule out other types of pathology, such as brain lesions or thyroid abnormalities, particularly if a patient's symptoms are atypical or the patient exhibits other clues.

Consider the Case

Mx. Starr is a 25-year-old genderqueer adult who presents as a new clinic patient despite already having a psychiatrist who treats them for major depressive disorder and PTSD. They describe a long history of family members forcing them to present and identify as male (the sex they were assigned at birth), as well as traumatic encounters when they were targeted for their gender identity. Since they moved out of their parents' house 7 years ago, their previous psychiatrist had been helping with mood- and trauma-related symptoms. However, about 6 weeks ago, their mood began to worsen, and they began to develop frequent abdominal pain. Mx. Starr is now looking for a new psychiatrist because they have become increasingly convinced that their psychiatrist no longer wants to help and has been prescribing their medication in such a way that the pharmacy replaces it with something else. They stopped taking their medication 3 weeks ago because of a concern that the pills could be poisonous.

The evaluating psychiatrist asks nonconfrontational questions about how these concerns arose, what evidence has led the patient to this conclusion, and how they are thinking about it now, as well as questions about Mx. Starr's recent experiences. The psychiatrist concludes that the patient has previously been mistreated in medical settings, perhaps predisposing them to this type of concern, but that their current concerns are not based in evidence or logic. Mx. Starr does not appear to have any other symptoms of psychosis. Their mood has been low for several weeks, but they do not meet full criteria for a major depressive episode. They report using alcohol socially, averaging one drink per week, and otherwise deny substance use including nicotine or alcohol. There have been no recent changes in their physical health, and they are continuing to work full-time.

Although younger persons can develop delusional disorder, it is likely more prevalent in older persons; age at onset may serve as an important diagnostic clue. The prevalence and types of delusional disorders are very similar between both sexes, although delusional disorder, jealous type, may be more common in males.

The genetics of delusional disorder are not well studied, but family connections suggest genetic overlap with both schizophrenia and schizotypal personality disorder. As with all of these disorders, more time is sometimes necessary for diagnostic clarity: about one-third of people diagnosed with delusional disorder will likely receive a diagnosis of schizophrenia within the first 3 months of the initial diagnosis. This number drops precipitously 6–12 months after the initial diagnosis, at which point the diagnosis of delusional disorder tends to be stable.

As with any presentation that includes features of psychosis, it is essential to understand the cultural context in which these appear. A person who is functioning well in their community may be referred for psychiatric evaluation by a medical provider on the basis of a specific belief the person expresses. However, such beliefs cannot be deemed delusional if they are culturally normative.

Differential Diagnosis

Delusional disorder should be considered when a person experiences delusional thoughts in the absence of other features of psychosis or related conditions (outside of nonprominent hallucinations that relate to the delusion). Substance/medication-induced psychotic disorder, delirium, and major neurocognitive disorders (dementia) should be appropriately ruled out. If the person meets Criterion A of schizophrenia, then delusional disorder should not be diagnosed. Delusional disorder typically produces less impairment than schizophrenia in social and occupational functioning, and the impairment is typically directly related to the delusion (e.g., legal difficulties for one's aggressive pursuit of a celebrity at the center of an erotomanic delusion).

Individuals with delusions should also be screened for mood disorders because unipolar depression and bipolar disorder (either with depression or manic episodes) might feature delusions as part of the presentation. For example, grandiose or erotomanic delusions could easily occur in the midst of a manic episode with mood-congruent psychosis.

Finally, persons with body dysmorphic disorder or OCD can appear to have severely distorted thoughts that may initially appear to be delusions. Appropriate clinical correlation and careful examination may be helpful.

Summary

- The presence of a fixed false belief in a person who does not meet the other criteria for schizophrenia may represent a diagnosis of delusional disorder.
- Rule out medical conditions, neurocognitive disorders, and delirium in anyone with psychotic symptoms. Appropriate cognitive screening and testing may be helpful.
- Delusions can occur in the midst of a depression or manic episode and should be considered part of the mood disorder episode instead of delusional disorder.
- External informants and collateral data are useful to determine if a patient has a delusion rather than a belief that is part of their culture or religion.

IN-DEPTH DIAGNOSIS: BRIEF PSYCHOTIC DISORDER

Ms. Baker is a 38-year-old woman who is brought to the emergency department by her sister. Ms. Baker has not been bathing or cooking meals for the past several days, and she was seen staring at a wall for hours while talking to herself. Her sister explains that Ms. Baker's husband of many years told Ms. Baker that he was pursuing a relationship with another woman. He then left her and their three children, and his whereabouts are currently unknown (the children are currently safe with the patient's mother). Ms. Baker has been a stay-at-home parent, has no independent source of income, and recently spent the last of her money paying bills. She has no known history of mental illness, including episodes of mood or psychotic symptoms. She denies any substance use, which is corroborated by urine toxicology, and her medical examination is unremarkable.

On examination, Ms. Baker is alert and oriented, with intermittent eye contact. She reports no thoughts of suicide. She states that she hears the voice of her grandmother trying to help her. She further explains that her grandmother's voice is very clear, and she feels her presence near her. Ms. Baker is admitted to the psychiatric hospital for observation. Several days later, these concerns have resolved, and her sister agrees that she is back to her baseline. Although she received low-dose antipsychotic medication early in her hospitalization, this was discontinued, and the only other interventions were attending groups and speaking to a social worker. No psychotic symptoms were evident at discharge, and no medications were prescribed. An outpatient therapist appointment was made for follow-up care. Eight months later, Ms. Baker has shown no further evidence of psychosis or a mood disorder.

Ms. Baker presented with sudden hallucinations and disorganized, possibly catatonic, behavior. These symptoms occurred when she was under significant stress because her husband left her and she faced a sudden financial crisis. It is extremely helpful that her sister can provide collateral information, especially about the recent onset of the symptoms and behavior. The psychotic symptoms did not appear to occur in the midst of a depressive or manic episode. Medical or substance causation is unlikely without a history of either and with normal lab results and toxicology screens. Likewise, Ms. Baker's intact orientation effectively rules out a delirium. The presumed diagnosis at admission is brief psychotic disorder, with marked stressors. Brief psychotic disorder often responds to interventions such as supportive care with individual or group therapy. By definition, the symptoms of brief psychotic disorder must last at least 1 day and less than 1 month. If the symptoms continue past 30 days, other diagnoses must be considered.

Approach to the Diagnosis

A sudden onset or brief history of psychotic symptoms compels clinicians to consider the diagnosis of brief psychotic disorder. The first task is to confirm the presence of one or more of the diagnostic symptoms, which include all of those seen in schizophrenia except for negative symptoms. Often, individuals are so confused by their symptoms that they cannot or will not be able to provide a detailed history. Collateral information from coworkers, friends, and family can be extremely helpful. Once the symptoms are identified, the duration must be determined. If the best estimation is less than 1 month, brief psychotic disorder remains a possibility. However, because of the brief nature of the symptoms and lack of past history, it is especially important to consider other causations. For example, any fluctuation in sensorium could indicate an intoxication or delirium. A careful evaluation of cognition, including a formal screen of cognitive capacity, can be illustrative. Reviewing past medical history, vital signs, lab results, electrocardiogram, toxicology screen, and any brain imaging obtained may indicate an organic cause of the psychotic symptoms. If these are all negative, then the differential of a psychotic disorder is most likely.

Sedative or antipsychotic medications may help calm an agitated person and allow a more detailed history to be obtained. Mood disorders with psychotic features can be seen in both mania and depression. Current and past mood episodes should be screened for carefully. Eliciting a marked stressor may help confirm the diagnosis of brief psychotic disorder, although the diagnosis may be indicated without a stressor as well. Possible stressors include loss of a loved one, witnessing or personally experiencing a traumatic event, or extreme financial hardship.

Getting the History

Mrs. Jones is a 43-year-old woman who presents to the psychiatry clinic with her wife because she has been hearing voices for the past week. They are baffled by her symptoms but note that they have been very worried about their son, who is deployed with the military overseas. The psychiatrist begins the interview by trying to empathize and build an alliance with Mrs. Jones: "It must be very hard to not know what is happening with your son."

Next, the psychiatrist takes a brief but comprehensive approach to the history and mental status examination and orders lab tests, a thyroid test, and a toxicology screen. The psychiatrist asks more questions, one at a time, to identify the types of symptoms present, such as, "What do the voices say? Are they inside your head, or do you hear them with your ears? Is it one or more voice? Are they voices that you recognize? Do they ever tell you to harm yourself or anyone else? Has anything like this ever happened to you before?" They also screen Mrs. Jones for other psychotic symptoms, such as delusions: "Do you ever worry that you're being watched or followed? Have you ever believed anything so strongly that you were sure you were right, even when others didn't believe you? Do you ever feel like your thoughts aren't private?"

Over the course of the intake interview, the psychiatrist asks questions about possible mood disorder symptoms: "Do you get depressed or sad? How have you been eating and sleeping recently? Do you ever have periods where you're so energetic that you don't need much sleep? Has any of this ever made you feel like life was not worth living?" Additional symptoms of depression or mania could be elicited if present.

The psychiatrist also carefully inquires about substance use: "How much alcohol do you drink? Do you smoke cigarettes or use other nicotine products? What about cannabis, cocaine, or other substances? What medications are you taking?" Inquiring about substance use is important because substance/medication-induced psychotic disorders commonly manifest with these presenting symptoms. Inquiring about physical health, obtaining lab results, and conducting a brief cognitive screen can help rule out delirium. With Mrs. Jones' permission, the psychiatrist gets additional perspective by asking her wife about these symptoms as well.

Mrs. Jones is seen in several follow-up appointments. The psychotic symptoms resolve about 3 weeks after their onset. She is seen over the next year and never has such symptoms again. In retrospect, the psychiatrist decides that the patient had brief psychotic disorder. They further determine that her son's deployment overseas was an acute stressor. Her wife continues to be a strong source of support and agrees with this assessment.

The age at onset and duration of symptoms are important. For example, if the symptoms last longer than 1 month, brief psychotic disorder cannot be diagnosed, and the clinician may decide whether another disorder, such as schizophreniform disorder, schizoaffective disorder, or schizophrenia, is more appropriate to explore.

Tips for Clarifying the Diagnosis

- Investigate the possibility of delirium first because this could be caused by an underlying condition warranting urgent treatment.
- Obtain collateral sources of information to develop a timeline of the symptoms, stressors, and events in the person's life.
- Mood disorders with psychotic features are much more common than other types of psychotic illnesses. Screen for these disorders, carefully taking into account the potential for suicidality.
- Brief psychotic disorder symptoms last for 1 day or up to a maximum of 1 month.
- Consider the diagnosis of schizophreniform disorder if the symptoms persist beyond 1 month.
- Often the diagnosis of brief psychotic disorder is made in retrospect and may be diagnosed as unspecified schizophrenia spectrum and other psychotic disorder until the picture becomes clearer.

Consider the Case

Ms. Norman is a 45-year-old woman who is brought to the hospital by the police, who found her running in the street wearing only a nightgown at 3:00 A.M. Neighbors called 911 when Ms. Norman knocked loudly on their door, yelling that she was being chased by assassins. Her speech was reportedly rapid and nonsensical. While in the emergency department, Ms. Norman tries to escape, saying that the doctors and security officers are trying to kill her, and she tries to strike staff members when they approach. She is given olanzapine to keep her and others safe. Her toxicology screen is negative, and her initial medical workup is unremarkable. Although she is not able to provide much history, the psychiatrist reaches her husband, who relates that Ms. Norman has no significant psychiatric, substance use, or medical history, although she had "always been a worrier" and frequently sought reassurance from the imam at their mosque. As the matriarch of a Black Muslim family living in a low-income area, she particularly worries about her sons being victims of hate crimes or police shootings, but her husband had not noticed her seeming particularly anxious recently or noticed anything out of the ordinary until 2 days ago, when she began to speak about being followed, in a way that did not make sense to her family.

Within an hour after receiving medication, she is feeling much calmer and ultimately sleeps for several hours. By the morning, she appears to be at her baseline, and her husband, who has never been concerned about her being a safety risk to herself or others, feels comfortable taking her home with close outpatient follow-up. She is discharged with a limited quantity of low-dose olanzapine to take only if needed. She meets with a new therapist several days later and describes that any symptoms of psychosis had fully resolved within 2 days of her initial presentation and without additional use of medication.

Ms. Norman was diagnosed with brief psychotic disorder, without marked stressors. She presented to the emergency department with a severe psychotic event. Her symptoms warranted an urgent workup, including a toxicology screen and laboratory studies. Even when the presence of psychosis seems clear, putting it into the context of the person's life is essential to appropriately elicit and clarify the symptoms. For example, if the psychiatrist evaluating Ms. Norman were a White Christian male, he may not have a full understanding of how aspects of her identity (Black, Muslim, female) inform her presentation. It is tempting to believe that the psychiatric interview transcends racial and other aspects of identity. However, approaching such situations with humility—asking questions, validating difficult experiences, and acknowledging one's own differences—both comforts the patient and helps the clinician gather the most accurate information. The psychiatrist might acknowledge to Ms. Norman that it must be very difficult to have to worry so much about her sons. In turn, Ms. Norman may feel reassured and comforted by the psychiatrist explicitly acknowledging that, as someone with a more privileged identity, he does not have the same stressors that she does but that he wants to understand her experience better.

In Ms. Norman's case, collateral information proved helpful in ruling out diagnoses that should be considered. Her lack of mood symptoms effectively rules out bipolar disorder or major depressive disorder with psychotic features. History and laboratory findings argue against a medical or substance-induced cause. This leaves a primary psychotic disorder as being most likely, and the time course—full resolution of symptoms and return to baseline functioning after a few days—leads to the diagnosis of brief psychotic disorder.

The epidemiology of brief psychotic disorder is largely unknown. Some investigators believe that it occurs most commonly in the third or fourth decade of life. It occurs more commonly in females than in males, and some personality vulnerabilities may confer risk.

Differential Diagnosis

The differential diagnosis of brief psychotic disorder includes psychosis from other causes, such as schizophrenia; delusional disorder; and mood disorders such as major depressive disorder with psychotic features or bipolar I disorder, current episode manic, with mood-congruent psychotic features. The examiner should also carefully exclude delirium and substance/medication-induced psychotic disorder. Personality disorders such as paranoid personality disorder and schizotypal personality disorder should also be considered. In some settings, particularly if the symptoms are atypical and well circumscribed, the possibility of a patient misrepresenting their symptoms for primary or secondary gain (i.e., factitious disorder or malingering, respectively) must be considered.

The time course of the development of a disorder is important to consider when formulating a differential diagnosis. For example, an acute or abrupt onset of confusion, disorientation, and bizarre behavior may indicate a delirium or acute neurological event. Mood disorders can be recurrent and often have a positive family history. Schizophrenia and schizophreniform disorder have both positive and negative symptoms and a much longer duration of symptoms. Personality disorders such as schizotypal (personality) disorder and paranoid personality disorder endure throughout a person's life span.

Summary

- The diagnosis of brief psychotic disorder requires the presence of one or more of the following symptoms: delusions, hallucinations, disorganized speech, or grossly disorganized or catatonic behavior. This list does not include symptoms that are culturally sanctioned.
- The duration for brief psychotic disorder is at least 1 day and less than 1 month, with a return to a premorbid level of functioning.
- Delirium, substance/medication-induced psychosis, and psychosis secondary to another medical condition should be carefully screened for and ruled out.
- A mood disorder such as major depressive or bipolar disorder with psychotic features must not be the cause of symptoms.
- Schizophreniform disorder or schizophrenia criteria must not be met, particularly the duration of symptoms criterion.
- Symptoms must not be the result of another mental health condition, including personality disorder, malingering, or factitious disorder.
- Symptoms may occur with or without a marked stressor.

SUMMARY: SCHIZOPHRENIA SPECTRUM AND OTHER PSYCHOTIC DISORDERS

The diagnoses of schizophrenia spectrum and other psychotic disorders underwent subtle but important changes in DSM-5 and have remained essentially unchanged in DSM-5-TR.

Diagnosing schizoaffective disorder has been difficult in the past because of the ambiguity of what was meant by having a mood disorder for a "substantial" period of time, which experts have described as ranging from 15% to 50%. DSM-5 changed this criterion to the "majority" of time, which led to much less ambiguity, and this change has remained stable in DSM-5-TR. It will still be a challenge, however, to determine the length of treated time because so many patients continue taking antidepressants whether they need them or not.

Brief psychotic disorder has remained essentially the same since DSM-IV and still relies on carefully determining that the illness interval is less than 1 month. Likewise, schizophreniform disorder remains a time-limited diagnosis that will either resolve or evolve to schizophrenia or another psychiatric disorder. Delusional disorder continues to identify persons with unfounded beliefs that have a limited effect on overall behavior and functioning. Note that DSM-5 eliminated shared delusional disorder, historically called *folie à deux*. DSM-5-TR further clarified this in the "Other Specified Schizophrenia Spectrum and Other Psychotic Disorder" section by changing "delusional symptoms in partner" to "delusional symptoms in the context of relationship."

Psychotic disorders due to another medical condition or substance/medication-induced psychotic disorder are continuing reminders that psychotic symptoms may have medical or substance-based etiologies. Finally, nearly all these diagnoses can have a catatonia specifier. The definition of catatonia is provided in this chapter of DSM-5-TR, and the catatonic features specifier includes symptoms such as stupor, catalepsy, mutism, and echolalia, which have been updated slightly for DSM-5-TR.

ELEMENTS TO CONSIDER IN THE CULTURAL FORMULATION

- A belief or experience cannot be classified as a hallucination or delusion if it is culturally normative. Collateral information from family members, religious or community leaders, or others who know the patient well may be helpful in distinguishing what is culturally normative.
- Interviews must be interpreted with particular care when not conducted in a patient's native language or when conducted through an interpreter. It is easy to mistake unfamiliar metaphors for delusions or disorganization, or language-based difficulties for alogia or negative symptoms. Using scales and instruments that have been validated in the relevant population and communicating with trained medical interpreters can mitigate these risks.
- These considerations are particularly important because members of marginalized immigrant and refugee communities are at increased risk of developing schizophrenia when experiencing immigration-related stressors or living in areas with few members of their ethnic or cultural group.
- A patient from a marginalized group may present as guarded in a medical setting because of past mistreatment that they or their family members have experienced; this may be misinterpreted as paranoia or alogia.

- Additionally, unconscious bias on the part of the evaluating psychiatrist may lead to misdiagnosis. Multiple studies have shown that identical symptoms are often interpreted differently based on the patient's race or ethnicity.

DIAGNOSTIC PEARLS

- Determining the presence of psychosis (with hallucinations, delusions, or disorganized speech) is the first task in diagnosing individuals in this category.
- The length of time a person has exhibited psychotic or negative symptoms drives the decision-making process for many cases: brief psychotic disorder < schizophreniform disorder < schizophrenia or schizoaffective disorder.
- The diagnosis of schizoaffective disorder requires two critical elements: a diagnosable mood disorder must exist for more than 50% of the time that a person has any symptoms (even if treated successfully), and a period of psychotic symptoms (Criterion A of schizophrenia) must last for at least 2 weeks in the absence of mood episodes.
- People from different cultural backgrounds and from marginalized communities are at increased risk of misdiagnosis. This risk can be mitigated by interpreting the symptoms in the appropriate context (e.g., suspicion may be warranted, and not evidence of psychosis) and by being aware of one's own implicit biases. Mental health providers may unconsciously associate schizophrenia (or substance-induced psychosis) with Black, Indigenous, and people of color (BIPOC) patients and jump to this diagnosis without adequately exploring other possibilities (particularly psychosis secondary to mania or depression).
- The relationship between substance use and schizophrenia is complex. Many substances (including some prescribed medications) can cause psychosis, but this typically resolves after any period of acute intoxication or withdrawal. Substance/medication-induced psychosis may persist far beyond this period, but it is more common for individuals to meet criteria for both a primary psychotic disorder and a substance use disorder. Prolonged periods without the substance(s) are often necessary to tease this apart.
- Individuals with schizophrenia-spectrum illnesses are typically oriented to person, place, and time, although orientation may be disrupted in a severe acute exacerbation of psychosis or if catatonia is present. Disorientation and confusion are more commonly associated with intoxication or withdrawal (either of which may also cause a substance-induced psychosis) or delirium, and these should always be considered.
- Many people who experience psychosis or have significant cognitive limitations may have difficulty following complex, multipart questions; questions should typically be asked one at a time.
- Autism spectrum disorder (ASD) can be confused with this category. ASD is usually an earlier-age phenomenon. Individuals with ASD are not expected to experience long-enduring hallucinations or delusions.

- A *hallucination* is a perception-like experience with the clarity and impact of a true perception but without the external stimulation of the relevant sensory organ.
- A *delusion* is a false belief based on incorrect inference about external reality that is firmly held despite what almost everyone else believes and despite what constitutes incontrovertible and obvious evidence to the contrary.
- The feeling that innocuous or coincidental external events have a particular and unusual meaning that is specific to the person is called an *idea of reference*. These may be more or less plausible: a person may pass a group of strangers and believe the strangers are talking about them, or they may believe that a news reporter is communicating coded messages directly to them through the television. A sufficiently fixed belief may be called a *referential delusion* or a *delusion of reference*.
- *Pressured speech* refers to speech that is increased in amount, accelerated, and difficult or impossible to interrupt. Usually, it is also loud and emphatic. Often, the person talks without any social stimulation and may continue to talk even if no one is listening. It is common for learners to conflate "fast" and "pressured," but speech that is difficult to interrupt is a more specific indicator.

SELF-ASSESSMENT

Key Concepts: Double-Check Your Knowledge

What is the relevance of the following concepts to the various schizophrenia spectrum and other psychotic disorders?

- Psychosis
- Delusions
- Hallucinations
- Negative symptoms
- Mood in psychotic disorders
- Timing or duration of symptoms in psychotic disorders

Questions to Discuss With Colleagues and Mentors

1. A significant change in the diagnosis of schizophrenia was the elimination of the subtypes (e.g., paranoid, disorganized) in DSM-5. Were these subtypes useful? Were they stable over time? Will not having them change practice?
2. How difficult is it to determine the differences among brief psychotic disorder, schizophreniform disorder, and schizophrenia? Are prodromal and attenuated symptom intervals reliably measured?
3. DSM-IV allowed a single symptom from Criterion A for the diagnosis of schizophrenia if the delusions were bizarre or the hallucinations consisted of either commenting voices or two or more voices conversing. In clinical practice, how often is this exemption problematic when making a diagnosis of schizophrenia?

Case-Based Questions

PART A

Mr. Jenkins, a 19-year-old man, is brought to the emergency department after being found incoherent by the police. According to paramedics, he was sitting on a street curb and appeared disoriented and confused. His identity was unknown at this time. Witnesses told police that he appeared to be yelling at someone and he acted as if someone were chasing him. Intravenous fluid was started at the scene, and the paramedics transported the man to the hospital. In the emergency department, Mr. Jenkins is drowsy, with a blood pressure of 180/98 and a heart rate of 148. His urine drug screen is positive for cocaine and cannabis. His pupils are dilated. One hour later, a medical student is examining his dirty clothes and his neck, where he had a tattoo of a crucifix, when the patient suddenly jumps up and screams. He believes that ghosts in the hospital and dead people are trying to choke him. He tears the intravenous line loose from his arm. He is immediately sedated with antipsychotic medication and later admitted to the intensive care unit for observation and monitoring of his unstable vital signs. He is found to be agitated because of hallucinations and delusions but is oriented to time, place, and person.

What is the most likely diagnosis for Mr. Jenkins? Do the circumstances leading to his hospitalization need to be considered?   Mr. Jenkins has signs and symptoms consistent with substance/medication-induced psychotic disorder. He is alert and oriented, which helps rule out the possibility of delirium. The patient also has autonomic symptoms and a urine drug screen result consistent with cocaine and cannabis intoxication. At this point, it is not possible to distinguish whether the symptoms were preexisting or only due to the ingested substances.

PART B

Three days after admission, Mr. Jenkins is calmer and medically stable. He is transferred to the psychiatric unit at the hospital and gradually becomes alert and oriented to all spheres. The hallucinations of ghosts also resolves. He watches television on the unit and talks with other patients. His affect is mostly flat. The nurses state that he has been seen talking to himself and responding to things in the room that were not there. On the eighth hospital day, he tells the psychiatrist, "It was now about the sixth hour, and darkness came over the whole land until the ninth hour, for the sun stopped shining. And the curtain of the temple was torn in two." Nobody understands this statement until a medical student queries the phrase on the internet and discovers it is a verse from the Bible. Mr. Jenkins continues to exhibit bizarre behavior and speech patterns. He stands in place for hours with a blank stare and has to be reminded to eat. He believes that he is a "prophet from the Gospels" and that he is here to "cure the evil of all men." He believes that his mind can move the sun and the moon. When asked about his past, he states that he was born on Saturn and that Uranus was his home. He cannot maintain a proper discourse for very long and laughs inappropriately while discussing the size of his feet and genitals. A nurse who used to work at another hospital states that she knew Mr. Jenkins from a previous psychiatric hospitalization 10 months earlier and that he had acted exactly like this. She is sure that he was not using drugs then. His mother is eventually located. She says that she has never observed any manic or depressive symptoms in her son, that he has been psychotic for the past year, and that he had never used drugs before this incident.

Is the persistence of this patient's psychotic symptoms important for making a definitive diagnosis? Mr. Jenkins remains psychotic for several days after using cocaine and cannabis. Although the effects of such drugs can persist, the psychiatrist should begin to suspect an underlying psychotic mental illness aside from the established diagnosis of substance abuse, especially given the nurse's observation that she had seen him in a similar mental state 10 months earlier. Because Mr. Jenkins has never had an episode of mania or depression and his psychotic symptoms have lasted for more than 6 months without the use of drugs, the diagnosis of schizophrenia is eventually made.

Short-Answer Questions

1. What are common substances that can cause psychotic symptoms?
2. Does it matter what type of hallucinations or delusions a person has in order to receive a diagnosis of substance/medication-induced psychotic disorder?
3. How can a clinician detect if a person with a substance/medication-induced psychotic disorder has another major mental illness, such as major depression or schizophrenia?
4. What are the symptoms of Criterion A for schizophrenia in DSM-5-TR? Which Criterion A symptoms must be present for at least 1 month in order to make the diagnosis of schizophrenia? What is the diagnosis if the symptoms of Criterion A for schizophrenia last only 20 days?
5. What are the symptoms of Criterion B for schizophrenia?
6. Is hearing voices of a running commentary or experiencing third-person hallucinations diagnostic of schizophrenia?
7. What is the diagnosis if a patient has symptoms consistent with schizophrenia for several years and then suddenly has a manic episode?
8. Does the duration of the prodromal and attenuated form of schizophrenia count toward the 6 months needed for a diagnosis of schizophrenia?
9. Do the DSM-5-TR criteria for delusional disorder allow for bizarre delusions?
10. What are the two time criteria critical to making a diagnosis of schizoaffective disorder?

Answers

1. Common substances that can cause psychotic symptoms are cocaine, amphetamines, cathinones, lysergic acid diethylamide (LSD), mushrooms, cannabis, medications, phencyclidine (PCP), alcohol, inhalants, sedatives, hypnotics, and anxiolytics.

2. No. It does not matter what type of hallucinations or delusions a patient has in order for them to receive a diagnosis of substance/medication-induced psychotic disorder, which can easily look like schizophrenia.

3. Generally, a clinician cannot detect another major mental illness and must either rely on outside sources, records, and informants or wait for the substance/medication-induced state to clear first.

4. Criterion A symptoms for schizophrenia include delusions, hallucinations, disorganized speech, grossly abnormal psychomotor behavior (including catatonia), and negative symptoms (e.g., diminished emotional expression or avolition). At least one of the following Criterion A symptoms for schizophrenia must be present for at least 1 month: hallucinations, delusions, or disorganized speech. If the symptoms of Criterion A for schizophrenia last only 20 days, the diagnosis is brief psychotic disorder.

5. Criterion B for schizophrenia requires that the current level of functioning in one or more major areas (e.g., work, interpersonal relations, or self-care) be markedly below the level achieved before the onset.

6. No single symptom is diagnostic for schizophrenia. Other criteria are also required. The symptoms noted in the question may also occur in other types of psychosis, such as during a manic episode or from substance use.

7. Several diagnoses should be considered in the context of an enduring psychotic disorder and the emergence of a new set of symptoms consistent with a disruptive mood. Medical and substance-related factors should be explored. The possibility that the patient has schizoaffective disorder may be evaluated as a clinical hypothesis.

8. Yes. Under Criterion C, the duration of the prodromal and attenuated form of schizophrenia counts toward the 6 months needed for a diagnosis of schizophrenia.

9. Bizarre delusions by themselves do not rule out delusional disorder, but these delusions cannot have a significant effect on functioning, and behavior cannot be odd or bizarre.

10. The two time criteria critical to making a diagnosis of schizoaffective disorder are 2 weeks of symptoms from schizophrenia Criterion A without a mood disorder and more than 50% of the time with a mood disorder (including treated intervals).

RECOMMENDED READINGS

Copeland JRM, Dewey ME, Scott A, et al: Schizophrenia and delusional disorder in older age: community prevalence, incidence, comorbidity, and outcome. Schizophr Bull 24(1):153–161, 1998 9502553

Di Forti M, Quattrone D, Freeman TP, et al: The contribution of cannabis use to variation in the incidence of psychotic disorder across Europe (EU-GEI): a multicentre case-control study. Lancet Psychiatry 6(5):427–436, 2019 30902669

Lauriello J, Pallanti S (eds): Clinical Manual for Treatment of Schizophrenia. Washington, DC, American Psychiatric Publishing, 2012

Lewis-Fernández R, Aggarwal NK, Hinton L, et al (eds): DSM-5 Handbook on the Cultural Formulation Interview. Washington, DC, American Psychiatric Publishing, 2016

Tandon R: Getting ready for DSM-5: psychotic disorders. Curr Psychiatr 11(4): E1–E4, 2012

REFERENCES

American Psychiatric Association: Diagnostic and Statistical Manual of Mental Disorders, 2nd Edition. Washington, DC, American Psychiatric Association, 1968

American Psychiatric Association: Diagnostic and Statistical Manual of Mental Disorders, 4th Edition. Washington, DC, American Psychiatric Association, 1994

American Psychiatric Association: Diagnostic and Statistical Manual of Mental Disorders, 4th Edition. Text Revision. Washington, DC, American Psychiatric Association, 2000

American Psychiatric Association: Diagnostic and Statistical Manual of Mental Disorders, 5th Edition. Arlington, VA, American Psychiatric Association, 2013

American Psychiatric Association: Diagnostic and Statistical Manual of Mental Disorders, 5th Edition, Text Revision. Washington, DC, American Psychiatric Association, 2022

CHAPTER 7

Bipolar and Related Disorders

Laura Weiss Roberts, M.D., M.A.

Max Kasun, B.A.

"I feel like a million bucks—I can do anything!"

"When he starts talking this fast, I know he is going off…"

- Bipolar I Disorder
- Bipolar II Disorder
- Cyclothymic Disorder
- Substance/Medication-Induced Bipolar and Related Disorder
- Bipolar and Related Disorder Due to Another Medical Condition
- Other Specified Bipolar and Related Disorder
- Unspecified Bipolar and Related Disorder
- Unspecified Mood Disorder

Adapted from Ketter TA, Miller S: "Bipolar and Related Disorders," in *Study Guide to DSM-5*. Edited by Roberts LW, Louie AK. Washington, DC, American Psychiatric Publishing, 2015, pp 99–112.

Bipolar and related disorders are common, recurrent, frequently debilitating, and in many instances tragically fatal illnesses, and they are characterized by oscillations in mood, energy, and ability to function (Table 7–1). The "Bipolar and Related Disorders" chapter in DSM-5-TR (American Psychiatric Association 2022) appears after the "Schizophrenia Spectrum and Other Psychotic Disorders" chapter and before the "Depressive Disorders" chapter in recognition of the place of bipolar disorders as a bridge between the schizophrenia spectrum and the depressive disorder categories in terms of symptoms, family history, and genetics.

Cultural factors may affect the prevalence of bipolar and related disorders. As stated in DSM-5-TR, "countries with reward-oriented cultural values that place significance on individual pursuit of reward have a relatively higher prevalence of bipolar disorder" (p. 147). Attunement to cultural influences on symptom prevalence and presentation is critical for making an accurate diagnosis of bipolar and related disorders. For example, delay in receiving health services in underserved populations may contribute to higher rates of bipolar disorder and more severe symptom presentations at the time of the diagnosis. Moreover, cultural and linguistic misunderstanding (e.g., misinterpretation of cultural mistrust as paranoia) can contribute to a misinterpretation of symptoms and risk of misdiagnosis.

Patients with bipolar I disorder have experienced at least one manic episode. The manic episode must not be better explained by schizoaffective disorder and must not occur on top of an existing diagnosis of schizophrenia, schizophreniform disorder, delusional disorder, or other specified or unspecified schizophrenia spectrum and other psychotic disorder. Manic episodes last at least 1 week (or briefer if hospitalized) and require elevated, expansive, or irritable mood, accompanied by increased energy or activity and at least three additional symptoms (four if the mood is merely irritable), such as inflated self-esteem, decreased need for sleep, overtalkativeness, racing thoughts, distractibility, increased goal-directed activity, and impulsivity. Manic episodes are, by definition, severe; they may entail psychosis, hospitalization, or severe impairment of occupational or psychosocial function. Patients with bipolar II disorder have experienced at least one hypomanic episode and at least one major depressive episode, but no manic episode. Hypomanic episodes are defined similarly to manic episodes, but they do not include psychotic symptoms, hospitalization, or severe functional impairment, and they have shorter minimum duration (a minimum of 4 days rather than 7 days).

Major depressive episodes are characterized by sadness or anhedonia, accompanied by additional symptoms to yield a total of at least five pervasive symptoms for at least 2 weeks. The specific additional symptoms include weight change, sleep disturbance, psychomotor agitation or retardation, poor energy, poor self-esteem or guilt, poor concentration (inability to focus), and suicidality. Although most patients with bipolar I disorder also endure major depressive episodes, such episodes are not required for the diagnosis of bipolar I disorder.

Some patients present with features of both mania or hypomania and major depression. These so-called mixed states require the presence of at least three symptoms of major depression in the context of a hypomanic or manic episode. Thus, patients with mixed bipolar disorder might experience dysphoria and feelings of worthless-

TABLE 7–1. Episode types in selected DSM-5-TR mood disorders

	Manic episode	Hypomanic episode	Major depressive episode	Chronic, episodic, subthreshold mood elevation symptoms	Chronic, episodic, subthreshold depressive symptoms
Bipolar I disorder	R	C	C	C	C
Bipolar II disorder	X	R	R	C	C
Cyclothymic disorder	X	X	X	R	R
Unipolar major depressive disorder	X	X	R	X	C
Persistent depressive disorder (dysthymia)	X	X	X	X	R

Note. Manic, hypomanic, and major depressive episodes may be with or without mixed features.
C=common (but not required); R=required; X=not permitted.

ness while feeling energized, impulsive, and having racing thoughts. Mixed state bipolar disorder can be difficult to diagnose because the mood states overlap.

Cyclothymic disorder is characterized by a chronic, fluctuating pattern of numerous periods of subsyndromal mood elevation and depression symptoms for at least 2 years (1 year in children and adolescents) without any interruption lasting longer than 2 months. In addition, the mood symptoms are present for at least half the time. If a major depressive episode, manic episode, or hypomanic episode occurs during the mood disturbance, cyclothymic disorder is not diagnosed because the chronic subsyndromal mood swings may be considered to be on the spectrum of bipolar disorder.

Substance/medication-induced bipolar and related disorder is characterized by the ingestion of or withdrawal from a substance or medication. In DSM-5-TR, a full manic or hypomanic episode emerging during antidepressant treatment (e.g., medication or electroconvulsive therapy) and persisting beyond the physiological effect of that treatment is sufficient evidence of a manic or hypomanic episode. Substance/medication-induced bipolar and related disorder is more common in patients with mixed features and rapid cycling.

As stated in DSM-5-TR, the prevalence of substance/medication-induced bipolar disorder "will depend on substance availability and level of substance use in a society; for example, countries with cultural prohibitions against alcohol or other substance use may have a lower prevalence of substance-related disorders" (p. 165). Bipolar and related disorder due to another medical condition is a function of the direct physiological effects of another medical condition (most often neurological or endocrine). It is more common in patients with mixed features and rapid cycling and is particularly common among older adults because of the high prevalence of medical disorders in that age group. In some instances, concurrent, overlapping influences of treatments and their underlying medical conditions may make it challenging to definitively determine whether mood symptoms represent substance/medication-induced bipolar and related disorder or bipolar and related disorder due to another medical condition.

Other specified bipolar and related disorder and unspecified bipolar and related disorder apply to people experiencing significant manic or hypomanic and depressive symptoms that do not meet diagnostic criteria of any other bipolar or depressive disorder and are not attributable to the direct physiological effects of a substance/medication-induced or general medical condition. The DSM-5-TR description of other specified bipolar and related disorder includes specific presentations that do not meet criteria for specific bipolar and related disorders, including the following:

- Major depressive episodes and short hypomanic episodes (lasting 2–3 days; i.e., with insufficient duration for full hypomanic episodes)
- Major depressive episodes and hypomanic episodes with insufficient symptom count for full hypomanic episodes
- Hypomanic episode without prior major depressive episode
- Short-duration cyclothymia (<2 years in adults or <1 year in children or adolescents)

TABLE 7–2. Key changes from DSM-5 to DSM-5-TR

Median age at onset for bipolar I disorder has been updated to approximately age 22 in the United States. Peak age at onset is between ages 20 and 30. Age at onset does not reliably distinguish between bipolar I and II.

Childhood adversity has been added as a risk factor for bipolar I disorder.

Specifiers applicable to manic episodes (mild, moderate, severe) have been added.

The unspecified bipolar and related disorder designator is used in situations in which clinicians choose *not* to specify the reason that criteria are not met for a specific bipolar and related disorder and includes presentations in which there is insufficient information to make a more specific diagnosis (e.g., in emergency department settings).

Individuals with bipolar and related disorders present much more commonly with depression than with mood elevation. Thus, all persons presenting with depression need to be questioned directly about any history of episodes of mood elevation, which they may experience as periods of irritability and agitation rather than elation. Individuals may focus mainly on periods of depression, at the cost of paying sufficient attention to periods of mood elevation, because they perceive periods of depression as subjectively distressing and as driving functional impairment. They may be less concerned about the subjective but significant other experiences and negative consequences of periods of mood elevation. Clinicians can foster the therapeutic alliance with these persons by acknowledging the important subjective and functional implications of periods of depression, but they need to balance this acknowledgment with eliciting and discussing corresponding information regarding periods of mood elevation from patients and their significant others; the latter may prove to be more sensitive observers of mood elevation. Key changes between DSM-5 and DSM-5-TR diagnostic criteria are listed in Table 7–2.

IN-DEPTH DIAGNOSIS: BIPOLAR I DISORDER AND BIPOLAR II DISORDER

Police bring Mr. Ross, a 38-year-old writer, to the emergency department after he created a disturbance at a computer store. His mood is irritable and expansive as he boastfully reports smashing a computer on the floor after the store manager refused to hire him as an advertising consultant (a job that had not been posted). Mr. Ross demonstrates pressured speech, flight of ideas, and distractibility while describing how the advertising campaign that he devised in the prior week will revolutionize not only the marketing of computers but also that of all other consumer goods. He denies drowsiness despite sleeping only 2 hours each night for the past week, but he admits that for the past few days he has been hearing the voice of Steve Jobs suggesting ideas for a computer advertising campaign. Mr. Ross admits to a month-long major depressive episode during high school, which was successfully treated with psychotherapy. He admits to a history of some binge drinking and weekend use of cannabis as a freshman in college but denies any use of alcohol or drugs in the past 3 months. His father was briefly hospitalized for an unspecified psychiatric disorder in his twenties and died in a single motor vehicle crash in his mid-thirties.

Mr. Ross meets the criteria for bipolar I disorder with a current manic episode with psychotic features. In addition to the presence of psychosis (i.e., auditory hallucinations and grandiose delusions), his behavior has been disturbed enough to result in his being transported to the emergency department by the authorities, indicating severe functional impairment and, therefore, representing a manic episode rather than merely a hypomanic episode. Male sex, onset in early adulthood, a possible family history of bipolar disorder, presence of psychotic features, and occurrence of a major depressive episode are all common risk factors but are not required for a diagnosis of bipolar I disorder.

Approach to the Diagnosis

Bipolar disorders may be more often underdiagnosed (e.g., in individuals with bipolar disorders who view themselves as merely having depression) than overdiagnosed (e.g., in persons with Cluster B personality disorders such as narcissistic personality disorder and borderline personality who have mood instability but not well-defined and more persistent mood cycles). Correct diagnosis of bipolar disorders crucially depends on the ability to accurately detect sustained episodes of mood elevation or irritability (i.e., hypomanic or manic episodes). Affected people more frequently present with, and are more sensitive observers of, symptoms of depression than of mood elevation, making distinguishing bipolar disorders from unipolar major depressive disorder (by detecting episodes of mood elevation) a particularly important challenge. Individuals may use the terms *mood swings*, *racing thoughts*, or even *mania* or *hypomania* with meanings that differ from the DSM-5-TR definitions, thus potentially causing confusion.

Manic episodes are severe (i.e., they may entail psychosis, hospitalization, or severe functional impairment) and must occur in patients with a diagnosis of bipolar I disorder. A history of bankruptcy, incarceration, and multiple occupational or relationship failures related to episodes of mood elevation might suggest that at least one such episode may have been severe enough to be considered manic rather than merely hypomanic. Hypomanic episodes are not as severe (i.e., they do not entail psychosis, hospitalization, or severe functional impairment). Function during hypomanic episodes may improve, rather than deteriorate, which makes detection more challenging. Decreased need for sleep ought to be distinguished from insomnia; it highly suggests episodes of mood elevation, although it is not a required symptom. Stressors that are either positive (e.g., occupational promotion, new romantic attachment) or negative (e.g., performance demands, relationship termination) can trigger episodes of hypomania, mania, or major depression. Manic and hypomanic episodes with mixed features may be reported by some persons as depressions. Because patients are at greater risk to fail to recognize past as opposed to current episodes, irritable as opposed to euphoric episodes, episodes with as opposed to without mixed features, and hypomanic as opposed to manic episodes, their detection is more challenging.

Major depressive episodes occur in bipolar II disorder and unipolar major depressive disorder and most often occur (but are not required) in bipolar I disorder. Distinguishing prior and even current major depressive episodes with mixed features, which may occur in both bipolar and related disorders and unipolar major depressive disorder, from hypomanic episodes, which may occur in the former but not in the latter, can be particularly challenging. Collateral history from significant others, particularly regarding the possibility of prior manic or hypomanic episodes and the extent of mood elevation symptoms during major depressive episodes, can help enhance diagnostic accuracy.

Distinguishing episodes of mood elevation related to bipolar I disorder or bipolar II disorder as opposed to episodes triggered by antidepressants or illicit substances can be challenging. Substance/medication-induced bipolar and related disorder tends to occur within 3 months of introduction of a substance or medication or a dose increase, and it tends not to persist once the person has discontinued and their body has fully withdrawn from the potentially implicated substance or medication. Sociocultural factors may also influence the pattern of comorbid conditions in bipolar disorder. For example, cultures that encourage or are more permissive toward alcohol or other substance use may have a higher prevalence of substance use comorbidity. Common comorbid conditions such as anxiety, substance use, personality, eating, and pediatric disruptive behavioral (e.g., ADHD, oppositional defiant disorder, and conduct disorder) disorders can distract clinicians, patients, and their families from detecting episodes of mood elevation.

In making a possible diagnosis of bipolar disorder, the timeliness and accuracy of the differential diagnosis is crucial and should include assessment of possible suicidal ideation or intent. As stated in DSM-5-TR, "the lifetime risk of suicide in individuals with bipolar disorder is estimated to be 20- to 30-fold greater than in the general population.... A past history of suicide attempt and percent days spent depressed in the past year are associated with greater risk of suicide attempts or completions" (p. 148).

Getting the History

Ms. Wright, an 18-year-old college sophomore, complains of having had depression for the past month in the setting of academic stress (upcoming final examinations). The interviewer determines that Ms. Wright has pervasive sadness, anhedonia, insomnia, poor concentration (trouble focusing on schoolwork), and passive thoughts of death. Ms. Wright comments that most of these symptoms are particularly prominent in the morning and persist into the afternoon. The interviewer then asks, "Is your mood much different in the late afternoon and in the evening?" and Ms. Wright responds that she is more irritable than sad in the late afternoons and evenings. The interviewer next asks, "How do you spend your time in the evenings?" and the patient responds that she stays up late cramming on her schoolwork (i.e., has increased goal-directed activity), attempts to multitask but is not able to complete homework (i.e., has distractibility), has trouble keeping up with her thoughts (i.e., has flight of ideas), frequently gets up from her desk and paces (i.e., has psychomotor agitation), and has been spending most of the rest of the night having sexual relations with a married graduate student (i.e., impulsivity). When asked, "How much sleep are you getting?" Ms. Wright responds that she is getting only 3 hours of sleep each night, which is substantially less than her baseline of 8 hours each night. The interviewer asks, "Are you sleepy during the day?" and she states that she is wide awake throughout the day and not napping (suggesting decreased need for sleep) and denies using caffeine or other substances. The interviewer asks, "How long have your late afternoons and evenings been like that?" and Ms. Wright states that this has been going on for a month. In response to further inquiry, Ms. Wright denies any lifetime history of psychosis, psychiatric hospitalization, or severe consequences related to the aforementioned symptoms of mood elevation. Finally, the interviewer asks, "Does anyone in your family have bipolar disorder or manic depression?" Ms. Wright responds that her father had intermittently taken lithium for several years before running off with his secretary when the patient was 13 years old.

Ms. Wright presents with complaints of depression and meets criteria for a major depressive episode but also meets criteria for a hypomanic episode. With more limited assessment, a clinician might determine only a current major depressive episode (or possibly a major depressive episode with mixed features), consistent with a diagnosis of unipolar major depressive disorder. However, with additional careful questioning, it becomes apparent that Ms. Wright also meets criteria for a hypomanic episode, consistent with a diagnosis of bipolar II disorder. Mixed symptoms of depression and mood elevation may involve ultradian cycling (i.e., mood changes occurring within a day), as seen in Ms. Wright, or more continuous, simultaneous mixed symptoms. DSM-5-TR indicates that patients with concurrent major depressive and manic episodes, in view of the severity requirement for manic episodes, ought to be diagnosed with a manic episode with mixed features.

Tips for Clarifying the Diagnosis

- Carefully assess all patients presenting with depression for a history of manic or hypomanic episodes—specifically ask about prior episodes of mood elevation immediately preceding or following depressive episodes. Encourage patients prospectively to chart their mood symptoms to help clarify the diagnosis.
- Carefully ensure that full criteria (including the minimum 4-day duration requirement) for hypomanic episodes are met in order to limit the risk of overdiagnosing bipolar II disorder (as opposed to other specified bipolar and related disorder, unspecified bipolar and related disorder, and unipolar major depressive disorder).
- In view of overlapping symptoms, carefully distinguish major depressive episodes with mixed features, which *may* occur in unipolar major depressive disorder and bipolar and related disorders, from manic or hypomanic episodes, which *must* occur in bipolar I or bipolar II disorder and *must not* occur in unipolar major depressive disorder.
- Obtain collateral history from significant others, particularly regarding the possibility of prior manic or hypomanic episodes and the extent of mixed features during major depressive episodes.

Consider the Case

Ms. Lee, a 20-year-old single Asian American woman, complains of depression with prominent hypersomnia, increased appetite, and lethargy that have worsened since she stopped taking bupropion about 1 month ago. She reports that during the prior year, she had experienced three similar depressive episodes, as well as three 4-day episodes of increased irritability accompanied by excessive energy, overtalkativeness, distractibility, decreased need for sleep (3 hours rather than her usual 9 hours), physical agitation, and impulsivity. Ms. Lee reports a history of Hashimoto's thyroiditis, occasional use of "diet pills," and worsening of mood symptoms around her menstrual periods, but she denies ever being psychotic or hospitalized for psychiatric reasons. She reports a history of treatment with sertraline, during which she developed suicidal ideation, and with bupropion, during which she developed increased irritability. Among her family, her mother received a diagnosis of bipolar I disorder with psychotic mania, and her sister was diagnosed with bipolar II disorder.

Ms. Lee's symptoms meet criteria for bipolar II disorder with a current major depressive episode and rapid-cycling course (at least four episodes in the prior year). Hypomanic episodes have a shorter minimum duration (4 days rather than 7 days) as compared with manic episodes and do not entail psychosis, psychiatric hospitalization, or severe social or occupational dysfunction. Diagnosis of bipolar II disorder requires the occurrence of at least one major depressive episode and at least one hypomanic episode. Compared with bipolar I disorder, bipolar II disorder is associated with more anxiety and substance use disorder comorbidity, somewhat later onset, and, in clinical samples, more association with female sex. Hypomanic episodes in females with bipolar II disorder are more likely to entail mixed features than those in males. In individuals with bipolar disorder who are undergoing rapid cycling, it is important to assess for confounding effects of substances or medications and medical disorders, which may indicate the presence of a substance/medication-induced bipolar and related disorder or a bipolar and related disorder due to another medical condition.

Ms. Lee's Asian American ethnicity could influence her presentation: data suggest that Asian American and Hispanic American individuals with bipolar II disorder may be less likely to present at bipolar disorder specialty clinics than their White counterparts, perhaps because of stigma.

Differential Diagnosis

Because the differential diagnosis of bipolar disorder includes disorders induced by a medication or substance (e.g., alcohol or illicit drugs) or due to another medical condition (most commonly neurological and endocrine disorders), it is important to perform a careful substance use and medical assessment. Unipolar major depressive disorder is the most common misdiagnosis. Individuals presenting with depression need to be carefully assessed for a history of prior manic or hypomanic episodes (including collateral history from significant others). Depressed patients with onset prior to age 25; a history of multiple, rapidly emerging, and rapidly resolving depressions; a history of psychotic depressive episodes, particularly prior to age 40; untoward experiences with antidepressants (e.g., worsening of depression or switching into mood elevation); and a family history of bipolar disorder are at increased risk for having bipolar disorder. Because manic episodes in bipolar I disorder and major depressive episodes in bipolar I or bipolar II disorder can have psychotic features, psychotic disorders such as schizophrenia must be ruled out—in the psychotic disorders, psychotic symptoms are more chronic and prominent than mood symptoms.

Bipolar II disorder is distinguished from bipolar I disorder primarily in that the latter, but not the former, entails severe episodes of mood elevation (with psychosis, hospitalization, or severe social or occupational dysfunction). Symptoms of cyclothymic disorder may overlap those of Cluster B personality disorders, but instability of mood is more prominent than disturbance of identity or interpersonal relationships. ADHD is most common in male children and adolescents and involves chronic (rather than episodic) problems related to disturbance of attention and behavior (rather than mood). Because anxiety can be accompanied by irritability or psychomotor activation (resembling mood elevation) or by demoralization or psychomotor retardation (resembling depression), it is important to distinguish anxiety disorders and PTSD from bipolar and related disorders. Also, use of certain substances can yield mood elevation symptoms, whereas discontinuation of such substances can yield depressive symptoms, making it important to distinguish substance use disorders from bipolar and related disorders.

Finally, patients with bipolar and related disorders commonly have comorbid anxiety disorders, ADHD, or substance use disorders, so it is important to consider the possibility of any comorbid disorders. See DSM-5-TR for additional disorders to consider in the differential diagnosis. Also refer to the discussions of comorbidity and differential diagnosis in their respective sections of DSM-5-TR.

Summary

- Bipolar disorders are common and chronic and involve recurrent episodes of mood elevation and (most often) depression that can be challenging to distinguish from unipolar major depressive disorder.
- Bipolar disorder diagnoses are made on the basis of both current and past clinical phenomena.
- Individuals with bipolar disorder more commonly present with depression than with mood elevation and may have difficulty recognizing past (or even current) periods of mood elevation.
- Bipolar I disorder requires at least one manic episode, which may entail psychosis, hospitalization, or severe functional impairment.
- Bipolar II disorder requires (in addition to at least one major depressive episode) at least one hypomanic episode that did not entail psychosis, hospitalization, or severe functional impairment, and no prior manic episode.

SUMMARY: BIPOLAR AND RELATED DISORDERS

As many as one in four people with depression have bipolar and related disorders. Thus, all depressed patients should be screened for a lifetime history of bipolar and related disorders by detecting prior (or current) episodes of mood elevation. Patients are less likely to recognize or report episodes that occurred in the past and involved irritability, mixed features, or hypomania, and they are more likely to report episodes that are current, involve euphoria or mania, and are without mixed features. Collateral information from significant others can be valuable in detecting such prior episodes of mood elevation. Common comorbidities include substance use and anxiety disorders, as well as pediatric disruptive behavioral disorders (e.g., ADHD, oppositional defiant disorder, and conduct disorder), Cluster B personality disorders (e.g., borderline personality disorder), and eating disorders. In patients with comorbid psychiatric disorders, bipolar disorders are commonly the current main focus for treatment, although on occasion comorbid disorders may represent more prominent current problems than bipolar disorders.

ELEMENTS TO CONSIDER IN THE CULTURAL FORMULATION

- Racial bias in diagnosis may lead to underappreciation of affective symptoms in bipolar and related disorders.
- Individuals who present with psychotic features should be assessed for bipolar I disorder as part of the differential diagnosis.
- Reward-oriented cultural factors can affect the prevalence of bipolar I disorder.

DIAGNOSTIC PEARLS

- Bipolar disorder is diagnosed on the basis of both current and past clinical phenomena.
- For a diagnosis of bipolar disorder to be made, the patient's mania and hypomania symptoms must not be better explained by schizoaffective disorder and must not occur on top of an existing diagnosis of schizophrenia, schizophreniform disorder, delusional disorder, or other specified or unspecified schizophrenia spectrum and other psychotic disorder.
- Unipolar major depressive disorder is a crucial differential diagnostic possibility and the most common misdiagnosis that people with bipolar disorder receive.
- Common comorbidities such as substance use, anxiety disorders, pediatric disruptive behavioral disorders, eating disorders, and Cluster B personality disorders can make diagnosing bipolar disorder more challenging.
- Bipolar disorders have complex, variable phenomenology with different subtypes, mood states, courses, and age-dependent presentations.
- Bipolar I and bipolar II are distinct diagnoses but do not necessarily differ in severity.
- During episodes of mood elevation, mood may be irritable rather than euphoric, making recognition of such episodes more challenging.
- Individuals with bipolar disorder more commonly present with depression than with mood elevation and may have difficulty recognizing past (or even current) periods of mood elevation.
- Collateral information from significant others can enhance accuracy in diagnosing bipolar disorder.

SELF-ASSESSMENT

Key Concepts: Double-Check Your Knowledge

What is the relevance of the following concepts to the various bipolar and related disorders?

- Bipolar I disorder versus bipolar II disorder
- Manic episode versus hypomanic episode
- Major depressive episode with mixed features versus without mixed features
- Manic or hypomanic episode with mixed features versus without mixed features
- Concurrent hypomanic and major depressive episodes
- Rapid cycling and non–rapid cycling
- Bipolar family history
- Early onset mood disorder (prior to age 25)
- Treatment-emergent affective switch (e.g., antidepressant-triggered hypomania or mania)

Questions to Discuss With Colleagues and Mentors

1. Do you screen all individuals with depression for bipolar and related disorders?
2. How do you distinguish bipolar and related disorders from unipolar major depressive disorder?
3. How do you distinguish bipolar I disorder from bipolar II disorder?
4. How do you distinguish bipolar and related disorders from Cluster B personality disorders?
5. How do you distinguish bipolar and related disorders from ADHD?
6. What are the diagnostic implications of antidepressant-induced hypomania or mania?
7. How important is a family history of bipolar and related disorders in a patient presenting with depression?

Case-Based Questions

PART A

> Mrs. Ramirez is a 26-year-old graduate student who complains of anxiety with physical discomfort when teaching. She reports increased social anxiety since becoming a teaching assistant 6 months ago. She gives a history of problems with social anxiety (e.g., shyness with dating, dreading being called on in class, avoiding parties) since she was 16 years old that responded partially to individual psychotherapy. She states that for the past 6 months her social anxiety has been increasing, and she admits that for every class she taught during the past 2 weeks, she has dreaded receiving poor assessments from her students (some of whom are older than she is), and she has been anxious to the point of physical discomfort (e.g., with flushing and sweating). She reports that she increased her individual psychotherapy to weekly 1 month ago and added group psychotherapy 2 weeks ago.

What other assessment is indicated at this time? Anxiety, mood, and substance use disorders commonly co-occur, and if one such disorder is detected, the possibility of the other two ought to be assessed as well. Co-occurrence of anxiety, mood, and substance use disorders is associated with earlier-onset age of mood problems and worse longitudinal outcome.

PART B

On direct questioning (e.g., "Have you been feeling down lately? For how much of the time?"), Mrs. Ramirez reports subsyndromal depressive symptoms during the past 2 weeks. Her symptoms include current pervasive anhedonia, low self-confidence, and difficulty concentrating, but she denies current sadness, insomnia, fatigue, appetite disturbance, psychomotor disturbance, and suicidal ideation. The clinician asks, "In the past have you felt down most of the time for a couple of weeks? Were your sleep, appetite, energy, concentration, and desire to live also affected?" Mrs. Ramirez reports a single lifetime major depressive episode at age 24 that occurred after the termination of a romantic relationship and was treated with increased psychotherapy. She denies any lifetime history of psychosis, suicide attempts, psychiatric hospitalization, or treatment with psychotropic medications. On direct questioning (e.g., "Tell me about alcohol and drug use in your teens and early 20s"), she reports past binge drinking and limited weekend use of cannabis as an undergraduate but denies any other lifetime drug use, although she admits to increasing her alcohol consumption to three drinks per day over the past 2 weeks. She reports that her mother and older brother have both struggled with social anxiety and depression and responded to citalopram. She also reports that her father struggled with alcoholism, which he managed through a 12-step program.

What other assessment is indicated at this time? Individuals with a history of a major depressive episode should be assessed for a history of manic or hypomanic episodes. Collateral information from significant others can be valuable because they may be more sensitive observers of symptoms of mood elevation (e.g., irritability) and their consequences (e.g., marital tension).

PART C

At the next visit, Mrs. Ramirez's brother accompanies her and provides important collateral information. The brother reports that for a time when Mrs. Ramirez was 24 years old, she had less social anxiety and embarked on her first lifetime romantic relationship with a male classmate, but she then began covertly dating the classmate's younger brother as well. When the classmate learned of Mrs. Ramirez's actions, he terminated the relationship, and she "crashed" into a 3-month depression. On careful direct questioning, Mrs. Ramirez and her brother agree that this all happened after the patient had a 1-month period of bright mood, increased activity, energy, self-confidence, rapid thoughts, increased social activity (joining three clubs on campus), and increased alcohol consumption (five or more alcoholic beverages each Friday and Saturday night). Mrs. Ramirez's brother adds that their paternal grandfather had had several affairs followed by depressions.

What is Mrs. Ramirez's diagnosis? Mrs. Ramirez appears to have social anxiety disorder (currently the main focus of treatment), as well as bipolar II disorder, with current subsyndromal depressive symptoms. Alcohol abuse must also be ruled out.

Short-Answer Questions

1. What is the minimum duration of manic versus hypomanic episodes?
2. What are the severity criteria for manic versus hypomanic episodes?
3. What sex differences are encountered in bipolar disorders?
4. What age differences are encountered in bipolar disorders?
5. Bipolar and related disorder due to another medical condition results most often from what kind of medical disorders?
6. What type of psychiatric medication most often triggers substance/medication-induced bipolar and related disorder?
7. Which psychiatric disorders may include major depressive episodes with mixed features?
8. Which psychiatric disorders may include hypomanic episodes with mixed features?
9. Which psychiatric disorders may include manic episodes with mixed features?
10. How many episodes per year are required for a rapid-cycling course?

Answers

1. Seven days is the minimum duration for a manic episode (or any duration if hospitalization occurs), versus 4 days for a hypomanic episode.

2. Manic episodes require (and hypomanic episodes prohibit) psychosis, hospitalization, or severe functional impairment.

3. Females with bipolar disorder experience more depression, rapid cycling, mixed states, and possibly bipolar II disorder compared with males.

4. Children and adolescents may present with disruptive behavioral disorders (e.g., ADHD, oppositional defiant disorder, and conduct disorder), whereas older adults may present with bipolar and related disorder due to another medical condition.

5. Bipolar and related disorder due to another medical condition most often results from neurological and endocrine disorders.

6. Antidepressants most commonly trigger substance/medication-induced bipolar and related disorder.

7. Bipolar I disorder, bipolar II disorder, and major depressive disorder may include major depressive episodes with mixed features.

8. Bipolar I disorder or bipolar II disorder (but not major depressive disorder) may include hypomanic episodes with mixed features.

9. Bipolar I disorder (but not bipolar II disorder nor major depressive disorder) may include manic episodes with mixed features.

10. Four episodes per year are required for a rapid-cycling course.

REFERENCE

American Psychiatric Association: Diagnostic and Statistical Manual of Mental Disorders, 5th Edition, Text Revision. Washington, DC, American Psychiatric Association, 2022

CHAPTER 8

Depressive Disorders

Bruce A. Arnow, Ph.D.

Raquel Osorno, Psy.D.

Tonita E. Wroolie, Ph.D.

Sanno E. Zack, Ph.D.

"Nothing will get better. What's the use of trying?"

"He doesn't even smile at our grandson anymore."

- Disruptive Mood Dysregulation Disorder
- Major Depressive Disorder
- Persistent Depressive Disorder
- Premenstrual Dysphoric Disorder
- Substance/Medication-Induced Depressive Disorder
- Depressive Disorder Due to Another Medical Condition
- Other Specified Depressive Disorder
- Unspecified Depressive Disorder
- Unspecified Mood Disorder

The cardinal symptoms of major depressive disorder (MDD), the most common of the depressive disorders, are sad or low mood and/or anhedonia. Other symptoms may include significant weight loss or change in appetite, insomnia or hypersomnia, psychomotor agitation or retardation, fatigue or loss of energy, feelings of worthlessness or excessive guilt, impaired concentration or indecisiveness, and recurrent thoughts of death, suicidal ideation, or a suicide attempt or plan. Symptoms must be present most of the day, nearly every day, for at least 2 weeks. Criteria for MDD require a total of five symptoms, one of which must be depressed mood or anhedonia. It is important to note that MDD is also a feature of bipolar disorder and that individuals meeting criteria for MDD must never have experienced a manic or hypomanic episode (unless the mania or hypomania is substance induced or is attributable to the physiological effects of another medical condition).

Although the symptomatic criteria of persistent depressive disorder overlap somewhat with those of MDD, with depressed mood being a hallmark, the key feature of persistent depressive disorder is chronicity—that is, the depressed mood must have been present for a period of at least 2 years in adults. In children, the minimum duration is 1 year, and mood can be predominantly irritable. Persistent depressive disorder requires fewer total symptoms than MDD (i.e., three vs. five) and must be present for more days than not, rather than nearly every day. A large percentage of individuals who meet criteria for persistent depressive disorder may meet criteria for MDD during the course of illness. Diagnosis of persistent depressive disorder is accompanied by specifiers clarifying the extent of overlap with MDD.

Premenstrual dysphoric disorder (PMDD) involves mood changes that arise during the final week before the onset of menses, subsequently improve within a few days following menses onset, and become minimal or absent in the week postmenses. Key symptoms of PMDD include at least one of the following: affective lability, irritability, anger, depressed mood, hopelessness, and anxiety. Other symptoms may include decreased interest in usual activities, difficulty concentrating, lack of energy, changes in appetite or food cravings, sleep difficulty, a sense of being overwhelmed, or physical symptoms including breast tenderness, bloating, or muscle pain. A total of five of the aforementioned symptoms is required to meet the diagnostic criteria. Symptoms must have been present for most menstrual cycles during the year preceding diagnosis.

Disruptive mood dysregulation disorder (DMDD) must be distinguished from other childhood disorders, including pediatric bipolar disorder. The key symptom in DMDD is severe, persistent irritability in response to everyday stressors. Individuals with DMDD present frequent (on average, three or more times weekly) temper outbursts, which may be verbal or behavioral (e.g., physical aggression toward people or property). Children must also manifest persistently negative mood between outbursts. The child must be age 6 or older, onset must be prior to age 10, and the diagnosis is not used if the patient is older than age 18. Symptoms must be present for at least 12 months.

A diagnosis of substance/medication-induced depressive disorder is appropriate when the symptoms of depression developed in conjunction with exposure to a medication that is known to cause such symptoms or in close temporal proximity to substance intoxication or withdrawal. Depressive disorder due to another medical condition is appropriate when there is evidence that the depressive symptoms are

TABLE 8–1.   Key changes between DSM-5 and DSM-5-TR

Persistent depressive disorder is no longer referred to as dysthymia.

Specifiers of persistent depressive disorder were updated.

Prevalence, risk and prognostic factors, sex- and gender-related issues, and culture-related issues were updated according to new research.

Validity for disruptive mood dysregulation disorder (DMDD) has been established in children ages 6–18 years (updated from ages 7–18 years).

Although prevalence of DMDD continues to be higher in males in clinical samples, consistent sex differences are not reported in community samples.

Greater prevalence of major depressive disorder in females may be partially explained by their being disproportionately affected by factors that increase depression risk, including higher likelihood of experiencing sexual abuse and interpersonal trauma, as well as hormone changes characteristic of reproductive life stages.

best explained by a medical condition (e.g., hypothyroidism). Three other depressive disorders are included in DSM-5-TR (American Psychiatric Association 2022):

- Other specified depressive disorder involves symptoms of depression with accompanying clinically significant distress or impairment, without full criteria being met for any of the previously noted depressive disorders. The clinician must specify the reason(s) why criteria for a depressive disorder are not met (e.g., short episode duration).
- Unspecified depressive disorder is similar to other specified depressive disorder except that the clinician does not have to document a specific reason why the individual does not meet full criteria for another depressive disorder. In many instances, they may not have sufficient information to specify a reason.
- Unspecified mood disorder, which was not included in DSM-5 (American Psychiatric Association 2013) but appears in DSM-5-TR, is appropriate when the symptoms are consistent with a mood disorder but do not fulfill criteria for any disorder in either the depressive or bipolar areas.

DSM-5 and DSM-5-TR distinguish the depressive disorders from the bipolar and related disorders. In DSM-IV (American Psychiatric Association 1994), they were grouped together as mood disorders. Persistent depressive disorder is now designed to incorporate cases of chronic major depressive episode and includes specifiers to delineate the relationship between symptoms of persistent depressive disorder and MDD over the prior 2-year period. In DSM-5-TR, pervasive depressive disorder is no longer referred to as "dysthymia," and a number of the persistent depressive disorder specifiers were removed (Table 8–1). PMDD, which in DSM-IV was listed as a diagnosis requiring further study, is a separate diagnosis grouped with the depressive disorders in DSM-5 and DSM-5-TR. DMDD, which first appeared in DSM-5, addresses concerns about previous overdiagnosis of bipolar disorder in children; those meeting criteria for DMDD are more likely to develop unipolar depression or anxiety as adolescents or adults, rather than bipolar disorder.

IN-DEPTH DIAGNOSIS:
MAJOR DEPRESSIVE DISORDER

Ms. Smith, a 26-year-old single woman, presents to her internist complaining of insomnia. She reveals that she is also experiencing depressed mood, her ability to concentrate is diminished, she is not finding pleasure in activities that are usually fun for her, her energy and appetite are diminished, and she has recently been having thoughts that she would be better off dead. She denies having a suicide plan but says "if something were to happen, I don't think I would care." Symptoms arose 2 months ago following a breakup with her boyfriend. She reports having been depressed in her early twenties, also following the end of a romantic relationship. Ms. Smith notes that she is a "worrier"—that is, she is anxious about a number of issues, particularly her job performance, although she has never had a negative job performance review. Medical tests are negative. Ms. Smith does not abuse substances and denies a history of mania or hypomania.

People experiencing depression often present to physicians with complaints such as insomnia or low energy. While medical problems must be ruled out, it is important in presentations like this one to ask questions that may reveal the presence of a mood disorder. Ms. Smith meets criteria for six of nine possible symptoms of depression, and among those six are the hallmark symptoms of low mood and anhedonia. The risk of depression is higher in females than males, and although MDD may arise at any age, its peak incidence is during the twenties. Ms. Smith has had one prior episode; the presence of environmental stressors, such as the breakup with her boyfriend, is more likely in early depressive episodes than in later or subsequent episodes. Anxiety disorders are often comorbid with MDD, and Ms. Smith's self-designation as a worrier may indicate the presence of a co-occurring generalized anxiety disorder.

Approach to the Diagnosis

Depressed mood for brief periods of time is common in everyday life. The criteria for MDD involve at least a 2-week period during which the individual experiences either depressed mood or diminished interest or pleasure in nearly all activities most of the day, nearly every day for that period of time. Therefore, it is important to establish the length of time the patient has experienced depressed mood. Given that the diagnosis requires the presence of at least five of nine symptoms, including sleep difficulties, psychomotor agitation or retardation, fatigue or loss of energy, and suicidal ideation, it is helpful to inquire about each of the potential symptoms. The diagnostic criteria also require that the symptoms cause clinically significant distress or impairment in key areas of functioning, so it is important to ask how the symptoms are interfering with the person's life and in which domains (e.g., family, work, social).

Because depression is the most important risk factor in suicide, it is critical to inquire about suicidal thoughts. A suicide risk assessment should be carried out with every patient meeting criteria for MDD. Questions in such an assessment may include "Are you feeling hopeless about the present or the future?" and "Have you had thoughts of taking your life?" If the answer to such questions is "yes," additional questions should be asked, such as "How recently have you had such thoughts?"; "Have you ever tried to take your own life?"; and "Do you have a specific plan to take your life?" Among the factors associated with high risk of suicide are male sex, social isolation, substance abuse, hopelessness, previous suicide attempts, and availability of a lethal method. Females are more likely to attempt suicide, but males are more likely to complete suicide.

Getting the History

Ms. Allen arrives for an initial appointment, reporting depressed mood. The therapist asks, "How long have you been feeling this way?" If Ms. Allen responds in an uncertain or vague manner, it may be helpful to go back to a salient event over the past year (e.g., a birthday or a holiday such as Thanksgiving) and ask whether she was feeling this way then or whether her mood was different. The therapist also asks a question designed to determine how persistent the depressed mood might be: "Do you feel this way every day, or is it more that the feeling comes and goes?" The therapist next asks specifically about each of the other symptoms of depression. "Since you've been feeling this way, have there been changes in your sleep pattern? Have there been changes in your appetite, either where you have a larger or smaller appetite? Have you either lost or gained weight? Do you notice that you are agitated or slowed down?" On this latter symptom, for Ms. Allen to meet the criterion for psychomotor agitation or retardation, the symptoms would have to be severe enough for others to notice. In this case, she responds that she has felt her movement is slowed down. However, when the therapist asks whether others have noticed or commented on this, she says that no one has. The therapist suggests that she specifically ask her roommate during the coming week whether she has noticed such a change.

As opposed to depressed mood, which people often do report, individuals rarely report anhedonia, that is, loss of interest or pleasure in previously enjoyed activities, without prompting. The therapist may want to ask, "Are you able to enjoy the things you normally enjoy?" If Ms. Allen is unsure, the therapist can say, "Tell me about some of the activities you enjoyed when you were not feeling depressed." Ms. Allen says, "Well, I enjoyed family dinners with my children." The therapist can then ask her to think back to the most recent family dinner and to reflect on whether her enjoyment was consistent with how she felt in the past or whether there might have been a change. Other recent family dinners can also be discussed to determine whether there might be a pattern consistent with anhedonia.

Females are at increased risk for interpersonal violence across the life span, which may account for their increased prevalence of MDD. Furthermore, they have an increased risk for MDD during specific reproductive phases, including premenstrual, postpartum, and perimenopausal periods. Females also report more atypical symptoms of depression such as hypersomnia, increased appetite, and leaden paralysis, and report higher levels of impairment in their relationships than depressed males.

Tips for Clarifying the Diagnosis

- Does the patient report either depressed mood or loss of interest or pleasure in activities that were previously engaging or enjoyable?
- In addition to these symptoms, does the patient report a total of five symptoms of depression?

- How long have the symptoms persisted? Have the symptoms been present for at least 2 weeks?
- What domains in the individual's life are impacted by the depressive symptoms?
- Have physiological effects of a substance (e.g., drug of abuse, medication) been ruled out as a cause of the symptoms?
- Has other medical illness (e.g., thyroid illness) been ruled out as a cause of the depressive symptoms?

Consider the Case

Mr. Calhoun, an 85-year-old widower, presents to his internist during a routine visit with slowed movement, weight loss, and diminished grooming, as compared with his usual presentation. A variety of in-office and laboratory tests are completed, all of which are negative. At a second visit to review the medical data, he reveals a lack of pleasure in activities that had previously been enjoyable ("I don't even have fun when I see my grandchildren anymore"), despondency, hypersomnia, impaired concentration, and reduced appetite. He denies suicidal ideation or plan but indicates, "I feel that I don't have a reason to go on." He reports feeling poorly throughout the day but worse in the morning upon awakening. His wife died 3 years earlier, and although he was very sad for approximately 1 year, he has since recovered. Several of his close friends have also died in the previous 5 years. Mr. Calhoun does not have a history of depression, and he is not taking any medications that would account for his symptoms.

Onset of major depression can occur at any age. Mr. Calhoun did not have a history of MDD earlier in his life. The onset of depression in late life is frequently associated with an accumulation of losses, such as those Mr. Calhoun has experienced. He describes a lack of purpose and an absence of goals going forward, which is also common in late-life depression. Symptoms that are worse in the early morning and involve either a loss of pleasure in all or almost all activities or a lack of reactivity to normally pleasurable stimuli, combined with psychomotor retardation and weight loss, are indicative of MDD with melancholic features. Excessive or inappropriate guilt may also be observed in cases of melancholic depression. As occurred in this case, it is important to rule out medical illness that might account for such symptoms.

Culture accounts for variation in symptom manifestation, prevalence, and course. Symptoms that may vary by culture include somatic complaints, social isolation, crying, and anger. Symptoms of MDD may be underreported or underrecognized, leading to misdiagnosis, especially in populations facing discrimination. In the United States, Black and Caribbean Black individuals experience increased MDD chronicity compared with non-Latinx White persons, possibly because of increased incidence of racism, discrimination, and sociocultural barriers to care.

Differential Diagnosis

One of the most important psychiatric disorders to differentiate from MDD is bipolar disorder. Indeed, many individuals with bipolar disorder are incorrectly diagnosed with unipolar depression and do not receive appropriate treatment. People who appear depressed but have experienced a manic or hypomanic episode should be diagnosed with bipolar disorder. Thus, any person who presents with depression should be queried about whether there has ever been a period in which they experienced decreased need for sleep, pressured speech or unusual talkativeness, risky behavior that is unusual for them (e.g., buying items they cannot afford), or other symptoms of mania or hypomania. It is also important to note that certain medications can be associated with manic-like symptoms; people with symptoms attributable to medication effects would not receive a diagnosis of bipolar disorder. Substance use may be associated with symptoms similar to depression (e.g., cocaine withdrawal); if the person's symptoms are fully attributable to the effects of substance use or withdrawal, then another diagnosis would be appropriate. For example, in the case of depressed mood associated with cocaine withdrawal, the diagnosis would be cocaine-induced mood disorder with depressive features, with onset during withdrawal.

Major depression is frequently comorbid with other psychiatric illnesses. For example, anxiety disorders and substance use disorders commonly coexist with major depression. Individuals with depression frequently present in medical settings with somatic symptoms such as insomnia and fatigue. This presentation occurs in all cultures but is more widespread in cultures in which it is explicitly considered more acceptable to present physical symptoms rather than psychiatric ones.

The possibility of suicidal behavior exists at all times during major depressive episodes. The most consistently described risk factor is a past history of suicide attempts or threats, but it should be remembered that most completed suicides are not preceded by unsuccessful attempts. Among features associated with an increased risk for completed suicide include male sex, being single or living alone, prominent feelings of hopelessness, and availability of lethal means including firearms.

Summary

- Hallmark symptoms of MDD involve depressed mood or loss of interest or pleasure in all or almost all activities.
- Symptoms must occur almost all day, nearly every day for at least 2 weeks.
- In addition to at least one of these symptoms, the individual must also have a total of five of nine symptoms of depression to qualify for a diagnosis of MDD.
- The symptoms must also cause significant distress or impairment in key social, occupational, or other areas of functioning.
- General medical conditions or use of substances as a cause of depressive symptoms should be ruled out.

IN-DEPTH DIAGNOSIS: PERSISTENT DEPRESSIVE DISORDER

Ms. Atkins is a 28-year-old woman whose boyfriend suggested that she seek a psychiatric evaluation. He told her that she seemed "down most of the time" and that she might be depressed. During the interview, Ms. Atkins reveals experiencing depressed mood "for as long as I can remember." On more detailed questioning, the onset of her depression dates to about 8 years of age. She denies anhedonia; she is active in recreational athletics and continues to enjoy them as well as other social activities. Some days are better than others, although she indicates that her depressed mood is present more days than not. She also reports generally low self-esteem and low energy. Sometimes she has difficulty making decisions, and she struggles with overeating. Her family history is remarkable for the death of her mother when Ms. Atkins was 7 years old. She reports that her father raised her, and she describes him as "usually depressed." She notes that she was about 8 years old when she fully grasped that her mother was "gone from my life" and that she was thus different from her peers in a way that caused her to feel deficient. She reports experiencing an episode of major depression during her late adolescence, which in addition to depressed mood included anhedonia, suicidal ideation, impaired concentration, and insomnia with early morning awakenings. The symptoms lasted for as long as 2 years, but she adds that they resolved by the time she was 20 years old.

Several issues in Ms. Atkins's case are typical of presentations of persistent depressive disorder. Persistent depressive disorder is more common among females than among males. Ms. Atkins's case typifies early onset; indeed, a large percentage of persistent depressive disorder cases have an onset in childhood or adolescence. A history of childhood adversity—in this case, parental loss—is also common among those with persistent depressive disorder, as is a family history of depression. The symptoms Ms. Atkins presents—depressed mood, low self-esteem, low energy, overeating, and difficulty making decisions—are chronic, but their intensity is lower compared with the symptoms of MDD (e.g., depressed mood is present more days than not rather than nearly every day). At the same time, her case typifies the observation that the vast majority of individuals with persistent depressive disorder experience MDD during their lifetime.

Approach to the Diagnosis

Persistent depressive disorder is by definition a chronic disorder, persisting for at least 2 years in adults and 1 year in children or adolescents. At the same time, the severity of symptoms may be milder than those of MDD. Patients cannot be free of symptoms for more than 2 months during the previous 2 years. Thus, both symptom persistence and severity are key issues in the diagnosis. People with "pure" persistent depressive disorder—that is, those who have never met criteria for MDD—are rare. The specifiers "with pure dysthymic syndrome," "with persistent major depressive episode," "with intermittent major depressive episodes, with current episode," and "with intermittent major depressive episodes, without current episode" are designed to describe the relationship between persistent depressive disorder and MDD for each patient. Impairment is marked and may be seen in marital, family, interpersonal, and occupational domains. Psychiatric comorbidity is common and may include anxiety disorders, substance use disorders, or others. Association between early onset persistent depressive disorder and Cluster B and C personality disorders is particularly high.

Getting the History

Ms. Crawford, a 33-year-old married woman, seeks a consultation for depressed mood. She reports that she functions tolerably at work and carries out tasks expected of her within her marriage but feels "weighed down by sadness and depression" and is often "not at my best." She also endorses fatigue, low self-esteem, and poor concentration but denies suicidal ideation. To determine how intense the symptoms are, the provider asks, "Do you feel this way every day, or is your mood more variable from day to day?" Ms. Crawford indicates that her mood varies somewhat from day to day. When asked approximately how many days per week on average she feels sad, down, or depressed, she responds, "about 4 days." The provider begins to inquire more closely about onset. To the question of how long she felt this way, Ms. Crawford answers, "I'm not sure; it's been a really long time." The provider prompts her further: "When was the last time you felt that you were *not* sad or depressed most of the time?" Ms. Crawford continues to be uncertain, so the provider begins to ask about prominent events in her life. She was married 6 years ago, did she feel depressed at the time she was married? She answers, "No, that was a very happy time." Did she feel depressed at the time of her first anniversary? Her first birthday after the wedding? Upon further inquiry, Ms. Crawford begins to realize that the symptoms came on about 3 years ago when, after a year of trying unsuccessfully to conceive a child, she began to worry that she and her husband would not be able to conceive. Thus, her onset was approximately 3 years ago.

One useful tool for establishing the intensity of depressed mood is to inquire how variable the symptoms are from day to day and from week to week. It is often useful to ask, "On average, how many days per week do you feel this way?" If persistent depressive disorder is suspected, inquire about all possible symptoms (e.g., poor appetite or overeating, sleep disturbance, hopelessness) and about specific symptoms of depression that are not included in the diagnostic criteria, such as anhedonia and suicidal ideation, to help differentiate persistent depressive disorder from MDD. With respect to onset, orienting the patient to prominent life events—for example, birthdays, anniversaries, and holidays—is often useful for establishing how long the symptoms have been present. A history of mania, hypomania, or mixed episode precludes diagnosis of persistent depressive disorder and must be ruled out. Symptoms also must cause distress or impairment, so it is important to ask how the symptoms affect the individual in key areas such as occupational, social, and family settings.

Tips for Clarifying the Diagnosis

- Has the patient experienced depressed mood for most of the day, more days than not, for 2 years or longer (1 year for children)?
- Has there been no more than a 2-month period during the past 2 years during which the individual was free of symptoms?
- Use specifiers to describe whether, and to what extent, major depression has been present for the previous 2 years.
- In addition to depressed mood, at least two additional symptoms must be present (e.g., low energy, poor concentration).

Consider the Case

Mr. Johnson is a 42-year-old man. He is casually dressed and moderately overweight. He decided to seek a psychiatric consultation after reading in the newspaper about a medication study for depression and wondering whether the agent mentioned in the article might be helpful to him. He is single and works as an engineer. He reports depressed mood most of the day, almost every day, over the past 15 years. In addition, he reports pervasive feelings of hopelessness about his life, low self-esteem, and frequent insomnia with early morning awakenings. He denies anhedonia, appetite disturbance, suicidal ideation, poor concentration, and other symptoms of MDD. He admits to drinking too much alcohol—reportedly three glasses of wine each evening. He denies any history of citations for driving under the influence, blackouts, or drinking alcohol during the day. He has never been married. He dated when he was younger but has not done so for the past several years. He says that he functions well at work but that his social life is limited and that his symptoms of depression have reduced his motivation for social contact. He doubts he would make a good husband, even if he were to meet "the right person." Mr. Johnson was raised in an intact family. He denies any history of abuse and loss but reports that his parents were distant and not attuned to him and that he did not feel particularly close to them. He does not know if either of them experienced depression. The interview reveals at least two clear episodes of MDD, one when he was about 32 years old and the other when he was 36.

Persistent depressive disorder, although more common among females, is also encountered in males. It is associated with significant functional limitations. Mr. Johnson is successful at work, but he leads a socially circumscribed life. His current symptoms are not sufficient in number or severity to qualify for an MDD diagnosis. Although he has no history of outright abuse or loss, Mr. Johnson came from an emotionally impoverished home and experienced emotional neglect, which is not uncommon in cases of persistent depressive disorder. He has also experienced episodes of MDD in the past. Patients with persistent depressive disorder who do not experience MDD at some point in their lifetime are the exception rather than the rule. Mr. Johnson has comorbid alcohol abuse, and substance-related disorders are among those that more frequently coexist with persistent depressive disorder. Underreporting of symptoms (e.g., suicidal ideation, alcohol abuse) may be observed in both sexes, but males are particularly known to underreport symptom severity. Careful and detailed questioning is imperative in making an accurate diagnosis and assessment of risk.

Differential Diagnosis

Both MDD and persistent depressive disorder are characterized by depressed mood. Differences between them involve number and severity of symptoms, how long the person has experienced them, or the specific symptoms themselves. Threshold criteria for persistent depressive disorder require only three symptoms lasting 2 years for adults and 1 year for children and adolescents. For an MDD diagnosis, at least five symptoms must be present for at least 2 weeks. Persistent depressive disorder must occur "more days than not," whereas for MDD, depressed mood must be present "nearly every day." Note also that there are some differences in the symptoms that are required for these disorders (Table 8–2).

Anhedonia, psychomotor agitation or retardation, and feelings of worthlessness or guilt are not among the criteria for persistent depressive disorder. On the other hand, low self-esteem and hopelessness, which are among the symptoms that may be encountered in people with persistent depressive disorder, are not noted as criteria for MDD. Some episodes of MDD do become chronic—that is, they last for 2 years or longer. In most cases, individuals with chronic MDD will meet criteria for persistent depressive disorder, with the specifier "with persistent major depressive episode."

TABLE 8–2.   Symptoms for major depressive disorder and persistent depressive disorder

Symptom	Major depressive disorder	Persistent depressive disorder
Depressed mood	X	X
Anhedonia	X	
Appetite change	X	X
Sleep change	X	X
Motor change	X	
Low energy or fatigue	X	X
Worthlessness	X	
Concentration	X	X
Suicidal ideation	X	
Low self-esteem		X
Hopelessness		X

An additional feature that distinguishes persistent depressive disorder from MDD is its insidious onset. Persistent depressive disorder often, but not always, begins prior to age 21 (early onset) and not infrequently can be traced back to childhood or adolescence.

Summary

- Persistent depressive disorder is a chronic disorder in which depressed mood has been present for at least 2 years.
- The symptoms have been persistent—that is, the individual has not been free of symptoms for a period longer than 2 months over the previous 2 years.
- Onset is typically insidious.
- A minimum of three symptoms (depressed mood plus two others) is required to meet the threshold for diagnosis.
- The vast majority of patients with persistent depressive disorder meet criteria for a major depressive episode sometime in their lives.

IN-DEPTH DIAGNOSIS: PREMENSTRUAL DYSPHORIC DISORDER

Ms. Sawyer is a 34-year-old married mother of two children, ages 3 years and 5 years. She presents with complaints of significantly increased irritability that began after the birth of her second child. She reports that prior to her first pregnancy, she noticed feeling more sensitive and frustrated a few days before her period. Once menses began, however, she was quickly "back to her old self." The symptoms did not interfere with her schoolwork or relationships, but she noticed a pattern over time. Ms. Sawyer's pregnancies were uneventful; both children are healthy, and she enjoys being a mother. She describes having a stable marriage, ample childcare, and support from friends and family. She is confused about what she calls her "Jekyll and Hyde" personality. Each month she experiences intense "mood swings" that begin about 10 days before her menses. During this time, she has difficulty sleeping and feels exhausted during the day, has trouble concentrating, and feels more disorganized than usual. Ms. Sawyer reports being most upset about the effect that her "monthly personality change" has on her family and her weight. She becomes extremely irritable and often feels "out of control and overwhelmed." She finds she yells at her children over the smallest things. She craves carbohydrates and gains 1–2 pounds per month. Her symptoms finally subside 2–3 days after her menstrual flow begins: "It is as if a toxin leaves my body, and then I'm back to my old self again for about 20 days."

Ms. Sawyer experiences monthly mood changes that begin during the luteal phase of her menstrual cycle and remit within the first few days after her menstrual flow begins. She experiences classic PMDD symptoms, including carbohydrate cravings, irritability, mood lability, feeling easily overwhelmed, and low frustration tolerance. In particular, she is distressed by how irritable she becomes and the effect this has on her behavior and relationships. Irritability is the most common symptom of PMDD in American females. Less well-known PMDD symptoms include cognitive complaints. Ms. Sawyer has a history of premenstrual symptoms that worsened after having children, and females with premenstrual symptoms often report progression to full criteria of PMDD following childbirth.

Approach to the Diagnosis

Patients with PMDD have a distinct pattern of severe and distressing symptoms. Mood lability, irritability, dysphoria, and anxiety symptoms typically peak around the time of menses and remit around the onset of menses or soon after. Patients may report difficulty with concentration; sleep problems, such as hypersomnia or insomnia; appetite changes, particularly overeating or food cravings; loss of interest; and lethargy. Symptoms must have been present during most menstrual cycles over the past year and must cause significant impairment in functioning for the diagnostic criteria to be met. Behavioral and physical symptoms also may be present, but without the mood or anxiety symptoms, a diagnosis of PMDD should not be given.

In addition to mood or anxiety symptoms, females with PMDD may experience significant behavioral disturbances. They may avoid social situations because of diminished interest. Decreased efficiency and productivity may cause problems at work, at school, or in keeping up with household responsibilities. Relationships with their spouse or partner, friends, and family may be negatively affected by the behavioral manifestations of mood swings, sudden irritability, hyperattention to dysphoric stimuli, rejection sensitivity, and increased response to stress.

Getting the History

Ms. Ford reports premenstrual symptoms that worsened after the birth of her children. She is particularly distressed by her irritability and the effect it has on her behavior and relationships. The physician explores the type and severity of her symptoms, asking questions such as "Do you feel as though your moods are out of control? Are you having any sleep difficulties or experiencing appetite changes or cravings? Are you more tired than usual around your menstrual periods? What other symptoms do you experience?" The physician evaluates Ms. Ford's level of distress and suicide risk. To determine the impact her symptoms have on her functioning, they ask, "How do your symptoms affect your ability to carry out your usual activities?" Psychotic symptoms are rare with PMDD, but the physician explores the existence of such symptoms. To clarify whether Ms. Ford is having a sustained mood episode or her symptoms are associated strictly with her menstrual cycle, they ask when her symptoms begin and whether they stop or significantly lessen once her period starts. The physician inquires whether Ms. Ford has a history of mood disorder or has experienced mood symptoms with oral contraceptive use as well as her risk factors for PMDD, such as current stressors, substance use, medical disorders, and a family history of affective disorders.

The physician performs a thorough evaluation of Ms. Ford's symptom profile and attempts to get a clear picture of the relationship between her symptoms and her menstrual cycle. Mood lability and irritability are prominent in PMDD and may coincide with physical symptoms related to hormone changes during the menstrual cycle. Minimization or complete remission of symptoms before or shortly after menses begins is necessary for a diagnosis of PMDD. Symptom pattern is shown to be stable across menstrual cycles in females with PMDD, and documenting daily symptom ratings prospectively over several months will help confirm the diagnosis.

Tips for Clarifying the Diagnosis

- Do symptoms begin in the luteal phase of the menstrual cycle and improve or remit in the follicular phase?
- Is there a history of hormone sensitivity (increased symptoms with some oral contraceptives, postpartum mood disturbances)?
- Is there a family history of PMDD or mood disorders?
- Does exercise or stress reduction improve symptoms?
- Does alcohol worsen symptoms?

Consider the Case

Ms. Jackson is a 43-year-old single woman with a family history (mother and sister) of severe, recurrent major depression who presents with complaints of mood lability over the past year. She has a long history of feeling more emotional before the onset of her menses, but in the past year, these symptoms intensified and include feeling very depressed and anxious, having difficulty with memory and concentration, and feeling easily overwhelmed. Currently, she experiences night sweats throughout the month that increase in frequency during the luteal phase. She also complains that all month long, her days are "ruined by constant fatigue." Ms. Jackson was promoted to an executive position at work and has been under a great deal of stress over the past several months. Her gynecologist diagnosed her with perimenopause and recommended an oral contraceptive to "even out her hormones." While taking the oral contraceptive, Ms. Jackson felt bloated and even more emotional. After 2 months, she stopped taking them. Ms. Jackson states that because of fatigue she stopped her daily aerobic exercise.

She also started drinking one to two glasses of wine per night because she feels so "keyed up" before her period. In the past month, Ms. Jackson has been feeling very depressed; she experiences decreased enjoyment in her activities, guilty ruminations, memory and concentration problems, and passive suicidal ideation. These symptoms do not remit with her menstrual flow.

As in Ms. Jackson's case, females with PMDD often report increased symptoms during menopause transition, and PMDD is a risk factor for perimenopausal depression. Family history of affective disorders is more common among females with PMDD than among healthy control subjects. Because ovulation triggers PMDD, oral contraceptives may be given to patients with PMDD to prevent ovulation. In addition, oral contraceptives sometimes are prescribed for females in perimenopause as estrogen replacement therapy. However, many oral contraceptives are associated with increased PMDD. Ms. Jackson is under more stress while transitioning into menopause because of increased work demands. Because of the fatigue associated with PMDD and the menopause transition, she gave up the exercise that might help manage stress and increased her alcohol consumption to relieve her symptoms. Both stress and alcohol are shown to increase PMDD symptoms, and Ms. Jackson now also appears to meet criteria for MDD.

PMDD is associated with regular cyclical hormonal fluctuations during reproductive age. Symptom worsening is often reported during menopause transition, at which time hormone levels are fluctuating erratically. Symptoms subside at menopause, although cyclical hormone therapy may trigger re-expression of symptoms. PMDD has been observed in the United States, Brazil, Europe, Nigeria, India, and Asia. Its manifestation, frequency, and intensity of symptoms and their management may be significantly influenced by cultural and social factors, including differences in attitudes toward menstruation, poor social support, and history of interpersonal violence or sexual abuse.

Differential Diagnosis

The symptoms of PMDD are more severe and debilitating than those of premenstrual syndrome, although both are associated with hormonal changes during the menstrual cycle. PMDD has a short, fluctuating course that differs from the chronic symptoms of persistent depressive disorder. Several other disorders share similar symptoms to PMDD. In MDD, the depressed mood or anhedonia with at least four additional symptoms of depression last for at least 2 weeks and are not specifically associated with a particular menstrual phase. The most commonly reported symptom in PMDD is mood lability and irritability, whereas in MDD depressed mood and diminished interest or pleasure are most prominent. The fact that the mood cycling in cyclothymia generally does not follow a regular menstrual pattern is a critical differential diagnostic criterion. Its cyclical irritability with distractibility and sleep disturbance can resemble PMDD, but PMDD is not characterized by increased goal-directed activity, grandiosity, or pressured speech. Both PMDD and binge eating disorder are characterized by increased consumption of food (often carbohydrates), and although binge eating disorder may increase during the luteal phase in some females, it is not confined to that phase.

It is not uncommon for females with PMDD to have a history of mood disorder or other psychiatric disorders. Mood and behavioral symptoms in affective or other psychiatric disorders may increase during the luteal phase ("premenstrual exacerbation"), but they do not remit around the onset of menstruation. Chronic medical conditions such as anemia or thyroid deficiency may complicate the clinical picture and should be ruled out. The premenstrual phase has been considered by some to be a risk period for suicide.

Summary

- PMDD is a cyclical mood disorder that occurs in females of reproductive age.
- Mood lability, irritability, and depressive symptoms begin after ovulation and remit or lessen in the early follicular phase of the menstrual cycle each month.
- Symptoms are associated with significant distress.
- Symptoms increase with stress, lack of exercise, and alcohol consumption; following childbirth; during the menopause transition; and, in some females, with oral contraceptive use.

IN-DEPTH DIAGNOSIS: DISRUPTIVE MOOD DYSREGULATION DISORDER

Richard, a 9-year-old boy, is referred by his pediatrician to a child psychiatrist because of concerns regarding chronic irritability and outbursts of rage. Richard's parents report that he is constantly angry, lashing out at his parents and siblings with little provocation, and is frequently in trouble at school for whining, pushing others, and refusing to complete homework. They describe temper tantrums that last for hours, during which time Richard screams, cries, and throws items such as schoolbooks and toys, often breaking them. At times he will hit his parents, younger brother, or family pets. These tantrums occur five or six times per week, and during the outbursts, Richard is unable to be soothed or redirected. Outbursts typically occur in response to nonpreferred activities, such as requests to complete homework or chores, or when Richard loses at games or perceives that others are being favored. Outbursts are worse when he is tired or hungry. His parents and pediatrician describe him as having been a difficult and colicky infant and report that he received a diagnosis when he was 4 years old for oppositional defiant disorder and symptoms of ADHD, but his difficulties have progressed over the past 2 years into chronic irritability and anger. Richard's parents became particularly concerned when he recently grabbed a knife during one tantrum and threatened to stab himself. He has no history of elevated or euphoric mood, pressured speech, flight of ideas, or goal-directed activity. His sleep is unremarkable. Distractibility is chronic for Richard and not mood related.

Parents, teachers, and peers typically identify children with DMDD as irritable, moody, or difficult to get along with. Although problems with sad, irritable, or angry mood must present across multiple settings for diagnosis, more severe tantrums are often observed in one setting, such as the home, as is the case for Richard. Recurrent temper outbursts are frequently in response to common stressors, such as a demand to complete chores or homework or a conflict with siblings or peers. However, the response is grossly disproportionate for both the situation and the child's developmental level. In this case, Richard's tantrums are excessive in both intensity and severity, lasting for hours at a time and escalating to hitting others, throwing and breaking household items, and threatening self-harm. Outside of these episodes, this child is chronically irritable and angry. Chronicity is an important feature that helps differentiate DMDD from the episodic mood events that occur in bipolar disorder. Like Richard, most children with DMDD are male, have premorbid difficulty with behavior and attention before meeting full criteria for DMDD, and present to mental health clinics because of the severity of their symptoms and the negative impact on families and classrooms. Richard also has historically presented with symptoms of ADHD. DMDD is most common from ages 6 years to 12 years and cannot be diagnosed if the patient is younger than 6 or older than 18.

Approach to the Diagnosis

Occasional temper outbursts are common for all children, especially those who are younger or developmentally immature. The criteria for DMDD require not only frequent (three or more times per week) outbursts of temper but outbursts that are grossly out of proportion in intensity and duration to the situation or provocation. Thus, it is important to establish the frequency, duration, and intensity of these outbursts as well as the triggers. In DMDD, triggers tend to be common stressors (e.g., not getting one's way, competing for attention with siblings) and occur across a variety of domains, not only in one specific situation. Symptoms must occur in at least two settings, although they may be more severe in one; clinicians should inquire whether outbursts occur in multiple settings, such as at home, school, sports practices, or other extracurricular activities, or with peers. When assessing any mood disorder, it is helpful to first establish an index mood and time course. DMDD requires a minimum 1-year time course characterized by chronic mood disturbance. Between temper outbursts, the child displays persistently negative affect (e.g., angry, irritable, or sad mood). This criterion distinguishes DMDD from bipolar disorder, which presents with episodic as opposed to chronic mood disturbance and in which mood may be euthymic between episodes. Inquire whether the negative mood is observable to others, including family, teachers, and peers, and establish that there has been no more than 3 months without symptoms. Because DMDD is a risk factor for dangerous behavior, including aggression, suicide, and other behaviors warranting psychiatric hospitalization, it is critical to inquire about suicidal thoughts and plans, actions that are a threat to others, or any other areas of risky or dangerous behavior. Both the child and the child's caregivers should be interviewed. Teachers are also an important source of information.

Getting the History

Arnold, an 8-year-old boy, is brought by his caregivers for an initial appointment with a child psychiatrist because of concerns about severe mood dysregulation. The psychiatrist asks Arnold's caregivers when they first started to have concerns about his mood, and they respond by describing severe temper tantrums that began after they enrolled Arnold in kindergarten at age 6. The psychiatrist asks, "Can you describe the tantrums in detail? What does Arnold do or say? How long do the tantrums last? Has he ever hurt himself or someone else or destroyed property?" His caregivers answer that Arnold typically yells and screams for a half hour to an hour and will break classroom items and sometimes destroy other students' possessions. They explain that these events typically happen "a few times per week," which the psychiatrist attempts to clarify—"How often is 'a few'? Would you say three or four? More?"—and then asks about Arnold's mood between outbursts: "Tell me what Arnold's mood is like on the days between these outbursts." The caregivers respond that he is generally sad and irritable. The psychiatrist then asks Arnold whether he agrees with this description, clarifying that Arnold knows what *mad* and *sad* mean by eliciting examples, such as "What sorts of things make you feel sad or mad? Sometimes kids get so mad that they want to yell or break things," and asking what sorts of things make him mad. The psychiatrist asks whether Arnold's teachers or friends also notice that he is sad and mad a lot. Having established that the outbursts are severe and have been occurring four times per week over the past year with sad and angry mood in between, the psychiatrist rules out instances of mania by asking whether Arnold has ever had times when he was "so happy or high or excited that he didn't seem like himself or got into trouble," to which both Arnold and his caregivers respond in the negative. Given Arnold's irritable mood, the psychiatrist also inquires about other symptoms of mania (e.g., decreased need for sleep, unusual talkativeness, grandiosity).

Clinicians should interview both the caregivers and the child regarding the child's symptoms. Frequently, caregivers are better reporters of externalizing symptoms, and children and adolescents of internalizing symptoms. However, in the case of DMDD, the child's sad, irritable, or angry mood must be observable to others, so caregiver report is particularly important, and corroboration by their teachers is also helpful. Parental report of "tantrums" is insufficient for diagnosis. The clinician must ascertain the frequency, intensity, duration, and severity of tantrums, such as by asking for examples of the behaviors that occur during the temper outbursts (e.g., yelling, throwing items), how long they last, the degree to which school and family routines are disrupted, the consequences (including injury to others or destruction of property), how the outbursts end (e.g., being sent to the principal at school, parents having to restrain the child), and whether caregivers feel the outbursts are markedly more intense than those of siblings, peers, or other children. Obtaining information about the child's presenting mood between the temper outbursts is of equal importance to the diagnosis.

Tips for Clarifying the Diagnosis

- Does the caregiver report temper outbursts that are grossly disproportionate to the situation?
- Are the outbursts occurring three times per week or more, and are they observable to others?
- Between outbursts, is the child's mood persistently negative (i.e., sad, irritable, or angry)?

- How long have the symptoms persisted? Have the symptoms been present for at least 12 months with no more than 3 months without symptoms?
- Is the onset of the symptoms between ages 6 and 10?
- Has mania or hypomania lasting more than 1 day been ruled out?

Consider the Case

> Cora is a 12-year-old girl whose parents bring her to the pediatrician with concerns about her sad and withdrawn mood, low frustration tolerance, and periodic "melt-downs" during which she will yell, destroy projects and favorite trinkets, or hit herself. Cora has had long-standing difficulties with peers because of her poor communication skills and negative mood, and her meltdowns are further exacerbated by social rejection from peers. In the classroom, Cora is described as generally sad and withdrawn, saying little and keeping to herself. According to her teachers, when peers tease her or she is unable to complete assignments to her satisfaction, she will rip up her paper, run out of the classroom, sob loudly, or scream at classmates who provoke her. This disruption occurs on average three times per week and results in considerable disturbance to the classroom. Cora's parents report similar struggles for her at home and add that if she is working on an art activity that is not coming out the way she wants, she will frequently have crying fits to the point that she is curled up on the floor, flailing, hitting herself, and calling herself stupid. If they attempt to intervene, she lashes out at them verbally. Onset is over the past year. No clear changes in appetite, sleep, or concentration are associated with Cora's symptoms, although she does endorse low self-worth.

Sex differences for DMDD in the general population have not been consistently reported, but it is observed less commonly in females than males in clinic samples. For Cora, the disorder presents with signs of possible comorbid anxiety or perfectionism and depression, conditions that commonly emerge in young females during adolescence. Cora's mood is chronically sad, and her temper outbursts are directed more at herself than toward others, occurring when she is frustrated with projects or with schoolwork not meeting her standards. Temper outbursts that are internally, as opposed to externally, oriented are more common among adolescent females than among males. However, when provoked, Cora also lashes out at peers and her parents. Cora's behavioral manifestations, such as running out of the classroom or curling up into a ball on the floor, are developmentally inappropriate, representing behavior more typical of a younger child. The severity (e.g., hitting herself) is also beyond what would be expected for a frustrated almost-adolescent. Cora's age at diagnosis is somewhat atypical because her onset is at the upper age range for the disorder. Her presentation may progress to MDD as she moves into adolescence, but at this time she does not meet the full criteria for MDD, and her temper outbursts suggest DMDD.

Data on culture-related influences for DMDD are limited but suggest that sociocultural factors including violence, racism, and discrimination impact the presentation of core features of the disorder, including emotion and behavior dysregulation and impulsivity. Care should be taken when screening for DMDD to distinguish between core features of this disorder and adaptive responses to adversity that may be specific to context.

Differential Diagnosis

The most important psychiatric disorder to differentiate from DMDD is bipolar disorder. The primary difference is that bipolar disorder manifests as delineated mood episodes with a discrete time period during which a change in mood is accompanied by four or more additional symptoms (e.g., racing thoughts, pressured speech). In bipolar disorder, as in DMDD, irritability may be the index mood; however, in DMDD, the irritability is pervasive and continuous, whereas in bipolar disorder patients have periods of time between mood episodes during which their mood may be euthymic. In addition, elevated or euphoric mood is characteristic of mania in bipolar disorder and is not typically seen in DMDD. If a child exhibits more than 1 day of manic-like symptoms, the child should not be diagnosed with DMDD. Thus, any child who presents with DMDD should be queried along with caregivers about whether the child has ever experienced a period in which they had a decreased need for sleep, pressured speech or unusual talkativeness, or grandiosity; engaged in risky behavior that is unusual (e.g., running into the street, hypersexuality, atypical "daredevil" activities); or demonstrated other symptoms of mania or hypomania. Intermittent explosive disorder is also exclusionary for DMDD because children with intermittent explosive disorder do not show persistent negative mood between outbursts.

It is important to identify the source that triggers temper outbursts. If these outbursts occur exclusively in a single context (e.g., medical appointments, classroom presentations, or when a preferred routine is disrupted), the tantrums might be better accounted for by specific phobia, social anxiety disorder, or autism spectrum disorder, respectively, and DMDD should not be diagnosed. However, co-occurrence of these disorders with DMDD is also possible. Evidence documenting suicidal behavior and aggression, as well as other severe functional consequences, in DMDD should be noted when evaluating children with chronic irritability.

Summary

- The hallmark symptom of DMDD is severe, recurrent temper outbursts.
- Outbursts can manifest verbally or behaviorally but are grossly disproportionate in intensity or duration to the situation and inconsistent with developmental level.
- Outbursts occur three times per week or more.
- Between outbursts, mood is persistently irritable, angry, or sad, and others observe this presentation.
- Symptoms must be present at least 12 months, with no more than a 3-month absence.
- Onset must be prior to age 10, but the diagnosis should not be assigned if the child is younger than 6 or older than 18.
- The child should at no time have presented mania or hypomania lasting more than 1 day.

SUMMARY: DEPRESSIVE DISORDERS

The diagnoses grouped under the depressive disorders in DSM-5-TR present considerable heterogeneity in onset, chronicity, and symptom presentation. MDD and persistent depressive disorder have the greatest overlap in symptoms; both feature depressed mood, with differences in onset, intensity, and persistence. Persistent depressive disorder is, by definition, a chronic disorder. MDD, although it requires sustained symptoms be present for as little as 2 weeks, can become chronic. Most patients with chronic major depression likely will meet the criteria for persistent depressive disorder. PMDD may or may not manifest with depressed mood; anxiety, irritability, and mood lability may manifest as key features of the disorder. DMDD, which is characterized by chronic and severe irritability, including frequent and developmentally inappropriate temper outbursts and angry mood, is the only one of these disorders that is specifically a disorder of childhood, with an onset between ages 6 and 10 years. However, MDD and persistent depressive disorder may manifest during childhood.

ELEMENTS TO CONSIDER IN THE CULTURAL FORMULATION

- Development and course of depressive disorders may be significantly impacted by sociocultural adversity, including marginalization, racism, and other forms of discrimination.
- Different cultures may have differing perspectives on, understanding of, or tolerance for symptoms of depressive disorders that may lead to over- or underdiagnosis or impact symptom detection and treatment acceptability.
- Members of some cultures may present with more somatic complaints of depression than reported feelings of sadness.
- Individuals can be asked directly if aspects of their background or identity contribute to their experience of depression.
- People often understand symptoms in their own way, which may be similar to or different from how clinicians describe them. Individuals can be asked to describe their symptoms in their own words.
- People have various ways of dealing with symptoms and can be asked directly about what they have done to cope.

DIAGNOSTIC PEARLS

- The depressive disorders class includes disorders with a chief feature of anhedonia (major depressive disorder [MDD]) or depressed mood (MDD, persistent depressive disorder, premenstrual dysphoric disorder [PMDD]), as well as affective lability (PMDD) and irritability (PMDD, disruptive mood dysregulation disorder [DMDD]).
- Symptoms attributable to MDD must be distinguished from those caused by specific medical conditions (e.g., reduced energy in people with untreated thyroid illness, weight loss associated with untreated diabetes, fatigue with anemia).

- MDD is also a feature of bipolar disorder in children or adults. A single episode of mania or hypomania triggers a diagnosis of bipolar disorder, rather than MDD, and ruling out mania is critical for making a diagnosis of MDD.

- Persistent depressive disorder may manifest with symptoms that are less severe and intense than symptoms of MDD. However, the vast majority of people with persistent depressive disorder meet criteria for MDD at some point during their lives. Diagnosis of persistent depressive disorder includes specifiers designed to describe its relationship to MDD over the previous 2-year period.

- Epidemiological findings reveal that MDD and persistent depressive disorder are approximately twice more common in females than in males.

- Symptoms of PMDD must be minimal or absent in the week postmenses.

- The onset of DMDD must occur by age 10 years.

- Take care to differentiate between true symptoms of depressive disorders and adaptive responses to systemic adversity such as racism, marginalization, and discrimination that may be context-specific.

- Depressive disorders increase risk for suicidal behaviors. Although past history of suicide attempts or threats is the most consistently described risk factor for suicide, most completed suicides are not preceded by unsuccessful attempts.

SELF-ASSESSMENT

Key Concepts: Double-Check Your Knowledge

What is the relevance of the following concepts to the various depressive disorders?

- Anhedonia
- Mood lability
- Frequent temper outbursts
- Double depression
- Symptom peak
- Excessive or inappropriate guilt
- Severe, persistent irritability
- Recurrent thoughts of death or suicidal ideation
- Chronic angry mood
- Insidious onset
- Early versus late onset
- Symptom-free follicular phase

Questions to Discuss With Colleagues and Mentors

1. When a patient presents with symptoms of depression, do you screen for other medical problems that may explain the symptoms?

2. Do you routinely use any validated short screens for depression in your practice?
3. Are there differences in the way you treat major depression versus persistent depressive disorder?
4. In cases in which premenstrual dysphoric disorder is suspected, do you incorporate prospective daily mood, anxiety, or irritability ratings across the menstrual cycle? If so, what sort of measure or log do you use?
5. What are your personal reactions to patients who meet criteria for disruptive mood dysregulation disorder? How do you manage these reactions in yourself?

Case-Based Questions

PART A

Ms. Frank is a 24-year-old woman whose internist refers her to a psychiatrist for treatment of depression. The results of her medical workup are negative. She reports that she has experienced symptoms of depressed mood for "many years" but that her mood problems exacerbated 3 months ago when she was fired from her job. Since then, she has developed severe insomnia, awakening several hours earlier than normal without being able to go back to sleep. She has difficulty enjoying activities such as social gatherings and church functions, which she previously looked forward to. She experiences reduced energy, her ability to concentrate has worsened, she feels worthless, and she now has thoughts of ending her life, although she does not have a specific plan. She has never sought treatment or a psychiatric evaluation before. The psychiatrist asks her about times when she experienced symptoms of mania or hypomania and is able to rule these out.

Given this information, does Ms. Frank meet the criteria for a major depressive episode?   Ms. Frank does meet criteria for a major depressive episode, having both depressed mood and anhedonia, as well as insomnia, diminished energy, impaired concentration, feelings of worthlessness, and suicidal ideation. There is no evidence that the episode of major depressive disorder (MDD) is related to bipolar disorder, and her symptoms are not attributable to other medical illness. However, the fact that she reports having had chronically depressed mood for many years before the onset of MDD causes the psychiatrist to ask questions that would establish whether the MDD might be superimposed on persistent depressive disorder.

PART B

The psychiatrist asks more specifically how long Ms. Frank experienced depressed mood before the onset of the major depressive episode. She is able to recall that the depressed mood began when she was a junior in high school. She reports that along with the depressed mood, she experienced difficulty concentrating and low self-esteem, and although these symptoms were chronic, the insomnia, anhedonia, and suicidal ideas were not present prior to the past 3 months.

Given the information regarding chronicity, what is the appropriate diagnosis?   Ms. Frank's prior symptoms and their chronicity are consistent with persistent depressive disorder beginning before age 21. Thus, she meets criteria for persistent depressive disorder, early onset, with alternative course, with current major depressive episode.

Short-Answer Questions

1. What is the minimum duration of the symptoms to meet criteria for major depressive disorder (MDD)?
2. What is the minimum duration of symptoms for adults to meet criteria for persistent depressive disorder?
3. What is the minimum duration of symptoms for children and adolescents to meet criteria for persistent depressive disorder?
4. Name the two hallmark symptoms of MDD—that is, the two symptoms of which at least one must be present to meet diagnostic criteria.
5. Define early onset and late onset for persistent depressive disorder.
6. What is the fewest number of symptoms necessary for a diagnosis of persistent depressive disorder?
7. Name the four hallmark symptoms of premenstrual dysphoric disorder (PMDD)—that is, the four symptoms of which at least one must be present to meet criteria for the diagnosis.
8. Describe the course of key symptoms of PMDD during the menstrual cycle.
9. How long must symptoms have been present to meet criteria for PMDD?
10. In disruptive mood dysregulation disorder (DMDD), onset must be before what age in a child?
11. How frequent must temper outbursts be to meet criteria for DMDD?
12. How long must temper outbursts have been present to meet criteria for DMDD?

Answers

1. The minimum duration of symptoms is 2 weeks to meet criteria for MDD.

2. The minimum duration of symptoms is 2 years for adults to meet criteria for persistent depressive disorder.

3. The minimum duration of symptoms is 1 year for children and adolescents to meet criteria for persistent depressive disorder.

4. The hallmark symptoms of MDD are depressed mood and loss of interest or pleasure in most activities.

5. In persistent depressive disorder, early onset is prior to age 21 and late onset is age 21 or older.

6. At least three symptoms are necessary for a diagnosis of persistent depressive disorder.

7. Mood lability, irritability, dysphoria, and anxiety are the hallmark symptoms of PMDD.

8. In PMDD, symptoms present in the final week before the onset of menses, improve after the onset of menses, and are minimal or absent in the week postmenses.

9. Symptoms must have been present for 1 year to meet criteria for PMDD.

10. Onset of DMDD must be before age 10 years.

11. Temper outbursts must occur an average of three or more times weekly to meet criteria for DMDD.

12. Temper outbursts must have been present for at least 12 months to meet criteria for DMDD.

RECOMMENDED READINGS

Abela JRZ, Hankin BL (eds): Handbook of Depression in Children and Adolescents. New York, Guilford, 2008

Gold LH, Frierson RL: The American Psychiatric Association Publishing Textbook of Suicide Risk Assessment and Management, 3rd Edition. Washington, DC, American Psychiatric Association Publishing, 2020

Gotlib IH, Hammen CL (eds): Handbook of Depression, 3rd Edition. New York, Guilford, 2015

Nemeroff CB, Rasgon N, Schatzberg AF, et al (eds): The American Psychiatric Association Publishing Textbook of Mood Disorders, 2nd Edition. Washington, DC, American Psychiatric Association Publishing, 2022

REFERENCES

American Psychiatric Association: Diagnostic and Statistical Manual of Mental Disorders, 4th Edition. Washington, DC, American Psychiatric Association, 1994

American Psychiatric Association: Diagnostic and Statistical Manual of Mental Disorders, 5th Edition. Arlington, VA, American Psychiatric Association, 2013

American Psychiatric Association: Diagnostic and Statistical Manual of Mental Disorders, 5th Edition, Text Revision. Washington, DC, American Psychiatric Association, 2022

CHAPTER 9

Anxiety Disorders

Alan K. Louie, M.D.

Laura Weiss Roberts, M.D., M.A.

"I'm going to make a fool of myself."

"My heart suddenly goes so fast that I can't breathe, but my doctor can't find anything wrong."

- Separation Anxiety Disorder
- Selective Mutism
- Specific Phobia
- Social Anxiety Disorder
- Panic Disorder
- Agoraphobia
- Generalized Anxiety Disorder
- Substance/Medication-Induced Anxiety Disorder
- Anxiety Disorder Due to Another Medical Condition
- Other Specified Anxiety Disorder
- Unspecified Anxiety Disorder

The diagnostic class of anxiety disorders relates to the states of fear, worry, and anxiety that are quite familiar to most, if not all, people. Certainly, such states can be key to people's survival by preparing, alerting, and mobilizing them against hazardous situations. Absence of any fear would be unhealthy—similar to the absence of pain, which would allow a person to touch a flame without flinching. Nevertheless, fear, worry, and anxiety can become too great—out of proportion or unreasonable—given the actual "hazards" of an individual's life. This extreme reaction can negatively affect the person's ability to fulfill the roles they have taken on, to enjoy healthy relationships, and generally to live a complete life. For instance, a mother understandably worries about her young child getting to school safely on the school bus. However, this same worry may be considered excessive as the child grows older, shaping the experience of the child and preoccupying the mother. When fear, worry, or anxiety causes unnecessary distress or adversely influences how the person leads their life, a diagnosis in the anxiety disorder class may apply. Some affected individuals may seek out counselors, clinicians, or others to whom they can describe their concerns and symptoms, in hopes of reassurance, commiseration, or treatment. Other individuals, however, may be too timid or embarrassed or so limited by their anxiety that they feel they cannot disclose their symptoms to anyone and instead experience them in silence.

The basic emotion that is most prominent in the diagnostic class of anxiety disorders is fear. Fear is often closely associated with an external entity or physical context. Most people remember having such fears as children—for instance, fear of the dark or of particular animals. The disorder of specific phobia involves fear of a specific thing or circumstance that is severe enough in the person's life to cause distress and to have an adverse effect on how they live—for example, by avoiding situations in which they might encounter the feared thing or circumstance. Other phobic disorders may focus on more abstract situations. For instance, social anxiety disorder results from a fear of social encounters in which a person believes that they will be assessed by others. Separation anxiety disorder relates to a fear of being disconnected from a place or person to which the individual feels close. Agoraphobia includes a fear of being out in various public places and away from home by oneself. With these disorders, patients experience fear when exposed to the respective entity or circumstance. In the context of an anxiety disorder, fear is often coupled with behaviors that allow the person to avoid the feared entity or circumstance.

Panic attacks occurring in panic disorder also involve fear—but the hallmark in these situations is having sudden bouts of fear or the physical reactions associated with fear that then become upsetting and frightening—and at least some of these bouts of fear or the physical reactions are unpredictable and seem to occur with no clear explanation. Panic disorder is distinct from phobias because it does not require an external entity or circumstance to bring on the fear. Without an external factor required in panic disorder, what is causing the fear symptoms? Investigators continue to research this question. Some posit that the person's fear system is firing off aberrantly, like a "false alarm," because of abnormal neuronal activity. Others have suggested that internal, not external, stimuli are inducing the panic attacks. These stimuli might be physiological sensations (e.g., shortness of breath, palpitations), with or

TABLE 9–1.   Key changes between DSM-5 and DSM-5-TR

No major changes in diagnostic criteria for any anxiety disorder.

Social anxiety disorder is no longer called social phobia.

Association with suicidal thoughts or behavior has been added to most anxiety disorders. For example, a shift from suicidal thoughts to attempts is correlated more with panic disorder, generalized anxiety disorder, and specific phobia, rather than with other anxiety disorders.

Prevalence, development, and course of anxiety disorders have been updated in keeping with best evidence. For example, in some countries, the prevalence of social anxiety disorders seems to be rising.

Culture-related diagnostic issues have been updated, including the potential role of racism.

Diagnostic markers and risk and prognostic factors have been updated, including genetic and physiological factors, such as greater sensitivity to CO_2 inhalation in panic disorder.

without the patient's conscious awareness, that set off fear but that are not external or readily observed by others.

In generalized anxiety disorder (GAD), the prominent symptom is worrying. DSM-5-TR describes worry as "apprehensive expectation"—usually that adverse things are going to happen relating to several issues and areas of daily living (American Psychiatric Association 2022). This kind of relentless and widespread worrying is different from what is experienced by those who feel fear in the narrower context of a phobia. Additionally, the worry is generalized to several life issues and areas and may spread to more; therefore, it is not as circumscribed in a person's life as specific phobias.

Of note in DSM-5-TR is that agoraphobia, GAD, separation anxiety disorder, specific phobia, and social anxiety disorder require symptoms to occur during a period of at least 6 months to meet diagnostic criteria in adults. This duration specification excludes more transient episodes of symptoms and results in greater consistency in DSM-5-TR with regard to the time requirement across diagnoses in this diagnostic class.

Some DSM-IV (American Psychiatric Association 1994) disorders were removed from and others added to the anxiety disorders diagnostic class in DSM-5 (American Psychiatric Association 2013) and DSM-5-TR. For instance, OCD, PTSD, and acute stress disorder were moved from the DSM-IV anxiety disorders into other DSM-5 diagnostic classes. This reorganization emphasized certain unique features of the diagnoses, such as compulsive behaviors in OCD and exposure to a traumatic event in PTSD. Separation anxiety disorder and selective mutism, which had been part of the DSM-IV chapter "Disorders Usually First Diagnosed in Infancy, Childhood, or Adolescence," were moved into the DSM-5 anxiety disorders class. See Table 9–1 for changes made between DSM-5 and DSM-5-TR.

Additional disorders in the DSM-5-TR anxiety disorders diagnostic class include substance/medication-induced anxiety disorder, anxiety disorder due to another medical condition, other specified anxiety disorder, and unspecified anxiety disorder.

IN-DEPTH DIAGNOSIS: PANIC ATTACK AND PANIC DISORDER

Ms. Brown, a 20-year-old soldier, presents to a military hospital complaining of the abrupt start of "feeling like my heart is pounding" and "feeling out of breath." This is the fourth episode she has experienced like this in a couple of weeks. She is trembling and extremely scared about what is wrong with her body. The doctor runs several tests and notes that she is medically fine. Ms. Brown has recently been deployed, and this is her first time away from her hometown. She has not yet been in combat, and she has not been exposed to any traumatic experiences. She remarks that she cannot understand how this could be happening to her because she is in excellent shape, having just finished boot camp. She has not had problems with anxiety before and generally has not thought of herself as an excessively anxious person. She does not use alcohol or other substances, nor does she take substances or medications that may cause anxiety. She denies having homicidal or suicidal ideation, intent, or plans.

Young adults with panic attacks may present to emergency facilities with concerns that they are experiencing an acute medical problem. This interpretation of acute and extreme anxiety as a physical health complaint is a familiar presentation of panic attacks in an otherwise healthy person. If medical illness has been ruled out and the person meets the criteria for panic attacks, a diagnosis of panic disorder may be considered. Such a diagnosis might fit with Ms. Brown's recurring panic attacks starting in early adulthood and the attacks being unpredictable. Being female increases her risk of the diagnosis. If she has panic disorder, her reaction to and acceptance of this diagnosis in the context of the military culture should be discussed. Referral to psychiatry should be considered.

Approach to the Diagnosis

Many patients report anxiety symptoms and may even describe them as "panic attacks." Encouraging uniformity, DSM-5-TR purposely provides criteria for use of the term *panic attack*, defining it as symptoms that increase in minutes from low levels to a crescendo at a very high level, like a surprise attack. Purported "attacks" that gradually build over hours (e.g., "I worked myself into a panic attack throughout the day thinking about the evening date") do not meet the panic attack requirement for either a sudden onset or quick crescendo. Panic attacks must manifest four or more symptoms from a list that includes ones that are somatic (e.g., sweating) and others that are mainly psychological (e.g., fear of dying). Some patients may have fewer than four symptoms during attacks. These attacks, called *limited-symptom attacks* in DSM-5-TR, may be attenuated panic attacks or progenitors and will perhaps subsequently become part of a panic disorder. DSM-5-TR also describes nocturnal panic attacks that occur related to sleeping.

Bear in mind that the terms *panic attack* and *panic disorder* are not synonymous. Panic attacks are the key symptom in panic disorder, and panic disorder requires the presence of panic attacks. However, not everyone with panic attacks has panic disorder. The criteria for panic attacks and panic disorder are different. In DSM-5-TR, panic attack is not a disorder but is instead a specifier that may be added to DSM-5-TR disorders when panic attacks are noted in the context of a disorder. Thus, this specifier may be added to a variety of psychiatric or general medical disorders.

DSM-5-TR states that at least some of the panic attacks in panic disorder must be recurrent and unexpected. "Unexpected" refers to panic attacks that do not seem to be produced or generated by any stimuli and thus occur without warning. Patients experiencing unexpected panic attacks in panic disorder often describe their attacks as completely coming from "out of nowhere." Such spontaneous attacks have encouraged some researchers to look for an endogenous cause, including an endogenous chemical circulating in the body and dysregulated pulmonary measures.

Determining whether unexpected panic attacks are present may be subject to some interpretation because every patient (and culture) has different views on the causality of behaviors. For example, DSM-5-TR notes that, when asked in retrospect, older adults may be more prone than younger individuals to attribute anxiety symptoms to various events in the environment; this may result in less reporting of "unexpected" panic attacks.

Evaluation for the panic disorder diagnosis additionally requires ascertaining if trepidation about future panic attacks and behaviors to avoid panic attacks have developed. These secondary manifestations of panic disorder should be seen as distinct symptoms from panic attacks.

With regard to suicide, DSM-5-TR cites studies suggesting that panic disorder may be a risk factor for suicidal behaviors, and that suicidal thoughts may associate with cognitive symptoms of panic attacks while suicidal behaviors may associate with physical ones.

Getting the History

A 27-year-old patient reports having problems with "anxiety." The interviewer asks open-ended questions to determine whether the patient has "attacks" of anxiety "that come from nowhere" and that include four of the symptoms listed in the criteria for panic attacks. The exact mix of symptoms may vary, but the patient should have at least four of the symptoms during any given attack. The interviewer might seek clarification by asking, "Were the anxiety symptoms set off by something, or did they seem to come spontaneously? How long was the time between the start of the anxiety symptoms to their highest level?" The patient may respond that the symptoms were unexpected and the time was within a few minutes. The interviewer might ask, "Do you remember the very first attack ever?" and get a description and the context. The interviewer wants to know an estimate of the frequency and pattern of attacks since they started.

The interviewer then questions, "When you are not having a panic attack, do you have any other symptoms?" The interviewer wants to know if the patient notes anxiety about having future attacks. This would be a different type of anxiety than the panic attack symptoms. The interviewer wants to know: "How do these symptoms affect your daily activities? Are you not doing certain things because of the symptoms?" The patient may note avoiding various public places. The interviewer asks about the patient having homicidal or suicidal thoughts, intent, or plans; alcohol and other substance use; use of substances or medications that may cause anxiety; and signs and symptoms of medical disorders.

This patient describes symptoms that may meet criteria for panic attacks and has had several attacks, some without any trigger or warning. Symptoms are extreme, sudden in onset, and hit the highest point in minutes. The interviewer ascertains whether the patient has frequent concerns about when the next panic attack will strike or what will happen to the patient during an attack. The interviewer assesses if the patient is avoiding going places because of the panic attacks, perhaps because they will not be able to easily escape or get help in these places or because attacks have occurred in these places previously. A medical workup, history of alcohol and other substance use, and history relevant to suicide and homicide are obtained. Referral to psychiatry is considered.

Tips for Clarifying the Diagnosis

- Ask the individual who reports being "anxious" or "nervous" to describe their exact experience, including physical sensations, thoughts, feelings, and behaviors.
- Clarify the time course of the symptoms: how quickly do they start, crescendo, and then tail off?
- Quantify how often panic attacks occur.
- Investigate whether any of the panic attacks occur without warning or cause.
- Evaluate whether the individual has other types of anxiety, such as trepidation about having future panic attacks.
- Determine whether any behaviors (e.g., not going to places) have developed to avoid panic attacks. If so, ask how often and long these behaviors have been occurring.

Consider the Case

Mr. Young, a 35-year-old Navajo man, presents to a primary care physician in the Indian Health Service. He had received a diagnosis of panic disorder in his early twenties. He sometimes has one or more panic attacks each day. The longest he has gone without panic attacks is a few months. Panic disorder has greatly affected his quality of life, and he has not been able to work or to participate in the ceremonies and dances that have been an important part of his life and role in his community. He has started to be concerned about when the next panic attack will strike and has stopped spending time at some public places. The places in which he feels comfortable have become progressively limited. For the past few years, he has had trouble leaving his tribal land, and now his home has become the only truly comfortable place. Recently, he has even had some panic attacks in this home. His symptoms cause him to experience low self-esteem. For the past couple of years, he has felt "depressed." His primary care physician says they have ruled out any medical disorder. He denies using substances other than alcohol or taking substances or medications that may cause anxiety. He is unclear about his alcohol use. He denies having homicidal or suicidal ideation, intent, or plans.

Beginning in early adulthood, panic disorder can be a chronic disorder that adversely affects people during what should be their most productive years. It may remit, but it often recurs. In addition to having the panic attacks, Mr. Young began to be anxious about when the next panic attack would occur. He also found that he was not going to many places because of panic attacks, and eventually he had trouble going anywhere outside his home. A comorbid major depressive disorder may now be complicating his condition. The clinician should explore Mr. Young's alcohol use further, consider the possible diagnosis of alcohol use disorder, and continue to check regularly if Mr. Young is having homicidal or suicidal ideation, intent, or plans. Some people use alcohol to ease their panic attacks. The risk for alcohol use disorder and suicide are of note in this case. The clinician will want to understand how Mr. Young's symptoms are viewed and managed within the dynamics of his family. Referral to psychiatry should be considered.

Differential Diagnosis

The differential diagnosis of panic disorder is quite broad because the hallmark of panic disorder is having panic attacks, which may occur in the context of many other disorders. Possible diagnoses may be divided into nonpsychiatric and psychiatric disorders. The former include several general medical disorders (e.g., cardiac arrhythmias, asthma), which necessitates appropriate medical workup. Panic attacks may also be seen in many psychiatric disorders, such as other anxiety disorders. If the panic attacks occur only in relation to symptoms of another anxiety disorder, then the other anxiety disorder is given diagnostic priority. For instance, if panic attacks happen solely in social circumstances that induce fear because of social anxiety disorder, then the diagnosis of social anxiety disorder takes priority; panic attacks might be used as a specifier, and the diagnosis of panic disorder would not be recorded. In other words, these are expected panic attacks in social circumstances in a patient with social anxiety disorder.

In cases of comorbid panic disorder and another disorder that may be associated with panic attacks, the clinician would look for evidence of at least some panic attacks that are not restricted to the context of the other disorder, that are unexpected, and that are attributable solely to the panic disorder. This pattern is important because panic disorder is highly comorbid with several disorders, such as other anxiety disorders, major depressive disorder, and bipolar disorder.

Patients may experience both panic disorder and agoraphobia. As noted in DSM-5-TR, the onset of panic attacks or panic disorder may antedate that of agoraphobia, as described by 30% of people with agoraphobia in community samples and at least 50% of those in clinical samples. Conversely, panic disorder may appear to follow agoraphobia in other cases. A diagnosis of agoraphobia is made if its criteria are met, regardless of whether panic disorder is present.

See DSM-5-TR for additional disorders to consider in the differential diagnosis. Also refer to the discussions of comorbidity and differential diagnosis in their respective sections of DSM-5-TR.

Summary

- When clinically significant anxiety symptoms are present, the clinician should determine whether the symptoms meet criteria for panic attacks and with which disorders these panic attacks might be associated.

- If panic attacks are present and some occur repeatedly and without warning, then the clinician should evaluate for panic disorder, including the patient's trepidation about subsequent panic attacks and their behaviors to avoid panic attacks.
- A careful history going back to the first anxiety symptoms should be taken to assess the frequency and natural course of the symptoms.
- The differential diagnosis of panic disorder includes the careful ruling out of a wide range of psychiatric disorders (including other anxiety disorders and substance use disorders) and general medical conditions.

IN-DEPTH DIAGNOSIS: SOCIAL ANXIETY DISORDER (SOCIAL PHOBIA)

James, a 14-year-old Hispanic teen, is seen for an outpatient evaluation at a pediatric clinic in the southeastern United States. He has consistently become very anxious when interacting with others. His parents encourage him to "hang out" with kids in their neighborhood, but he cannot make himself do this. Every social circumstance feels overwhelming to him, even if his parents are present. During the evaluation, he does not have any problems with speaking. He wants to participate in high school activities and to go out with friends, but he has not pursued any of these activities for fear that he will make a fool of himself and become embarrassed. He says that he thinks he will not be seen as "macho"—he wants to be "machismo" but thinks he will be teased for being "nervous" instead. He says he cannot be "in public." He mainly stays at home, surfs the internet, and does his homework. He aspires to go to a professional school of some sort, but recently he has begun to worry about whether he can even finish high school because of his nervousness. He denies any physical symptoms, and the results of his recent medical workup were normal. He does not use alcohol or other substances and does not take substances or medications that may cause anxiety. He denies having homicidal or suicidal ideation, intent, or plans.

James has always been an anxious child in social circumstances, including those with other children. Apparently, he experiences this anxiety even if his parents are present, and thus it does not seem related to separation anxiety. He never had a childhood period of not speaking in social situations and thus did not have symptoms of selective mutism. Now in high school, he is finding that his life is greatly limited by his social anxiety, and he and his parents are finally seeking professional help. As an adolescent, he is able to describe his major concern, which is that he will make a fool of himself in front of other adolescents who will then reject him. The clinician might explore how his desire to be "macho" plays a role in his social anxiety and whether there is any cultural basis for it. Referral to psychiatry should be considered.

Approach to the Diagnosis

Individuals with social anxiety disorder fear assessment and disapproval by others. They fear they will in some way appear foolish and feel shame. This fear may include concern that people will see overt signs of their social anxiety disorder, particularly blushing. A diagnosis of social anxiety disorder involves fear that is disproportionate to the real risk of embarrassment.

People with social anxiety disorder avoid social circumstances that may be potentially embarrassing, resulting in an inability to function in social roles, such as an unwillingness to go to job interviews, doctor's appointments, or family gatherings. This disorder often starts before adulthood. Children may become tearful or upset when faced with going to school. When forced to attend social activities, the person may fret in advance and report significant distress during the activity. During the event, they may act bashful and reserved and hardly speak. The effects of avoiding social situations may be evidenced by difficulty with working, dating, or forming romantic relationships. For these reasons, social anxiety disorder may become extremely disabling.

Getting the History

During a routine physical examination, a 20-year-old patient reports rarely leaving the house. The physician asks in an open-ended and nonjudgmental manner, "Why don't you leave your house?" They explore whether the patient fears going places, being away from home, or having a panic attack in public. The patient expresses fears about interacting with people but does not say why. The physician pursues the issue further: "Are you afraid someone will hurt you or that you will embarrass yourself?" The patient quietly nods to the latter several times with shame but does not voluntarily elaborate. After a pause, the physician asks, "Are you afraid of doing things in front of other people such as saying the wrong thing or doing something wrong?" The physician evaluates whether any of these fears seem delusional or simply suggest a concern that others will be critical of the patient in social contexts, and tries to ascertain whether the patient has symptoms of a major depressive disorder, autism spectrum disorder, or other disorders. Moving on, the physician asks, "Would you have interest in leaving the house and in socializing if it weren't for these anxiety symptoms?" and inquires how long the patient has had the symptoms and whether they have lasted longer than 6 months. The physician checks for whether the patient has homicidal or suicidal ideation, intent, or plans; meets criteria for alcohol and other substance use disorders; is taking substances or medications that may cause anxiety; or has signs and symptoms of medical disorders. Next, the physician carefully revisits why the patient is reluctant to leave the house, bearing in mind that social anxiety may make talking about this difficult (e.g., fearing the physician's disapproval). They also consider other psychiatric conditions that may be responsible for the symptoms, such as agoraphobia, or the possibility that the patient stays at home because they lack interest in seeing other people.

The physician questions the patient about duration to determine if it meets the time criterion. If an adult patient says that their symptoms began 6 months ago, this duration would meet the criterion but would indicate first onset in adulthood. Adult onset is unusual and would put the diagnosis of social anxiety disorder in some question. The criteria are only guidelines, however, and must always be applied in the context of good clinical common sense and judgment. Of note, the physician checks for whether the patient has homicidal or suicidal risks. Referral to psychiatry should be considered.

Tips for Clarifying the Diagnosis

- Establish whether the person has relatively predictable anxiety symptoms in social circumstances in which others may assess them and be disapproving.

- In children, determine whether the symptoms are evident in social circumstances with other children.
- Determine how long these symptoms have been occurring (6 months is required).
- When social anxiety occurs only in public speaking or performance circumstances, the DSM-5-TR "performance only" specifier may apply.

Consider the Case

Mr. Andrews is a 52-year-old single Black man who seeks evaluation by a psychiatrist via a telemedicine program in the rural southern United States. His internist set up this evaluation to help with the patient's anxiety, which prevents him from going out socially. Talking over a telemedicine connection, Mr. Andrews recollects the gradual development of relatively consistent anxiety in social situations; he is unsure when it began exactly. In high school, he was too anxious to socialize with others. He was able to finish high school but kept to himself because he feared that others would laugh at him for doing or saying something wrong. He has always wanted to have friends and to be social. Now, he would like to start going out with coworkers after work but is afraid he will make a fool of himself in various ways. He is able to decrease his anxiety when interacting with people only by drinking alcohol. He has been unsuccessful in trying to stop drinking several times. His internist says he is medically healthy. He does not use substances other than alcohol nor does he take substances or medications that may cause anxiety. He denies homicidal or suicidal ideation, intent, or plans. He has been reluctant to go to a mental health clinic because of the stigma of mental illness in his culture and the possibility that a clinician will diagnosis him as "crazy."

Mr. Andrews began to have difficulties with anxiety early in life. His social anxiety had a gradual onset, as in many cases; in contrast, some people will report a precipitating event that usually involves becoming embarrassed. He appears to have experienced chronic symptoms of social anxiety disorder ever since his youth, and these symptoms are still limiting his lifestyle. He very much wishes to have friends, so the anxiety clearly is causing problems in his life. In social circumstances, he intentionally drinks alcohol to lessen his social anxiety. He is having trouble stopping his drinking and needs to be assessed for alcohol use disorder; consultation with an addiction psychiatrist should be considered. Some patients may appear to use alcohol or other substances to manage their social anxiety disorder. The clinician should explore whether the use of a telemedicine connection helps or hinders the interview for this socially anxious patient. The issue of stigma and the influences of rural culture, racial or ethnic identity, and racism need to be addressed.

Differential Diagnosis

DSM-5-TR includes many disorders in the section on differential diagnosis; social anxiety disorder may be parsed out by determining whether fear about potential assessment and disapproval is the primary reason for these symptoms. If present, alternative causes of this fear require examination. Such a fear may be part of an avoidant personality disorder. Concern with disapproval may indicate poor self-esteem and a major depressive disorder; in such cases, other symptoms of depression should also be present. The social anxiety disorder diagnosis is most clear when extreme fear of social assessment is the central—and perhaps the only—symptom when the person is exposed to potential assessment by others.

Many patients do experience social anxiety disorder along with other disorders. In some instances, these co-occurring disorders (e.g., major depressive disorder, substance use disorder) appear after the onset of social anxiety disorder, which suggests—but does not prove—a secondary relationship. Differentiating avoidant personality disorder from social anxiety disorder can be complicated because of their overlapping symptoms.

See DSM-5-TR for additional disorders to consider in the differential diagnosis. Also refer to the discussions of comorbidity and differential diagnosis in their respective sections of DSM-5-TR.

Summary

- Individuals with social anxiety disorder fear assessment and disapproval in social situations.
- Social anxiety disorder often starts before adulthood; initial onset in adulthood is uncommon.
- Social anxiety disorder can result in significant dysfunction.
- Social anxiety disorder must be differentiated from several psychiatric disorders that have an impact on socialization. Additionally, it must be separated from normative bashfulness and avoidant personality disorder.
- Social anxiety disorder may be comorbid with a number of other disorders.

IN-DEPTH DIAGNOSIS: GENERALIZED ANXIETY DISORDER

Ms. Armstrong, a 35-year-old woman, is seen in a medical clinic on a military base in the southern United States. Her husband is an active-duty serviceman. She tells her primary care physician about muscle aches and tension that inhibit her from doing many activities. Later, she also admits to worrying "day and night." She has been this way since adolescence and had assumed that everyone felt this way until her friends began to point out that she is a "worrier." She worries about anything that comes up in her daily life, and as soon as one thing turns out okay, she will move on to worry about something else. She denies symptoms of other types of anxiety disorders. She does not take substances or medications that may cause anxiety and does not use alcohol or other substances. She denies having homicidal or suicidal ideation, intent, or plans. The results of a complete medical workup are normal, and the symptoms do not appear to be caused by a medical condition or a side effect of a medication.

After determining that the patient has no medical issues that might be producing her muscle aches, tension, and other symptoms, the physician evaluates whether these physical symptoms might be associated with an anxiety disorder. This line of questioning leads Ms. Armstrong to reveal that she has been a "lifelong worrier" and that her friends have noticed that she is always worrying. It is a way of life for her. Worry is ever present, associated with one life task after another, and wears her down with muscle tension and always being vigilant for peril. Further psychiatric evaluation should investigate whether Ms. Armstrong meets the full criteria for GAD. The presence of a comorbid major depressive disorder should be considered. The influences of both her southern and military family cultures on the patient's perception of her symptoms should be examined. Referral to psychiatry should be considered.

Approach to the Diagnosis

Comparing the DSM-5-TR criteria for GAD with those of the other anxiety disorders, readers will note an emphasis on symptoms of excessive worry, rather than fear. Worry is described in DSM-5-TR as "apprehensive expectation." Worrying has a pervasive nature that lingers and is always in the back of the person's mind. These qualities of the constant "worrier" are key to this diagnosis.

Getting the History

A 50-year-old patient seeing a psychotherapist complains of "nervousness." The therapist says, "People sometimes mean different things when they use that term. Tell me more about what you are experiencing." The patient describes broad-spectrum symptoms of worrying. The therapist subsequently asks, "Please give me a specific example of something you were worried about—for instance, what did you worry about this morning?" The patient describes a variety of everyday concerns across different areas of living that the patient magnifies in terms of the risk of adverse outcomes. The therapist asks more questions to rule out that the worrying is not focused on panic attacks; social anxiety; an obsession; separation from someone close to the patient; body image or weight; physical complaints, illness, or abnormalities; a past trauma; or other causes. To determine whether their worry occurs to a delusional extent or is related to other disorders, such as a mood disorder, they ask, "How does this worrying impact your life? Does it cause you to live a certain way?" The patient denies having homicidal or suicidal ideation, intent, or plans; does not use alcohol or other substances; and does not take substances or medications that may cause anxiety. No medical problems are identified.

The therapist immediately realizes that the patient needs to be more specific in reporting their symptoms and does not automatically assume knowledge of what the patient means when they use the term "nervousness." The therapist asks open-ended questions regarding the patient's experience of their symptoms and then asks more focused questions to obtain specific examples of the symptoms and the contexts in which they occur. Asking patients to describe specific examples of their worries helps the therapist determine whether the patient meets the diagnostic criteria for GAD. The therapist methodically rules out other anxiety disorders, mood disorders, psychotic disorders, and other potential diagnoses (e.g., substance/medication-induced anxiety disorder, anxiety disorder due to another medical condition) and checks whether the patient is having homicidal or suicidal ideation, intent, or plans. Finally, using a very open-ended and nonjudgmental question, they inquire how the patient's life is affected by their symptoms and subsequently explore for any abnormal behaviors associated with the patient's anxiety. The therapist considers referring the patient to a psychiatrist.

Tips for Clarifying the Diagnosis

- Ask whether the person experiences pervasive worrying that is hard to manage.
- Find out whether the worrying involves several issues and areas of life.
- Quantify how often the person worries and how long worries last.

Consider the Case

> Robert, an 11-year-old boy, has been "super" nervous, so his parents made an appointment with his pediatrician. He tells the pediatrician that he feels "tense" and restless all the time. He is a terrific student, but he worries about day-to-day schoolwork, club activities, and athletic contests. He finds that he cannot stop worrying. As his pediatrician takes more history, they learn that Robert has also been quite sad and may be experiencing a major depressive episode. Robert denies having homicidal or suicidal ideation, intent, or plans. He denies use of alcohol or other substances and does not take substances or medications that may cause anxiety. The results of a careful workup do not provide a medical diagnosis to explain the symptoms.

Although Robert may have GAD, the diagnosis is not clear and the mean age at onset tends to be older. His symptoms are relatively nonspecific and, as noted in DSM-5-TR, clinicians must be careful about making this diagnosis too readily in children. He describes several symptoms that may relate to GAD, including feeling tense and restless and worrying about day-to-day stresses. Nevertheless, the clinician must be sure that these symptoms are not better explained by other conditions that may manifest with anxiety (e.g., OCD). Robert may also be experiencing a major depressive episode, which further complicates the diagnostic picture. His anxiety symptoms may all be related to the major depressive disorder. The diagnosis of GAD is not made if the anxiety symptoms occur only in the presence of a major depression—if this is the case, then the anxiety symptoms are considered part of the depressive disorder, and an additional diagnosis of GAD is not recorded. The GAD diagnosis may be considered if there has been a time when the anxiety symptoms were present and major depression was not. Robert is referred to psychiatry for careful evaluation and diagnosis.

Differential Diagnosis

Many disorders include symptoms of worrying. Patients with major depressive disorder, bipolar disorder, and psychotic disorders frequently experience some anxiety and worry. When the worrying is present only during episodes of these disorders, an additional diagnosis of GAD should not be made. Worrying not only is frequent in other disorders but also is a normal state from time to time for most people. Thus, GAD is more likely in individuals who demonstrate more general worrying in isolation from other disorders and whose worrying is more extreme, extensive, and chronic than "normal" worry.

GAD is quite often comorbid with other disorders, such as mood disorders. To ensure the relative separateness of GAD and another disorder, symptoms of GAD should be seen during some periods when the other disorder is not present.

See DSM-5-TR for additional disorders to consider in the differential diagnosis. Also refer to the discussions of comorbidity and differential diagnosis in their respective sections of DSM-5-TR.

Summary

- In GAD, the symptoms picture emphasizes pervasive worrying about multiple issues and areas of daily life.
- Worrying is associated with certain specified symptoms (see DSM-5-TR criteria).
- The symptoms of GAD are often chronic, with waxing and waning courses.
- Worrying is so frequent in both normal and pathological states that the diagnosis of GAD should not be made unless its symptoms clearly depart from normal levels and cause dysfunction.
- GAD is often comorbid with mood disorders.

SUMMARY: ANXIETY DISORDERS

Anxiety is ubiquitous; at times the experience of anxiety is expected and adaptive, and at other times it can be pathological. The diagnostic class of anxiety disorders includes disorders with fear, panic attacks, worry, or anxiety, and it may include behaviors to avoid these states. This grouping suggests some commonality across these disorders, which in DSM-5-TR are considered to be distinct from OCD and PTSD. Despite these commonalities among the disorders in this diagnostic class, they are certainly heterogeneous, for example with regard to age at onset. Some disorders in this class are relatively common and can cause significant distress and impact on the person's life, along with an increased risk of suicide attempts and ideation in some cases.

ELEMENTS TO CONSIDER IN THE CULTURAL FORMULATION

- U.S. multicultural subpopulation–reported prevalence figures for social anxiety disorder, panic disorder, and GAD, from higher to lower, are as follows: White> Hispanic≈Black>Asian (Asnaani et al. 2010).
- Cultural explanatory models of bodily symptoms can influence the presentation of anxiety disorders. For example, the Cambodian idea that neck soreness is caused by dangerous "wind" inside the body may result in neck soreness triggering panic attacks.
- Many anxiety disorders are more common in females than in males.
- Exposure to racism may be a risk factor or associated feature in social anxiety disorder, panic disorder, and GAD.

DIAGNOSTIC PEARLS

- In separation anxiety disorder, specific phobia, social anxiety disorder, and agoraphobia, different entities or circumstances external to the individual bring on symptoms of fear or anxiety.

- In panic disorder, bouts of fear (panic attacks) occur repeatedly and unpredictably (without clear external cause).

- In generalized anxiety disorder, a core symptom is worrying, described in DSM-5-TR as "apprehensive expectation," about several issues and areas of daily living.

- Among anxiety disorders, separation anxiety disorder is the most common anxiety disorder among people younger than 12.

- In selective mutism, the person does not speak in certain social circumstances, even though their speech is quite normal otherwise, for instance at home with family members.

- The anxiety disorders diagnostic class includes disorders with prominent symptoms of fear, panic attacks, worry, or anxiety. In DSM-5-TR, some disorders with similar symptoms (e.g., OCD, PTSD) are seen as diagnostically separate from this class and have been put in other classes.

- A necessary consideration is whether the symptoms of anxiety disorders may be caused by substances or medications or be due to another medical condition; each possibility has its own diagnostic code in DSM-5-TR. These disorders may also co-occur with anxiety disorders.

- In many anxiety disorders, individuals may develop behaviors to avoid entities or circumstances that they associate with anxiety symptoms (e.g., staying away from social events).

SELF-ASSESSMENT

Key Concepts: Double-Check Your Knowledge

What is the relevance of the following concepts to the various anxiety disorders?

- Agoraphobic situations
- Avoidance behaviors
- Excessive worry
- Performance only
- Phobic objects and situations
- Public scrutiny and negative evaluation
- Recurrent and unexpected panic attacks
- Restlessness and muscle tension
- Selective mutism
- Worries about panic attacks

Questions to Discuss With Colleagues and Mentors

1. Do you screen all new patients for anxiety disorders, and if so, what questions do you use to screen for each disorder? For example, how do you screen for panic attacks?
2. If a patient has symptoms of fear or worry, what laboratory tests and medical workup do you pursue?
3. What are your typical reactions (e.g., feeling anxious yourself, becoming impatient, wanting to comfort) when you are with anxious people, and how do you manage your reactions in the therapeutic setting?

Case-Based Questions

PART A

Ms. Butler, a 36-year-old woman, describes having had anxiety problems for more than 10 years that have progressively worsened and for which she has never received treatment. She is so "nervous" that she does not go out of her house. She has meals delivered to her and cannot visit her doctor. She has never been able to work. Her family doctor makes a home visit to her in a rural area of the Pacific Northwest. She tells them, "I worry all the time, and I have anxiety that lasts all day long." The results of her current medical workup are normal. She denies using alcohol or any other substances or taking any substances or medications that may cause anxiety. She denies having homicidal or suicidal ideation, intent, or plans. Her family doctor has asked her to see a psychiatrist.

Assuming she has one or more anxiety disorder(s), what are reasons why she does not leave the house?   With the limited history obtained at this point, the clinician might think of a variety of reasons for her not leaving the house, including having agoraphobia, being afraid of having panic attacks away from home, or fearing social anxiety if she encounters people.

PART B

Ms. Butler says she does not leave the house because she fears having a panic attack outside the house when she is by herself. Further discussion reveals that she meets DSM-5-TR criteria for panic disorder. Even at home, she worries all the time.

How do you ascertain if she has generalized anxiety disorder (GAD) in addition to panic disorder?   In GAD, the concerns should not be about having another panic attack. She should have anxiety about issues and areas in daily life and have symptoms of GAD during times when she does not have panic disorder symptoms.

Short-Answer Questions

1. In adults, at least how long must the duration be for a diagnosis of specific phobia, social anxiety disorder, generalized anxiety disorder, agoraphobia, and separation anxiety disorder?

2. Rank in order from youngest to oldest the age at onset for panic disorder, specific phobia, and social anxiety disorder.
3. What are two characteristics required of at least some of the panic attacks in panic disorder?
4. During a panic attack, what is the typical length of time from the onset of symptoms to the maximum level of symptoms?
5. Why do social situations make patients with social anxiety disorder anxious?
6. Worrying is the cardinal feature of which of the following disorders: agoraphobia, generalized anxiety disorder, panic disorder, or social anxiety disorder?
7. In both separation anxiety disorder and agoraphobia, individuals may fear being alone. Contrast the reasons for not wanting to be alone in these two disorders.
8. List a substance that may be associated with substance-induced anxiety disorder, either during intoxication or withdrawal.
9. What is the relationship between panic disorder and suicide attempts or suicidal ideation?
10. May patients with social anxiety disorder have other DSM-5-TR disorders at the same time?

Answers

1. The duration must be 6 months in adults for these diagnoses.

2. The rank order for age at onset is as follows: specific phobia (median ages 7–11 years) < social anxiety disorder (median age 13) < panic disorder (median ages 20–24).

3. Panic attacks required in panic disorder are repeated and unpredicted.

4. Symptoms of a panic attack peak usually within a few minutes.

5. People with social anxiety disorder fear possible assessment and disapproval by others.

6. Worrying is a key feature of generalized anxiety disorder.

7. Individuals with separation anxiety disorder fear being disconnected from a person to whom they are close, whereas people with agoraphobia fear being in places where they will not be able to flee or get help.

8. The following are examples of substances that may be associated with substance-induced anxiety disorder: intoxication from alcohol, cocaine, caffeine, cannabis, hallucinogens, inhalants, and phencyclidine or withdrawal from alcohol, opioids, cocaine, sedatives, hypnotics, and anxiolytics.

9. A diagnosis of panic disorder is related to a greater risk of suicide behaviors and suicidal thoughts.

10. Yes. Not uncommonly, patients with social anxiety disorder may also meet criteria for other DSM-5-TR disorders, such as substance use disorders and major depressive disorder.

REFERENCES

American Psychiatric Association: Diagnostic and Statistical Manual of Mental Disorders, 4th Edition. Washington, DC, American Psychiatric Association, 1994

American Psychiatric Association: Diagnostic and Statistical Manual of Mental Disorders, 5th Edition. Arlington, VA, American Psychiatric Association, 2013

American Psychiatric Association: Diagnostic and Statistical Manual of Mental Disorders, 5th Edition, Text Revision. Washington, DC, American Psychiatric Association, 2022

Asnaani A, Richey JA, Dimaite R, et al: A cross-ethnic comparison of lifetime prevalence rates of anxiety disorders. J Nerv Ment Dis 198(8):551–555, 2010 20699719

CHAPTER 10

Obsessive-Compulsive and Related Disorders

Elias Aboujaoude, M.D., M.A.

Robert M. Holaway, Ph.D.

Richa Bhatia, M.D.

"I know I shouldn't but I can't stop pulling out my eyebrows."

"His hands are raw because he washes his hands so many times during the day."

- Obsessive-Compulsive Disorder
- Body Dysmorphic Disorder
- Hoarding Disorder
- Trichotillomania
- Excoriation (Skin-Picking) Disorder
- Substance/Medication-Induced Obsessive-Compulsive and Related Disorder
- Obsessive-Compulsive and Related Disorder Due to Another Medical Condition
- Other Specified Obsessive-Compulsive and Related Disorder
- Unspecified Obsessive-Compulsive and Related Disorder

The obsessive-compulsive and related disorders in DSM-5-TR include obsessive-compulsive disorder (OCD, the organizing "anchor" and the condition that has been given the most research attention), body dysmorphic disorder (BDD), hoarding disorder, trichotillomania (hair-pulling disorder), and excoriation (skin-picking) disorder (American Psychiatric Association 2022). Other diagnostic entries in this category involve presentations attributable to substance use (substance-induced obsessive-compulsive and related disorders), medical etiologies (obsessive-compulsive and related disorder due to another medical condition), other specified obsessive-compulsive and related disorder (e.g., nail biting, lip biting, cheek chewing), and atypical manifestations (unspecified obsessive-compulsive and related disorder). In DSM-5-TR, olfactory reference disorder (olfactory reference syndrome) has been added to other specified obsessive-compulsive and related disorder and is characterized by the persistent preoccupation that one emits a foul or offensive body odor that is unnoticeable or only slightly noticeable to others, often accompanied by repetitive and excessive behaviors such as repeatedly checking for body odor, showering excessively, or seeking reassurance. There are differences as well as overlap among these disorders with regard to diagnosis and treatment. Given their comorbidity and relatedness to each other, individuals presenting with any of the conditions listed here should also be screened for the others in the group.

As with any disorder, a thorough clinical assessment is crucial to an accurate diagnosis and effective treatment and requires a review of the various elements of the case history, including the chief complaint; history of present illness; stressors and precipitants; medical and psychiatric histories and comorbidities; current and past medications; developmental, cultural, and social backgrounds; family history; review of systems; mental status examination; and distress, time consumed, and impairment in functioning caused by the presenting symptom—personally, academically, and professionally.

When assessing someone with suspected OCD, specifically, it is important to recognize that although the symptoms can be highly unique and variable, they typically fall under a limited number of general themes. The most common obsessional themes include contamination fears, pathological doubt, somatic concerns, symmetry worries, and disturbing thoughts, images, or impulses of an aggressive, sexual, or religious nature. Similarly, the most common compulsive themes include checking, cleaning, counting, reassurance seeking, repeating, and mental rituals. The "Approach to the Diagnosis" section in the main discussion of OCD later in this chapter provides more details and specific examples.

Other obsessive-compulsive and related disorders warrant specifically tailored questions. In an individual with suspected hoarding disorder, for example, the clinician should investigate the meaning of the person's collections, the function they might fulfill, their impact on the safety and "health" of the living space, and the balance of input into and output from that space. In an individual with suspected BDD, excoriation disorder, or trichotillomania, the clinician should explore whether cosmetic surgery, extreme self-grooming, and dermatological interventions are misunderstood and overvalued as shortcuts to "perfection." Inquiry into deeper self-esteem deficits that may be manifesting with a somatic fixation is also important.

TABLE 10–1. Key changes between DSM-5 and DSM-5-TR

Olfactory reference disorder has been added to other specified obsessive-compulsive and related disorder.

Section on OCD now includes sensory phenomena (e.g., physical sensations, just-right sensations, and feelings of incompleteness that tend to precede compulsions and are common in OCD).

Cultural considerations have been updated to better incorporate cultural factors because they can significantly affect presentation and diagnosis.

Sex- and gender-related and genetic factors have been updated to reflect recent evidence. For body dysmorphic disorder, the heritability is thought to be as high as 37%–49%.

Association with suicidality has been updated. Suicidality is highly prevalent in OCD and is particularly linked with severity of OCD, with having unacceptable thoughts, and with severity of comorbid depressive and anxiety disorders. Body dysmorphic disorder is thought to confer a higher likelihood of suicidal ideation than OCD, eating disorders, or anxiety disorders.

While assessing for possible obsessive-compulsive and related disorders, the clinician should consider questions about the sociocultural context within which the problem is occurring. For example, in a religious individual who spends many hours daily in prayer, when do the religious thoughts become an intrusive "symptom," and when does ritualized praying become a mental compulsion? In a superstitious individual who was raised in a superstitious culture, when does rigid avoidance of certain anxiety-producing stimuli become a treatable OCD symptom and when should it be viewed as part of that individual's cultural norm? In the person whose family has survived famine and war, when does the accumulation of food and other necessities become a hoarding compulsion worthy of urgent clinical attention, and when is it a self-protective and justifiable reaction to a history of loss and deprivation? And given society's body image fixation and saturation with body-enhancing interventions, when do individuals with heightened appearance anxiety or excessive grooming behaviors cross the threshold into pathological BDD, trichotillomania, or excoriation disorder? A careful examination of the larger sociocultural space within which the repetitive thoughts or behaviors are arising, as well as attention to any associated negative consequences, helps answer these questions. Please see Table 10–1 for suicidality in OCD and for other recent updates in the diagnosis and prevalence of obsessive-compulsive and related disorders.

IN-DEPTH DIAGNOSIS: OBSESSIVE-COMPULSIVE DISORDER

Ms. Hansen is a 35-year-old university librarian. She presents to her first psychotherapy visit for help with intrusive thoughts focused on a form of contamination fear that she has struggled with since her early 20s. Back then, for no apparent reason, Ms. Hansen began worrying that the water supply in the house she shared with her three college roommates was contaminated by the sewer system. As a result, she started having trouble drinking the water at her house and started avoiding using the bathroom for fear she might worsen the problem and contaminate her housemates' potable water. Since then, this concern has forced Ms. Hansen to relocate numerous times, but each move would give her only a brief respite before her fears recurred, typically a few months after each move, causing significant anxiety and prompting yet another relocation. Over the years, Ms. Hansen has sought reassurance through numerous expensive consultations and inspections with plumbers, architects, and general contractors, as well as several laboratory tests meant to test water quality. None of these measures, however, provided sustained relief.

Ms. Hansen currently spends 3 hours per day worrying about cross contamination between the clean water and waste systems in her house or seeking reassurance that the two have not become somehow linked. She blames her preoccupation with this problem on her limited social life and absence of romantic relationships. Except for moderate depression that typically follows each move, Ms. Hansen has not experienced other psychiatric symptoms, including tics. She has been physically healthy all her life. She drinks alcohol rarely and has never used other substances. When asked by her new therapist to describe the problem that caused her to seek help, Ms. Hansen gives this preface to her answer: "I know this is crazy and makes absolutely no sense, but I can't help worrying about it."

Based on this brief history, Ms. Hansen's symptoms would appear to meet the DSM-5-TR criteria for OCD. She has recurrent, bothersome, intrusive thoughts focused on contamination fears (the obsession) and multiple attempts at obtaining reassurance through inspections and laboratory tests (the compulsion). Her life has been significantly affected as a direct result of her symptoms: the multiple moves have undoubtedly created much instability for her, and her time-consuming preoccupations and self-reassuring actions have precluded a meaningful social or romantic life. Because she has no other medical, psychiatric, or substance use problems that might explain her symptoms, her presentation cannot be attributed to causes other than OCD. Moreover, despite her inability to control her symptoms on her own, Ms. Hansen clearly realizes the irrationality of her symptoms. As such, she would be characterized as having "good insight" into her condition.

Approach to the Diagnosis

Most people have habits that they perform in set or unusual ways or have intrusive worries that may strike another person as odd or irrelevant. Yet most individuals do not have OCD. The key to making the OCD diagnosis is to evaluate the degree of negative effect or impairment the behaviors have on the person's life and how consuming and distressing these behaviors and thoughts are—not their mere presence.

A comprehensive interview should help the clinician arrive at an accurate diagnosis and implement a successful treatment plan. An empathetic, nonjudgmental approach is crucial, along with a systematic effort to cover all important elements of the presentation, including the chief complaint, history of present illness, stressors and precipitants, medical and psychiatric histories, medication history, developmental and social backgrounds, family history, review of systems, mental status examination, and consequences of the presenting problem to the person's life.

When approaching a person with suspected OCD, the clinician must keep in mind that individual obsessions or compulsions can vary greatly among people but that they generally fall under a limited number of themes. Tables 10–2 and 10–3 cover common obsessional and compulsive themes seen in OCD, with examples of each. The clinician should ask questions that explore the various themes, how individual obsessions and compulsions may have changed over time, and whether one or more symptoms are currently occurring. Along with these themes, sensory phenomena, which can be described as physical sensations, just-right sensations, and feelings of incompleteness, are common in OCD and should be explored.

The clinician should remember that the content of obsessions or the details of rituals can be highly embarrassing and heavily guarded secrets, adding to the stigma many people feel about seeking psychiatric care or divulging symptoms. An open mind, nonjudgmental attitude, and empathetic approach are therefore indispensable if people are to feel at ease sharing information about their obsessions and compulsions and if mental health professionals are to succeed in helping them.

Importantly, suicidal thoughts occur at some point in nearly half of individuals with OCD, and suicide attempts have been reported in up to one-quarter. The increased risk for suicidality is substantial, even after adjusting for psychiatric comorbidities. Severity of comorbid depressive and anxiety symptoms, severity of OCD, unacceptable-type thoughts, and a history of suicidality have been linked to suicide risk in OCD. Some research also suggests that comorbidity with substance use disorder, PTSD, personality disorders, and impulse control disorders may also increase the risk of suicidality in OCD.

Cultural formulation is a crucial aspect of the assessment, diagnosis, and treatment of obsessive-compulsive and related disorders. When considering a diagnosis of OCD, the clinician should aim to understand individuals within their larger cultural contexts and consider what might be a culturally sanctioned norm for the "symptom." The term *culture* incorporates the processes through which an individual assigns meaning to experiences. It draws from the values, orientations, knowledge, and practices of the person's social, ethnic, religious, or other groups. Some factors affecting a person's perspective include age, sex, gender, social class, place of birth and growing up, migration history, language, religion and spirituality, sexual orientation, disability, socioeconomic status, and ethnic or racial background. The severity and meaning of the distressing experience should be assessed in relation to these contexts. Some cultures are considered more superstitious, for example, and some incorporate more ritualistic practices. Heterogeneity and subcultural or regional differences can be present even within the same culture. Therefore, persons who appear to have the same cultural background may still differ in ways that are significant and relevant to care. Finally, causal attributions of OCD (e.g., biological, psychological, social, spiritual) may vary among groups and subgroups. Elements of the cultural formulation and why they deserve attention are explored later in the chapter.

Getting the History

Ms. Silva is a 34-year-old woman who reports not allowing chicken meat into her kitchen because of fear of contracting salmonella. She worries that she is depriving her children and husband of a nutritious food that they might enjoy because of her fear. To assess for any logical explanation for her worry, the physician asks, "Have you or a

TABLE 10–2. Obsessional themes in obsessive-compulsive and related disorders

Obsessional theme	Example
Contamination fear	A young person has a consuming fear of catching a prion illness from coming across human waste.
Pathological doubt	A young woman spends several work hours daily worrying whether she has run over someone during her morning commute.
Somatic worries	A physically healthy middle-aged man frequently worries that he may spontaneously stop breathing.
Symmetry	A husband worries that if objects in his environment are not arranged symmetrically, something bad may happen to his wife.
Aggression	A law-abiding teacher with no history of violence or other psychiatric symptoms worries they may suddenly "lose control" and assault a student.
Sexuality	An adult son experiences repetitive, intrusive, and highly distressing images of him having a sexual encounter with his mother.
Religion	While in church, an observant Catholic parishioner experiences repetitive sacrilegious urges to desecrate a crucifix.

TABLE 10–3. Compulsive themes in obsessive-compulsive and related disorders

Compulsive theme	Example
Checking	A woman checks the locks on the front and back doors, as well as all of her windows, three times before she can leave the house.
Cleaning/washing	To avoid contracting a virus, a salesperson washes their hands for 15 minutes each time they shake hands with a customer.
Counting	A retired man who no longer drives counts the number of footsteps he takes whenever he walks anywhere.
Need to confess/seek reassurance	An administrative assistant frequently worries they may have hurt a recipient's feelings by not using the appropriate greeting in an email, often prompting the assistant to send several follow-up emails to seek reassurance and apologize.
Repeating	A carpenter experiences a need to have their left hand repeat all movements performed by their right hand.
Mental rituals	A nonreligious person says a silent prayer in reverse whenever they come across the number two because they associate it with bad luck.

loved one had salmonella or other foodborne poisoning before, or do you tend to undercook food?" When Ms. Silva answers no, the exaggerated nature of the worry becomes more confirmed. The physician then asks, "Do you have decontaminating rituals that you have to perform if you think you have been exposed to chicken? Do you avoid going to or eating in certain places because of this?" Ms. Silva responds that she relies on her husband for her grocery shopping, or if she absolutely must go to the store herself, she will skip the meat section and will engage in 2-hour showers once she returns home. She also has a special pair of shoes that she stores outside the house and reserves for trips to the grocery store, and she has unsuccessfully tried to lobby her husband to do the same. "How has this affected your marriage and family life?" the physician asks. Ms. Silva reports that her husband is very frustrated and her children have called her excessive worry "crazy." The physician then tries to determine the onset and timeline of her symptoms and identify any recent stressors, other obsessions and compulsions that she may have experienced, and any associated mood or other psychiatric symptoms. Further questions explore her medical, family, and social history.

The physician carefully explores the roots of this irrational fear, its extent, and its spillover effects. They try to elicit any associated symptoms, such as other obsessions and compulsions or non-OCD psychiatric symptoms. By asking about any decontaminating rituals or other avoidance behaviors that may be present, they gently allow Ms. Silva to divulge potentially embarrassing details, including her avoidance of grocery stores, her cleaning rituals, and her request that her husband wear special shoes when he goes to the store on her behalf. The interview begins by focusing on the chief complaint and then broadens in a way that elucidates the complaint, investigates its consequences, and identifies the presence of other linked or independent pathological findings worthy of clinical attention.

Tips for Clarifying the Diagnosis

- When a person "self-diagnoses" with OCD, investigate whether there are sufficient negative consequences to the person's life to warrant a clinical diagnosis.
- Ask these important questions: What is the time course of the symptoms? How have the symptoms changed over time? Are there symptom-free periods?
- Determine whether both obsessions and compulsions are present.
- Question whether symptom intensity correlates with stress or negative mood.
- If multiple obsessions or compulsions are present, clarify which are the most time-consuming and anxiety provoking.
- Assess how much control the individual has over the symptoms. Ask what their success rate is when attempting to self-distract from the obsession or to delay acting on the compulsion.

Consider the Case

Ms. Webb is a 75-year-old grandmother and retired university administrator who has never before visited a mental health professional. Over the past 15 months, she has become gradually withdrawn, lost weight, and developed insomnia. She has also voiced suspicions to her concerned neighbors about her downstairs tenants, complaining that they mean to harm her, including through poisoning her water supply by introducing a lethal substance into the pipes supplying her house. When her neighbors try to reassure her that her tenants are good people who are upstanding members of the community, Ms. Webb questions her neighbors' motives for "covering up for them." Because of her fear, Ms. Webb now refuses to drink the water at her house and only very reluctantly uses it to shower or for cleaning purposes. As a result, she has become dehydrated, compounding the weight loss she has sustained and making her vulnerable to serious medical complications.

Ms. Webb has developed a type of contamination fear involving her water supply, and her fear has led to medically compromising avoidance behavior. However, the concomitant presence of other symptoms makes it less likely that OCD is the root cause of her problem. The fear of being poisoned by her tenants is most likely a paranoid symptom. In addition, late onset of symptoms is less likely to be a feature of OCD. Delirium, a major depressive episode with psychotic features, or a dementia-related syndrome with psychosis are more likely explanations than late-onset OCD.

This case illustrates how OCD-like symptoms can occur in a wide range of psychiatric illnesses. A broad psychiatric "review of systems" and careful history taking help delineate whether the symptoms are the result of OCD or if an alternative diagnosis may better explain them. Naturally, treatment success depends highly on diagnostic accuracy.

Differential Diagnosis

Because OCD symptoms can be so variable and partially overlap with several other diagnostic categories, a broad differential diagnosis should be entertained when approaching someone with suspected OCD, and the diagnosis of OCD should be made only after other candidate conditions have been ruled out. Patients whose OCD symptoms meet the specifier "with absent insight/delusional beliefs" should not be assumed to have a primary psychotic disorder. Anxiety disorders as well as trauma- and stress-related disorders should be explored when an OCD diagnosis is being considered in a person who has significant worry about a particular trigger or who seeks the temporary calming effects of performing a ritual. For example, anxious avoidance of a specific location may not be provoked by OCD superstitions associated with it, but rather may result from PTSD that has linked the place with a trauma in the person's history.

The particular nature of the obsession or compulsion can also point to other diagnostic possibilities. In someone with rigid eating patterns, excessive attempts to lose weight, and chronic body image concerns, an eating disorder might be the more appropriate diagnosis. In the case of a child with social reciprocity challenges, below-average IQ, peculiar interests, and some repetitive motor behaviors, an autism spectrum disorder might better explain the observed deficits. Similarly, someone who checks their email and social networking accounts relentlessly and unnecessarily but has no other checking behaviors, compulsions, or obsessions might be better considered to have some pathological relationship with the digital world. Individuals with rigidly defined ways of performing tasks, who are convinced they are right, want others to adopt their patterns, and see no problem with their behavior despite functional impairment in one or more life domains might be more appropriately diagnosed with obsessive-compulsive personality disorder.

Finally, when a person derives pleasure or gets a thrill from performing a repetitive act (e.g., skin picking, hair pulling, pathological gambling) as opposed to seeking a temporary reduction in anxiety, the somewhat "ego-syntonic" nature of the behavior might point to a diagnosis of a behavioral addiction or impulse-control disorder rather than to OCD, in which obsessive thoughts are unwanted and intrusive, often cause significant distress or anxiety, and are not pleasurable. See DSM-5-TR for additional disorders to consider in the differential diagnosis. Also refer to the discussions of comorbidity and differential diagnosis in their respective sections of DSM-5-TR.

Summary

- OCD is a common, often disabling condition that can manifest with a great variety of obsessions or compulsions that typically fall under a limited number of themes.
- Many people describe performing some repetitive behaviors or having obsession-like thoughts, images, or urges. A diagnosis of OCD can be made only if symptoms are consuming and result in significant impairment.
- A careful history should be taken to assess the natural course of symptoms, context within which they occur, and resulting consequences and complications.
- Diagnosing OCD requires carefully ruling out a wide range of psychiatric and other disorders that can masquerade as OCD.

IN-DEPTH DIAGNOSIS: BODY DYSMORPHIC DISORDER

Ms. Thompson is a 28-year-old married former high school teacher. When she was 22, following her parents' surprising divorce, she started worrying that her face was asymmetrical. More specifically, she felt that the left side of her jaw was higher than the right side by about a half inch. Ms. Thompson had sustained no injury and had no malformation that might explain this "defect." Shame over her appearance led to drastic efforts to hide the perceived asymmetry, including using creative hairstyling and wearing scarves to partially cover her cheeks. When no technique worked, Ms. Thompson left her teaching job, convinced that her students were mocking her appearance, and gradually withdrew from social interactions. Reassurances by her husband that her jawline was entirely normal do not allay her anxiety, and neither have a number of professional consultations with dentists. Ms. Thompson is now researching oral surgeons in the hopes of finding one who can rid her of this problem by operating on her jaw. She exhibits no other psychiatric symptoms, including any concerns about body weight or body fat composition. She has no history of medical conditions and does not use substances. She does see herself as debilitated by her symptoms but does not view the cause as psychiatric. Instead, Ms. Thompson is convinced that a jaw malformation, treatable by surgery, is at its root.

Ms. Thompson is preoccupied by a nonexistent body defect, and this preoccupation has caused her severe impairment, including causing her to quit work and to withdraw from society. She does not appear to have insight into her problem; she is not relieved by reassurances from her husband or from dental professionals that her jaw is normal, and she is so convinced of this flaw that she is seeking painful and potentially dangerous corrective surgery in order to fix it. As such, her presentation is most consistent with the DSM-5-TR criteria for BDD with absent insight/delusional beliefs.

Approach to the Diagnosis

People with BDD will often only reluctantly present for mental health evaluation and treatment. They may feel egregiously unattractive and think that only an experienced plastic surgeon or dermatologist—not a therapist or psychiatrist—can assuage their misery. This resistance to seeking care is more likely to soften if the mental health professional adopts a caring, nonjudgmental approach, fully acknowledging the distress and pain caused by the perceived defect even as they decline to acknowledge the presence of the defect itself.

Observing the person's appearance is crucial to ruling out the presence of a defect. In some cases in which a defect can be seen, it is important to explore whether the visible defect was self-induced and resulted from an attempt to fix a perceived defect (e.g., scarring from excessive self-excoriation meant to erase a blemish). Anxious affect and poor eye contact can point to self-consciousness and social avoidance linked to BDD. Other clues in the patient's appearance can suggest compensatory measures meant as camouflage (e.g., unusual, big, or awkward accessories or clothing, sometimes strategically positioned to hide certain areas).

In addition to the usual components of a comprehensive interview needed to make an accurate diagnosis, some questions are uniquely important when assessing a patient with suspected BDD. Family history is valuable; studies of adolescent and young adult twin cohorts indicate relatively high heritability for BDD. Inquiry into the degree of "corrective" measures sought, including invasive procedures from other specialists, is crucial. Should the patient consent, contact with those specialists is important to coordinate care and provide psychoeducation. Professionals in other disciplines may have little awareness of BDD (as well as trichotillomania and excoriation disorder) and the psychological underpinnings of some people's body-focused complaints. It is often the mental health care provider's role to educate both the person and the other providers about these conditions and about how a nonpsychiatric treatment approach is rarely curative and may in fact exacerbate the condition. Collaboration with other providers serves to present a united front to patients about the primacy of mental health treatment in their situation, prevents "splitting," avoids reinforcing symptoms, and helps increase awareness.

As the clinician narrows down the diagnosis and tailors the interview questions, they should pay particular attention to other conditions that share features with BDD, especially other obsessive-compulsive spectrum disorders (in which repetitive behaviors or mental acts are a hallmark) and eating disorders (in which anxiety about body weight is often a defining feature). Patients' appearance-focused symptoms should be appreciated within their larger cultural context; for example, a fixation on BMI and biceps size in a young bodybuilder with suspected muscle dysmorphia should exceed the broad societal dictate to work out and develop muscular physiques and should cause the individual more distress and impairment than is typically experienced by similar avid bodybuilders in the same age group and with the same cultural background.

Finally, suicide risk should be carefully assessed. As summarized in DSM-5-TR, meta-analytic data suggest that individuals with BDD are significantly more likely to have experienced suicidal thoughts compared with healthy control subjects and with individuals with eating disorders, OCD, and any anxiety disorder.

Getting the History

> The therapist welcomes a patient, Ms. Fleming, into their office. They are struck by her avoidant gaze and by one element in her appearance: she is sporting extremely long bangs that cover her forehead and partially her eyes. "It was my husband's idea for me to come here. I don't think I need this kind of help," the 32-year-old woman tells the therapist. "I am glad to meet you, even if it seems as though you hesitated about coming here," the therapist answers. "May I ask a few questions to see if I can help you?"
>
> The therapist asks her to explain what has been bothering her. Ms. Fleming opens up about feeling "deformed" because her eyebrows are asymmetrical. She lifts her bangs to reveal a pair of eyebrows that appear normal and symmetrical to the therapist. "See?" she says, pointing to her forehead, her finger anxiously trembling. "I look like a freak! I can't be seen in public looking like this! Please don't be like my husband and tell me they look normal. Give me your honest opinion!"
>
> "I'm very sorry this is causing you so much pain," the therapist answers. "My opinion is that your eyebrows look fine, but I also understand that the anxiety they cause you is very real and overwhelming, and I want to help you deal with it and help you feel better in your own skin."

Ms. Fleming presents as anxiety-ridden over the appearance of her eyebrows and as actively employing strategies meant to hide the embarrassing part of her body. She expresses reluctance about mental health care, likely because of poor insight into the psychological roots of her problem. She has received reassurance, at least from her husband, that her eyebrows look normal, but it seems to have done little to help her symptoms. The therapist avoids getting into a tug-of-war with Ms. Fleming about the symmetrical nature of her eyebrows, giving their honest opinion when directly asked but also focusing on the downstream effects of the patient's faulty conviction—namely, the intolerable anxiety she is feeling, which is something on which they both agree. Such an approach can help start building the therapeutic alliance, which is absolutely crucial for getting someone with little or no insight into their BDD diagnosis to accept mental health care and to heed treatment recommendations.

Tips for Clarifying the Diagnosis

- Consider whether the person is preoccupied with a body part's appearance or with perceived ugliness. Preoccupation with a body part, if not focused on looks or appearance, cannot be the basis for a diagnosis of BDD.
- Inquire about repetitive behaviors (e.g., mirror checking, excessive grooming, reassurance seeking) or repetitive mental acts (e.g., comparing one's appearance with that of others) as a consequence of the preoccupation.

- Assess the patient's level of insight, including whether they are completely convinced of their views about personal appearance. Explore any delusional dimension to the symptoms.

- Inquire about any dermatological or cosmetic interventions that have been performed or are being sought to try to remedy the perceived problem. Ask about other strategies used to hide the perceived problem (e.g., wearing heavy makeup, particular types of clothes, or other accessories).

- Screen for muscle dysmorphia, especially in men who engage in excessive bodybuilding or use anabolic steroids, because they may be responding to a baseless worry that they are insufficiently muscular or too small.

Consider the Case

Ms. Thompson, the 28-year-old former high school teacher discussed earlier, continues to be unhappy about her "malformed" jaw. She underwent "corrective" surgery abroad when no licensed local surgeon would agree to operate on her. Following surgery, Ms. Thompson felt self-confident and began socializing more, but this self-confidence proved short-lived as a new, all-consuming worry overtook her about 2 months later. For no reason and without any precipitant, Ms. Thompson began worrying that her nose was significantly asymmetrical, leading her to undergo a procedure to modify it. Around the same time, she started worrying that her skin is too pale and now has begun to frequent tanning salons excessively to try to develop a darker skin tone.

This case shows that the physical feature that is the source of the fixation in BDD may change over time because the illness can "migrate" from one area of concern to another. It also shows that the desperate and expensive interventions people sometimes seek—cosmetic, surgical, dermatological, and so on—are rarely curative and can serve to validate an unnecessary worry that should instead be confronted according to established treatment guidelines. Notably, BDD can affect all ethnic groups, and discomfort with skin color (e.g., "too dark," "too pale") is not an uncommon symptom. Any success derived from nonpsychiatric treatments for BDD tends to be temporary, with the appearance-based anxiety often returning, either with the same focus or a different one.

Differential Diagnosis

In a society often described as being obsessed with appearances, it is important to differentiate people's run-of-the-mill, culture-concordant worries about their looks from the pathological preoccupations of BDD. For a diagnosis of BDD to be made, the person's worry must be excessive and significantly impair their functioning. On the other hand, if the physical defect is clearly noticeable or disfiguring, the worry it generates cannot be attributed to BDD.

The intrusive physical appearance–based thoughts of BDD—and the repetitive mirror checking, grooming, or reassurance seeking that frequently go with them—are reminiscent of other obsessive-compulsive and related disorders, such as excoriation disorder or trichotillomania. When the skin picking or hair pulling is intended as a grooming behavior meant to correct a perceived defect, a diagnosis of BDD is more appropriate. The typically poorer insight seen in BDD and the narrower fixation on appearance help distinguish it from OCD. Similarly, in a person with an eating disorder, worries about being fat or overweight are more likely to be part of the eating disorder, although an eating disorder can be comorbid with BDD.

The poor or absent insight seen in some patients with BDD can reach a delusional degree, with patients completely convinced that their view of their appearance is accurate and undistorted. However, the focus on appearance and the absence of disorganized thinking or hallucinations help distinguish BDD from a primary psychotic illness. Also of note is *Koro*, a culturally related disorder that usually occurs in epidemics in Southeast Asia. These cases consist of a fear of the penis (or occasionally of the labia, nipples, or breasts) shrinking and disappearing into the body, often with the associated belief that death will result. The focus on death rather than perceived ugliness helps differentiate it from BDD.

See DSM-5-TR for additional disorders to consider in the differential diagnosis. Also refer to the discussions of comorbidity and differential diagnosis in their respective sections of DSM-5-TR.

Summary

- BDD is an often-disabling condition defined by a preoccupation with a nonexistent or slight body defect, repetitive actions or thoughts meant to reduce the associated anxiety, and variable degrees of insight into the psychological roots of the illness.
- The societal message to meet certain narrow beauty standards is strong and inescapable. Patients with BDD have an appearance-derived anxiety that far exceeds society's "epidemic" of unease with one's body image.
- A careful history is needed to assess the natural course of symptoms, their larger context, the resulting consequences (including, but not limited to, depression, suicidal ideation, and social withdrawal), and any complications (e.g., from personal attempts at correcting "defects" or from unnecessary dermatological or surgical interventions).
- Making the diagnosis of BDD requires carefully ruling out a wide range of psychiatric and other disorders, such as OCD, eating disorders, social anxiety disorder, and psychotic illnesses.

IN-DEPTH DIAGNOSIS: TRICHOTILLOMANIA (HAIR-PULLING DISORDER)

Ms. Gonzalez is a 28-year-old woman currently working on a doctorate in mathematics. She has a 12-year history of pulling hair from her scalp and eyebrows, a behavior that has waxed and waned over the years but has become progressively worse since she began working on her dissertation and studying for her comprehensive examinations 3 months ago. Her first episode of hair pulling occurred when she was 16 years old, when she first began tweezing her eyebrow hairs for aesthetic purposes. She remembers continuing to pull from her right eyebrow well beyond what was aesthetically justifiable and recalls enjoying the feeling that followed plucking each hair. However, the initial pleasurable experience was followed by shame and embarrassment because she had to use makeup to conceal the patch of missing hair. Thereafter, she engaged in similar, sporadic episodes of right eyebrow hair plucking, usually using her right thumb and index finger, most often during times of stress or other intense emotional experiences.

Over time, Ms. Gonzalez began pulling hair from both of her eyebrows and from her scalp. When her parents eventually noticed the patches of missing hair, they took her for evaluations with her pediatrician and a dermatologist, who determined that the hair pulling was not the result of an undiagnosed skin or other medical condition. Numerous therapists unsuccessfully focused on Ms. Gonzalez's "lack of self-control" and questioned whether she had body image issues for which she was attempting to compensate. Currently, Ms. Gonzalez has a small bald spot on the vertex of her head that she attempts to hide by pulling her hair back. She no longer goes to her usual hair salon because she fears having to explain her bald patch to a stylist or hearing a lecture on how she is intentionally damaging her hair.

Although Ms. Gonzalez has attempted to stop this behavior on numerous occasions, she has never been able to maintain complete cessation for more than a few weeks. She currently engages in hair pulling from her eyebrows or her scalp for at least 1.5–2 hours each day, with an average of 50 hairs pulled daily. She finds that she engages in pulling with little awareness, usually while engrossed in reading for her comprehensive exams or at the computer working on her dissertation. In addition, Ms. Gonzalez reports that she has been "playing" with the pulled hairs; although previously she would immediately discard them, she now finds herself either rolling the hair between her fingers after pulling it or chewing on the root bulb. She does not know exactly why she started playing with the pulled hairs but reports significant shame about these new behaviors.

Because she does not want people to notice her bald spots, Ms. Gonzalez has been spending less time with friends, even though she acknowledges that social support would help mitigate her stress. She has also discontinued swimming because she finds it difficult to hide the bald spot on her head when her hair is wet. Without the outlet of exercise and social activities, her mood has become increasingly depressed, which she believes further exacerbates her hair pulling and decreases her motivation to engage in alternative behaviors.

Ms. Gonzalez appears to meet DSM-5-TR criteria for trichotillomania. Her hair pulling has had a chronic course since onset, although the location and function of her pulling has changed over time. She repeatedly engages in pulling hair from her eyebrows and scalp despite efforts to control the behavior. She no longer finds the effects of pulling pleasurable, does not pull for purposes of correcting perceived imperfections, and most often engages in the behavior with little awareness. Ms. Gonzalez is experiencing significant distress from her inability to control her hair pulling and from the effects the behavior is having on her physical appearance and life. She endorses depressed mood, social withdrawal, shame, and embarrassment—all stemming from her pulling. Medical and dermatological evaluations suggest that her pulling behavior is not attributable to a medical condition, and no other DSM-5-TR disorder would better explain this presentation.

Approach to the Diagnosis

Patients with trichotillomania often present for treatment with a significant amount of shame and embarrassment. They may not only be self-conscious of the effects of their pulling (e.g., bald spots, missing eyebrows) but also feel shame and fear judgment for engaging in a behavior that family, friends, or previous providers have indicated is within their control. Thus, they may present as self-conscious and socially avoidant during the initial consultation. Providers must maintain an empathetic and nonjudgmental approach and offer a supportive and understanding environment during the initial assessment and throughout treatment.

When conducting a comprehensive interview, it is important to assess the nature and extent of hair-pulling behaviors with respect to their location, frequency, and function. Some patients may not be completely forthcoming when reporting all the sites from which they pull hair, particularly sites that might be embarrassing to discuss, such as pubic areas. Thus, asking patients about pulling from locations they did not initially mention is important. With regard to the function of the pulling, many patients with trichotillomania experience it as an automatic and out-of-awareness activity that happens during times of stress or intense focus. Others report engaging in focused pulling to remove a coarse hair, alleviate an uncomfortable sensation or emotion, or produce a pleasurable sensation.

On the other hand, hair pulling that is not excessive and functions to improve someone's appearance may be best considered normative hair removal. Excessive hair pulling that serves to correct a perceived imperfection may be better accounted for by BDD. Pulling that serves to alleviate a chronic itch or skin irritation may suggest an undiagnosed dermatological condition, and hair pulling that functions as a symmetry ritual may be best captured by OCD.

In addition to asking about the function of the hair pulling, it is important to ask what the person does with each pulled hair. Most individuals with trichotillomania discard the hairs following removal. Others may keep an occasional hair to roll between their fingertips or use it to caress their lips or cheek. However, some will put a pulled hair in their mouth to play with it with their tongue, chew on the root bulb, or swallow it, and they may be reluctant to endorse these behaviors because of embarrassment. It is important to assess for the presence of such behaviors because they can result in significant health problems, including dental issues and trichobezoars (hairballs in the stomach or intestines).

Getting the History

During her initial evaluation, Ms. Lowe, a 28-year-old woman, reveals that she frequently plucks individual hairs from her eyelashes or eyebrows whenever she feels stressed out and is intensely focused on completing a homework assignment or studying for an exam. "I know what you're thinking," she says. "I'm destroying my appearance and could stop—but I'm *choosing* not to, right?"

"I think what you're going through is extremely difficult," the therapist responds. "And I'm sure you've tried everything you can think of to stop pulling but have found this to be a very difficult disorder to gain control of. If you don't mind, I'd like to ask you some additional details about your pulling. For example, what do you do with each hair after you pull it?"

Ms. Lowe replies that she discards most hairs immediately after pulling them but does frequently chew on the ends of those with large root bulbs and eventually swallows them. "In addition to pulling from your eyebrows and eyelashes, do you ever pull from your scalp, arms or legs, or pubic area?" the therapist asks. Ms. Lowe expresses embarrassment but reports occasionally pulling hair from her pubic region when using the bathroom or lying in her bed reading.

Ms. Lowe expresses an initial concern that her therapist will be critical of her hair pulling and judge her for not exercising better self-control. The therapist empathizes with how difficult it must be to live with this disorder and acknowledges that the patient has probably tried everything in her power to stop pulling her hair. With their empathetic and nonjudgmental approach, the therapist obtains the information necessary to make an accurate diagnosis by helping Ms. Lowe feel understood and supported and allowing her to be open about the specifics of her disorder. By building rapport and assessing for behaviors that Ms. Lowe did not initially reveal, the therapist develops a thorough view of the extent of Ms. Lowe's hair pulling, including behaviors that put her at risk for possible medical problems (e.g., consuming hair).

Tips for Clarifying the Diagnosis

- Assess the frequency and location(s) of hair-pulling behaviors, including locations that may be embarrassing for individuals to discuss.
- Clarify the function of the hair pulling. Does it largely occur outside of awareness or feel out of control, and does it serve the purpose of regulating an uncomfortable sensation or emotion? Does it coincide with a preoccupation with the person's appearance and serve the purpose of correcting a perceived imperfection? Does the function of the hair pulling suggest that it may be better accounted for by another disorder, such as BDD or OCD?
- Assess the ways in which the person has attempted to conceal the effects of hair pulling, the effect the pulling has had on their health, and the ways in which the behaviors have affected their social and occupational functioning.
- Inquire about what the person does with each hair following removal. Is each hair immediately discarded, or are the hairs sometimes consumed?
- Consider whether the individual has a medical or dermatological disorder that may cause hair pulling as a way to alleviate physical discomfort.

Consider the Case

Ms. Davis is a 22-year-old single woman with a 10-year history of compulsively removing hair from various locations of her body using her fingers or tweezers. In general, Ms. Davis reports that she finds body hair disgusting and can tolerate hair on her head and face only if it looks perfect. She engages in hair pulling for approximately 1 hour each day and commonly focuses on hair that is visible to those with whom she interacts. She denies having episodes of pulling that are automatic and out of her awareness; rather, she endorses focused pulling that serves the function of removing hairs that look "ugly and unattractive." She indicates that she stands in front of a mirror and pulls or tweezes "unsightly" hairs from her eyelashes and eyebrows almost daily to maintain their "perfect appearance." Several times throughout the day, especially while sitting in class or riding public transportation, she uses her fingers to pluck any visible hairs from her arms and hands because she finds hair in these areas to be repulsive and unattractive. Although she regularly shaves her legs and armpits, she reports that she frequently examines these areas with her hands for new hair growth and will use tweezers to remove any hairs she finds that are long enough to be pulled. In addition, she reports that she is intolerant of having pubic hair and frequently uses tweezers to remove any new hair growth.

Although Ms. Davis has a long history of engaging in focused hair pulling across several sites on her body, the function of these behaviors appears to be exclusively aesthetic and is motivated by her desire to remove unsightly hair and maintain a perfect appearance. She finds the presence of hair in most regions of her body "ugly and unattractive" and engages in hair pulling to correct these perceived imperfections. Thus, her hair pulling would be better accounted for by a diagnosis of BDD than of trichotillomania. This case illustrates the potential similarities in presentation among the obsessive-compulsive and related disorders and the importance of understanding the function of seemingly similar symptoms and behaviors during assessment to determine an accurate diagnosis and treatment plan.

Differential Diagnosis

To accurately differentiate trichotillomania from other disorders, it is necessary to understand the function of the hair-pulling behavior. For example, hair pulling that is meant to correct a perceived physical imperfection, such as "ugly" arm hair, may be better accounted for by BDD. OCD may better describe hair pulling that functions as a superstitious ritual (e.g., a person who pulls a hair from the top of his head whenever he hears the word *cancer* to prevent becoming sick). Hair pulling that serves to alleviate a chronic itch, skin irritation, or other discomfort may suggest a dermatological condition. Finally, hair pulling in response to a delusion or command auditory hallucination is likely best explained by a psychotic disorder.

Behaviors associated with trichotillomania occur frequently in individuals who do not meet criteria for this or any other disorder. Many cultures engage in normative hair removal for grooming purposes; for example, people may use tweezers to remove hairs from the eyebrows to improve their appearance. It is also common for individuals with longer hair to play with their hair by twisting, twirling, or tugging it. Such hair-based behaviors do not point to a pathological condition. See DSM-5-TR for other disorders to consider in the differential diagnosis. Also refer to the discussions of comorbidity and differential diagnosis in their respective sections of DSM-5-TR.

Summary

- Trichotillomania is a serious condition characterized by repeated pulling of one's hair that often results in bald spots, hair damage, and attempts to conceal the consequences.
- Trichotillomania is associated with shame and embarrassment because of the perception that the person should be able to refrain from self-inflicted harm to their body.
- Trichotillomania can include focused pulling (targeting a hair because of a tactile sensation or the desire to produce a pleasurable sensation), automatic pulling (en-

gaging in hair pulling out of the person's awareness, usually while engrossed in a specific task), or a combination.

- A careful assessment is necessary to differentiate pathological hair pulling from normative grooming and from other psychiatric disorders that share similar features, such as BDD and OCD.

SUMMARY: OBSESSIVE-COMPULSIVE AND RELATED DISORDERS

Like many psychiatric conditions, illnesses grouped in the obsessive-compulsive and related disorders diagnostic class are extreme manifestations of common, everyday experiences. Exactly at what point repetition, collecting, appearance-focused anxiety, and self-grooming cross into the pathological realm and become clinical entities requiring treatment is a question mental health care providers are often called on to answer. This determination requires a deep understanding of individuals and their lives and consideration of empirically defined criteria, such as those offered in DSM-5-TR, for what constitutes a diagnosis.

Repetition is an important common feature that helps unite the disparate conditions listed in the obsessive-compulsive and related disorders class—but important differences exist. For example, the contamination fear and anxious collecting seen in OCD and hoarding disorder are usually accompanied by a dysphoria and frustration that contrast with the pleasurable feelings sometimes reported by people with trichotillomania and excoriation disorder. Such distinctions and other nuances are beyond the scope of this chapter but should be pursued by interested readers (see "Recommended Readings" at the end of this chapter). More advanced reading will reveal that these conditions—diagnosable and potentially highly impairing as they are shown to be here—are also treatable in a large percentage of patients.

ELEMENTS TO CONSIDER IN THE CULTURAL FORMULATION

- Cultural identity of the individual (e.g., age, sex/gender, ethnoracial background, religion and spirituality, socioeconomic status, place of birth and growing up, migration history, sexual orientation, other) may influence interpersonal relationships and developmental and current challenges, conflicts, and predicaments.
- Differences in cultural background, language, education, and social class between the patient and the clinician, treatment team, or institution may influence perception during assessment, potentially leading to a misunderstanding of the cultural and clinical significance of experiences and to difficulty building rapport.
- Social determinants of health, such as exposure to racism, discrimination, institutional stigmatization, and social marginalization or exclusion, may contribute to the presentation or affect the establishment of trust and a sense of safety during the clinical encounter.

- Cultural concepts of distress may affect symptom expression and presentation, content of obsessions or compulsions, help-seeking behaviors, and perceived seriousness of the illness.
- Migrants' varying degrees of identification with the cultural context of origin and the present cultural context may affect symptom expression and presentation, content of obsessions or compulsions, help-seeking behaviors, and perceived seriousness of the illness.

DIAGNOSTIC PEARLS

- Although the obsessive-compulsive and related disorders diagnostic class has been separate from the anxiety disorders since DSM-5 (American Psychiatric Association 2013), anxiety remains a prominent feature of many conditions within this class.

- Overlap exists among conditions within the obsessive-compulsive and related disorders diagnostic class and disorders in other diagnostic classes. Careful history taking and familiarity with diagnostic criteria are necessary to clarify the diagnosis.

- There is much misunderstanding within the medical profession and society at large about the obsessive-compulsive and related disorders. Increasing awareness and psychoeducation are part of the clinician's role in addressing these problems.

- The details of individuals' unusual worries and behaviors are often embarrassing to them and laden with stigma. An open mind and an empathetic, nonjudgmental approach are needed to put individuals at ease and to maximize diagnostic accuracy and treatment success.

- Information on cultural, subcultural, and familial contexts should be elicited to help determine whether a particular concern or behavior is pathological or within the expected norm for the person being evaluated. Nuanced cultural factors may significantly influence the expression and manifestation of symptoms.

SELF-ASSESSMENT

Key Concepts: Double-Check Your Knowledge

What is the relevance of the following concepts to the various obsessive-compulsive and related disorders?

- Intrusive thoughts, urges, or images
- Repetitive behaviors or mental acts
- Purpose of repetitive behaviors or mental acts
- Time-consuming nature of obsessions or compulsions
- Perceived body defect or flaw

- Muscle dysmorphia
- Range of insight in body dysmorphic disorder
- Trichotillomania
- Hair pulling or loss that is secondary to a medical condition

Questions to Discuss With Colleagues and Mentors

1. Do you systematically screen patients for disorders in the obsessive-compulsive and related disorders diagnostic class? If so, what questions do you use for each disorder? For example, how do you define *obsession* or *compulsion* to people in your screenings?
2. How do you manage your reaction when you are faced with disturbing symptoms of obsessive-compulsive and related disorders (e.g., hearing about an obsession to stab someone from a patient who has no desire or intent to do so, or meeting a disheveled, hoarding person whose collections have created unsanitary conditions at home and have visibly affected their personal hygiene)?
3. How do you determine whether OCD (or any condition in this diagnostic class) is the "best explanation" for a person's symptoms?
4. How do you assess "insight" in patients diagnosed with a condition in the diagnostic class of obsessive-compulsive and related disorders?

Case-Based Questions

PART A

Ms. Lee is a 45-year-old business accountant at a software firm. While still in college at age 20, and for no apparent reason, an anxiety that struck her as peculiar suddenly hit her: she started worrying that she may have inadvertently stepped on a baby during her morning jog. She could not say how the baby would have materialized on the isolated riverside trail where she ran, or how she might have tripped over a baby, but her need to verify was so intense that she started to follow her jog with a slow-paced hike during which she would comb the trail for any evidence of her "crime." As a result of this time-consuming pattern, Ms. Lee had to miss morning classes, but once the ritual was completed, she could focus on afternoon lectures and on doing her homework in the evening.

Is Ms. Lee experiencing OCD?   Ms. Lee's symptom can be described as a repetitive, intrusive thought that she recognizes as unusual and that involves having inadvertently hurt someone. She has associated checking behaviors meant to provide reassurance and reduce anxiety. Her life was negatively affected in that her school performance worsened. This picture is consistent with a diagnosis of OCD.

PART B

After graduating from college, Ms. Lee stopped jogging because the corporate job she chose did not accommodate late-morning starts. Two decades later, her more sedentary lifestyle has contributed to weight gain and early blood pressure problems. However, giving up on running did not eradicate the compulsions or the anxiety triggering them.

Her worry changed over the years but did not go away. Ms. Lee's commute today involves a 20-minute drive from home to work. Depending on her level of anxiety, that trip is sometimes followed by another drive during which she retraces her route to ascertain that she did not run over a baby on her first attempt to get to work. On what she calls her "bad days," she even has to check her tires for additional reassurance.

What does the evolution of symptoms in this case history so far tell us about the course of OCD?   OCD is often a chronic illness with a waxing and waning course. Whether the symptoms vary within the same general theme (as in this example) or take on different themes, individual symptoms often change. Their toll is cumulative over time, in this case indirectly contributing to medical problems.

PART C

Throughout her years of struggling with OCD, Ms. Lee was able to raise two healthy children and draw reasonable satisfaction from work. Until very recently, Ms. Lee had never sought professional help for her symptoms and says she learned to "adapt" to them, setting aside a certain amount of time on some days to "calm them down."

Why did Ms. Lee delay seeking care?   Although symptoms of OCD often manifest early, it is not unusual for individuals to delay treatment or not seek it at all. Reasons include lack of access to care, embarrassment about divulging symptoms, the stigma of a psychiatric diagnosis, the ability in some situations to adapt to the illness, inadequate knowledge of the pathological nature of the symptoms, and a tendency to view symptoms as peculiar personality traits.

Short-Answer Questions

1. Are both obsessions and compulsions required for a diagnosis of OCD?
2. Define obsessions in OCD.
3. Define compulsions in OCD.
4. What specifier would the clinician use in the OCD diagnosis for a person who is totally convinced that their fears of catching a very rare prion illness are well founded and that their associated cleaning rituals to prevent this outcome are entirely legitimate?
5. Would people who are preoccupied with essential body functions (e.g., adequate breathing, regular pulse rate, number of bowel movements) meet criteria for body dysmorphic disorder (BDD)?
6. Could people who have an actual body defect meet criteria for BDD?
7. Could patients with alcohol use disorder receive a primary diagnosis of BDD?
8. What form of BDD is much more common in men?
9. Does a person's excessive twirling of their hair along with frequent massaging of the scalp constitute trichotillomania?
10. An older male is having difficulty navigating his home because of excessive clutter, which has created a risk of falling. He collects and saves unnecessary things because "he might need them some day." No other obsessions or compulsions are evident. What is the most likely diagnosis?

Answers

1. No. Obsessions and compulsions are not both required for a diagnosis of OCD.

2. OCD obsessions are recurrent and persistent thoughts, urges, or images that are experienced, at some time during the disturbance, as intrusive and unwanted and that cause marked anxiety or distress in most individuals.

3. OCD compulsions are repetitive behaviors (e.g., hand washing, ordering, checking) or mental acts (e.g., praying, counting, repeating words silently) that individuals feel driven to perform in response to an obsession or according to rules that must be applied rigidly.

4. The individual would be diagnosed with OCD with absent insight/delusional beliefs.

5. No. These people do not meet criteria for BDD unless they are also preoccupied with the appearance of a body part.

6. Yes. People who have an actual body defect can meet criteria for BDD, but the defect in question must be minor and the preoccupation and distress caused by it disproportionately larger.

7. Yes. Patients can have alcohol use disorder and still receive a primary diagnosis of BDD.

8. The muscle dysmorphia form of BDD (i.e., the belief that the person's body build is too small or insufficiently muscular) is more common among men.

9. No. The criteria for a trichotillomania diagnosis require recurrent hair pulling with resulting hair loss.

10. The most likely diagnosis is hoarding disorder.

RECOMMENDED READINGS

Aboujaoude E: Compulsive Acts: A Psychiatrist's Tales of Ritual and Obsession. Berkeley, University of California Press, 2008

Koran LM: Obsessive-Compulsive and Related Disorders in Adults: A Comprehensive Clinical Guide. New York, Cambridge University Press, 1999

REFERENCES

American Psychiatric Association: Diagnostic and Statistical Manual of Mental Disorders, 5th Edition. Arlington, VA, American Psychiatric Association, 2013

American Psychiatric Association: Diagnostic and Statistical Manual of Mental Disorders, 5th Edition, Text Revision. Washington, DC, American Psychiatric Association, 2022

CHAPTER 11

Trauma- and Stressor-Related Disorders

Cheryl Gore-Felton, Ph.D.

"I can't watch the news—the memories come flooding back."

"I am numb inside."

- Reactive Attachment Disorder
- Disinhibited Social Engagement Disorder
- Posttraumatic Stress Disorder
- Acute Stress Disorder
- Adjustment Disorders
- Prolonged Grief Disorder
- Other Specified Trauma- and Stressor-Related Disorder
- Unspecified Trauma- and Stressor-Related Disorder

Adapted from Gore-Felton C, Koopman C: "Trauma- and Stressor-Related Disorders," in *Study Guide to DSM-5*. Edited by Roberts LW, Louie AK. Washington, DC, American Psychiatric Publishing, 2015, pp 177–194.

Trauma- and stressor-related disorders explicitly have exposure to a traumatic or stressful event as a diagnostic criterion and include reactive attachment disorder, disinhibited social engagement disorder, posttraumatic stress disorder (PTSD), acute stress disorder, adjustment disorders, other specified trauma- and stressor-related disorder, unspecified trauma- and stressor-related disorder, and the recently added prolonged grief disorder (PGD; see Table 11–1 for summary of differences between DSM-5 and DSM-5-TR). How individuals respond to traumatic or stressful events varies; some individuals may respond with increased anxiety, whereas others may respond with increased fear, anhedonia, dysphoria, dissociation, externalizing anger and aggression, or a combination of symptoms. Cultural syndromes and idioms of distress also may influence how people respond to traumatic or stressful events and therefore must be considered when establishing a diagnosis.

The clinical expression of reactivity to trauma varies across the life span. For instance, children older than 6 years are more likely to express intrusion symptoms through repetitive play in which themes or aspects of their trauma are expressed, whereas adults may experience prolonged psychological distress in response to involuntary and distressing memories of the traumatic event. Social neglect or environments that prevent secure attachments to caregivers are a diagnostic requirement for reactive attachment disorder and disinhibited social engagement disorder. Reactive attachment disorder is considered an internalizing disorder and is moderately associated with depression and withdrawn behavior. In contrast, disinhibited social engagement disorder resembles an externalizing disorder and may be marked by disinhibition (e.g., reduced reticence when approaching or engaging with unfamiliar adults). Children with reactive attachment disorder have a lack of or incompletely formed attachments to caregiving adults, whereas children with disinhibited social engagement disorder may or may not have established attachments, including secure attachments. A child must have a developmental age of at least 9 months to receive a diagnosis of reactive attachment disorder because they must be developmentally able to form selective attachments. Diagnostic assessments should include multiple sources of input to support that the symptoms occur across different contexts.

The necessary feature of PTSD is the development of characteristic symptoms following exposure to one or more traumatic events. Exposure to a traumatic event that qualifies as Criterion A (i.e., the stressor criterion) can occur by directly experiencing the event, witnessing it, learning that it occurred to a close relative or close friend, or experiencing repeated contact with aversive details of the event (e.g., as for first responders). The responses to these events constitute a disorder when the stressor is extreme (i.e., exposure to actual or threatened death, serious injury, or sexual violation) and when symptoms of intrusion, avoidance, negative alterations in cognitions (e.g., inability to recall important aspects of the traumatic event; persistent and exaggerated beliefs or expectations about oneself, others, or the world) and mood (e.g., persistent negative state; diminished interest or ability to experience happiness, satisfaction, or loving feelings), and marked alterations in arousal and reactivity (e.g., irritable behavior, angry outbursts, exaggerated startle responses, problems with concentration, or sleep disturbance) begin or worsen *after* the traumatic event occurs. For individuals older than 6 years, PTSD requires one or more intrusion symptoms, at least one

TABLE 11–1. Differences between DSM-5 and DSM-5-TR

DSM-5-TR added the new diagnosis of prolonged grief disorder. This diagnosis reflects the continued presence of intense yearning for or persistent preoccupation with thoughts of a deceased loved one, along with other grief-related symptoms such as emotional numbness, intense emotional pain, and avoidance of reminders that the person is deceased. Symptoms must persist for at least 12 months after the death and cause significant impairment in psychosocial functioning.

Adjustment disorders now include two duration specifiers: acute (symptoms last for <6 months) and persistent (chronic; symptoms last ≥6 months in response to a chronic stressor or enduring consequences of a stressor).

The "Association With Suicidal Thoughts or Behavior" section was added to the adjustment disorders diagnosis, highlighting the increased risk of suicide attempts and suicide associated with adjustment disorders.

Persistent complex bereavement was removed from the "Other Specified Trauma- and Stressor-Related Disorder" section because the symptoms are better characterized by the new prolonged grief disorder diagnosis.

The "Risk and Prognostic Factors" section for disinhibited social engagement disorder was expanded to include a "Temperamental" subsection based on research in the United States that found blunted reward sensitivity and decreased inhibitory control are associated with indiscriminate social behavior. A subsection on genetic and physiological factors also was added based on evidence that neurobiological factors have been associated with symptoms of the disorder.

persistent avoidance symptom, two or more symptoms of negative alterations in cognitions and mood, and two or more symptoms of alterations in arousal and reactivity (e.g., hypervigilance, exaggerated startle response). For children ages 6 and younger, PTSD requires at least one symptom of intrusion, at least one symptom of persistent avoidance or negative alterations in cognitions and mood, and at least two symptoms of alterations in arousal and reactivity. For all individuals, the duration of these symptoms must be longer than 1 month after exposure to the trauma, and they must cause clinically significant distress or impairment in social, occupational, or other important areas of functioning.

Acute stress disorder has the same essential feature as PTSD (Criterion A) in requiring exposure to a traumatic event. Individuals must experience the presence of nine or more symptoms in any category of intrusion, negative mood, dissociation, avoidance, or arousal. The symptoms must be present for at least 3 days up to 1 month following the traumatic event and must cause clinically significant distress in social, occupational, or other important areas of psychosocial functioning.

Adjustment disorders can be distinguished from acute stress disorder and PTSD in that the type of stressor is not considered traumatic (i.e., actual or threatened death, serious injury, or sexual violence), yet the distress exceeds what would be considered culturally and contextually appropriate given the type of stressor (e.g., termination of a romantic relationship, marital problems) present. Adjustment disorders have the following specifiers: with depressed mood, with anxiety, with mixed anxiety and depressed mood, with disturbance of conduct, with mixed disturbance of emotions and conduct, and unspecified (i.e., maladaptive reactions that cannot be classified with the aforementioned specifiers). Stressors can be single events (e.g., loss of a job) or multiple events (e.g., death of a pet and a marital problem). Adjustment disorders begin within 3 months of the onset of the stressor, and symptoms must not persist more than an additional 6 months following termination of the stressor or its consequences. Symptoms that persist for less than 6 months are specified as acute. If the stressor or its consequences persist for a prolonged period (i.e., longer than 6 months), the adjustment disorder may become persistent or chronic (e.g., financial and emotional difficulties resulting from a divorce).

In DSM-5-TR (American Psychiatric Association 2022), persistent complex bereavement disorder was removed from the chapter "Conditions for Further Study" where it appeared in DSM-5 (American Psychiatric Association 2013). PGD was introduced in DSM-5-TR to recognize that although grief, despair, and general dysphoria are often part of the normal grieving process after the death of a loved one, some people experience these emotions for an abnormally excessive amount of time or intensity. The necessary feature of PGD is that the death of a person who was close to an adult bereaved individual must have occurred at least 12 months ago. For bereaved children and adolescents, the death must have occurred at least 6 months ago. Since the death, one or both symptoms of intense yearning or longing for the deceased person or preoccupation with thoughts or memories of the deceased person (in children and adolescents, the preoccupation may focus on the circumstances of the death) must have been present. Additionally, since the death, at least three of the following symptoms must have been present:

- Identity disruption (e.g., feeling as though part of oneself has died)
- Marked sense of disbelief about death
- Avoidance of reminders that the person is dead (in children and adolescents this may be characterized as efforts to avoid reminders)
- Intense emotional pain (e.g., anger, bitterness, sorrow) related to the death
- Difficulty reintegrating into one's relationships and activities
- Emotional numbness
- Feeling that life is meaningless as a result of the death
- Intense loneliness as a result of the death

Furthermore, all of the symptoms must have been present nearly every day for at least the past month, and the disturbance must cause significant distress or impairment in social, occupational, or other important areas of functioning. It is important to consider whether the nature, duration, and severity of the bereavement reaction exceeds expected social, cultural, or religious norms for the individual's culture and context.

The diagnosis of other specified trauma- and stressor-related disorder refers to conditions in which an individual's trauma- and stressor-related symptoms cause impairment in several domains of life and psychosocial functioning but do not meet the full criteria for any of the other disorders included in this diagnostic class. Clinicians must indicate the specific reason why an individual's symptoms do not meet another set of criteria; for example, a person who experiences most symptoms of PTSD for several years but does not experience at least one symptom of intrusion might receive a diagnosis of persistent response to trauma with PTSD-like symptoms. Other specified trauma- and stressor-related disorders may include cultural syndromes, chronic presentations of adjustment disorder without prolonged exposure to stressors, and other presentations that do not meet the full criteria for other specific disorders in the trauma- and stressor-related disorders class. In cases in which the full criteria for this class of disorders are not met and clinicians either choose not to specify the reason why symptoms do not meet criteria or have inadequate or insufficient information to support another diagnosis in this class, the diagnosis of unspecified trauma- and stressor-related disorder may apply.

Other disorders involving clinically significant anxiety that are not in the trauma- and stressor-related disorders diagnostic class include anxiety disorders, obsessive-compulsive and related disorders, and somatic symptom and related disorders (including illness anxiety disorder). Although similarities exist across these diagnoses, the diagnostic classes have been developed based on unique characteristics of the respective disorders that set them apart from one another. For instance, panic disorder may include symptoms of avoidant behavior and fear-based anxiety; however, a person given this diagnosis is not experiencing these symptoms following exposure to a traumatic event, and such exposure is required for a diagnosis of PTSD.

Working with individuals who have trauma- and stressor-related disorders requires an empathetic, validating, and accepting clinical stance. For individuals who have experienced trauma, a sense of safety and control are primary psychiatric needs that affect their mood, cognition, behavior, and interpersonal relationships. For patients with a history of childhood sexual or physical abuse, interpersonal boundaries may be distorted such that relationships are too enmeshed or too disengaged. Thus, clinicians must accurately assess each patient's comfort with setting, enforcing, and maintaining healthy interpersonal boundaries across different relationships (e.g.,with colleagues, supervisors, children, romantic partners, parents, siblings, and strangers). Moreover, they must assess how their own background and identity may influence their therapeutic engagement with patients experiencing trauma-related symptoms. A great deal of the distress experienced by childhood trauma survivors occurs within interpersonal relationships because these individuals attempt to feel safe and secure but do not know how to establish healthy boundaries with others. An essential skill clinicians need to master when providing trauma-focused therapy is the ability to establish healthy interpersonal boundaries that facilitate a sense of safety and security.

IN-DEPTH DIAGNOSIS: ACUTE STRESS DISORDER AND PTSD

Ms. Benitez, a 28-year-old married Hispanic woman who lives with her husband and 3-year-old daughter, presents to an outpatient mental health clinic with complaints of experiencing a "weird sensation, like I'm floating and not myself" whenever her husband kisses her. The sensation is so distressing that she pulls away from her husband,

and at times she has even felt nauseated. During the initial evaluation, the therapist learns that 3 weeks earlier, Ms. Benitez had been robbed by a man who walked up behind her in a parking lot, put a knife to her throat, and demanded her purse as she was getting into her car. Without turning around, she handed the man her purse, and while taking it from her, the man licked her cheek, leaving saliva on her face. Since the incident, she has tried not to think about it and to "put it behind me." However, she has been experiencing disturbing dreams about the incident, and several times at work she had been bothered by "seeing the knife in my mind" while working on tasks that required concentration. She does not feel comfortable driving by herself anymore, and she has not gone back to the store where the incident occurred. She reports sleep disturbance and feels "jumpy all the time." Toward the end of the evaluation, she says, "Since that day, I just haven't been myself. I don't have patience with my daughter as I used to. I get angry really fast and just don't want to be around people anymore."

It is not uncommon for individuals who are victims of a violent crime to want to forget about it and to avoid reminders of the incident. Ms. Benitez's symptoms are in response to a traumatic event and are within the time frame (3 days to 1 month) required to meet criteria for acute stress disorder. If her symptoms continue beyond 1 month, she should be reassessed to determine whether she meets criteria for PTSD. Consistent with clinical presentation of acute stress disorder, she has a dissociative presentation (i.e., floating sensation) combined with a strong emotional and physiological reaction (i.e., pulling away from her husband when kissed and feeling nauseated) to a reminder of the traumatic event (i.e., being licked). Ms. Benitez should be monitored over time because acute stress disorder and PTSD are more prevalent across the life span among females than among males. Additionally, in the United States, higher rates of PTSD have been found among people of Hispanic, Black, and Native American race/ethnicity compared with White persons.

Approach to the Diagnosis

When evaluating symptoms for a diagnosis of acute stress disorder or PTSD, the clinician must first make sure that a qualifying traumatic event, in accordance with DSM-5-TR, accounts for the symptoms. Such symptoms can include those that result from experiencing repeated or extreme exposure to aversive details of the traumatic event through electronic media, television, movies, or pictures, but only if the exposure is work related (e.g., for first responders, police officers). The criteria that define traumatic events are now narrowly specified so that even if a person experiences a life-threatening illness, unless it is a life-threatening medical emergency (e.g., acute myocardial infarction, anaphylactic shock) or a particular medical treatment that evokes catastrophic feelings of terror, pain, helplessness, or imminent death (e.g., waking during surgery, debridement of severe burn wounds, emergency cardioversion), then the illness would not meet criteria for what constitutes a traumatic event. Being bullied may qualify as a traumatic event when there is a credible threat of serious harm or sexual violence. For children, sexually violent events may include developmentally inappropriate sexual experiences without physical violence or injury.

To be diagnosed with acute stress disorder, an individual must endorse a minimum of nine symptoms from any category of intrusion, negative mood, dissociation, avoidance, and arousal that began or worsened after the traumatic event. For PTSD, it is important to examine the number of symptoms within each category. For individuals older than 6 years, a PTSD diagnosis requires at least one intrusion symptom, at least one avoidance symptom, at least two symptoms of negative alterations in cognitions and mood associated with the traumatic event, and at least two symptoms of arousal and reactivity. For children ages 6 and younger, a PTSD diagnosis requires at least one symptom of intrusion, at least one symptom of either avoidance or negative alterations in cognition, and at least two symptoms of arousal. There are some differences in how the symptom criteria are defined for children versus adults; for example, intrusion symptoms may be expressed as play reenactment in children. Also, acute stress disorder and PTSD require duration of disturbance criteria to be met, which is 3 days to 1 month for acute stress disorder and more than 1 month for PTSD.

As stated in DSM-5-TR, "traumatic events such as childhood abuse or sexual trauma increase an individual's suicide risk in both civilians and veterans. PTSD is associated with suicidal thoughts, suicide attempts, and death from suicide" (p. 311). Thus, it is critically important that providers who see patients with a history of childhood abuse or sexual trauma assess suicidal risk and use therapeutic approaches that stabilize acute suicidal risk as well as reduce suicidal ideation and corresponding behaviors.

Getting the History

Ms. Keane, a 28-year-old woman, is referred by her primary care physician to a psychotherapist because she is having difficulty sleeping after being in a head-on car crash in which a fatality occurred. When conducting an initial evaluation, the therapist asks, "Can you tell me when you had the car accident?" to which Ms. Keane responds "Yes, 2 weeks ago." The therapist then asks Ms. Keane when she began to experience difficulty sleeping, and Ms. Keane responds that it began about a week after the car accident. "I would like to understand more about your difficulty sleeping," the therapist says. "Can you describe for me—with specific examples, if you can—what sleep difficulty you are experiencing?" Ms. Keane describes nightmares of reexperiencing the car accident that awaken her and disrupt her sleep. To understand what other symptoms may be present, the therapist inquires whether the accident has affected other parts of Ms. Keane's life, such as how she behaves, how she interacts with others, how she feels, or how she thinks; when these additional symptoms started; and how long they have lasted. The therapist asks about any head trauma that may have occurred in the accident and, if the answer is positive, follows up with questions to rule out neurocognitive symptoms related to a traumatic brain injury such as headaches, dizziness, sensitivity to light or sound, irritability, or concentration deficits (such symptoms were previously termed *postconcussive*). The therapist also asks about the history of other traumatic experiences to understand Ms. Keane's risk for ongoing trauma-related symptoms that may lead to her developing PTSD.

The therapist uses a combination of 1) direct, closed-ended questions to ascertain the timing of the traumatic event and the duration of symptoms and 2) open-ended questions to gain an understanding of the types of symptoms that are present and the degree to which they are interfering with Ms. Keane's psychosocial and physiological functioning. To develop an effective treatment plan, the therapist must rule out other comorbid diagnoses, such as depression or anxiety disorders. Given the strong emotional response that may be activated by questions about the traumatic event, the therapist needs to pace Ms. Keane through the process by attending to her nonverbal responses and assessing her ability to regulate her emotional response to questions. For example, the therapist may notice Ms. Keane's breathing becomes rapid when she recalls traumatic memories and may interrupt her by asking, "How are you doing? I noticed your breathing is getting rapid."

Caretaking on the part of the therapist may also be welcomed by the patient and validates that the therapist understands how difficult the situation is for the person to discuss. The therapist might ask "Would you care for any water?" or "Would you like to take a break?" Depending on the type of trauma experienced, the evaluation may need to occur over multiple sessions. To facilitate a safe environment for discussing horrific experiences, therapists whose patients have trauma-related symptoms must maintain an open, compassionate, and nonjudgmental stance.

Tips for Clarifying the Diagnosis

- Determine whether the individual experienced one or more of the following as described in DSM-5-TR: actual or threatened death, serious injury, or sexual violence.
- Consider whether the person directly experienced the traumatic event, witnessed the traumatic event, learned that a traumatic event happened to a close relative or close friend in which the actual or threatened death was violent or accidental, or experienced repeated or extreme exposure to aversive details of the event.
- Assess whether the symptoms began after exposure to the traumatic event.
- Clarify whether the symptoms lasted at least 3 days and not more than 1 month (acute stress disorder) or longer than 1 month (PTSD).
- If stress reactions are in response to a stressor that is not considered severe or extreme, consider adjustment disorder as the more appropriate diagnosis.

Consider the Case

Mr. Cooper, a 32-year-old single man, describes an injury he experienced while doing construction work as a U.S. civilian in Iraq during Operation Iraqi Freedom. He was in his office talking with coworkers and laughing at a joke when he heard a loud boom and sirens. He heard someone yell to get into the bunker, and then everyone started running. While running toward the bunker, he fell to the ground, got up, and started running again. Once in the bunker, he heard muffled voices that slowly became louder, and he soon realized people were talking to him. He remembers saying "I'm fine," and the next thing he remembers is waking in a hospital with bandages around his neck, arms, and legs. He had been shot multiple times, and shrapnel had been embedded in his neck, affecting his ability to speak. Mr. Cooper has undergone several surgeries, and a few more are scheduled, to remove the remaining shrapnel. It has been 8 months since the attack, and he reports that recently he started feeling "panicky and jumpy." He describes severe sleep disturbance with nightmares about the attack. He says everything around him seems surreal, as though he is "an actor in a play" that he is watching. He finds loud noises particularly disturbing, causing panic attacks that make it difficult for him to leave his apartment. He reports no previous trauma history, and his childhood experiences are what would be considered normative and healthy.

Mr. Cooper describes the type and duration of symptoms that are consistent with a diagnosis of PTSD with delayed expression. PTSD is characterized by the development of particular symptoms following exposure to events that involve actual or threatened death, injury, or sexual violence. In this case, Mr. Cooper experienced the threat of injury and actual injury. The delay of symptoms at least 6 months after the event (i.e., 8 months in this case) is atypical. Given Mr. Cooper's complaints of derealization (e.g., he feels as though he is an actor in a play), a clinician will have to evaluate his symptoms to determine whether they are persistent or recurrent and require the diagnosis to include the specifier "with dissociative symptoms." They also will need to evaluate any negative alterations in cognition and mood he may have that are associated with the traumatic event and need to be addressed in therapy. Furthermore, Mr. Cooper describes having panic attacks, but the symptoms to which he is referring are not clear. Therefore, a thorough evaluation of these symptoms is needed, and if they occur following exposure to traumatic reminders, then the PTSD diagnosis is warranted. An additional diagnosis of panic attacks may be warranted if Mr. Cooper experiences panic attacks in circumstances beyond reminders of the traumatic event. According to DSM-5-TR, rates of PTSD are higher among individuals whose jobs increase the risk of traumatic exposure, which is the case for Mr. Cooper. Thus, his job puts him at higher risk for developing PTSD.

In adults, it is expected that the content of recurrent, involuntary intrusive distressing memories will be related to the traumatic event. However, symptoms of intrusion vary across human development; as such, young children may start to experience nightmares that are not specific to the traumatic event.

Differential Diagnosis

Many life stressors can result in psychiatric symptoms that are acute or chronic, and not everyone who is exposed to an extreme stressor or traumatic event will meet all the criteria for a diagnosis of PTSD or acute stress disorder. The diagnosis of adjustment disorders is used in these instances. A patient may be experiencing a high-conflict divorce that invokes feelings of panic, sleep disturbance, and dissociative symptoms. Although these symptoms are also found in individuals with PTSD and acute stress disorder, the event (i.e., divorce) does not meet the diagnostic criteria for a traumatic event.

Acute stress disorder can be differentiated from PTSD because the symptoms for acute stress disorder must occur within 4 weeks of the traumatic event, whereas PTSD is diagnosed when symptoms persist for longer than 1 month.

Other posttraumatic disorders and conditions should be considered instead of PTSD if symptoms are not preceded by trauma exposure. Also, if symptoms that occur in response to a severe stressor meet criteria for another mental disorder, then the other diagnosis is given instead of or in addition to PTSD. In OCD, patients may have recurrent thoughts similar to the reexperiencing symptoms in trauma-related disorders, but these thoughts are not related to a traumatic event. Similarly, the arousal and dissociative symptoms of panic disorder and the avoidance, irritability, and anxiety of generalized anxiety disorder are not associated with a specific traumatic event.

In separation anxiety disorder, the symptoms associated with separation are not considered to be a traumatic event. Major depression may or may not be preceded by a traumatic event and should be diagnosed if full criteria have been met. Importantly, major depressive disorder does not include the Criterion B (i.e., intrusion) or Criterion C (i.e., avoidance) symptoms required for PTSD. Also, several of the Criterion D (i.e., alterations in cognitions and mood) and Criterion E (i.e., marked alterations in arousal and activity) symptoms found in PTSD are absent in major depressive disorder. If full criteria for PTSD and major depression are met, then both diagnoses should be given.

ADHD and PTSD may each include difficulties in attention, concentration, and learning, but ADHD symptom onset must occur prior to the person reaching age 12, whereas in PTSD the onset of symptoms follows exposure to a traumatic event. Personality disorders are expected to occur independently of trauma exposure; interpersonal difficulties that developed or were exacerbated by exposure to a traumatic event or multiple traumatic events may indicate PTSD rather than a personality disorder. Dissociative symptoms such as those seen in dissociative amnesia, dissociative identity disorder, and depersonalization/derealization disorder can be preceded by a traumatic event and may have co-occurring PTSD symptoms. When the full criteria for a PTSD diagnosis are met, then PTSD with dissociative symptoms should be considered.

Functional neurological symptom disorder (conversion disorder) may be better diagnosed as PTSD if the somatic symptoms occur after exposure to a traumatic event. Flashbacks or the reexperiencing of traumatic events found in PTSD must be differentiated from illusions, hallucinations, and other perceptual disturbances that occur in schizophrenia, brief psychotic disorder, and other psychotic disorders; depressive and bipolar disorders with psychotic features; delirium; substance/medication-induced disorders; and psychotic disorder due to a medical condition. Acute stress disorder flashbacks are directly related to the traumatic event and occur in the absence of other psychotic or substance-induced features.

Patients who experience a traumatic event (e.g., military combat, child physical abuse, intimate partner violence, motor vehicle or other accidents) that results in a TBI may develop symptoms of acute stress disorder and PTSD. It may be possible to differentiate PTSD from neurocognitive disorder symptoms by the presence of a distinct presentation. For example, symptoms of reexperiencing and avoidance are characteristic of PTSD and acute stress disorder, whereas persistent disorientation and confusion are more specific to TBI. Moreover, TBI-related memory problems are usually attributed to an inability to encode information, whereas PTSD-related memory problems are usually reflective of dissociative amnesia.

Feelings of panic are common in acute stress disorder. Panic disorder should be diagnosed only if the panic attacks are unexpected and the person has anxiety about future panic attacks occurring or engages in maladaptive behaviors in an effort to thwart what they believe to be disastrous consequences of a panic attack (e.g., death, severe embarrassment).

Acute stress disorder is distinguished from PTSD because the symptom pattern in acute stress disorder must resolve within 1 month of the traumatic event. If the symptoms persist for more than 1 month and the criteria for PTSD are met, the diagnosis is changed from acute stress disorder to PTSD. See DSM-5-TR for additional disorders to consider in the differential diagnosis. Also refer to the discussions of comorbidity and differential diagnosis in their respective sections of DSM-5-TR.

Summary

- Acute stress disorder and PTSD require exposure to an event involving actual, threatened, or witnessed death, serious injury, or sexual violation. In cases of actual or threatened death of a family member or friend, the event(s) must have been violent or accidental.
- Exposure to the traumatic event can occur in one or more of the following ways: directly experiencing the trauma, witnessing it, learning that it occurred to a close relative or close friend, or being repeatedly exposed to aversive details of an event that is work related (e.g., first responder).
- In acute stress disorder, nine or more symptoms must occur in any of the following five categories: intrusion, negative mood, dissociation, avoidance, and arousal.
- In PTSD, individuals older than 6 years must experience one or more intrusive symptoms, one or more avoidance symptoms, two or more negative alterations in cognitions or mood, and two or more arousal symptoms. Children ages 6 years and younger must experience one or more intrusion symptoms, one or more symptoms of avoidance or negative alterations in cognitions or mood, and two or more arousal and reactivity symptoms.
- The duration of symptoms is 3 days to 1 month for acute stress disorder, and longer than 1 month for PTSD.
- In acute stress disorder and PTSD, the symptoms cause significant distress or impairment in social, occupational, or other important psychosocial areas of functioning.
- In acute stress disorder and PTSD, the symptoms are not associated with the direct physiological effects of a substance or medical condition.
- Variability in the expression of symptoms in reaction to traumatic events may be influenced by age, cultural syndromes and idioms of distress, co-occurring traumatic brain injury, preexisting mental health disorders, and medical conditions.

IN-DEPTH DIAGNOSIS: ADJUSTMENT DISORDERS

Ms. Meyers, a 48-year-old married woman who was diagnosed with breast cancer 6 weeks ago, is referred to an outpatient mental health clinic for an evaluation of what her oncologist describes as "anxiety symptoms." She has two children, ages 10 and 13. During the psychiatric intake evaluation, she describes having difficulty sleeping since her diagnosis. She also reports experiencing a racing heart, sweating, and nausea when she has to see her oncologist, resulting in several missed appointments. When asked what stage of breast cancer she has, she is unable to answer, replying, "I don't know. There are stages?" When asked what treatment her physician is recommending, she replies, "I don't know; he said something about surgery." She has a difficult time recalling her conversations with her physician and states that she often "goes blank" when she is in his office, resulting in her not engaging with her physician regarding her care and experiencing difficulty recalling recommendations. She reports feeling "down" since the diagnosis and being unable to stop thinking about having cancer. She stopped going to her job of more than 15 years and has been unable to take her children to school, stating she has been "too depressed." She cannot turn to her husband for support because she does not want to upset him.

Ms. Meyers has developed emotional and behavioral (e.g., missing appointments) symptoms in response to her cancer diagnosis within 3 months of learning about it. The symptoms are clinically significant such that she is experiencing significant impairment in her occupational role (e.g., not going to work) and social relationships (e.g., disengaging from family responsibilities and from her husband emotionally). Her symptoms have features consistent with adjustment disorder with mixed anxiety and depressed mood. Her experiences of "going blank" when she is in her doctor's office and not recalling her physician's recommendations can be viewed as dissociative symptoms associated with a diagnosis of PTSD, except that a diagnosis of breast cancer does not meet DSM-5-TR criteria for a traumatic event. Adjustment disorders can complicate the course of illness and influence medical outcomes. In this case, Ms. Meyers is missing appointments and experiencing significant distress during appointments with her physician that interfere with her ability to recall information received during visits, which prevents her from engaging in her treatment.

Approach to the Diagnosis

The key to diagnosing adjustment disorder is to evaluate the presence of an *identifiable* stressor. The onset of emotional or behavioral symptoms must occur within 3 months of exposure to the stressor. The symptoms must meet a clinical threshold as indicated by distress that exceeds what would be expected, or the patient must have significant impairment in psychosocial functioning (e.g., social, occupational). The stressor must not meet criteria for another specific psychiatric disorder and not be an exacerbation of a preexisting psychiatric disorder. The symptoms do not represent normal bereavement and are not better explained by PGD. Also, they do not persist for more than 6 months once the stressor or its consequences are no longer present.

Adjustment disorder can be specified with depressed mood, anxiety, mixed anxiety and depressed mood, disturbance of conduct, mixed disturbance of emotions and conduct, or unspecified (e.g., maladaptive reactions that do not fit the other specific subtypes, such as physical complaints, social withdrawal, or academic problems). It can accompany many other psychiatric diagnoses, such as depressive or bipolar disorders and any medical illness.

An adjustment disorder can be acute if the symptoms are present for less than 6 months or persistent (chronic) if they persist for 6 months or longer. Symptoms cannot persist for more than 6 months after the stressor is no longer present; however, this does not mean that an initial stressor cannot lead to other stressful events, resulting in a continuous or chronic course. For example, the death of a spouse may lead to financial stress, which may in turn lead to the loss of a home; if warranted, the diagnosis of adjustment disorder can continue to be given during this sequence of events.

Because adjustment disorders are fairly common in clinical practice, and most individuals respond well to psychotherapy, it can be easy to miss the fact that, as stated in DSM-5-TR, "adjustment disorders are associated with an increased risk of suicide attempts and suicide" (p. 321). Best practice should include an assessment of suicidality for all individuals with an adjustment disorder diagnosis to ensure appropriate treatment and care.

Getting the History

> Darryl, a 10-year-old boy, is brought to the clinic by his mother because he has been suspended from school for vandalism. Darryl has been carving his name into the desks at school and was found using markers to write on the walls in the bathroom. He has also been disobeying his teachers, and his excessive talking in class is disruptive to the other students. He has been picking fights with his 7-year-old sister and engaging in frequent angry outbursts with his mother. Two months ago, Darryl's mother started having discipline problems with Darryl at home shortly after she separated from his father and moved with Darryl and his sister into a new home. The recent move meant Darryl had to attend a different school across town from the friends with whom he had grown up.

When evaluating a young child, the clinician needs to conduct a comprehensive assessment of the child's medical and psychiatric history with the parents or guardians to understand the nature, duration, and scope of the emotional and behavioral problems. It is important to rule out any medical basis for the symptoms and make sure the symptoms are not an exacerbation of a preexisting psychiatric diagnosis.

In Darryl's case it may be difficult to determine whether the stressor was the separation of the parents, the transfer to a new school, both, or some other related stressor. Stressors can be concurrent and may be multiple. The stressors in this case do not meet criteria for a traumatic event; however, Darryl is definitely experiencing marked distress that is causing serious emotional and behavioral disruptions. The stressors of his parents' separation and his subsequent move have both occurred recently, so if Darryl's behavioral symptoms have arisen in reaction to one or both of these stressors, the diagnosis of adjustment disorder could be made because the onset of the symptoms would clearly be within 3 months of the onset of the stressor(s). It would be important to inquire about the meaning of these stressors to Darryl to understand how they are linked to his functioning. Given Darryl's behavior at school and home, it would also be important to determine whether the criteria are met for adjustment disorder with disturbance of conduct.

Tips for Clarifying the Diagnosis

- Establish that the individual's symptoms are in response to an identifiable stressor that is not considered a traumatic event.
- Verify that the individual has developed symptoms within 3 months of the onset of the stressor.

- Assess whether the symptoms exceed what would be expected within the context of cultural or religious norms.
- Consider whether the symptoms persist for less than 6 months once the stressor and its consequences cease.
- Individuals who have not been exposed to a traumatic event but otherwise have the full symptom profile of either acute stress disorder or PTSD should be given a diagnosis of adjustment disorder.

Consider the Case

> Ms. Carter is a 32-year-old woman seeking services at an outpatient mental health clinic for her feelings of irritability and anxiety. At times, she engages in verbal rages with co-workers and her boyfriend, followed by feelings of sadness and hopelessness. Recently, she received disciplinary action at work for her disrespectful communication and excessive absences. Ms. Carter has been working at a midsize company for the past 5 years where she has been quite successful, working her way up from an entry-level administrative position to a program manager position in a relatively short period of time. She says that she was recently named "employee of the year" and has won numerous awards for excellence at her job. This changed 2 months ago when Ms. Carter was not selected for a director position at her company. The person who was promoted was someone whom she had trained. Ms. Carter states that she is constantly thinking about not getting the promotion and replaying in her mind the day she learned she did not get the position. During the intake interview, Ms. Carter states that she has been thinking that "my life is falling apart, and it would be so much easier if I wasn't around." She is convinced that if things do not change, she will lose her job and her boyfriend.

After someone devotes a great deal of time and effort to their career, it is understandable that when promotions or advancements do not occur, feelings of anger, sadness, disbelief, and irritability can develop. However, when symptoms persist beyond what would be expected, causing profound impairment in social, occupational, or other important areas, the person may have an adjustment disorder. Assessing the length of time since the stressor occurred is important because, to meet the criteria for adjustment disorder, the symptoms must develop within 3 months of the onset of the stressor and persist for less than 6 months once the stressor and its consequences have ended. Additionally, the stressor must not be a traumatic event as defined by DSM-5-TR.

In this case, Ms. Carter is experiencing marked impairment in her occupational and interpersonal relationships. Her reaction is clinically significant and out of proportion to the severity or intensity of the stressor (i.e., not getting promoted). A thorough mental health history will be needed to ensure that her symptoms are not an exacerbation of a preexisting psychiatric disorder. The nature, meaning, and experience of the stressor for Ms. Carter will be important to understand because other factors (e.g., social, cultural) may be contributing to her distress.

In the United States, adjustment disorder is often the most common diagnosis in hospital psychiatric consultation settings, frequently reaching 50%. Adjustment disorders are associated with an increased risk of suicide and suicide attempts and therefore require a thorough risk assessment and plan. This is particularly true in this case because Ms. Carter has expressed a cognitive belief consistent with suicide ideation that requires a thorough assessment, evaluation, and treatment plan to ensure her safety.

Differential Diagnosis

In DSM-5-TR, the symptom profile for major depressive disorder, even in response to a stressor, differentiates it from adjustment disorder. Therefore, if a person meets criteria for major depressive disorder, they would not be diagnosed with adjustment disorder.

Adjustment disorder can be differentiated from PTSD and acute stress disorder by the type of stressor. In adjustment disorder the stressor does not meet the Criterion A requirements found in PTSD and acute stress disorder. Moreover, adjustment disorders can be diagnosed immediately and persist up to 6 months after exposure to the stressor, whereas acute stress disorder occurs 3 days to 1 month after a traumatic event and PTSD is diagnosed 1 month after exposure to a traumatic event.

Differentiating personality disorders from an adjustment disorder requires a thorough evaluation of the patient's lifetime psychiatric symptoms and functioning. To diagnose an adjustment disorder when a personality disorder is present, it is important to assess whether the symptoms for adjustment disorder are met. Also, the distress response must exceed what may be attributable to maladaptive personality disorder symptoms.

Specific psychological symptoms, behaviors, and other factors can precipitate, exacerbate, or put an individual at risk for medical illness. In contrast, an adjustment disorder is a psychological reaction to a stressor (e.g., having a medical illness). Adjustment disorder can accompany any medical illness and may complicate the course of a medical illness; therefore, behaviors such as missing appointments, noncompliance, and complicated interactions with medical staff may warrant an assessment for this disorder.

Adjustment disorder can be distinguished from normative stress reactions by assessing the magnitude of the distress. Clinicians should evaluate whether the distress response (e.g., alterations in mood, anxiety, or conduct) exceeds what would normally be expected in response to the stressful event. Considerations of cultural factors are important when making determinations of normative reactions. See DSM-5-TR for additional disorders to consider in the differential diagnosis. Also refer to the discussions of comorbidity and differential diagnosis in their respective sections of DSM-5-TR.

Summary

- In adjustment disorders, symptoms develop in response to identifiable stressors that do not meet criteria for a traumatic event.
- Symptoms occur within 3 months of exposure to the stressors.
- Symptoms are characterized by marked distress in excess of what would be considered normative and culturally appropriate.

- Symptoms do not persist for more than 6 months after termination of the stressor or its consequences.
- The persistent specifier is used to indicate the presence of symptoms lasting longer than 6 months that occur in response to a chronic stressor that has enduring consequences.

IN-DEPTH DIAGNOSIS: PROLONGED GRIEF DISORDER

Mr. Smith is a 71-year-old retiree whose wife of 45 years died 2 years ago. He has three children, ages 37, 41, and 43, and six grandchildren who range in age from 2 years to 13 years. He is referred to an outpatient clinic by his primary care physician, who has become concerned about Mr. Smith since he lost his wife. Mr. Smith reports that he thinks about his wife "every day, all day." He says that he will sometimes walk into the kitchen thinking she will be there. He wishes that they had experienced their "golden anniversary" of 50 years together, and he says he cannot imagine himself happy without her at any point in the future.

Mr. Smith continues to eat well ("My wife would want me to keep eating") and denies sleep problems. He denies feeling suicidal but acknowledges that he "can understand it for some people." He shows no evidence of psychotic symptoms. The primary care physician referred him for evaluation of the following symptoms: paying inconsistent attention to personal hygiene; declining to visit his children and grandchildren or go to the coffee shop with his neighbor, as he did in the past; expressing the feeling that life lacks meaning without his wife; choosing not to answer calls from longtime friends; and expressing the idea he wants to join his wife. During his previous appointment, he told his physician he would not need his blood pressure medication anymore. Aside from high blood pressure and some osteoarthritis, he is in good physical health.

Approach to the Diagnosis

A diagnosis of PGD requires that a person who was close to the bereaved individual has been deceased for at least 12 months for adults and 6 months for children or adolescents. Persistent grief since the death is characterized by intense yearning or longing for the deceased person or preoccupation with thoughts or memories of the deceased person (in children and adolescents, preoccupation may be with the circumstances of the death). Also, at least three of the following symptoms have been present during that time: identity disruption (e.g., feeling as though part of oneself has died), a marked sense of disbelief about death, avoidance of reminders that the person is dead, intense emotional pain related to the death, difficulty reintegrating into one's relationships and activities, emotional numbness, feeling that life is meaningless, and intense loneliness. The symptoms are present most days to a clinically significant degree and have occurred nearly every day for at least the past month, and their duration and severity exceed expected social, cultural, or religious norms. The symptoms must cause significant distress or impairment in the person's social, occupational, or other important areas of functioning. They cannot be better explained by another mental disorder, such as major depressive disorder, PTSD, or psychosis, and are not caused by substance use or a medical condition.

Individuals whose symptoms of PGD develop following a violent loss (e.g., homicide, suicide, accident) are at greater risk for suicidal ideation, "even after adjustment for the effect of major depression and PTSD" (DSM-5-TR, p. 326). In addition, "individuals who experience the death of a child, especially if the child is younger than 25, are more likely to develop prolonged grief disorder symptoms that are associated with suicidal ideation" (p. 326). Consistent with other trauma- and stress-related disorders, the clinical approach to individuals with symptoms of PGD should include an assessment of suicidality, and if warranted, treatment should focus on reducing suicidal ideation and corresponding behaviors.

Getting the History

> Shayla is 5 years old and is brought into the clinic by her mother. Since Shayla's grandmother died 8 months ago, Shayla has been having difficulty sleeping, has been wetting the bed, and has lashed out whenever her mother does not care for her exactly the way her grandmother did. Shayla has also been complaining of stomach pains that seem to be getting worse. On most days, Shayla will sob and state she wants her grandmother to come home. She is having difficulty concentrating at school and often sits alone during recess. Recently, Shayla was found walking on the sidewalk with a bag full of her favorite things. Her mother asked her where she was going, and Shayla replied, "To be with Grandma." When asked where her grandmother was, she replied, "In heaven." Shayla's parents divorced when she was 1 year old. Shayla's grandmother moved in with Shayla and her mother after the divorce, stepping into a primary caregiver role.

As with all psychiatric disorders, clinicians need to conduct a comprehensive assessment of children's and adolescents' medical and psychiatric history with the parents or guardians to understand the nature, duration, and scope of the emotional and behavioral problems. It is important to rule out any medical basis for the symptoms and to confirm that the child's symptoms are not an exacerbation of a preexisting psychiatric diagnosis.

In Shayla's case, her grandmother was someone with whom she had a close relationship and who died at least 6 months ago. Since her grandmother's death, Shayla has experienced symptoms related to grief associated with losing a primary caregiver. It will be important to determine if Shayla's symptoms have occured nearly every day for at least the past month. She is also experiencing significant impairment in her functioning at school. Children tend to experience somatic manifestations of grief such as disturbances in sleep, eating, digestion, and level of energy. Shayla is experiencing sleep disruption, which is often associated with PGD, and has started wetting the bed, which may be indicative of developmental regression. The loss of a primary caregiver for children may be particularly traumatic because of the disorganizing effects of the caregiver's absence. Young children may protest or become angry when daily care activities are performed differently than by the deceased, which is marked by Shayla lashing out at her mother when her mother does not do something exactly the way her grandmother used to do it. They may also express that they want to physically reunite with the deceased to overcome painful physical separation (e.g., Shayla wanting to be with her grandmother in heaven).

Tips for Clarifying the Diagnosis

- Establish that the symptoms have developed in response to the death of a person who was close to the bereaved individual and who died at least 12 months ago for adults and at least 6 months ago for children and adolescents.
- Verify that the symptoms have been present most days to a clinically significant degree for at least the past month.
- Assess whether the symptoms cause significant distress or impairment in social, occupational, or other important areas of functioning.
- Consider whether the duration and severity of the bereavement reaction exceed expected social, cultural, or religious norms for the individual.
- Confirm that the symptoms are not better explained by another mental disorder, such as major depressive disorder or PTSD, and are not attributable to substance use or a medical condition.

Consider the Case

Ms. Liu is a 61-year-old widow whose husband died 13 months ago from an unexpected heart attack. Ms. Liu has been relying on her adult children (ages 30, 35, and 37) to buy her groceries, cook, clean, and take her to her doctor's appointments because she "just hasn't felt like doing it herself" since her husband died. Prior to her husband's death, she used to get together with friends on the weekends, but she no longer "feels like it." She tells her children she wants to join their father and feels as though she has died too.

Ms. Liu's symptoms are associated with impairment in her social functioning because she is withdrawing from social engagement with friends and has a marked reduction in her daily living activities (e.g., cooking, cleaning). PGD has a higher prevalence following the death of a spouse, partner, or child compared with other kinship relationships. Among children, the death of a caregiver increases the risk of developing PGD. If the unexpected death of Ms. Liu's husband has led to persistent stressors (e.g., financial problems), her symptoms may meet criteria for adjustment disorder with depressed mood, persistent, as well as for PGD, underscoring the importance of getting a complete and thorough history of the onset, severity, and duration of her symptoms.

Individuals with symptoms of PGD are at increased risk for suicidal ideation. Given that Ms. Liu has expressed the desire to join her husband, a thorough assessment and evaluation are needed to develop an appropriate treatment plan that ensures her safety and well-being.

Differential Diagnosis

PGD is differentiated from normal grief by the presence of severe grief reactions that persist for at least 12 months (6 months in children or adolescents) following the death of a person who was close to the bereaved individual. The severe grief symptoms must interfere with the individual's capacity to function; exceed cultural, social, or religious norms; and be present for most days over the past month. It is not unusual to notice marked increase in grief symptoms around dates that are reminders of the loss (e.g., anniversary of death, birthdays, wedding anniversaries, holidays); however, in the absence of persistent grief at other times, this temporary increase is not considered PGD.

Although PGD shares several symptoms with major depressive disorder and persistent depressive disorder, the distress in PGD is caused by feelings of loss and separation from the deceased loved one rather than being reflective of a generalized low mood. Individuals who experience bereavement following a violent or accidental death may develop both PTSD and PGD. Both conditions have symptoms of intrusive thoughts and avoidance. However, in PTSD, the intrusions are associated with the traumatic event (e.g., people, places, circumstances associated with the loss), and individuals with PTSD avoid memories, thoughts, or feelings that remind them of the loss. In PGD, on the other hand, symptoms are focused on the relationship with the deceased, including positive aspects of the relationship and distress over the separation, and individuals with PGD avoid reminders that the loved one is no longer present (e.g., activities shared with the deceased loved one). Reexperiencing memories in PTSD tends to feel as though the memory is occurring in the "here and now," which is not the case in PGD. A PGD diagnosis requires that the person feel a yearning for the deceased, which is absent in PTSD.

Differentiating separation anxiety disorder from PGD requires evaluation of the attachment figure who is the source of distress. Separation anxiety disorder is characterized by anxiety about separation from current attachment figures, whereas distress in PGD is caused by separation from a deceased loved one or caregiver. For a psychotic disorder diagnosis, someone with PGD must also endorse symptoms such as delusions, disorganized thinking, or negative symptoms (e.g., diminished emotional expression or avolition). See DSM-5-TR for additional disorders to consider in the differential diagnosis. Also refer to the discussions of comorbidity and differential diagnosis in their respective sections of DSM-5-TR.

Summary

- In PGD, symptoms develop in response to the death of someone with whom the bereaved had a close relationship.
- The symptoms persist for at least 12 months (6 months in children and adolescents) following the death.
- The symptoms are present to a clinically significant degree nearly every day for at least the past month.
- The symptoms include marked distress characterized by yearning or longing for the deceased person; preoccupation with thoughts or memories of the deceased; and marked changes in cognitions, mood, and behavior directly associated with the relationship to the deceased.

SUMMARY: TRAUMA- AND STRESSOR-RELATED DISORDERS

Reactions to traumatic events and life stress vary depending on the type of stress, the person, and the cultural context. The diagnostic class of trauma- and stressor-related disorders includes disorders arising after traumatic, life-threatening events and those that develop in response to stressors that vary in severity. The key to diagnosing these disorders is that the symptoms reported have developed in response to stressors that are identifiable. Reactive attachment disorder and disinhibited social engagement disorder develop in response to having experienced a pattern of insufficient care during childhood, even if the child is currently being reared in a normative caregiving setting. Adjustment disorders occur when a person responds to a nontraumatic event in ways that are considered excessive or that cause impairment in social, occupational, or other domains of functioning. Acute stress disorder and PTSD occur in response to traumatic events. PGD occurs in response to the death of a loved one with whom the bereaved had a close relationship.

The trauma- and stressor-related disorders have similarities with anxiety disorders and obsessive-compulsive and related disorders but differ in the course and duration of symptoms, prevalence, and age at onset. Reactive attachment disorder and disinhibited social engagement disorder are diagnosed in children and adolescents and are relatively rare. Childhood abuse, sexual trauma, adjustment disorders, and PGD are associated with increased risk of suicide. All of the trauma- and stressor-related disorders are serious and cause marked disruption in psychosocial functioning. For individuals with medical illness, these disorders can alter the course of their illness, thereby increasing morbidity and mortality.

ELEMENTS TO CONSIDER IN THE CULTURAL FORMULATION

- Research on reactive attachment disorders among children from diverse cultural backgrounds is scarce. Caregiving practices that are influenced by cultural norms and expectations may influence attachment behaviors that are quite different across diverse cultural settings. Diagnosing reactive attachment disorder in patients whose attachment styles have not been studied within their cultural contexts may result in misdiagnosis and poor treatment outcomes. To understand normative behavior in these circumstances, it will be necessary to assess cultural factors related to psychosocial functioning.
- Like reactive attachment disorders, disinhibited social engagement disorder should not be diagnosed in cases in which there is limited information on the influence of cultural expectations on children's social behavior. For children and adolescents, assessments should include cultural collateral information obtained from caregivers, teachers, and others who can assist the clinician in understanding the presenting problem.
- Exposure to traumatic events varies across different cultural, ethnic, and racialized groups, which may impact their response to the trauma and the severity of symptoms experienced. In addition to understanding the cultural factors associated with responses to trauma, clinicians must assess how their own background and identity may influence their ability to effectively diagnose and treat the patient's presenting problem.

- Cultural concepts of distress may influence dissociative responses, nightmares, avoidance, and somatic symptoms. Asking individuals what they think is happening to them and what the causes of their problems are allows them to describe their symptoms and problems in their own words.
- Grief responses may occur in culturally specific ways, such as seeing hallucinations of the deceased, having somatic symptoms, or engaging in poor self-care. Variations in mourning practices may lead to misdiagnosis because cultural norms can affect grief intensity, expression, and duration. Understanding how the patient's family, friends, and other community members perceive the presenting problem can help the clinician define the role of cultural factors and deliver effective treatment that is culturally relevant.

DIAGNOSTIC PEARLS

- The trauma- and stressor-related disorders diagnostic class includes disorders in which exposure to a traumatic or stressful event must precede the onset of symptoms. The response to such events may vary; some patients may develop anxiety- or fear-based symptoms, whereas others may experience anhedonic or dysphoric symptoms.
- In acute stress disorder and PTSD, traumatic events may be experienced directly or indirectly, threatened, or witnessed.
- Exposure to an event through electronic media, television, movies, or pictures does not meet criteria for an event that can trigger acute stress disorder or PTSD unless this exposure is work related (e.g., first responders).
- Acute stress disorder can be diagnosed 3 days after a traumatic event and may progress to a diagnosis of PTSD after 1 month if the symptoms persist.
- The symptoms associated with acute stress disorder and PTSD cause clinically significant distress or impairment in social, occupational, or other important areas of functioning.
- The absence of necessary and appropriate caregiving during childhood is a requirement for reactive attachment disorder and disinhibited social engagement disorder. The former diagnosis is expressed as an internalizing disorder with depressive symptoms and withdrawn behavior, whereas the latter is marked by disinhibition and externalizing behavior.
- Adjustment disorder can accompany any medical disorder and most psychiatric disorders.
- Prolonged grief disorder (PGD) is diagnosed when a person continues to experience clinically significant grief symptoms 12 months (6 months for children and adolescents) after the death of an individual with whom they had a close relationship.
- The symptoms of PGD must be present most days and occur nearly every day for at least the past month to a clinically significant degree.

SELF-ASSESSMENT

Key Concepts: Double-Check Your Knowledge

What is the relevance of the following concepts to the various trauma- and stressor-related disorders?

- Traumatic event
- Stressors
- Avoidance
- Negative alterations in cognitions and mood
- Hypervigilance
- Sleep disturbance
- Marked distress in excess of what would be expected
- Markedly disturbed and developmentally inappropriate attachment behaviors
- Intense yearning or longing for deceased loved one

Questions to Discuss With Colleagues and Mentors

1. How do you decide whether a response is normative or appropriate in different cultural contexts when trying to determine if a patient's symptoms meet criteria for adjustment disorder?
2. If adjustment disorder symptoms persist for more than 6 months and do not meet criteria for differential diagnoses, what diagnosis would you consider?

Case-Based Questions

PART A

Alton is 38 years old, identifies as nonbinary, uses they/them pronouns, and is HIV-positive. They describe using alcohol and cocaine since high school to "deal with stress." Alton describes "being on edge" all the time and "always jumping out of my skin." Between ages 5 and 9, Alton was sexually molested by an uncle. They report experiencing nightmares about the abuse and having difficulty trusting others. They often miss medical appointments because of not liking to be in a waiting room with "people I don't know." They describe their heart racing, palms sweating, and difficulty breathing when they are in the waiting room, and this happens whenever they are in a closed area around people they do not know. They are worried about the progression of their HIV and are afraid to be in a relationship because they do not want to transmit the virus to anyone. They avoid being around people and find it difficult to leave the house. They report feeling hopeless and "down" most days.

Thinking about the stressors Alton has experienced, what diagnosis or diagnoses might best capture the symptoms and behaviors they describe?   Alton may have PTSD associated with childhood sexual abuse and adjustment disorder with mixed anxiety and depressed mood associated with HIV.

Alton says they use alcohol and cocaine to cope with stress. It will be important to understand the signs, symptoms, and causes of Alton's "stress." Alton needs to be asked directly what they mean by "stress" and to describe their symptoms in detail. These questions are necessary to develop an understanding of the duration of their symptoms and the corresponding stressors that exacerbate them, as well as to appropriately diagnose Alton's condition.

PART B

Alton's CD$_4$ T-cells start declining, and their viral load increased. They are hospitalized with pneumonia. Once stabilized and released from the hospital, they begin to increase their alcohol and cocaine use to cope with the fear that the hospitalization evoked. After Alton enters into therapy that focuses on their childhood sexual abuse, panic symptoms subside, and they are able to attend medical appointments. As Alton begins to engage with their physician and understand HIV, they enter into a detox program. After completing detox, Alton is connected with a community organization for individuals living with HIV and begins attending a support group, which is helping to reduce isolation and improve skills to maintain sobriety.

Given that the co-occurrence of psychiatric symptoms and medical illness can complicate the course of both, how would you begin to work with Alton? Missing medical appointments that were necessary to manage their HIV compromised Alton's health. Their panic symptoms were in response to memories of sexual abuse (i.e., being in a closed area with people they did not know caused feelings of vulnerability, which triggered abuse memories). This case illustrates the complexity of childhood sexual abuse and comorbid medical illness. It can be difficult to know what the antecedent is to a particular stress response. A careful evaluation that explores the history of the symptoms, including the duration and contextual cues that elicit a stress response, is necessary for developing an effective course of treatment.

Short-Answer Questions

1. For acute stress disorder, what is the duration of symptoms following exposure to the traumatic event?
2. For PTSD, what is the duration of symptoms following exposure to the traumatic event?
3. True or False: Acute stress disorder and PTSD are more common among men than women.
4. For adjustment disorder, how long can the symptoms persist?
5. Acute stress disorder symptoms occur in five categories: intrusion, negative mood, dissociation, avoidance, and arousal. How many symptoms across any of these five categories are necessary to meet criteria?
6. How many symptoms of intrusion are required for PTSD?
7. How many symptoms of avoidance are required for PTSD in individuals older than 6 years?
8. For adults, how many symptoms of negative alterations in cognitions and mood are required for PTSD?

9. How many symptoms of arousal and reactivity are required for PTSD?
10. Adjustment disorders often complicate medical illness. What percentage of people in a hospital psychiatric consultation setting are typically diagnosed with an adjustment disorder?
11. True or False: For adults, prolonged grief disorder occurs when symptoms persist for at least 6 months after the death of a loved one who had a close relationship with the bereaved.

ANSWERS

1. In acute stress disorder, the duration of the symptoms following exposure to the traumatic event is 3 days to 1 month.

2. In PTSD, the duration of symptoms following exposure to the traumatic event is longer than 1 month.

3. False. Acute stress disorder and PTSD are more common among women.

4. In adjustment disorder, symptoms can persist no longer than 6 months.

5. Nine or more symptoms across any of the five categories are necessary to meet criteria for acute stress disorder.

6. One or more symptoms of intrusion are required for PTSD.

7. One or more symptoms of avoidance are required for PTSD in individuals age 6 years or older.

8. Two or more symptoms of negative alterations in cognition and mood are required for PTSD in adults.

9. Two or more symptoms of arousal and reactivity are required for PTSD.

10. As many as 50% of people in a hospital psychiatric consultation setting may be diagnosed with an adjustment disorder.

11. False. Symptoms must persist for at least 12 months following the death of a loved one for adults (at least 6 months for children and adolescents).

REFERENCES

American Psychiatric Association: Diagnostic and Statistical Manual of Mental Disorders, 5th Edition. Arlington, VA, American Psychiatric Association, 2013
American Psychiatric Association: Diagnostic and Statistical Manual of Mental Disorders, 5th Edition, Text Revision. Washington, DC, American Psychiatric Association, 2022

CHAPTER 12

Dissociative Disorders

David Spiegel, M.D.
Daphne Simeon, M.D.

"Sometimes I must have lapses of memory."

"Sometimes I feel as if I'm watching myself."

- Dissociative Identity Disorder
- Dissociative Amnesia
- Depersonalization/Derealization Disorder
- Other Specified Dissociative Disorder
- Unspecified Dissociative Disorder

The dissociative disorders all reflect a disruption of the normal integration of consciousness, memory, identity, emotion, perception, body representation, motor control, or behavior. This diagnostic class includes dissociative identity disorder (DID), dissociative amnesia, depersonalization/derealization disorder, other specified dissociative disorder, and unspecified dissociative disorder. Dissociative symptoms are experienced as intrusions into awareness and behavior, with loss of continuity in subjective experience (i.e., "positive" dissociative symptoms, such as identity disruption), or inability to access information or to control mental functions that normally are readily amenable to access or control (i.e., "negative" dissociative symptoms, such as amnesia or depersonalized detachment).

The dissociative disorders are more frequently observed in the aftermath of trauma, including childhood maltreatment such as sexual, physical, or emotional abuse. In keeping with such a history, many of the symptoms are deliberately hidden or confusing to individuals, making careful diagnostic evaluation critical. Stress often exacerbates dissociative symptoms. See Table 12–1 for key changes between DSM-5 and DSM-5-TR for dissociative disorders.

IN-DEPTH DIAGNOSIS: DEPERSONALIZATION/DEREALIZATION DISORDER

Ms. Day is a 20-year-old college freshman when she first presents to her school's mental health clinic complaining of feeling "very strange and out of it." She describes that over the past 5 months she has started to feel increasingly detached from her body, as though she has no self, and her mind feels blank. She goes about her daily activities like a robot, becoming less academically and interpersonally adept over time. At extreme moments she feels uncertain whether she is alive or dead, as though her existence is a dream; these experiences terrify her.

When asked by the school counselor, she denies any other unusual thoughts or experiences, hearing voices, or being fearful of others. She admits to feeling depressed over a recent breakup with her boyfriend. During that time, she first began to notice some feelings of numbness and unreality, but she did not pay much attention. As her low mood resolved over several months, she found herself becoming increasingly disconnected and became worried enough to finally seek help. She tells the counselor that her 6-month romantic relationship with her boyfriend had been very meaningful to her and that she had been planning to introduce him to her family soon.

Ms. Day denies ever having been depressed before, any history of hypomania or psychosis, and any other past psychiatric symptoms other than a time-limited bout of extreme anxiety and panic attacks in ninth grade precipitated by the psychiatric hospitalization of her mother. When her mother returned from the hospital, all of Ms. Day's symptoms cleared fairly rapidly. She also admits to several days of transient unreality symptoms in elementary school, when her parents separated, her father left, and Ms. Day lived alone with her mother, who had paranoid schizophrenia. This transient depersonalization in the context of her father's departure provides a framework for understanding her more severe depersonalization after the loss of her boyfriend.

Ms. Day's childhood was significant for pervasive aloneness and the sense that she not only raised herself but also had to parent her ill mother. Her mother did not abuse her but profoundly neglected Ms. Day's emotional needs and frightened her with her own limitations. Although Ms. Day largely kept to herself as a child, she did well in school and had a few close friends. She was deeply ashamed of her mother and rarely brought friends home; this boyfriend would have been the first to meet her mother. Ms. Day tells the school counselor that it feels as though a switch has gone off in her brain; she is so preoccupied by the seeming physicality of her symptoms that the counselor refers her for routine lab tests, otolaryngology and ophthalmology evaluations, a brain MRI, and an electroencephalogram (EEG). When all test results come back normal, she is referred to a psychiatrist. She also denies using any illicit substances, in particular cannabis, hallucinogens, ketamine, or salvia, and her urine toxicology result is negative.

Ms. Day's preliminary diagnosis is depersonalization/derealization disorder. She is experiencing various symptoms, such as detachment from her physical body, mind,

TABLE 12–1. Key changes between DSM-5 and DSM-5-TR

Although the diagnostic criteria for dissociative disorders did not change, the associated text was elaborated to better reflect the nuances of each disorder's presentation and to account for more recent literature.

Clarification has been added about similarities and differences between the dissociative disorders and other major psychiatric disorders, such as schizophrenia, bipolar disorder, depressive disorders, functional neurological disorders, and PTSD.

The importance of taking a careful trauma history and the impact of sexual abuse and child trafficking in the genesis of dissociative disorders is emphasized.

and emotions, and she has a pervasive sense of "no self," the cardinal symptom after which the disorder is named. Although she has had two previous minor bouts of such symptoms in her lifetime, those do not qualify for the diagnosis. The first bout was too short to meet criteria for "persistent or recurrent" symptoms; although DSM-5-TR does not specify a minimal duration for symptoms (American Psychiatric Association 2022), most clinicians follow the rough guideline of at least 1 month in duration. Ms. Day's brief bout was triggered by a severe emotional stressor, one of the more common precipitants of the disorder in large samples. The second bout of symptoms occurred in the context of escalating panic attacks probably meeting criteria for panic disorder, again precipitated by a severe emotional stressor. Although the symptoms were recurrent and occurred over a couple months, they did not meet criteria for depersonalization/derealization disorder because they occurred exclusively in the context of another psychiatric disorder and lifted with the resolution of that disorder. In contrast, Ms. Day's third bout was of several months' duration after the resolution of the short-lived depressive episode, increasing in intensity, distress, and impairment over time, and causes from medical conditions or illicit substances have been ruled out. Of note, her second bout of symptoms (during the panic disorder phase) was more heavily weighted toward derealization, whereas this third and clinically diagnostic bout is more heavily weighted toward depersonalization.

Approach to the Diagnosis

A very careful history of symptoms is central to making an accurate diagnosis of depersonalization/derealization disorder. Most patients with the disorder have been previously misdiagnosed. The symptoms are very subtle and subjective in nature, often with no observable signs, and individuals can find them very difficult to put into words. Clinicians need to encourage patients to describe their symptoms to the fullest, and they need to address patients' fears that they sound "crazy" and that they have never heard of or known of anyone with similar experiences. For clinicians who are not readily familiar with the whole range of symptoms, a thorough assessment scale (e.g., the Cambridge Depersonalization Scale) can be a very helpful guide. All major symptom domains need to be covered, including the sense of absence of core self and agency; the pervasive experience of unreality and detachment from self and surroundings; the numbing in the emotional and physical sphere; the disconnection and deadness of feelings; the detachment from mental content and thoughts; the perceptual alterations in all sensory modalities (visual, auditory, and tactile alterations are most common, but changes also occur in taste, smell, hunger, thirst, and libido); and the temporal disintegration (altered sense of time—past, present, and future; detachment from autobiographical memories as if they are not owned).

The onset and duration of symptoms must also be carefully assessed, as well as the frequency and duration of actual episodes and any change in all of these patterns over time. If there are psychiatric comorbidities, a thorough past and present history of the relationship of the depersonalization/derealization disorder symptoms to all other psychiatric symptoms must be assessed.

One important differential diagnosis to consider is that of a psychotic disorder or prodrome. This consideration is particularly important for Ms. Day because her mother experienced schizophrenia. There is no suggestion, however, that Ms. Day is experiencing a schizophrenia-spectrum disorder. Before the onset of her symptoms, she had a lifetime history of high academic and social functioning, unlike her mother. More importantly, there was no evidence of any schizophrenia-spectrum symptoms at presentation; the distortions in the experience of reality (rather than reality in and of itself) were only subjective in nature ("as if"), and Ms. Day had full cognitive awareness of this fact (intact reality testing). Finally, Ms. Day, like many others with this disorder, was initially strongly convinced of the "physical" nature of her distress. This focus on a physical source is a common feature of the disorder's presentation, but individuals never have a delusional elaboration on the nature of the physical source. In this context, such individuals commonly receive varying degrees of general medical and neurological workups, sometimes more extensive than is indicated, especially if they are young, with no atypical aspects to their presentation and no other pertinent risk factors. Such workups may be of value for their reassuring effect and may help individuals begin to come to terms with a psychiatric diagnosis that they may never have heard of and that is much less known than anxiety or depression.

Getting the History

The interviewer asks individuals to describe the nature of their symptoms, encouraging them to put their experiences into words and to elaborate as best they can because the symptoms of depersonalization/derealization disorder can be very difficult to describe. After asking open-ended questions, the interviewer inquires more specifically about symptoms in all the previously described domains, including unreality of self, unreality of surroundings, physical and emotional numbing, perceptual alterations, and temporal distortions. It is important to elicit the time frame for onset of symptoms and, especially if the symptoms were initially transient as can sometimes be the case, to find out when they became clearly persistent, recurrent, and associated with significant distress and dysfunction. All other past and present psychiatric history must be assessed in order to clearly ascertain the relationship of other psychiatric syndromes to the depersonalization/derealization syndrome, both in the past and in the present. If it is difficult to determine whether depersonalization/derealization disorder is the primary current diagnosis, the interviewer further teases out whether the comorbid conditions are largely resolved, are clearly of lesser magnitude than the de-

TABLE 12–2. Helpful prompts and questions for the clinical interview

I know these experiences are very hard to put into words. Do your best. You are doing a good job. Please say more.

Do you feel unreal, almost as if you no longer have a self or have lost yourself?

Do you feel detached from your emotions, numb, as if you cannot feel them even though you know you have them?

Do you feel disconnected from your mind as if it were blank or you have no thoughts?

Do you feel detached from parts of your body or your whole body?

Does your voice sound as if you are not the one speaking or choosing the words?

Do your past memories feel remote, colorless, and difficult to evoke?

Has your sense of passing time and its continuity been affected?

Do you feel robotic or as if you are on automatic pilot, going through the motions?

Do your bodily sensations feel dulled?

Do things around you look as if you are seeing them through a veil or fog, or as if they are dreamy or unreal?

Do things look different visually, such as too sharp or too blurry, two-dimensional or three-dimensional, too close up or far away, or otherwise distorted?

Does your sense of your body in space, your balance, or your movements feel off?

How do all these experiences make you feel? [After individual answers:] Sometimes people feel as if they are going crazy or losing their minds or as if they have some permanent brain damage.

Are these experiences causing you a lot of distress? In what ways?

Are these experiences affecting the way you relate to others, your interests and motivation to engage in life, or the ways you can focus and remember to do your work?

---

personalization/derealization disorder symptoms, or are clearly sequelae to the onset of depersonalization/derealization disorder. Table 12–2 provides some helpful prompts and questions, worded simply and in lay terms, to elicit more information.

As noted earlier, the following three aspects are crucial to the diagnosis:

1. Are the depersonalization/derealization disorder symptoms the predominant picture at the present time, equally or not more so than other psychiatric syndromes? In other words, are they clearly of greater proportion than any other associated psychopathology?
2. Are the depersonalization/derealization disorder symptoms frequent and severe enough to qualify as "persistent or recurrent," associated with significant distress or dysfunction, and not adequately accounted for by psychiatric comorbidity?
3. Are the depersonalization/derealization disorder symptoms clearly not due to any medical or neurological condition or to ongoing use of precipitating illicit substances?

Tips for Clarifying the Diagnosis

- Determine whether the patient has clear symptoms of unreality and detachment.
- Question whether the systems are persistent or recurrent, not just transient.
- Investigate whether the symptoms cause significant distress or impairment.
- Consider whether the symptoms are clearly independent or out of proportion in course and presence to other psychiatric symptoms.
- Rule out other medical conditions (e.g., seizures, brain injury or lesions).
- Make sure that the symptoms are not associated with ongoing use of alcohol or other substances, including illicit drugs, such as cannabis, hallucinogens, ketamine, ecstasy, or salvia.

Consider the Case

Mr. Rogers was 45 years old when he first started experiencing unusual symptoms, such as tightness in his head, tingling sensations over his scalp, "tuning out" to the extent that others thought he suddenly became noncommunicative, and experiences of his body floating and rotating in space. He denies feeling detached from his core sense of self, feelings, or agency over his actions. He does, however, admit to having his mind suddenly go blank, as if all thoughts have been sucked out. He is convinced that the cause of all his troubles is a defect in a specific right front part of his brain, which he thinks he can exactly pinpoint. The symptoms are very paroxysmal in nature and, although highly recurrent over the period of 1 year, typically last less than 1 hour. Mr. Rogers reports no other associated symptoms during these bouts. As a child, he had a history of febrile seizures, which had remitted by age 7; he also had a strong family history of epilepsy on his mother's side. The episodes have no clear precipitants, such as mood or anxiety states, severe stressors, or use of alcohol or other substances. He was a football player in high school and, during that time, experienced one severe concussion with loss of consciousness, a 3-day hospitalization and monitoring, and weeks of residual symptoms. He denies any other psychiatric or neurological history.

Mr. Rogers requires a comprehensive medical evaluation. His case necessitates careful consideration of the medical differential diagnosis. His symptoms of depersonalization/derealization disorder are rather atypical, highly physical, and suggestive of an underlying physical cause. Their duration is also quite short; although short episodes do occur in depersonalization/derealization disorder, typically episodes are either continuous (i.e., symptoms are ongoing in two-thirds of cases) or episodic but of longer duration (in one-third of cases). Additionally, Mr. Rogers has no identifiable acute precipitants for his symptom bouts; although lack of precipitants is not unusual for depersonalization/derealization disorder (in about one-half of cases), it does heighten the possibility of a medical differential diagnosis.

Mr. Rogers has a personal and family history of seizure disorders, and the brief duration and unusual symptoms with which he presents could suggest atypical seizures. The late age at onset of symptoms, which rarely begin after the third decade of life in depersonalization/derealization disorder, is also suspicious. The lack of any psychiatric comorbidity is very atypical. Finally, the history of a serious concussion, although historically remote, cannot be ignored, and very late–onset sequelae can occur.

In particular, mild traumatic brain injury (TBI) can go undiagnosed and can be difficult to detect, and the brain fog often associated with TBI highly mimics psychogenic derealization. For all these reasons, Mr. Rogers warrants a much more extensive workup than the usual patient presenting with depersonalization/derealization disorder. Brain imaging and a sleep-deprived EEG with temporal leads are strongly indicated. If the results are unremarkable, an extended ambulatory 3-day EEG recording examining the correlation between symptom bouts and brain events would assist in making a definitive diagnosis.

Differential Diagnosis

According to DSM-5-TR, depersonalization/derealization disorder cannot be diagnosed if the symptoms occur exclusively in the context of another mental disorder. Therefore, a very thorough present and past psychiatric history must be obtained so that the following five points become clear to the clinician:

1. If the person has had past episodes of another psychiatric disorder, such as major depressive disorder, panic disorder, social anxiety disorder, OCD, or psychotic disorders, these episodes have been treated or spontaneously remitted to an extent that the current depersonalization/derealization disorder symptoms clearly "have a life of their own" that unequivocally extends above and beyond any such comorbidity.
2. If the person is currently presenting with depersonalization/derealization symptoms as well as symptoms of other psychiatric disorders, particularly in the mood and anxiety spectrum, the depersonalization/derealization symptoms must be out of proportion to the other comorbid symptoms, and the comorbid symptoms must have later onset or be largely resolved.
3. The presence of depersonalization/derealization symptoms in an individual with PTSD most likely indicates the presence of PTSD with a dissociative subtype, rather than a separate diagnosis.
4. Depersonalization/derealization symptoms are common in various dissociative disorders, including DID. Therefore, before making a depersonalization/derealization diagnosis, other types of dissociative symptoms must be excluded.
5. Any suspected medical or ongoing substance use that may be causing the current depersonalization/derealization disorder symptoms must be excluded. Initial substance use that acutely precipitated the symptoms but is no longer occurring is not an exclusion (e.g., patient smoked cannabis 2 months ago, had a bad trip, and has had depersonalization/derealization disorder since without any subsequent substance use).

Summary

- In depersonalization/derealization disorder, a range of symptoms representing detachment and unreality from self or surroundings is present.
- The symptoms are persistent or recurrent; although there is no clear duration guideline in DSM-5-TR, a minimum of 1 month is a rough guideline.

- Significant medical conditions and comorbid psychiatric disorders must be ruled out. Another psychiatric disorder must have never been present; been present but be largely remitted; be clearly secondary to the depersonalization/derealization disorder symptoms; or, if still present, be clearly lesser in associated severity, frequency, and dysfunction to the depersonalization/derealization disorder.
- The depersonalization/derealization disorder symptoms must not be due to medical conditions or ongoing drug use.
- Affected individuals must be clear about the "as if" nature of the symptoms; psychotic elaborations must be absent.

IN-DEPTH DIAGNOSIS:
DISSOCIATIVE IDENTITY DISORDER

Ms. Moore, a 37-year-old divorced personal assistant, seeks psychiatric help because of gaps in her memory, suicidal thoughts, and relationship problems. She finds herself unable to account for things people say she has done. She also notices that even though she has just filled the gas tank in her car, it is half empty the next day, and miles have been added to the odometer. She is a hard worker, but her personal life is limited, and she spends much of her time alone. She mistrusts others and frequently feels taken advantage of in relationships. She is often sad but is able to put aside her dysphoria in the service of getting work done. Her marriage had ended at her insistence, and she has little interest in other relationships with men. She comes from a family that emphasized adherence to strict religious values but in which she had felt singled out and misunderstood. It later emerged that a relative had physically and sexually abused her over a period of years. She is highly critical of herself for not having run away from home. Further examination, including measurement of hypnotizability, indicates that she is highly hypnotizable. Ms. Moore has no history of substance use of any kind.

In the course of the initial examination, she suddenly switches among several identity states, one presenting the dysphoric persona, another that is angry and critical of the former, and a third that has a childlike personality.

Key features of Ms. Moore's presentation included gaps in memory, switching among identity states, and a history of sexual abuse. To make the diagnosis, the clinician does not need to observe the changes in identity. A history of memory gaps, reports by others of changes in identity, or evidence of behavior for which the person could not account provides evidence of dissociation. A history of sexual abuse is common in such cases, and individuals with DID are often dysphoric as well, but change in affect is usually a part of the dissociative process (one identity being primarily sad, another angry, and so forth). Structured shifting among identities, often facilitated with hypnosis, can help the person to understand and control the dissociation; other treatments include management of depression and suicidal ideation, psychotherapy aimed at stabilization, affect management, and then working through traumatic memories. Affected individuals are also prone to engage in activities that put them at risk for further mistreatment, so a therapeutic structure for protection is important. They also often expect further exploitation from caring figures in their life, including the therapist, so discussing and managing the "traumatic transference" is important.

Approach to the Diagnosis

The key to diagnosing DID is assembling a full picture of the person's history, behavior, memories, and mood that can encompass possible discontinuities in memory and affect. It is useful to be open, nonjudgmental, and exploratory in assembling information about the person's pattern of interpersonal interactions, mood changes, trauma history, and history of prior diagnosis and treatment. Such individuals may exhibit puzzlement, confusion, or guardedness in revealing their histories. They often feel guilty for traumatic experiences, blame themselves inappropriately for "allowing" mistreatment, or feel responsible for protecting family secrets. The information they present may be inconsistent. Persons with DID are often seen for medical and psychiatric treatment for 4–10 years before the diagnosis is made. Thus, their dissociative symptoms are likely to have been overlooked or discounted by previous diagnosticians. Such individuals are not likely to change from one personality state to another during early diagnostic interviews, although this change is possible, so a careful history of the person's experiences and reports of others are useful in determining whether there is discontinuity of identity, memory, or consciousness.

Standard assessments of hypnotizability, such as the Hypnotic Induction Profile or the Stanford Hypnotic Susceptibility Scale, can be useful in assessing both the likelihood of a dissociative disorder (high scores) and the potential for using hypnosis to identify and control the symptoms. Hypnotic and dissociative mental states are similar. Individuals with DID can learn to switch among identity states using hypnosis and eventually can begin to control spontaneous switching. Overt evidence of such dissociation is not damaging but rather presents a therapeutic opportunity for the clinician to clarify the diagnosis and teach the person how to understand and control the symptoms.

Because the disorder usually occurs in the wake of sexual or physical abuse, affected individuals often expect mistreatment by clinicians as well, so caution and respect for the person's tolerance of distress is crucial. The clinician can distinguish themselves from abusers by inquiring frequently about the person's response to questions or interventions and offering to change the course of the interaction to increase the person's comfort with it. Ultimately, the clinician's job is not to proliferate but to integrate dissociated elements of the individual's personality, to view these elements as a statement of distress, and to keep the focus on the whole person and on constructing the person's life story—which includes the scattered elements experienced by the person that may be seen as a problematic means of stress management.

As stated in DSM-5-TR (p. 334):

> Suicidal behavior is frequent. Over 70% of outpatients with dissociative identity disorder have attempted suicide; multiple attempts are common, and other self-injurious and high-risk behaviors are highly prevalent. Individuals with dissociative identity disorder have multiple interacting risk factors for self-destructive and/or suicidal behavior. These include cumulative, severe early- and later-life trauma; high rates of comorbid posttraumatic stress disorder (PTSD), depressive disorders, and substance use disorders; and personality disorder features. Dissociation itself is an independent risk factor for multiple suicide attempts....

Getting the History

A woman reports hearing a voice that is critical of her and that provides a running commentary on her mistakes and shortcomings. Such a symptom should raise questions regarding the possibility of schizophrenia as well as DID. Clarification of the differential diagnosis should include inquiring about the nature of the content of the hallucination: Is it bizarre or not? Does it have a consistent theme or is it disorganized? Other comorbid symptoms that would indicate schizophrenia include looseness of associations and flatness of affect. Individuals with DID would have alterations in identity and episodes of amnesia. The auditory hallucination would more likely take the form of a self-critical element of an individual's own fragmented personality structure. The differential diagnosis of DID from schizophrenia is especially important because the treatments are so different, and inappropriate use of neuroleptics with a dissociative disorder may not treat the target symptoms but instead flatten affect, delaying the appropriate diagnosis. Those individuals with DID may come to believe that there really are multiple identities within them, which could also be misinterpreted as a psychotic delusion and therefore another symptom of schizophrenia.

Clear differential diagnosis includes a careful history regarding the onset of the disorder. A history of trauma or abuse is more likely consistent with a dissociative disorder, and history of a decline in function in late adolescence or the early twenties without a marked traumatic origin is more consistent with schizophrenia. The interviewer should carefully ask about evidence for amnesia, including lost periods of time and inability to account for activities others witnessed. Sudden changes in personality and interpersonal behavior are more consistent with dissociation, whereas social withdrawal, a decline in planning and initiation of behavior, and persistent bizarre beliefs are more consistent with schizophrenia. A careful exploration of the use of substances is essential to ensure that the symptoms are not attributable to substance intoxication or withdrawal.

Tips for Clarifying the Diagnosis

- Ask the individual whether they or anyone else has noted sudden changes in their manner or identity.
- Ask whether they find clothing or other objects at home that they apparently purchased but cannot recall buying.
- Question whether they have noticed any gaps in their memory or periods of time for which they cannot account.
- Determine whether friends, family, or other people tell the person that they have said or done things that they cannot remember saying or doing. Such episodes must be differentiated from substance abuse.
- Establish whether the individual has engaged in dangerous or self-mutilative behavior that they cannot remember doing.
- Clarify whether the person has a history of sexual or physical abuse in childhood.

Consider the Case

> Mr. Smith is a 42-year-old gay man and veteran in a stable relationship who reports episodes of depression, personality change, time loss, and suicidal ideation. He has had repeated psychiatric hospitalizations and was previously diagnosed with borderline personality disorder and PTSD related to combat experiences. He has been aware for some time of his shifts in identities but views it as part of who he is and is more troubled by combat-related flashbacks. He shows evidence of self-mutilation, with scars on his forearms, and he has had intermittent depressive episodes. He is unable to keep a job because of poor attendance and memory gaps.

Mr. Smith has multiple comorbidities and is chronically impaired, but he has maintained a stable relationship. In fact, his partner is very accepting of Mr. Smith's shifting personality states. Because of his partner's perspective and Mr. Smith's concern about symptoms other than his dissociation, treatment will focus more on stabilization, safety, and affect management. Mr. Smith and his partner's shared sexual orientation place them in a stable relationship in a broader community that supports their bond, although they tend to be reclusive as a couple. Multiple psychiatric comorbidities present both a problem and a choice of clinical focus. In this case, Mr. Smith, his partner, and the clinician agree to emphasize treatment of PTSD and depressive symptoms rather than resolution of the dissociative disorder.

Differential Diagnosis

The mood of individuals with DID may fluctuate very rapidly in minutes or hours because of switching among different identities, which may include an active, upbeat personality state and another state that appears more depressed. Such shifts of mood can be mistaken for rapid-cycling bipolar disorder.

Psychotic disorders may appear to overlap with DID. Identity fragmentation can be confused with delusional disorder, and internal communication from dissociated identities can mimic auditory hallucinations in schizophrenia. Differential diagnosis from brief psychotic disorder should be guided by the predominance of dissociative symptoms and occasional amnesia for the episode.

Other considerations in the differential diagnosis of DID include the following: Posttraumatic flashbacks, amnesia, or affective blunting suggests a differential diagnosis of PTSD. Somatic symptoms involving alterations in sensory or motor functioning suggest a differential diagnosis of functional neurological symptom disorder (conversion disorder). A history of sexual abuse that results in conflicts over sexuality, body shape, and appearance may suggest a differential diagnosis of feeding and eating disorders and sexual dysfunctions. Questions regarding gender arising from differently gendered identities may suggest a differential diagnosis of gender dysphoria. DID may manifest with symptoms identical to those produced by some seizure disorders, especially complex partial seizures with temporal lobe foci. Symptoms associated with the direct physiological effects of a substance can be distinguished from DID by the fact that a substance (e.g., a drug of abuse or a medication) is judged to be etiologically related to the disturbance. Factitious disorder or malingering is also possible and is indicated by evidence of conscious manipulation of information about symptoms, as distinct from dissociative amnesia in regard to aspects of identity or experience.

Many individuals with DID have comorbid depressive symptoms, often sufficient to meet criteria for a major depressive episode. In major depressive disorder, most or all personality states are depressed. Individuals with DID often present with identities that comprise features of personality disorders, suggesting a differential diagnosis of personality disorder, especially borderline type. Comorbidity is also possible, especially when there is a severe trauma history in childhood and comorbid depression. PTSD is a common differential diagnosis and comorbid disorder.

Stabilization of dissociative and posttraumatic symptoms may be necessary before diagnosing a comorbid personality disorder.

See DSM-5-TR for additional disorders to consider in the differential diagnosis. Also refer to the discussions of comorbidity and differential diagnosis in their respective sections of DSM-5-TR.

Summary

- Individuals with DID exhibit failure of integration of aspects of identity, memory, or consciousness.
- Individuals with DID experience amnesia for daily as well as traumatic events.
- Disruption of personality or identity states occurs in individuals with DID.
- Trauma history is frequent among individuals with DID.

SUMMARY: DISSOCIATIVE DISORDERS

Dissociative disorders are a failure in function rather than an aberration in mental content; they involve the loss of integration of elements of identity, personality, memory, sensation, and consciousness, as well as depersonalization/derealization (e.g., detachment from the body, sense of self, or surroundings), amnesia for traumatic or other memories, and fragmentation of identity. These disorders occur typically in the aftermath of trauma, but unlike acute stress disorder and PTSD, a traumatic stressor is not a diagnostic requirement. There is a dissociative subtype of PTSD that involves depersonalization or derealization in addition to other dissociative symptoms of PTSD, such as flashbacks and amnesia. Neuroimaging data suggest that these dissociative symptoms of PTSD involve increased frontal and inhibited limbic activity—that is, an overmodulation of affective response. Symptoms may fluctuate, and many people with the disorder have limited awareness of the extent of their disabilities. Dissociative disorders are functional disorders, meaning that the ability to integrate elements of identity, recover memories, and reintegrate perception is compromised but remains, complicating diagnosis but offering opportunities for treatment.

ELEMENTS TO CONSIDER IN THE CULTURAL FORMULATION

- Culturally determined characteristics, such as those involving religious beliefs and practices, and the nature of altered states and their culture-bound interpretations, may appear more dysfunctional to outsiders despite being part of accepted religious practice.

- The nature of dissociation of identity in sociocentric cultures may take the form of intrusion by outside spirits rather than fragmentation in individual identity, which is more common in the West.
- Across cultures, predictors of dissociative pathology include earlier or more severe traumatic experiences; cumulative adversity; and social-political-economic adversity such as poverty, war, captivity, and trafficking.

DIAGNOSTIC PEARLS

- Dissociative disorders represent a discontinuity or failure of integration of common mental processes, including identity, memory, perception, and consciousness.
- Dissociative symptoms can constitute an intrusion into ordinary integrated functioning, such as identity disruption, or a failure of integrated function, such as amnesia or depersonalization.
- Dissociation is often related to a history of trauma, including physical and sexual abuse in childhood, as well as emotional abuse and neglect.
- Dissociative symptoms such as amnesia, flashbacks, and depersonalization/derealization can also be part of PTSD (including a new dissociative subtype) and acute stress disorder.
- Dissociative symptoms, including pathological possession and trance, occur in many cultures around the world.
- Dissociative symptoms are often hidden or unrecognized, requiring careful and informed evaluation. They tend to be underdiagnosed or misdiagnosed.
- Individuals should be evaluated in the context of their cultural milieu.
- Dissociative disorders must be inquired about in any new psychiatric evaluation. Basic questions covering all major dissociative domains must be asked.
- For a variety of reasons, including wariness and difficulty with verbalization, concerns over being deemed psychotic even though reality testing is intact, fearful attachment and mistrust, noncooperative alter states, and overall low symptom visibility, individuals with dissociative disorders are not always forthcoming in sharing their experiences with the clinician.
- While symptoms of dissociative disorders may appear to overlap with those of schizophrenia, bipolar disorder (especially Type II), borderline personality disorder, and PTSD, they should be evaluated in the context of the full range of symptoms present for each disorder.
- Because many individuals with a dissociative disorder are partially unaware of aspects of identity, memory, and consciousness or seek to suppress such awareness, it is very important to inquire carefully about suicidal thoughts or actions, which are common.

SELF-ASSESSMENT

Key Concepts: Double-Check Your Knowledge

What is the relevance of the following concepts to the various dissociative disorders?

- Dissociation and trauma
- Disintegration of identity
- Restricted memory access
- Impaired affect management
- Overmodulation of affect

Questions to Discuss With Colleagues and Mentors

1. What is the relationship between early life trauma and the development of dissociative disorders?
2. How can the clinician recognize dissociative symptoms of which the individual is not fully aware?
3. What accounts for fragmentation of identity?
4. How is dissociative identity disorder different from personality disorders?
5. How does the dysregulation of affect in dissociative disorders differ from that in mood and personality disorders?
6. What is the best way to clarify the potential role of other influences on the symptom picture, such as an emergent medical issue or effect of substances?

Case-Based Questions

PART A

Ms. Powell, age 29, is brought to the emergency department with deep lacerations on her forearm that were apparently self-inflicted. She reports having no memory of how it happened and acts in a fearful and tearful manner. She thinks she was running in the dark, tripped, and fell, cutting her arm on a piece of metal. This story, emotional but vague, does not fit the nature of the injury. She has in the past been diagnosed with bipolar disorder and antisocial personality disorder. Her presentation in the emergency department indicates some depression, no evidence of mania or hypomania, and no anger. The result of a urine toxicology screen is negative.

What should be considered in the differential diagnosis at this point? Ms. Powell may be deliberately concealing the history of her injury, either to avoid facing the consequences of self-harm or to avoid legal and interpersonal implications of accusing a family member or someone else of assault. This concealment could represent the minimization of adversity typical of mania, in which case elevated affect and pressured speech should accompany it. The appearance of anger, fear of abandonment, and manipulation may represent a demand for help coupled with interference in receiving it, which is typical of people with borderline personality disorder. If the patient has amnesia for the event, this amnesia could be caused by substance use, a cognitive disorder, postconcussive syndrome, or epilepsy. The amnesia could also indicate dissociative amnesia or dissociative identity disorder (DID). Inquiring about a recent or past trauma history can be helpful in clarifying the differential diagnosis.

PART B

> Ms. Powell agrees to assessment with hypnosis and proves to be highly hypnotizable. She is asked to relive, in hypnosis, the time just before her injury. In hypnosis, her affect and voice change markedly, and she says, "I wanted to be out, and she wouldn't let me, so I cut her so deep that she wouldn't want to be out and feel it. It was so deep that even I couldn't look at it, but it sure scared her." This dissociative picture, with amnesia of the self-inflicted wound, is consistent with a diagnosis of DID rather than depression with suicidal ideation or borderline personality disorder. This diagnostic interview provides a basis for future therapeutic work that can teach Ms. Powell to control her dissociation and negotiate conflicts among her dissociated identities.

How does this information clarify the diagnosis?   The fact that further information was retrievable with the assistance of hypnosis illustrates the type of amnesia typical of a dissociative disorder. A plausible explanation for Ms. Powell's wound was elicited, coupled with a sudden change in her affect and identity, which is typical of DID.

Short-Answer Questions

1. Describe two effects on brain activity during response to trauma-related stimuli in the dissociative subtype of PTSD, according to recent neuroimaging studies.
2. What is the relationship between hypnotic and dissociative mental states?
3. What would confirm the diagnosis of dissociative identity disorder (DID) during a diagnostic interview?
4. For what type of events may individuals with DID experience amnesia?
5. Depersonalization involves the psychological experience of feeling detached from what?
6. Derealization involves the psychological experience of feeling detached from what?
7. Dissociative fugue involves what two things?
8. What history do people with DID frequently have?
9. Dissociative symptoms and substance use disorder may be comorbid diagnoses under what circumstance?
10. Can auditory hallucinations be a symptom of DID?

Answers

1. **Neuroimaging data suggest that dissociative symptoms in PTSD involve increased frontal and inhibited limbic activity.**

2. **Hypnotic and dissociative mental states are similar, involving narrowing of focal attention and dissociation of awareness at the periphery. This shift in mental state is broader, less controlled, and more persistent in people with dissociative disorders.**

3. The occurrence of a dissociative switch during a diagnostic interview would confirm the diagnosis of DID.

4. Individuals with DID may experience amnesia for everyday or traumatic events.

5. Depersonalization involves the psychological experience of feeling detached from one's self or body.

6. Derealization involves the psychological experience of feeling detached from the surrounding world.

7. Dissociative fugue involves bewildered wandering coupled with dissociative amnesia.

8. People with DID frequently have a history of physical or sexual abuse.

9. Dissociative symptoms and substance use disorder may be comorbid diagnoses if the dissociative symptoms are not better accounted for by the substance abuse.

10. Yes. Auditory hallucinations may be a symptom of DID.

RECOMMENDED READINGS

Dorahy MJ, Middleton W, Seager L, et al: Dissociation, shame, complex PTSD, child maltreatment and intimate relationship self-concept in dissociative disorder, chronic PTSD and mixed psychiatric groups. J Affect Disord 172:195–203, 2015 25451418

Dorahy MJ, Lewis-Fernández R, Krüger C, et al: The role of clinical experience, diagnosis, and theoretical orientation in the treatment of posttraumatic and dissociative disorders: a vignette and survey investigation. J Trauma Dissociation 18(2):206–222, 2017 27673351

Dorahy MJ, Gold SN, O'Neil JA (eds): Dissociation and the Dissociative Disorders: Past, Present, Future, 2nd Edition. New York, Routledge, 2023

Killeen TK, Brewerton TD: Women with PTSD and substance use disorders in a research treatment study: a comparison of those with and without the dissociative subtype of PTSD. J Trauma Dissociation 24(2):229–240, 2023 36266949

Lebois LAM, Li M, Baker JT, et al: Large-scale functional brain network architecture changes associated with trauma-related dissociation. Am J Psychiatry 178(2):165–173, 2021 32972201

Lebois LAM, Harnett NG, van Rooij SJH, et al: Persistent dissociation and its neural correlates in predicting outcomes after trauma exposure. Am J Psychiatry 179(9):661–672, 2022 35730162

Menon V: Dissociation by network integration. Am J Psychiatry 178(2):110–112, 2021 33517751

Myrick AC, Webermann AR, Loewenstein RJ, et al: Six-year follow-up of the treatment of patients with dissociative disorders study. Eur J Psychotraumatol 8(1):1344080, 2017 28680542

Nester MS, Schielke HJ, Brand BL, Loewenstein RJ: Dissociative identity disorder: diagnostic accuracy and DSM-5 criteria change implications. J Trauma Dissociation 2021 Oct 18:1–13, 2021 34661505

Schlumpf YR, Nijenhuis ERS, Klein C, et al: Resting-state functional connectivity in patients with a complex PTSD or complex dissociative disorder before and after inpatient trauma treatment. Brain Behav 11(7):e02200, 2021 34105902

Vesuna S, Kauvar IV, Richman E, et al: Deep posteromedial cortical rhythm in dissociation. Nature 586(7827):87–94, 2020 32939091

Webermann AR, Brand BL, Chasson GS: Childhood maltreatment and intimate partner violence in dissociative disorder patients. Eur J Psychotraumatol 5:5, 2014 25279109

REFERENCE

American Psychiatric Association: Diagnostic and Statistical Manual of Mental Disorders, 5th Edition, Text Revision. Washington, DC, American Psychiatric Association, 2022

CHAPTER 13

Somatic Symptom and Related Disorders

Ann C. Schwartz, M.D.

Thomas W. Heinrich, M.D.

"They tell me I'm fine, but I know I'm not."

"None of the doctors can figure out why I have
so many things wrong with me."

- Somatic Symptom Disorder
- Illness Anxiety Disorder
- Functional Neurological Symptom Disorder (Conversion Disorder)
- Psychological Factors Affecting Other Medical Conditions
- Factitious Disorder
- Other Specified Somatic Symptom and Related Disorder
- Unspecified Somatic Symptom and Related Disorder

The somatic symptom and related disorders, when introduced in DSM-5 (American Psychiatric Association 2013), replaced DSM-IV's somatoform disorders (American Psychiatric Association 1994). Although the somatic symptom and related disorders remain in DSM-5-TR (American Psychiatric Association 2022) and continue to share the features of predominant physical symptoms associated with significant distress and subsequent functional impairment, there are some minor changes (Table 13–1). The somatic symptom and related disorders differ from DSM-IV's somatoform disorders by emphasizing the presence of distressing thoughts, feelings, and behaviors associated with physical complaints rather than focusing on the presence of medically unexplained somatic symptoms. Individuals with somatic symptom and related disorders integrate maladaptive cognitive, behavioral, or emotional valence(s) with their physical complaints. It is not the absence of an identified medical etiology for the individual's physical complaints but how the individual interprets and functions with these physical complaints that is the focus of the somatic symptom and related disorders. Indeed, individuals may present with both a diagnosed medical condition and abnormal behaviors and thoughts related to this identified illness and its associated physical symptoms and still meet the criteria for a somatic symptom disorder.

The diagnosis of somatic symptom disorder requires the manifestation of maladaptive feelings, thoughts, or behaviors related to physical symptoms. Individuals with somatic symptom disorder typically have multiple active and distressing physical complaints, although sometimes they may present with only one severe and persistent symptom. Emotionally, individuals experience significant worry and distress about their symptoms or illness. Cognitive features include an abnormal focus on physical symptoms and attribution of normal bodily sensations to the presence of an illness. Behavioral features may consist of the repeated seeking of medical help and reassurance. The presence of a concurrent medical illness, which may explain the person's somatic symptoms, does not rule out the diagnosis of a somatic symptom disorder.

A person with illness anxiety disorder experiences excessive concern about acquiring or preoccupation with having a serious, yet-undiagnosed medical illness. This is despite thorough medical evaluations that have failed to identify a medical condition to account for the individual's concern. Although the individual's fear may be derived from a physical sign or sensation, it does not originate primarily from the somatic complaint but instead from anxiety surrounding the significance of the symptom and the potential for an adverse etiology of the complaint.

In functional neurological symptom disorder (conversion disorder) (FNSD), the person experiences functional symptoms or subjective deficits affecting the voluntary motor or sensory nervous system. In addition, there is evidence that these deficits or symptoms are inconsistent with recognized neurological and medical diseases. If a recognized neurological, medical, or psychiatric disorder is present, the symptom must not be better explained by that disorder. FNSD differs from other somatic symptom disorders in that medically unexplained symptoms remain a key feature of this diagnosis. However, the diagnosis should not be made simply because investigations for an etiology yield normal results. There must also be evidence that the symptoms are functional in etiology, as demonstrated by internal inconsistency or incompatibility with a known disease process.

The disorder of psychological factors affecting other medical conditions is also included in the somatic symptom and related disorders category of DSM-5-TR. The essential feature of this disorder is the presence of clinically significant behavioral or psychological factors that adversely affect the management of a co-occurring medical condition, increasing the risk of poor medical or psychological outcomes. Factitious

TABLE 13–1. **Key changes between DSM-5 and DSM-5-TR**

Functional neurological symptom disorder (conversion disorder) is the new DSM-5-TR classification for DSM-5's conversion disorder (functional neurological symptom disorder).

Increased rates of suicidal thoughts and behaviors related to somatic symptom disorder and functional neurological symptom disorder are described.

Sex- and gender-related diagnostic issues have been clarified in somatic symptom disorder and factitious disorder.

Psychological factors affecting other medical conditions and factitious disorder have both been added to the diagnoses listed in the "Differential Diagnosis" section of somatic symptom disorder.

disorder, another diagnosis included within the somatic symptom and related disorders section of DSM-5-TR, addresses patients who intentionally falsify physical or psychological symptoms or signs of a disease or injury in the absence of external rewards.

IN-DEPTH DIAGNOSIS: SOMATIC SYMPTOM DISORDER

Ms. Thomas is a 32-year-old cisgender woman referred to the mental health clinic for a "second opinion" from her primary care physician. Ms. Thomas endorses a multiyear history of chronic headaches, pain in multiple joints, and intermittent abdominal pain complicated by occasional nausea. She reports that she has undergone numerous studies and seen multiple specialists to find a cause for her symptoms, but unfortunately, no clear etiology has been identified to date. Nothing has improved the chronic waxing and waning of these symptoms. She has not been able to hold a job for any length of time because of frequent and often lengthy medical hospitalizations for nausea. The patient further explains that her immediate family has grown tired of all her physical complaints and her intense and excessive focus on these symptoms. Despite what appears to be a comprehensive medical evaluation to date, Ms. Thomas feels that a few more tests may be warranted (she brought a list) to help find the medical cause of her "suffering." She is slightly "put off" by being referred to psychiatry. Although she is frustrated with the lack of explanation for her somatic complaints, she denies depression or significant anxiety. A careful review of her medical records reveals multiple negative studies, vague discharge summaries, numerous medication trials coupled with many medication "sensitivities," and many diagnoses from many providers.

Ms. Thomas displays multiple physical complaints that she finds quite distressing and that interfere with her daily life (i.e., the quality of her relationships with others and her ability to work). The physical symptoms of somatic symptom disorder could be related to a known medical condition or, as in this case, may be medically unexplained. The experience of somatic symptoms of unclear etiology is not in itself sufficient to make a diagnosis of somatic symptom disorder, however. These somatic symptoms must be complicated by excessive maladaptive thoughts, feelings, and behaviors.

Ms. Thomas also displays persistent and excessive concern about the seriousness of her symptoms, despite a thorough medical evaluation that failed to reveal a potential etiology to her multiple somatic complaints. She displays a chronic high level of anxiety or worry related to her physical symptoms. Her family reports that she is always, and overly, focused on her multitude of symptoms. Her health issues appear to dominate her life, leading to significant functional and social impairment.

Approach to the Diagnosis

Well-trained clinicians will keep somatic symptom disorder in mind when encountering individuals with one or multiple somatic complaints, such as pain, sexual problems, fatigue, or gastrointestinal problems. Individuals often present dramatically with lengthy and complicated past medical and surgical histories. Evaluation of a person with possible somatic symptom disorder starts with a thorough review of the medical records for appropriate medical evaluation and confirmation of the medical diagnoses. The presence of an identified concurrent medical illness, such as coronary artery disease, does not rule out the diagnosis of somatic symptom disorder. Collateral information, from a spouse, for example, may help clarify symptoms, functional disability, and previous evaluations or diagnoses (medical and psychological). Attention to the person's mental status for evidence of a mood or anxiety disorder is essential because these disorders are often comorbid with somatic symptom disorder and may complicate its presentation and subsequent treatment.

The clinician should carefully assess the person's attitude toward the somatic complaints and illness-related behaviors. Cognitive distortions may include catastrophic interpretations of normal bodily sensations. The maladaptive thoughts, feelings, and behaviors that they experience with the physical complaints tend to cause them to think the worst about their health, worry at high levels, and spend excessive amounts of time and energy devoted to their health concerns. Consequently, it is not uncommon for the physical symptoms to become central to the person's personality and to contaminate important interpersonal relations (e.g., family, professional, and health care).

The high level of somatically focused distress experienced by these individuals contributes to poor health-related quality of life. Their focus on somatic symptoms often also leads to increased use of health care resources. However, they obtain little associated long-term clinical benefit for their somatic complaints or health-related concerns. In addition, individuals with somatic symptom disorder often prove intolerant to various medications or other therapies meant to help address an identified pathology or the associated symptoms. As a result, they may experience their health care as frustrating or inadequate and will often seek multiple referrals and receive care from numerous medical providers in pursuit of a resolution.

Several specifiers are associated with the diagnosis of somatic symptom disorder, including the current severity (mild, moderate, or severe) and course (persistent) of the disorder. The severity is determined by tallying the patient's excessive thoughts, feelings, and behaviors, along with the severity and number of physical complaints they experience. In addition, defining features of the symptom presentation may be included in the diagnosis. For example, if the person's somatic focus is predominantly pain, it is often most appropriately coded with the specifier "with predominant pain."

Getting the History

Ms. Adams, a 27-year-old woman, is referred by her primary care physician for a mental health evaluation because she has multiple somatic symptoms without an identified "organic" cause. Ms. Adams is displeased that her primary care physician has referred her to a mental health provider because she believes that her problems have a physical etiology. Despite a degree of defensiveness in the patient, the clinician determines that Ms. Adams finds these symptoms "very distressing" and that they cause a significant level of functional impairment. During the interview, the physical symptoms tend to take "center stage," with most of her responses involving at least some mention of her somatic complaints.

The interviewer asks Ms. Adams, "Please describe your thoughts about your symptoms and what might be causing them." She answers that she has no idea what is causing these symptoms and implies that the physician should know the answer to that question. She adds that she is extremely frustrated with what she perceives as inadequate medical care and an unresponsive medical system. Next, the clinician asks a question to determine if the worrisome thoughts are excessive to her physical symptoms. Ms. Adams responds that despite many medical evaluations on both an inpatient and outpatient basis and multiple episodes of physician reassurance, her somatic worries and health-related concerns persist. She explains that these issues cause significant anxiety about her health. The clinician follows up with a query about how her somatic complaints may alter her behavior. Ms. Adams responds that she is afraid to engage in certain physical activities for fear of worsening her symptoms. When the interviewer inquires about the duration of her complaints, Ms. Adams states that she has been symptomatic for more than 6 years.

The history provided by Ms. Adams makes somatic symptom disorder the most likely clinical diagnosis. Ms. Adams exhibits a greater than 6-month history of somatic symptoms that she finds very distressing and that impair her quality of life. The history also reveals that she experiences maladaptive thoughts (e.g., catastrophic interpretations of her symptoms), intense health-related anxiety, and abnormal behaviors (e.g., avoidance of certain activities) related to her physical complaints. Ms. Adams's persistent focus on her myriad somatic symptoms is a primary feature of her presentation. Her intense attention to her physical symptoms and her illness anxiety dominate the interview and, most likely, her social and professional relationships.

Many individuals with somatic symptom disorder may meet referral to a mental health clinician with skepticism because they resist accepting that there is an underlying psychological problem. The somatic symptoms they experience may or, as in this case, may not be associated with a medical condition. Regardless of the etiology of the physical complaints, however, these individuals are truly distressed, often with very high levels of health anxiety and impairment.

Tips for Clarifying the Diagnosis

- Have the individual describe the somatic complaints, including organ system involvement and duration, along with aggravating and alleviating factors.
- What is their perception of the somatic symptom(s), including thoughts and feelings related to their physical complaint(s)?

- Do they exhibit maladaptive behaviors or cognitions related to their somatic complaints?
- What is their level of health care utilization?
- How have they responded to past reassurances, medical interventions, or pharmacotherapies?

Consider the Case

Mr. Knight is a 42-year-old cisgender man with a medical history significant for well-controlled hypertension and hyperlipidemia and a history of coronary artery disease and myocardial infarction. He presents to the mental health clinic on referral from his cardiologist for evaluation of depression following a recent medical admission for chest pain. He is somewhat disgruntled with the referral to a mental health provider. He has presented to the emergency department several times over the past 8 months with concerns that he may be having another "heart attack" after experiencing some chest discomfort. A thorough medical evaluation has not demonstrated progression of his underlying heart disease or another medical cause of his symptoms. His father died from a myocardial infarction in his mid-forties. Mr. Knight's wife reports that he is "very focused" on his risk factors for cardiac disease, measures his blood pressure multiple times a day, and gets very "antsy" if he forgets his cardiac medications. He admits that if he perceives any chest discomfort, he races to the emergency department because he fears that if he does not do so, it "may be too late." He denies any affective symptoms suggesting a major depressive disorder. He reports being relieved after receiving physician reassurance and when each successive test shows no more "muscle has died," but his excessive concern about the progression of his heart disease gradually returns.

Individuals with somatic symptom disorder often have multiple somatic symptoms, but some experience only one severe physical complaint, such as Mr. Knight's chest pain. The presence of an identified concurrent medical illness, such as coronary artery disease, does not rule out the diagnosis of somatic symptom disorder. Somatic symptom disorder differs from the DSM-IV somatoform disorders in that it does not require that the symptoms be medically unexplained. If a medical condition is present that may account for the somatic symptoms and health-related anxiety, the associated abnormal feelings, thoughts, and behaviors must be excessive. Mr. Knight demonstrates excessive maladaptive thoughts, feelings, and behaviors that are related to his complaint of chest pain and his associated health concerns of experiencing another myocardial infarction. His complaints and concerns are persistent and anxiety provoking, and he spends excessive time addressing these health concerns. Cognitive distortions may include catastrophic interpretations of normal bodily sensations. Health concerns, most often surrounding the somatic complaints, may assume a central role in the person's life, dominating interpersonal relationships and complicating psychosocial functioning. Individuals with somatic symptom disorder typically first present in the general medical setting rather than the mental health setting because their symptom focus is physical, not psychological. Studies have demonstrated that somatic symptom disorder is more common in females.

Several variables may contribute to the development of somatic symptom disorder, including physiological factors, such as the potential for a person to have a genetic vulnerability to an elevated level of sensitivity to pain. Cultural norms that often stigmatize psychological distress but not physical pain may influence the development of somatic symptom disorder. In these cases, it is often helpful to view the physical symptoms that may complicate the presentation of a psychiatric disorder as a marker of clinical distress that varies across cultures. In addition, the language used by individuals to explain their somatic complaints may differ among cultures, complicating the diagnosis for physicians who are unfamiliar with the person's culture. These factors interact to various degrees to influence how the person with somatic symptom disorder presents their distress to the clinician.

Differential Diagnosis

The differential diagnosis of somatic symptom disorder is extensive. It includes other psychiatric disorders and medical conditions with nonspecific, transient, and often multisystem involvement (e.g., autoimmune disorders such as systemic lupus). If another psychiatric disorder better accounts for the person's physical symptoms (e.g., the neurovegetative symptoms of major depression or the symptoms of autonomic arousal associated with panic disorder) and the diagnostic criteria for that disorder are fully satisfied, then that psychiatric disorder should be considered as an alternative diagnosis or a comorbid condition. Psychiatric disorders to consider in the differential diagnosis of somatic symptom disorder include anxiety disorders such as generalized anxiety disorder (GAD) and panic disorder. The anxiety in somatic symptom disorder is related to wellness concerns, not other more general or environmental sources of anxiety. The affective symptoms such as sadness and hopelessness and the negative cognitions of guilt and suicidal thoughts are absent in somatic symptom disorder, unlike in major depressive disorder. Individuals experiencing illness anxiety disorder have maladaptive anxiety about their health but lack significant associated somatic symptoms. FNSD is defined by a loss of function, whereas in somatic symptom disorder, the diagnostic focus is on bodily symptom–related distress. Somatic symptom disorder is differentiated from a delusional disorder because, in somatic symptom disorder, the somatic beliefs are usually realistic and not held with a delusional intensity. Unlike OCD, the recurrent ideas about illness or somatic symptoms in somatic symptom disorder do not have associated repetitive behaviors aimed at reducing anxiety. In body dysmorphic disorder, the person is preoccupied with a perceived defect in their physical features, not a somatic complaint related to a fear of an underlying medical illness. Malingering and factitious disorder should also be considered in the differential diagnosis when there is a concern that the patient may be deceiving the provider with their somatic presentation.

Summary

- The individual experiences one or more somatic symptoms that they find distressing or that result in significant disruption of daily function.
- Somatic symptom disorder may occur in the presence or absence of a medical condition accounting for the physical symptoms. However, if a medical condition is responsible for the physical complaints, the symptom-associated thoughts, feelings, and behaviors are disproportionate, excessive, and maladaptive.

- The person experiences chronic and excessive thoughts about the seriousness of the somatic symptoms.
- The somatic complaints and health concerns contribute to the person's substantial anxiety about their health or the significance of the associated symptoms.
- The individual with somatic symptom disorder may also spend excessive time or energy on the physical symptoms or related health concerns.
- The person must be somatically preoccupied for more than 6 months. The symptoms, however, may vary throughout the course of the illness.

IN-DEPTH DIAGNOSIS: ILLNESS ANXIETY DISORDER

Ms. Xavier, a 32-year-old woman, presented to the emergency department complaining of a mild headache and "floaters" in her vision. She appeared anxious and expressed concern that these were symptoms of a brain tumor. She underwent several tests, including head imaging, and was told that the headache was likely a tension headache. She declined pain medications, stating that the pain was minimal.

Ms. Xavier has presented to the emergency department and her primary care physician six times in the past few months with various somatic symptoms, including dizziness, headaches, and floaters in her eyes. Multiple medical evaluations have failed to identify a serious medical condition, but Ms. Xavier remains concerned that she has a brain tumor despite reassurance from her primary care physician. She has missed several days of work because of medical appointments and has difficulty completing tasks and concentrating because of anxiety. She states that the anxiety primarily revolves around her health concerns. Collateral history from her husband indicates a strain on the marriage because of her "obsession" with having a brain tumor.

Individuals with illness anxiety disorder may present to a medical setting with a high level of anxiety about having a serious illness (e.g., a brain tumor). Although Ms. Xavier is young and otherwise healthy, a complete medical workup must be completed to rule out a medical cause for the physical complaints. If medical illnesses are ruled out, and she fails to respond to reassurance, illness anxiety disorder should be considered. Ms. Xavier's age (middle adulthood) is consistent with illness anxiety disorder. Her symptoms are chronic (a minimum duration of 6 months is required for the diagnosis), and her anxiety is primarily related to health issues and worries. She exhibits excessive behaviors to check for illness, including repeatedly looking up symptoms of a brain tumor on the internet, which would be consistent with the specifier of care-seeking type. Individuals in the care-avoidant type rarely seek medical care because it can heighten their anxiety.

Approach to the Diagnosis

Individuals with illness anxiety disorder are preoccupied with, and fear having, a serious, undiagnosed medical illness. The minimum duration of this state of preoccupation is 6 months. A thorough medical evaluation fails to identify a serious medical condition that accounts for the individual's symptoms and concerns. Physical signs and symptoms may be present, but when they are, they are typically mild in intensity and are often a regular physiological sensation or a bodily discomfort not generally considered indicative of disease. If a physical sign or symptom is present (e.g., abdominal pain), the person's distress is largely from the fear of the suspected medical illness (e.g., colon cancer) rather than the physical complaint itself. If a medical condition is present, the anxiety and preoccupation are clearly excessive to the severity of the condition. Hearing about another's illness can cause anxiety because it heightens the person's health concerns.

There are two specifiers for illness anxiety disorder: care-seeking type and care-avoidant type. Individuals with the care-seeking type may perform excessive behaviors (e.g., examine themselves or seek information and reassurance repeatedly) or investigate their suspected and feared disease excessively (e.g., through medical appointments, internet searches). On the other hand, individuals with the care-avoidant type may not seek medical care because it heightens their anxiety, and they may avoid situations or activities (e.g., exercise) that they fear may endanger their health.

Getting the History

Mr. Zimmer reports having a several-month history of abdominal pain and requests a repeat colonoscopy. The interviewer determines that Mr. Zimmer has had an extensive medical workup over the past few months, including physical examinations, laboratory studies, X-rays, colonoscopy, and an abdominal CT scan, all of which yielded unremarkable results. The interviewer asks him to "describe the abdominal pain," and he further elaborates that his stomach feels "full" and appears to "rumble excessively." He also describes intermittent diarrhea. The interviewer asks Mr. Zimmer what he thinks is causing the symptoms, and he responds, "I am certain that it is colon cancer."

The interviewer asks Mr. Zimmer about his thoughts on the negative medical workup to date, to which he responds, "The tests must have missed the tumor, but I can feel a mass in my stomach, and it is getting larger." The interviewer asks how often he palpates the "mass" and whether he has checked for illness in any other way. He responds that he presses on his stomach several times a day and has conducted countless internet searches on the symptoms and treatments of colon cancer. The interviewer asks, "How do these symptoms impact your daily activities, and are you not doing things because of the symptoms?" Mr. Zimmer responds that he has been able to continue working as a teacher but has missed several days because of medical appointments. He fears he will have to take additional time off soon to pursue treatment when he is diagnosed with cancer. Mr. Zimmer also states that he feels preoccupied much of the day with thoughts about cancer, which has negatively impacted his teaching. However, he denies excessive worrying in other areas.

Mr. Zimmer describes a high level of anxiety about his physical symptoms, including abdominal fullness and rumblings. A complete medical workup should always be conducted; in this case, an extensive workup has been negative. The somatic symptoms appear to be mild and have begun to affect his work (e.g., missed days for appointments and preoccupation with illness at work). The anxiety relates to the fear of having colon cancer, rather than distress from the abdominal discomfort, and it also seems to predominantly revolve around illness concerns rather than multiple domains of activities or events. Mr. Zimmer also describes excessive behaviors related to the anxiety of having colon cancer, including frequently palpating his abdomen for masses and conducting frequent internet searches. In addition, he has sought frequent medical care for the symptoms. The interviewer will want to clarify how long these symptoms have been present—criteria require at least a 6-month duration for the state of being preoccupied with having the illness.

Tips for Clarifying the Diagnosis

- Is the person preoccupied with having or acquiring a serious illness?
- Does a thorough medical workup identify a medical condition that accounts for their symptoms and concerns?
- How long has the person been preoccupied with fears of having a serious illness?
- How do they respond to reassurance from physicians or to test results that indicate they do not have a serious medical condition?
- Does the person seek out medical care and information, or do they avoid medical care and situations around illness because these may heighten their anxiety?

Consider the Case

> Mrs. Best brings her 40-year-old husband to the office and reports that he is having difficulties with "anxiety." The interviewer determines that Mr. Best has episodes in which he experiences "a pounding heart," shortness of breath, difficulty swallowing, and the feeling that his heart "misses a beat." The episodes last approximately 10 minutes. The interviewer asks if there are any precipitants to these attacks. Mr. Best states that he was seen in the emergency department the previous week following an attack that started when he learned that a coworker was in the hospital with heart failure. He states that his father died of a myocardial infarction 2 years ago, and ever since, he has been sure that he also has cardiac problems. A routine visit to his doctor soon after his father's death yielded normal results, although he continues to worry that he will have a heart attack "any time now." Mr. Best has not returned to his primary care physician because he "just can't handle hearing any bad news." His wife reports he is "obsessed with thoughts about having heart trouble." He previously exercised regularly but has stopped exercising because he does not want to "stress" his heart or "drop dead." He has been avoiding certain colleagues at work, stating that he "can't handle" hearing about others' health problems. He denies misuse of substances.

Mr. Best likely has illness anxiety disorder, although a thorough medical workup is necessary to rule out a general medical disorder. This case is atypical because Mr. Best describes several symptoms of panic attacks. The attacks, however, appear to be precipitated by concerns about his heart. He is preoccupied with having cardiac disease like his father, although a medical workup to date has failed to reveal cardiac issues. Individuals with illness anxiety disorder may experience panic attacks triggered by illness concerns, in this case, worry about having a myocardial infarction. This case demonstrates illness anxiety disorder in a male, but the prevalence appears equal between males and females. At least one-quarter of individuals with illness anxiety disorder have an anxiety disorder, and a separate diagnosis of panic disorder could be made if some of the attacks are not triggered by worries about health.

Predisposing factors for illness anxiety disorder could include a history of childhood abuse and severe childhood illness. Major life stress also may precipitate the disorder, such as a serious threat to the individual's health that ultimately is benign or the death of a family member. Cultural factors must be considered, and the diagnosis of illness anxiety disorder should be made with caution in individuals whose ideas about disease are congruent with widely held, culturally sanctioned beliefs.

Mr. Best has features of the care-avoidant type. He avoids exercising because he fears that it might jeopardize his life. He also avoids seeing his primary care physician for fear of getting a negative report on his physical health. He is easily alarmed when he hears about others with health difficulties and avoids interactions with certain colleagues at work as a result. Clearly, a thorough medical workup is necessary to rule out a general medical disorder.

Differential Diagnosis

The first consideration in the differential diagnosis is an underlying medical condition. The presence of an underlying condition does not exclude the possibility of a coexisting illness anxiety disorder, but if a medical condition is present, the health-related concerns and anxiety are disproportionate to the medical diagnosis. Individuals with illness anxiety disorder fear having or acquiring a serious medical illness. Adjustment disorders should be considered if the health anxiety is related to a medical condition and is time-limited. Somatic symptoms are also present in somatic symptom disorder, but persons with this disorder are primarily focused on symptom relief and less concerned about having a serious illness and getting the proper diagnosis. The anxiety in illness anxiety disorder is limited to health-related concerns, which helps differentiate the disorder from other anxiety disorders, such as GAD and panic disorder. The anxiety in GAD could also include anxiety related to health, but that is only one of the domains about which persons with GAD worry. Individuals may experience panic attacks triggered by their illness concerns, but panic disorder should be considered in individuals who also have panic attacks that are not triggered by health concerns. Individuals with illness anxiety disorder may have intrusive thoughts about having a disease and may compulsively seek reassurance, whereas in OCD, the thoughts are typically focused on getting a disease in the future. Individuals with illness anxiety disorder are not delusional and are able to recognize the possibility that they do not have the feared illness. Persons with a major depressive episode may be preoccupied with illness, but a diagnosis of illness anxiety disorder should be considered if preoccupation with health concerns is present outside of a major depressive episode.

Approximately two-thirds of individuals with illness anxiety disorder have at least one other comorbid major psychiatric disorder. Comorbid psychiatric disorders include anxiety disorders such as GAD and panic disorder, OCD, and depressive disorders. In addition, individuals with illness anxiety disorder may have comorbid personality disorders.

Summary

- Illness anxiety disorder entails a preoccupation with having or acquiring a serious, undiagnosed medical illness. A thorough medical evaluation does not identify a severe medical condition accounting for the concerns.
- Somatic symptoms typically are not present, and if present, they are only mild in intensity. If a diagnosable condition is present, the individual's anxiety and preoccupation are excessive and disproportionate to the severity of the condition.

- The person has significant anxiety about health and disease, and their concerns do not respond to negative diagnostic test results and medical reassurance.
- Illness becomes a central feature of the individual's identity and self-image. They may examine themselves repeatedly and research their suspected illness excessively.

IN-DEPTH DIAGNOSIS: FUNCTIONAL NEUROLOGICAL SYMPTOM DISORDER (CONVERSION DISORDER)

Ms. Omni is a 31-year-old transgender woman brought to the emergency department by ambulance after an acute onset of right-sided weakness. A lawyer at a large law firm, she was at work in a meeting when she experienced numbness in her left hand and dizziness. She reports feeling lightheaded and dizzy and left the meeting to sit down. Over the next hour, her left hand became weak, and she could not hold her coffee cup. The weakness gradually spread to her lower extremity, and on presentation, she was unable to move her right leg. On physical examination, she appears anxious and states that, in the meeting, she was working on completing a big project with a looming deadline. On strength testing, Ms. Omni is unable to lift her right leg. However, her deep tendon reflexes have normal functionality. While supine, she is asked to raise her left leg against resistance while the doctor's hand cups her right heel. In this maneuver, the doctor feels downward pressure with the hand under her right heel, which she previously could not raise (positive Hoover sign). A CT scan of the brain is completed and reveals no acute process. Ms. Omni states that she does not use alcohol or other substances.

Patients with FNSD often present to emergency facilities, especially when the onset is acute. Although the symptoms may appear inconsistent with medical or neurological disease, a thorough medical workup must be completed. If a neurological cause for the presentation is ruled out, FNSD should be considered. Ms. Omni's weakness appears "non-physiological" in this case because it is inconsistent with an identified neurological cause. In addition, she exhibited a "positive sign" during the examination, as the Hoover test revealed inconsistent strength in hip extension, suggesting an FNSD. Finally, the stressful work environment appears to have been a precipitant in the onset of the symptoms.

Approach to the Diagnosis

The essential feature in FNSD in DSM-5-TR is the presence of symptoms or deficits affecting motor and sensory functioning that are inconsistent or incongruous with recognized neurological or medical conditions. The presenting symptoms can vary and may include motor symptoms, sensory symptoms, reduced or absent speech volume, or episodes resembling epileptic seizures. The symptoms are non-physiological or psychogenic, meaning that there is not a corresponding, recognized medical or neurological cause. An example would be a tremor that disappears with distraction when the person is asked to perform other tasks. Neurological and medical diseases must be excluded as a cause of the symptoms.

In DSM-IV conversion disorder, psychological factors were judged to be associated with the symptom or deficit. In DSM-5-TR's FNSD, such symptoms or conflicts may be present and may appear relevant to the development of the symptoms (e.g., a person develops dysphonia after witnessing an emotionally traumatic event); however, this is not required for this diagnosis because these stressors are not always apparent at the time of the initial diagnosis.

In DSM-IV, the diagnosis of conversion disorder required that the symptom or deficit not be intentionally produced or feigned. This criterion is not in DSM-5-TR for FNSD because clinicians may have difficulty reliably assessing the underlying motivation behind the production of the neurological symptoms. However, if there is evidence that the symptoms are intentionally produced, the diagnosis of FNSD would not be made, and factitious disorder or malingering should be considered. The presence of apparent secondary gain should not be used to make the diagnosis.

Specifiers include the symptom type, course, and presence of stressors. Symptom specifiers include with weakness or paralysis, abnormal movement, swallowing symptoms, speech symptom, attacks or seizures, anesthesia or sensory loss, special sensory symptom, or mixed symptoms. The course can be described as acute or persistent. With or without psychological stressor is an additional specifier.

Getting the History

> Mr. Henry presents to his primary care physician and reports a new-onset tremor in both hands. The physician asks about the symptoms' onset, severity, and duration. Mr. Henry states that the tremors started suddenly 2 months ago. The tremors are bothersome, and he has difficulty eating and drinking but is able to write without difficulty. The physician inquires about current medication, and Mr. Henry states that he is not taking any medications. The physician explores the family history, and Mr. Henry denies a family history of movement disorders. The physician asks about alcohol use, and Mr. Henry responds, "I used to have one or two beers on the weekend but haven't had anything to drink in over a month." The physician completes a physical exam, which yields normal results except for the bilateral tremor in both hands and an occasional jerking movement in the man's right arm. Because the tremor is not typical, the physician asks Mr. Henry to tap his toes and perform other strength maneuvers. While focused on these activities, the tremor diminishes and even disappears briefly. Finally, the physician asks, "Do you recall a particular stressor or event that may have precipitated these tremors?" Mr. Henry does not recall any precipitating event or stressor.

After a careful assessment, the physician did not identify a potential medical etiology for Mr. Henry's tremor. In addition, the physician observes that the tremor is inconsistent with a recognized neurological tremor and decreases when the patient is distracted. The physician then explores potential stressors or conflicts that may have precipitated the symptoms and determines that the patient has functional impairment from his symptoms. The physician should also be vigilant for clues on whether the symptoms may be purposely feigned because this would exclude the diagnosis of FNSD and raise concern about a factitious disorder or malingering.

Tips for Clarifying the Diagnosis

- Does the person have one or more symptoms that affect voluntary motor or sensory function?

- Are the symptoms inconsistent with a known neurological disorder?
- Has a medical or neurological source of the symptoms been ruled out?
- Is there an apparent psychological precipitant to the symptoms?
- Is there evidence on physical examination of a "positive sign" suggesting the presence of FNSD?

Differential Diagnosis

Individuals with FNSD present with neurological symptoms and signs, so the differential diagnosis includes neurological conditions that could explain the presentation. These individuals must have a thorough medical workup and may require repeated assessments, especially if the symptoms appear progressive. Mental health disorders to be considered include other somatic symptom disorders, dissociative disorders, body dysmorphic disorder, depressive disorders, panic disorder, factitious disorder, and malingering. If the diagnostic criteria of FNSD and another medical or psychiatric disorder are present, both diagnoses should be made. The distinction of whether the symptoms are feigned or falsified can be a difficult one. Individuals with FNSD are not intentionally producing the symptoms, whereas individuals with malingering and factitious disorder are deliberately and purposefully feigning the symptoms.

Summary

- Individuals with FNSD have one or more symptoms or deficits that affect voluntary motor or sensory function.
- There is positive evidence that the symptoms are inconsistent with a recognized neurological or medical disease.
- Medical and neurological diseases have been excluded and do not explain the symptoms or deficits.
- There may be identifiable psychological precipitants in the initiation or exacerbation of the symptoms, although such a precipitant is not required for the diagnosis because apparent stressors and trauma may not be identifiable.
- Positive evidence that the symptoms are feigned or falsified excludes a diagnosis of FNSD.

IN-DEPTH DIAGNOSIS: PSYCHOLOGICAL FACTORS AFFECTING OTHER MEDICAL CONDITIONS

Mr. Silver, a 52-year-old man with a medical history significant for hypertension and coronary artery disease, presents for a follow-up appointment. One month prior, he presented to the emergency department with exertional left-sided chest pain and was hospitalized for an acute myocardial infarction. At the follow-up visit, Mr. Silver's blood pressure is elevated. He has gained 6 pounds since his discharge. Collateral information from his wife reveals that Mr. Silver has been nonadherent with his medications and the exercise recommendations since his discharge. She states that he initially quit smoking after the hospitalization but recently restarted because smoking helps him cope with his stressful job as an executive of a large company. Mr. Silver admits to intermittent medication adherence, stating that he feels fine and is not sure he needs the medication.

Psychological and behavioral factors are adversely affecting Mr. Silver's medical condition. Many psychological factors may adversely influence medical conditions, including depression or anxiety, stressful life events, personality traits, and coping styles. In this case, chronic occupational stress increases Mr. Silver's risk for hypertension and coronary artery disease. An illness can evoke multiple emotional responses, including denial, anger, anxiety, fear, sadness, guilt, or shame. Mr. Silver's rejection of the severity of his illness may be adaptive in protecting him from being emotionally overwhelmed by his illness. However, it can also be maladaptive and prevent or delay diagnosis, treatment, and advantageous lifestyle changes.

Mr. Silver's medical nonadherence and maladaptive health behaviors, including his smoking and sedentary lifestyle, have significant adverse effects on the course of his medical condition and do not appear to have developed in response to the medical condition. It would be important to screen Mr. Silver for any comorbid psychiatric disorders affecting his adherence, including depression. In addition, it is vital to inquire about treatment-related factors, such as medication side effects that could be affecting his adherence.

The severity is moderate because Mr. Silver is engaging in maladaptive behaviors (i.e., smoking, poor diet, sedentary lifestyle) that are aggravating his medical illness (i.e., hypertension, coronary artery disease).

Approach to the Diagnosis

The presence of one or more clinically significant psychological or behavioral factors that adversely affect a medical condition is the essential feature of psychological factors affecting other medical conditions. These factors influence the course of the medical condition by increasing the risk for pain, death, or disability. Psychological or behavioral factors may adversely affect the course of the medical condition in one of four ways per Criterion B. It is important to differentiate the reason behind the delayed treatment, such as financial conditions, employment status, relationships, cultural differences, or the presence of a mental disorder. Abnormal psychological or behavioral symptoms may develop in response to a medical condition, but this would be classified as an adjustment disorder because it is a response to an identifiable stressor.

There are four specifiers for this diagnosis. In mild cases, psychological or behavioral factors increase medical risk. In moderate cases, the factors aggravate the underlying medical condition. Severe cases may result in medical hospitalization or emergency department visits, while extreme cases result in severe, life-threatening risk.

Getting the History

Mr. Jones, a 54-year-old man with a history of depression, anxiety, and asthma, presents to the emergency department with an asthma exacerbation. This is his fourth presentation in the past month. Mr. Jones has been homeless for approximately 1 year after being fired from his job at a fast-food restaurant. He reports feeling anxious "most of the day" and describes panic attacks "where I get short of breath and sweaty, and I feel like I'm dying." He states that his asthma has worsened since he became homeless, and asthma attacks often follow his panic attacks. He admits to intermittent adherence with his oral asthma medication and inhalers, stating that his medications have been stolen several times since he began living "on the streets."

Psychological or behavioral factors can adversely influence medical conditions. In this case, Mr. Jones's anxiety, stressful life events, and medication nonadherence likely exacerbate his asthma. Some degree of anxiety is likely to be experienced by patients with chronic medical conditions, and the degree of anxiety will differ according to the person and the situation.

It is important to note that nonadherence may be caused by factors other than psychological motivations. Social factors, including marital stress, poor social support, job strain, and disadvantaged socioeconomic status, may amplify the adverse effects of psychological factors on medical illness. In the case of Mr. Jones, the costs, side effects, and medication dosing schedules are treatment-specific factors that should be considered.

This case is severe because the inconsistent adherence and anxiety have affected the underlying diagnosis of asthma, resulting in emergency department visits.

Tips for Clarifying the Diagnosis

- Is a medical symptom or condition present?
- Is the medical condition causing the mental disorder through a direct physiological mechanism?
- Do psychological or behavioral factors exacerbate the medical condition?
- Are underlying psychological motivating factors affecting the medical condition?
- Does another mental disorder better explain these psychological and behavioral factors?

Consider the Case

Ms. Lopez, an 18-year-old woman with diabetes, is admitted to the medical unit for diabetic ketoacidosis. Ms. Lopez speaks Spanish, and the interview is conducted using a certified interpreter. This is Ms. Lopez's third admission in the past 2 months. She admits to "forgetting to take her insulin" at times and comments that she wishes she did not have this illness, stating, "I just want to be a normal teenager." Her father is present, and collateral information is obtained using an interpreter. Ms. Lopez lives with her father, but he states that she is often away from home for days with friends and has not followed his household rules. He states that he works long hours and has been unable to monitor her blood sugar levels or remind her to take her insulin.

In this case, difficulties in controlling Ms. Lopez's blood glucose may be attributed to her dislike of lifestyle restriction, tendency to rebel against her parents, denial of vulnerability, and wish to be "normal." These psychological issues undermine management through nonadherence with medication, diet, follow-up visits, and activity limitations. A lack of information about the illness or treatment should be investigated as a potential contributing factor to her nonadherence. Patient education should be provided in her primary language. It is also essential to understand patients' cultural and religious backgrounds, particularly their beliefs and values about health and illness.

Premature attribution to psychological factors may lead clinicians to overlook a medical explanation for a "treatment-resistant disease" and unfairly blame the patient. For example, difficulty in achieving stable glucose control in adolescents could result from hormonal lability rather than psychological factors. Investigating whether the patient may be manipulating their insulin dose to lose weight is also essential.

Ms. Lopez's case would be categorized as severe because her nonadherence led to a medical hospitalization.

Differential Diagnosis

A mental disorder due to a medical condition must be considered, particularly if there is a close temporal association between psychiatric symptoms and a general medical condition. In this diagnosis, the mental symptoms are the direct result of the physiological effects of the medical condition rather than affecting the course of the medical condition by psychological or behavioral factors.

If abnormal psychological or behavioral symptoms develop in response to a medical condition, an adjustment disorder should be considered. Somatic symptoms, psychological stress, and maladaptive health behaviors can also occur in somatic symptom disorder. However, in somatic symptom disorder, the excessive or maladaptive thoughts, feelings, or behaviors are the focus, rather than the worsening of the medical condition due to psychological factors. Illness anxiety disorder is characterized by an individual's worry about having a disease, whereas in psychological factors affecting other medical conditions, anxiety may be a relevant psychological factor adversely affecting a medical condition.

Summary

- Psychological factors affecting other medical conditions is diagnosed when a general medical condition is adversely affected by psychological or behavioral factors.
- The factors may precipitate or exacerbate the medical condition, interfere with treatment, or contribute to morbidity and mortality.
- A medical condition is not found to be causing the mental disorder through a direct physiological mechanism, and the factors are not part of another mental disorder (e.g., unipolar major depression).

IN-DEPTH DIAGNOSIS: FACTITIOUS DISORDER

Ms. Harlow is a 22-year-old cisgender woman whose past medical history is significant for recurrent abdominal pain and chronic headaches as a child (now resolved per report) who has been admitted to the hospital for recurrent cellulitis of a left forearm wound. Psychiatry is consulted to evaluate her for depression secondary to multiple readmissions.

The plastic surgery service thinks the wound is so severe that Ms. Harlow may eventually need a skin graft. A review of the medical records indicates that this is the fifth occurrence of the infection. Documentation from the home health service reveals a concern that she may have manipulated the occlusive dressing applied to protect the wound on multiple occasions. Ms. Harlow denies access to any other provider or hospital records. Since admission, although allowing intravenous antibiotics, the patient has refused to have the wound bandaged, and nurses have witnessed her manipulating the wound. She has not requested pain medication stronger than acetaminophen for discomfort.

On examination, the patient denies manipulating the wound. She states that in her experience as a nursing assistant, she learned that wounds need to "breathe," and that is why she is refusing to have her forearm bandaged by staff. Ms. Harlow denies any affective symptoms, anxiety, or depression. There is no evidence of a thought disturbance. Ms. Harlow further denies any legal or financial links to the nonhealing wound. She endorses a history of multiple hospitalizations as a child for intractable headaches or abdominal pain (sometimes both). When queried about her upbringing, Ms. Harlow reports that her stepbrother sexually abused her as a child and that her parents did not believe her when she revealed this to them.

Patients with factitious disorder most commonly present to medical hospitals. Patients may fabricate an illness through many mechanisms. For example, they may merely exaggerate existing symptoms, lie about the occurrence of symptoms, tamper with tests to produce false-positive results suggesting an illness, or cause harm to themselves leading to an actual disease state that requires medical attention. Some patients will do all four at various times throughout their illness. As a result, evidence of illness fabrication must often be derived from multiple sources: laboratory results, an implausible history, medical records, inconsistent physical examination, and direct evidence (e.g., tampering with tests, surreptitious medication administration).

It is essential to piece together the chronology of Ms. Harlow's illness using multiple sources of information. Potential clues to the diagnosis of factitious disorder include conflicting or misleading information, history of employment in health care, refusal to allow access to outside medical records, multiple presentations at several hospitals, atypical disease course, a demand for an unusual or invasive test or procedure, and unexpected or unexplained complications immediately before a planned discharge from the hospital.

An attempt should also be made to clarify Ms. Harlow's motivation for the suspected fabrication of the repeated infections. In this case, the lack of external motivations, such as financial gain, medications, or legal judgment, suggests the presence of factitious disorder.

Approach to the Diagnosis

Like many other somatic symptom and related disorders, the exact prevalence of factitious disorder is unclear but likely underdiagnosed. However, it is estimated that approximately 1% of patients seen by psychiatric consultation services in general hospitals have factitious disorder. Higher prevalence rates may be observed in specialty centers. For example, one study looking at patients evaluated in an occupational medicine setting found that 8% of patients exhibited findings consistent with the fabrication of an illness.

Factitious disorder is more commonly identified in females, with an onset in early adulthood. Many patients with falsified illness have a history of trauma or other childhood adversity. There also may be a history of frequent childhood illnesses, hospitalizations, and operations. Some studies have found that the perpetrators of factitious disorder imposed on another have a high incidence of somatic symptom and related disorders, including factitious disorder.

Getting the History

Consistent with other disorders discussed in this chapter, a thorough medical record review is critical to correctly diagnosing a factitious disorder and preventing potential iatrogenic harm. Establishing a longitudinal history of illness-inducing behavior or evidence of illness fabrication can be very helpful in narrowing the differential diagnosis. Multiple sources of evidence, all consistent with a factitious disorder, are often necessary to make a firm diagnosis and effectively rule out other possible explanations for the patient's presentation.

Maintaining a neutral, nonpunitive tone during the diagnostic interview is essential. The interview should focus on reviewing the patient's clinical course, understanding the illness and its clinical presentation, and assessing the varied risk factors of factitious disorder. At times, evidence of a factitious cause to the patient's presentation is discovered during the hospitalization. This may take the form of direct physical evidence of illness induction and laboratory or study results consistent with induction or falsification of illness. In the case of factitious disorder imposed on another (previously factitious disorder by proxy), video surveillance is sometimes used to capture the injurious behavior, and then steps can be taken to prevent further harm.

If the mental health clinician is serving as a consultant, it is essential that they collaborate with the primary team caring for the patient with factitious disorder, along with hospital administration, to provide quality clinical care, clear documentation, and appropriate discharge planning. Discussing the diagnosis of factitious disorder and subsequent treatment plan with the patient should be done with others present. The tone of the interaction should be supportive, nonjudgmental, and nonpunitive. The treatment plan should include the offer of ongoing support and behavioral health follow-up, although most patients decline such offers of care.

Tips for Clarifying the Diagnosis

- Identify evidence that the patient has been intentionally fabricating the signs and symptoms of illness in themselves or others.

- Clarify that external incentives for the illness-inducing behavior are absent from the presentation.
- In the case of factitious disorder imposed on another (previously factitious disorder by proxy), the diagnosis is given to the perpetrator.

Differential Diagnosis

Multiple sources of evidence are necessary to rule out medical or psychiatric conditions that are not intentionally produced or feigned and to diagnose factitious disorder. A thorough medical record review will likely reveal a longitudinal history of illness-inducing behavior and evidence of fabrication of illnesses.

Determining the patient's reason for illness fabrication is often tricky because many presentations include external and internal incentives for producing illness at various times over the course of the illness. In factitious disorder, the patient's reason for falsifying the illness may only be to assume the sick role and become the center of the treatment team's attention. Whereas, in malingering, external motivations are the primary motivation for the patient's manufacturing of the presenting illness.

The differential diagnosis for factitious disorder also includes Cluster B personality disorders and other somatic symptom and related disorders.

Summary

- In factitious disorder, physical and psychological illness is feigned or falsified by the patient.
- In patients experiencing factitious disorder imposed on self, the patient presents themselves as ill, impaired, or injured.
- In factitious disorder imposed on another, the perpetrator presents another as ill, impaired, or injured. It is not the victim that receives the diagnosis but rather the perpetrator of the falsification.
- In factitious disorder, external rewards are absent or do not explain the illness's fabrication.
- There is often no clear demarcation between factitious disorder and malingering, because the motivation for the patient's illness deception may be complex.

SUMMARY: SOMATIC SYMPTOM AND RELATED DISORDERS

The somatic symptom and related disorders all focus on somatic symptoms and their occurrence primarily in general medical rather than mental health care settings. They represented a new category of disorders in DSM-5 and remain in DSM-5-TR, replacing the somatoform disorder section in previous editions of DSM. The hallmarks of these disorders are the prominence of distressful somatic symptoms or illness belief associated with functional impairment. This approach emphasizes that the diagnoses are based on troubling somatic symptoms along with associated maladaptive thoughts, feelings, and behaviors rather than the absence of a medical explanation for the physical complaints. Several biological, sociocultural, and psychological factors contribute to the development and various presentations of these disorders. The somatic symptom and related disorders recognize that how a person interprets and adapts to the experience of somatic symptoms may be as important as the somatic symptom itself.

ELEMENTS TO CONSIDER IN THE CULTURAL FORMULATION

- In the context of the cultural interpretation of somatic symptoms, it may be helpful to conceptualize physical symptoms as an expression of emotional distress.
- Cultural factors, such as stigmatization of mental illness, often influence the emphasis placed on somatic complaints within the context of depression or anxiety and may account for some of the observed racial or ethnic differences in the reporting of somatic symptoms.
- It is not only the patient's culture that needs to be explored when interpreting a patient's presenting physical complaints and their response to these symptoms but also the provider's sociocultural background.
- The diagnosis of somatic symptom and related disorders should be made cautiously when a patient's beliefs regarding an illness or symptom are congruent with widely held cultural beliefs.

DIAGNOSTIC PEARLS

- Individuals with somatic symptom disorder respond to the presence of physical complaints and health concerns with excessive and maladaptive thoughts, feelings, or behaviors.
- These disorders are commonly associated with a markedly poor patient-rated self-assessment of health status.
- There is a significant increase in health care use among individuals with somatic symptom disorders.
- Individuals with somatic symptom and related disorders are most often found in the medical setting and less commonly encountered in mental health settings.
- It is not the absence of an identified medical etiology for the physical complaints that is the focus of the somatic symptom and related disorders but how individuals interpret and adapt to them.
- Functional neurological symptom disorder differs from other somatic symptom disorders in that a medically unexplained symptom of the voluntary motor or sensory nervous system remains a key feature of the diagnosis.
- In illness anxiety disorder, a person experiences intense concern about acquiring, or preoccupation with having, an undiagnosed medical illness.

- The essential feature of psychological factors affecting a medical condition is the presence of clinically significant behavioral or psychological factors that adversely affect the management of a co-occurring medical condition.
- Patients presenting with factitious disorder intentionally fabricate signs or symptoms of a psychological or medical condition without clear external incentives.
- It is imperative to understand the patient's somatic complaints and the associated beliefs and behaviors within the patient's sociocultural context.
- A distinctive feature of many of the disorders in this chapter is the emphasis on the presence of distressing symptoms and signs, not the absence of an identified medical etiology for the complaints.
- The collection of collateral information often proves helpful in clarifying the diagnosis.
- It is important to consider a team-based approach to assessment and treatment of somatic symptom disorders.

SELF-ASSESSMENT

Key Concepts: Double-Check Your Knowledge

What is the relevance of the following concepts to somatic symptom and related disorders?

- Preoccupation with somatic symptoms
- Most commonly present in general medical, rather than mental health, settings
- Cognitive misinterpretations of somatic symptoms
- Illness preoccupation
- Comorbid with anxiety and depressive disorders
- Medically unexplained symptoms
- Impaired professional and personal quality of life
- Marked impairment in self-reported health status
- Elevated rates of health care utilization
- High levels of illness anxiety
- Risk of iatrogenic harm

Questions to Discuss With Colleagues and Mentors

1. What is the best way to communicate a diagnosis of a somatic symptom disorder to the patient?
2. How can mental health providers serve as effective consultants to colleagues in other branches of medicine when caring for patients with somatic symptom and related disorders?
3. How does a provider determine if a person's health-related thoughts, feelings, and behaviors are excessive to the person's actual state of health or, as the case may be, illness?

4. What signs on physical examination suggest functional neurological symptom disorder?

5. How does one clinically differentiate illness anxiety disorder from another somatic symptom and related disorder?

6. What is the best way to engage individuals experiencing somatic symptom and related disorders in mental health care, given their inherent focus on physical health rather than mental health?

Case-Based Questions

PART A

Ms. James is a 36-year-old woman with a recent diagnosis of hypothyroidism who presents to the mental health clinic on referral from her primary care physician for evaluation of anxiety. The referral form indicates that Ms. James has had recurrent physical complaints (e.g., fatigue, dizziness, and palpitations) over the past 3 years. As a result of the workup of these symptoms, she was discovered to have clinical hypothyroidism. The hypothyroidism was successfully treated, but unfortunately the symptoms continued largely unabated. Further medical evaluation did not reveal any etiology for these continued symptoms. Her primary care physician referred her to endocrinology because of concern that her symptoms may be secondary to either over- or undertreatment of her hypothyroidism. The endocrinologist determined that she was clinically and physiologically euthyroid. Ms. James "no-showed" for her first scheduled mental health intake 2 weeks ago but arrived on time for her current appointment. She disagrees with the referral to a mental health provider.

What aspects of her history are consistent with somatic symptom and related disorders?   Ms. James presented initially to her primary care provider, a common occurrence in individuals with probable somatic symptom disorders. In addition, she has undergone a series of studies and a subspecialty medical referral to determine a possible etiology of her somatic symptoms. Increased use of health care resources is frequently encountered in somatic symptom and related disorders. Her missed appointment may signify hesitance to see a mental health care provider. Individuals with somatic symptom and related disorders may resist referral to mental health care because of the somatic, rather than psychological, focus of their symptomatology.

PART B

Ms. James reports that the somatic symptoms are very bothersome and prevent her from engaging in many activities she used to enjoy. She spends a lot of time searching the lay press for potential etiologies of her symptoms and natural remedies. Ms. James is profoundly frustrated and somewhat angered at the medical establishment for what she perceives as substandard medical care and attention to her symptoms. She is very focused on her physical complaints throughout the interview and wants to know how a mental health provider will help her "obviously physical" problems.

What aspects of Ms. James's presentation further support the diagnosis of somatic symptom and related disorders?   Ms. James's symptoms meet the criteria for somatic symptom disorder in that she has been experiencing one or more somatic symptoms for more than 6 months. These symptoms are distressing and disrupt her daily life. She also exhibits maladaptive and excessive thoughts and behaviors associated with her physical symptoms. The presence of an underlying medical disorder that may account for her symptoms (i.e., hypothyroidism) does not rule out somatic symptom disorder. She endorses significant health-related anxiety. Because of these beliefs, she spends excessive time searching for answers to her somatic symptoms. The somatic symptoms may become a central characteristic and defining aspect of her personality.

Short-Answer Questions

1. What is required of the individual's thoughts, feelings, and behaviors related to the somatic symptoms in somatic symptom disorder if the person has a medical condition that may account for those symptoms?
2. What is the minimum duration of the symptoms in somatic symptom disorder and the health preoccupation in illness anxiety disorder?
3. What are some examples of the maladaptive thoughts and feelings related to the somatic symptom focus present in somatic symptom disorder?
4. How does one differentiate somatic symptom disorder from illness anxiety disorder?
5. Describe some abnormal or excessive health-related behaviors that may be observed in individuals with somatic symptom disorder.
6. Individuals with functional neurological symptom disorder (FNSD) have one or more symptoms involving which parts of the nervous system?
7. How must psychological factors affect medical conditions to qualify for the diagnosis of psychological factors affecting other medical conditions?
8. Which somatic symptom and related disorder requires the individual to feign or produce symptoms or disease states?
9. What are the two specifiers in illness anxiety disorder, and how do they differ?
10. How does one differentiate illness anxiety disorder from generalized anxiety disorder?

Answers

1. **The associated maladaptive thoughts, feelings, and behaviors must be excessive.**

2. **The minimum duration is 6 months.**

3. **Cognitive features of somatic symptom and related disorders include intense attention to somatic symptoms, the ascription of normal bodily sensations to pathological disease states, and often fierce concern about physical health status.**

4. **In illness anxiety disorder, the person experiences intense worries about health, but the focus on co-occurring somatic symptoms is minimal.**

5. Behavioral features of somatic symptom disorder may include repeated checking for health-related abnormalities, high health care utilization, and avoidance of activities that may be thought to worsen health status.

6. Individuals with FNSD have functional deficits in the voluntary motor or sensory nervous system.

7. The psychological or behavioral factors must negatively impact the individual's underlying general medical condition.

8. In factitious disorder, the individual is purposely feigning or inducing symptoms and signs of disease to seek the sick role.

9. The two specifiers in illness anxiety disorder are care seeking and care avoidant. Individuals with the care-seeking type tend to have higher medical utilization rates and to perform excessive behaviors. Conversely, individuals with the care-avoidant type exhibit maladaptive avoidance and rarely seek medical care because it may heighten anxiety.

10. Preoccupation with illness is the primary concern in people with illness anxiety disorder. In generalized anxiety disorder, individuals worry about multiple events, situations, or activities, including health concerns.

RECOMMENDED READINGS

Hallett M, Aybek S, Dworetzky BA, et al: Functional neurological disorder: new subtypes and shared mechanisms. Lancet Neurol 21(6):537–550, 2022 35430029

Henningsen P: Somatic symptom disorder and illness anxiety disorder, in The American Psychiatric Association Publishing Textbook of Psychosomatic Medicine and Consultation-Liaison Psychiatry, 3rd Edition. Edited by Levenson JL. Washington, DC, American Psychiatric Association Publishing, 2019, pp 305–322

Jafferany M, Khalid Z, McDonald KA, et al: Psychological aspects of factitious disorder. Prim Care Companion CNS Disord 20(1):17nr02229, 2018 29489075

Löwe B, Levenson J, Depping M, et al: Somatic symptom disorder: a scoping review on the empirical evidence of a new diagnosis. Psychol Med 52(4):632–648, 2022 34776017

REFERENCES

American Psychiatric Association: Diagnostic and Statistical Manual of Mental Disorders, 4th Edition. Washington, DC, American Psychiatric Association, 1994

American Psychiatric Association: Diagnostic and Statistical Manual of Mental Disorders, 5th Edition. Arlington, VA, American Psychiatric Association, 2013

American Psychiatric Association: Diagnostic and Statistical Manual of Mental Disorders, 5th Edition, Text Revision. Washington, DC, American Psychiatric Association, 2022

CHAPTER 14

Feeding and Eating Disorders

Brittany Matheson, Ph.D.

Cara Bohon, Ph.D.

"My eating is out of control."

- Pica
- Rumination Disorder
- Avoidant/Restrictive Food Intake Disorder
- Anorexia Nervosa
- Bulimia Nervosa
- Binge-Eating Disorder
- Other Specified Feeding or Eating Disorder
- Unspecified Feeding or Eating Disorder

Feeding and eating disorders are characterized by the altered consumption or absorption of food that results in problems in physical health, psychological well-being, or both. This diagnostic class combines the previous DSM-IV (American Psychiatric Association 1994) diagnostic class of eating disorders with some of the childhood disorders, including feeding disorder of infancy or early childhood (redefined as avoidant/restrictive food intake disorder, or ARFID), pica, and rumination disorder. Additionally, binge-eating disorder (BED), which was previously included as eating disorder not otherwise specified and as a category for further study, is now included as an actual diagnosis. Together with anorexia nervosa and bulimia nervosa, these diagnoses capture commonly observed patterns of eating disturbance throughout the life span.

Pica is characterized by the eating of nonnutritive or nonfood substances of at least 1 month in duration that is not developmentally appropriate and is not culturally normative. Eating disturbance in pica does not necessarily result in food restriction or weight loss, although it can, and is not related to body image or shape and weight. Many individuals with pica have intellectual developmental disorder or developmental delay, and those without intellectual problems may be embarrassed or feel ashamed about their eating. Pica can also occur during pregnancy, with estimates suggesting one-third of pregnant individuals engage in pica.

Rumination disorder is characterized by the repeated regurgitation of food of at least 1 month in duration that is not better explained by any gastrointestinal or medical condition. All feeding and eating disorders other than pica take diagnostic precedence over rumination disorder, meaning that if the regurgitation occurs only during the course of anorexia nervosa, bulimia nervosa, BED, or ARFID, the other disorder is diagnosed instead of rumination disorder. Rumination disorder is most commonly diagnosed in children but can have onset at any age. The limited prevalence data available suggest rumination may occur in 1%–2% of grade school–age children, and not just among individuals with intellectual developmental disorder. Similar to other feeding and eating disorders, individuals with rumination disorder may feel ashamed of or secretive about the disorder, making it difficult to identify.

ARFID is the diagnostic term for the DSM-IV diagnosis of feeding disorder of infancy or early childhood. The change resulted in part from the prevalence of older children, adolescents, and adults who presented with similar eating disturbance and food restriction but did not meet criteria for other feeding and eating disorders. The disorder is characterized by avoidance or food intake restriction associated with significant weight loss, nutritional deficiency, health impact, dependence on oral supplements or tube feeding, or interference with psychosocial functioning. The eating disturbance is not part of an effort to control one's shape or weight, and no body image disturbance is present. The food restriction may result from an overall lack of interest in food or may be based on specific sensory characteristics of food, such as texture or smell. Additionally, some individuals are worried about aversive consequences of eating, such as upset stomach or choking. If criteria for anorexia nervosa or bulimia nervosa are met, those diagnoses take precedence over ARFID.

Anorexia nervosa is characterized by significantly low body weight due to food restriction, intense fear of weight gain, and disturbance in body image, such as the belief of being fat despite evidence of dangerously low weight. The fear of weight gain does not have to be explicitly articulated but could be presumed on the basis of persistent behavior that interferes with weight gain. Individuals with anorexia nervosa may or may not engage in binge-eating and purging behaviors. The diagnosis of anorexia nervosa supersedes all other eating disorder diagnoses because of the acute need for intervention. It is no longer required that postmenarcheal females have an absence of menstrual periods for three cycles to qualify for this diagnosis. This criterion was removed in light of evidence that females not missing their periods showed equivalent levels of impairment, as well as the difficulty assessing the criterion in females taking hormonal birth control. Additionally, the DSM-5-TR criteria no longer suggest what constitutes low weight, which allows professionals to use clinical data better matched to the individual, such as weight and medical history, to determine what would be minimally expected (American Psychiatric Association 2022).

Individuals presenting with bulimia nervosa engage in binge eating and compensatory behaviors at least weekly on average over the past 3 months. Additionally, they put undue emphasis on the importance of weight and shape. Binge eating occurs when an individual eats an amount of food in a discrete period of time (typically less than 2 hours) that most people would consider large under similar circumstances. Additionally, the eating is characterized by the sense of loss of control. In response to this increase in food intake, compensatory behaviors such as self-induced vomiting, laxative or diuretic misuse, fasting, or excessive exercise may constitute an effort to counter the effects of the binge episode on weight gain. The primary change from DSM-IV is a decrease in the frequency of binge eating and compensatory behaviors required to meet the diagnosis. Research showed significant impairment when individuals engaged in these behaviors once per week, which was less than the previous frequency of twice per week.

BED was previously included in DSM-IV as an eating disorder not otherwise specified until additional research could be conducted. Clinical utility and validity for the diagnosis have since been established. BED is characterized by recurrent binge eating, without compensatory behaviors, at least once weekly over the past 3 months. Disturbance in body image may or may not be present. Compared with anorexia nervosa and bulimia nervosa, BED tends to have a later age at onset, typically in early adulthood. Rates of BED are two to three times higher in females than males and are reported with a similar prevalence in most high-income industrialized countries. Individuals with BED are often overweight or obese and may have tried weight-loss treatments in the past with little success unless the treatment directly addressed binge-eating behavior.

Two new categories replaced the diagnosis of eating disorder not otherwise specified from DSM-IV:

- Other specified feeding or eating disorder includes specific variants of symptom presentation that do not fit the criteria for the other disorders in the diagnostic class. These include atypical anorexia nervosa (anorexia nervosa with a normal weight); bulimia nervosa of low frequency and/or limited duration (bulimia nervosa with binge eating and compensatory behaviors occurring less than once a week and/or for less than 3 months); binge-eating disorder of low frequency and/or limited duration (BED with binge eating occurring less than once a week and/or less than 3 months); purging disorder (recurrent purging in the absence of binge eating); and night eating syndrome (recurrent excessive eating after awakening from sleep or after the evening meal).
- Unspecified feeding or eating disorder is given as a diagnosis when symptoms of a feeding and eating disorder that cause significant distress or impairment do not meet full criteria for any other disorder in the diagnostic class. This is given if the

reason that the disorder does not meet full criteria for another diagnosis is not provided or there is insufficient information available.

Anorexia nervosa has the highest mortality rate and poses the greatest medical risk out of all the eating disorders. Thus, if criteria for anorexia nervosa are met in addition to other feeding and eating disorders, only a diagnosis of anorexia nervosa is made, in order to emphasize the need for treatment. Please see Table 14–1 for key changes to the feeding and eating disorders section between DSM-5 and DSM-5-TR.

IN-DEPTH DIAGNOSIS: PICA

Peter is a 6-year-old boy whose mother first noticed that the erasers from all the pencils were missing. Although she had not seen Peter eat any erasers, his older sister had reported the behavior to her. Peter had been diagnosed with autism spectrum disorder (ASD) when he was 3 years old, and his mother assumed that eating erasers was related to his developmental delay. She tried to keep erasers from him so that he would not eat them, but she then began to notice edges of books with bite marks, as well as missing feet from action figure toys with teeth marks along the end. Because of the communication difficulty related to his ASD, his mother had trouble explaining to Peter that he should not eat these things, and when she removed various items, he seemed to find new things to eat in their place. She sought treatment for him after a few months because she realized that his obsessive urge to eat objects was becoming disruptive, seemed to be related to his lack of interest in eating meals, and might be affecting his nutritional status.

Pica is often reported in children with a diagnosis of ASD or intellectual developmental disorder. Because these children have difficulty communicating, they often do not express concern about their eating behavior, and a parent provides information about the behavior. Siblings may have more information about the actual behavior because of their frequent proximity during play and the fact that children may hide the eating behavior from their parents for fear of discipline. Although some nonfood ingestion may occur in the context of ASD, diagnosis and treatment of pica are important if the eating behavior leads to potential medical problems, such as lack of adequate nutrition, poisoning, choking hazards, or bowel obstruction. In Peter's case, his mother was appropriately concerned that Peter's consumption of nonnutritive substances could be impacting his health and was above and beyond what would be expected for his age.

Approach to the Diagnosis

Many individuals with pica present for treatment on referral from a primary care physician after they have gastrointestinal complications from nonfood ingestion. Individuals may generally be secretive about their eating of nonfood items because either they feel guilt and shame or (for children) they have been disciplined in the past for eating nonfood items. Because of the disorder's secretive nature, assessment should include collateral information from parents or others in the home, if available, and all diagnostic interview questions should be posed sensitively and without judgment.

TABLE 14–1. Key changes between DSM-5 and DSM-5-TR

Culture-related diagnostic issues have been updated to reflect recent research estimates and to highlight disparity in treatment utilization based on ethnic group.

Prevalence estimates have been updated based on current research evidence.

The previous requirement of a persistent failure to meet nutritional and/or energy needs in avoidant/restrictive food intake disorder (ARFID) (Criterion A) was removed.

Significant impacts to family functioning, such as extreme accommodations to find foods from specific locations or restaurants, is enough to qualify as marked interference with psychosocial functioning (Criterion A4) in ARFID.

Differential diagnosis section for ARFID was updated to reflect potential rule out of obsessive-compulsive and related disorder due to pediatric acute-onset neuropsychiatric syndrome in individuals presenting with acute-onset symptoms, late age at onset, or otherwise atypical symptoms.

Association with suicidal thoughts or behavior has been added to binge-eating disorder (BED) and updated for anorexia nervosa and bulimia nervosa.

Updated estimates of suicidal ideation reflect severity and encourage thorough assessment of individuals presenting with eating disorders; approximately one-quarter to one-third of individuals with anorexia nervosa or bulimia nervosa and one-quarter of individuals with BED experience suicidal ideation.

Pica is diagnosed when an individual eats nonnutritive, nonfood substances (e.g., ice, dirt, chalk, paper, paint, hair) over a period of at least 1 month. Many individuals report that they typically ingest a primary type of nonfood, but some ingest a variety of items. It is important to ask about the duration and frequency of the nonfood eating, regardless of type. The developmental level of the individual is important to assess; as a result, pica is not often diagnosed in patients younger than 2 years. Because toddlers often put objects and nonfood items in their mouths, nonfood ingestion is not considered pica until teething and oral exploration have otherwise ceased. Additionally, when assessing a potential diagnosis of pica, the clinician needs in-depth understanding of cultural practices. If the eating behavior is supported by cultural norms, such as spiritual or medicinal practices, a diagnosis of pica is not met.

Finally, the presence of other mental disorders, such as ASD or schizophrenia, should be considered when assessing for pica. In adults particularly, pica often occurs alongside other mental disorders or intellectual developmental disorders. If the eating behavior is severe enough to warrant focused treatment outside the scope of the other disorder, then pica is diagnosed. This diagnosis is generally related to the severity and frequency of the nonfood ingestion and its influence on other aspects of functioning, such as obtaining adequate nutrition.

Getting the History

Julia, a 5-year-old girl, was referred after presenting to her primary care physician with an obstructed bowel from swallowing a sponge. In a sensitive and nonjudgmental manner, the interviewer asks whether she eats sponges often and whether she has any other things that she eats besides food. Julia appears shy and looks at her mother, who answers that she has noticed sponges missing in the past few weeks, and after doing laundry, she has noticed that the edges of Julia's blankets are frayed and chunks of the blankets are missing. After being reminded that she will not get in trouble for talking about what she has eaten, Julia admits that she ate the missing sponges and had been chewing pieces off the edge of her blankets. Because children are often poor reporters of the duration of a problem, the interviewer asks the mother to be specific about when she first noticed that sponges or pieces of blanket were missing or otherwise had suspicions about Julia's eating behavior. The interviewer asks about overall development, including language and social development, to assess for developmental delay or intellectual impairment, which is commonly comorbid with pica. The mother reports that Julia had delayed speech and did not make good eye contact. She has never been assessed for ASD. To determine whether nonfood ingestion is developmentally appropriate, the interviewer asks about related behaviors, such as mouthing toys. The mother reports that Julia had stopped placing other objects in her mouth approximately 2 years prior, which suggests that the current eating behavior is not developmentally appropriate. Finally, the interviewer asks about any cultural practices of the family that may include this type of eating. The mother reports that they do not have any such practices.

Because individuals with pica may not feel comfortable or be physically able due to intellectual impairments to discuss their eating behavior, information obtained from parents or other care providers is particularly important. Additionally, children may not be monitored constantly, so some nonfood ingestion may not be witnessed by others. Thus, reliance on other evidence of the behavior is important, such as missing objects or objects found in feces or by medical professionals when evaluating gastrointestinal problems. Some children may have been punished for eating objects in the past, so encouragement and reassurance that they will not be punished for talking about their behavior is important to obtain accurate information.

Tips for Clarifying the Diagnosis

- Evaluate the frequency and duration of ingestion of nonfood items in a sensitive manner, collecting collateral information as needed through medical records and caregiver report.
- Assess the patient's developmental level to ensure that the nonfood ingestion is not due to oral exploration or teething, which is common in toddlers and very young children.
- Evaluate the influence of cultural norms regarding eating of nonfood items.
- Explore the influence of other mental disorders on the nonfood ingestion, and evaluate whether the eating disturbance requires additional focused treatment to ensure health and adequate nutrition.

Consider the Case

Ms. Harrington is a 25-year-old pregnant woman. She has never experienced any disordered eating in her past, but during her pregnancy she has begun having strong urges to eat ice. She started filling cups with ice and then chewing the ice regularly for the first few months of her pregnancy. She became concerned about her teeth from the constant crunching and felt pain from cold sensitivity. However, she does not believe she could control her urges to eat ice. She also reports cravings for dirt and sand or anything gritty against her teeth. Ms. Harrington had a typical development and was of average intellectual functioning. She does not report any other mental disorders. She denies any cultural practices involving the ingestion of nonfood objects.

Although pica can occur throughout the life span, it is most commonly reported in children. The prevalence of pica is estimated to be 5% among school-age children and between 28% and 33% among pregnant and postpartum individuals worldwide.

Most adults with pica have intellectual developmental disorder, but pregnant individuals without intellectual developmental disorders may also engage in ingestion of nonnutritive or nonfood items. Pregnant individuals with limited access to nutritious foods during pregnancy may be at especially high risk for developing pica. Pica is diagnosed in these cases only if eating the nonfood items presents a medical risk. The relationship between pregnancy and nonfood ingestion is unclear, but some researchers theorize that the behavior is related to vitamin deficiencies during pregnancy. Little is known about the prevalence of pica in individuals of different ethnic backgrounds. Even if a person comes from a culture with a practice of nonfood ingestion, the behavior would qualify for a diagnosis of pica if they do not identify the eating behavior as equivalent to the cultural practice. Additional follow-up questions should be asked to determine whether the ingestion of nonfood items is socially normative.

Differential Diagnosis

Pica can be diagnosed simultaneously with other disorders, except these three main conflicting diagnoses: anorexia nervosa (if the ingestion of nonfood is used by the individual to control appetite), factitious disorder (if the nonfood ingestion is a means to feign symptoms of illness), and nonsuicidal self-injury (if the person swallows objects such as needles). Pica may be diagnosed in the presence of a gastrointestinal condition because some nonfood ingestion may lead to complications such as intestinal obstruction or mechanical bowel problems. In fact, medical complications are sometimes how which the disordered eating behavior is discovered. Pica is sometimes related to neglect or lack of supervision, and it is commonly associated with intellectual developmental disorder and ASD. It is also sometimes present in individuals with schizophrenia and OCD. Individuals with trichotillomania (hair-pulling disorder) or excoriation (skin-picking) disorder may eat their hair or skin, resulting in pica if the nonfood eating is severe enough to warrant clinical attention. Finally, pregnant individuals may develop pica in response to odd cravings or vitamin deficiencies during pregnancy.

Summary

- Pica is characterized by the eating of nonfood items that is severe enough to warrant clinical attention.
- Children younger than 2 years are not diagnosed with pica because eating nonfoods may be developmentally appropriate.

- Individuals with pica may have another diagnosis if the eating behavior is severe enough to warrant clinical attention directly.
- Pica is often comorbid with ASD and intellectual developmental disorder (intellectual disability).

IN DEPTH DIAGNOSIS: ANOREXIA NERVOSA

Angela is a 14-year-old Asian American woman presenting with a 20-pound weight loss over the past 3 months. She is currently in the 4th percentile for BMI, despite being in the 25th percentile throughout most of her childhood. She denies having a problem with her eating, reporting that her eating changes have simply been an effort to be healthy. She has cut out dairy products, stating that they make her stomach upset, and she has cut back on meat intake because she believes it is unhealthy. She refuses to eat what her mother prepares for dinner because it is "gross" and "greasy." Her daily food intake is often restricted to a small bowl of oatmeal, fruit, and a small salad without dressing. She runs cross-country at school but reports feeling more tired lately and unable to keep up with her team. When asked about fear of becoming fat, she denies it, but she refuses to increase her food intake, even of "healthy foods," suggesting discomfort with the prospect of weight gain.

A common presentation in anorexia nervosa is an adolescent who denies any problem with their behavior. Individuals with anorexia nervosa commonly experience a lack of insight into their symptoms. Individuals often present for treatment with concerned parents. Having information about the person's current weight, as well as their weight trajectory through childhood, can help determine the presence of the low body weight criterion. The DSM-5-TR criterion of fear of weight gain does not require that the person express such fear verbally; the person can instead show evidence of the fear via behavior and refusal to gain a healthy weight. Some individuals with anorexia nervosa may report gastrointestinal problems on which they blame food restriction, but the refusal to increase food intake of "safe" foods suggests that fear of weight gain is indeed present. Furthermore, the refusal to increase food intake is evidence that a person has not understood the seriousness of the low weight.

Approach to the Diagnosis

Individuals with anorexia nervosa often present for evaluation at the urging of parents or loved ones, rather than of their own accord. For this reason, consultation of previous records and interviews with family members or significant others is important for accurate representation of symptom presentation. Individuals must meet three specific criteria for the diagnosis, and specifiers of subtype and severity require additional information.

To assess for low body weight, the first criterion, it is important to know the person's current weight and height, lowest weight at the current height, and highest weight at the current height. Knowing the approximate dates of these weights is also helpful. If the person is still growing in height, it is important to know their typical growth trajectory to determine if the patterns are significantly changed. For adults, a general rule for low weight is a BMI less than 18.5 kg/m^2, but exceptions may exist. For children and adolescents, BMI below the 5th percentile for age and sex is typically considered low weight. Children presenting with a BMI greater than the median BMI for age should be assigned a diagnosis of other specified feeding or eating disorder (e.g., atypical anorexia nervosa) rather than anorexia nervosa. Severity specifiers for adults are based on body weight, as follows: mild, BMI $\geq$17 kg/m^2; moderate, BMI 16–16.99 kg/m^2; severe, BMI 15–15.99 kg/m^2; and extreme, BMI <15 kg/m^2. If an adult presents with a BMI of 19.0 kg/m^2 or greater, a diagnosis of other specified feeding or eating disorder (e.g., atypical anorexia nervosa) should be considered.

The second criterion is fear of weight gain, which can be elicited verbally and directly through questioning about the fear or can be assessed via the presence of persistent behavior that interferes with weight gain, suggesting a fear that is being alleviated through behavior. It can be helpful to ask the person how they would feel about gaining weight during treatment. Most individuals with anorexia nervosa will express resistance to weight gain regardless of whether they acknowledge a fear of weight gain.

The third criterion, overvaluation of shape and weight, can be assessed by inquiring where shape and weight fall in a ranking of the importance of aspects individuals use to evaluate themselves, such as work ethic and friendships. Individuals with overvaluation of shape and weight place those aspects toward the top of this ranked list. Disturbance of body image, or the lack of recognition of the seriousness of current body weight, can be assessed through questions about whether the person's current body weight is acceptable or what their ideal weight is. It can also be helpful to ask about body parts the person may believe are fat, despite their overall low weight. To determine subtype, the interviewer should ask the person to confirm the presence or absence of purging (self-induced vomiting or misuse of laxatives, diuretics, or enemas) or binge eating. If the person is hesitant to answer, family members should be asked if they have noticed bathroom trips after meals or excessive food wrappers in the trash.

Suicide risk is increased among individuals with anorexia nervosa, with rates reported to be 18 times greater compared with individuals without anorexia nervosa. Research suggests that one-quarter to one-third of individuals with anorexia nervosa experience suicidal ideation. Thus, it is important to thoroughly assess for suicidal ideation and risk factors for suicide in this patient population.

Getting the History

Jessica, a 15-year-old woman, reports weight loss but does not specify changes to eating. The interviewer asks explicitly about any changes. The patient replies that she was "really stressed out about finals and forgot to eat." The interviewer clarifies about the forgotten eating by asking if Jessica ate more at other times to make up for the missed meal. She replies, "No, I sort of liked the idea of being able to eat less. I felt in control of my hunger and could overcome it, unlike other people." The interviewer clarifies again, "So even though it seemed as if your eating changes were from stress, you kept restricting food intake because it made you feel good about yourself?" Additionally, the interviewer, needing to know about Jessica's feelings about weight and shape, asks, "Was weight loss important?" Jessica replies, "It didn't seem that way at first, but I guess I did like that I lost weight." The interviewer asks directly about the importance of the weight: "How important is your weight in dictating how you feel about yourself as a person? If you had to rank all the things you use to evaluate yourself, like how good you are at school or how good a friend you are, where would weight or shape fall in that list?" Jessica replies, "Well, I want to say that being a good friend is more important, but honestly, weight and shape matter a lot. Don't they to everyone?" The interviewer clarifies yet again: "So would you put weight and shape at the very top? If you had a scale of 0–6 and 0 meant that it didn't matter at all and 6 meant that it was the most important aspect of yourself, where would weight and shape fall?" Jessica replies, "Well, they're not the *most* important thing, but they're definitely a main aspect, so I would say 5."

When a person's initial food restriction does not obviously relate to a desire to lose weight, it is important to evaluate potential feelings about weight loss and body image. The initial weight loss may be from a change in eating habits or from stress; the key is evaluating the eventual intention of weight loss to the degree of low body weight currently presenting and what sort of value the patient places on weight and shape. If a patient reports that weight and shape are main aspects of self-evaluation, then that suggests an undue influence. Furthermore, if the initial food restriction has another cause, such as stress, but subsequent food restriction is an effort to continue weight loss, it still fits the criteria of anorexia nervosa.

Individuals with anorexia nervosa may appear sluggish and withdrawn due to poor nourishment and desire to refrain from social situations where food may be present. Obsessive thinking about food and weight are common, as are desires to cook for others. Individuals with anorexia nervosa also tend to be rigid, rule bound, and harm avoidant. Some individuals present with excessive exercise, which may precede the disorder. If they do not present for treatment earlier at the urgings of family, some patients will present medically due to bradycardia, orthostatic hypotension, or frequent bone breaks due to low bone density.

Tips for Clarifying the Diagnosis

- Ensure that the low weight criterion is met by consulting both normed growth charts and historical growth trajectories for the individual.
- Evaluate the patient's fear of weight gain directly or through questions about willingness to gain weight in treatment.
- Evaluate the patient's body image disturbance through questions about desired weight, thoughts about current weight, and level of importance of shape and weight on self-evaluation.
- For overvaluation of shape and weight, ask individuals to rank aspects of self that they use to evaluate themselves, and see where shape and weight fall in that list. If shape or weight is one of the main aspects, then this criterion is met.
- Access collateral information from significant others and past medical records.

Consider the Case

Mr. Miller is a 26-year-old man presenting for treatment after a 30-pound weight loss over the past 6 months. He denies having a history of food obsession, body image disturbance, or anxiety. He reports having changed to a vegan diet because his girlfriend was vegan and it was easier to eat with her if he changed the way he ate. He reports not liking a lot of vegan options for protein, so his diet has consisted primarily of steamed vegetables and rice. He lost weight quickly and lost energy to continue his usual hobbies, including sports. Mr. Miller reports having initially received compliments for his weight loss, which reinforced his eating changes. Over time, his eating has become more restrictive, and he has become obsessed with foods and calorie counts and has difficulty focusing on other things.

This case is atypical for a few reasons. Mr. Miller is male and his age at onset is past the prime adolescent years. Although older males with anorexia nervosa are less common, they do present for treatment and can meet criteria for the disorder. Furthermore, this patient's concerns about his body and general anxiety did not precede onset of the disorder, which is a less typical order of events; however, food restriction that occurs for a non-body-related reason, such as depression, stress, or a change in dietary preference, can result in body consciousness, often through reinforcing comments from others about initial weight loss. These individuals often deny obsession with food initially but report that, over time, they find it difficult to focus on other things and continually think about their next meal and how many calories to allow themselves to eat.

Anorexia nervosa is more commonly diagnosed in postindustrial countries, such as the United States, Australia, New Zealand, Japan, and countries throughout Europe. Research suggests that rates of anorexia nervosa are increasing in countries in Asia and the Middle East. Although anorexia nervosa occurs across all racial and ethnic groups in the United States, the prevalence appears to be lower in Latinx and Black Americans compared with non-Latinx White Americans. Anorexia nervosa appears to have a strong genetic association, and biological relations of individuals with anorexia nervosa are themselves at risk for developing anorexia nervosa as well as other eating disorders or psychiatric conditions.

Differential Diagnosis

Low body weight alone could indicate a number of diagnoses, including some general medical conditions. Individuals with low weight due to a medical condition, however, are typically aware of the seriousness of their low weight and would willingly gain weight if they were able. Major depressive disorder can be associated with loss of appetite and subsequent weight loss, but again, these individuals often desire weight regain and acknowledge the low weight as a problem. Schizophrenia and substance use disorders are sometimes associated with altered eating behavior or poor nutrition, but individuals with these disorders do not endorse a fear of weight gain. Social anxiety disorder (social phobia), OCD, and body dysmorphic disorder may have food- and body-related symptom presentations. If an individual meets criterion for anorexia nervosa and presents only the eating-related symptoms of social anxiety disorder or OCD, the second diagnosis is not made. If the body concerns in body dysmorphic disorder are unrelated to shape and weight (e.g., the person feels their nose is too big), an additional diagnosis should be made. Bulimia nervosa would be the proper diagnosis if binge eating and purging are present and body weight is not low. ARFID is the proper diagnosis if food restriction is not accompanied by body image disturbance.

Summary

- Anorexia nervosa is characterized by an inability to maintain normal weight due to the restriction of food intake.
- Also present is an intense fear of weight gain or behavior that suggests an underlying fear of weight gain, such as behavior that sabotages attempts to reach a healthy weight range, even if the individual will not verbalize a fear of weight gain.
- The diagnosis of anorexia nervosa requires that the person have an overvaluation of weight and shape, which entails placing a great emphasis on weight and shape when determining self-worth.
- The weight loss in anorexia nervosa is not just the consequence of a medical condition.
- Individuals with anorexia nervosa may or may not engage in frequent binge eating and purging. These subtypes should be specified when making a diagnosis.

SUMMARY: FEEDING AND EATING DISORDERS

The category of feeding and eating disorders includes symptom presentations characterized by a disturbance in typical eating patterns. This disturbance may consist of eating nonnutritive substances, as in pica; overall restriction of food intake, as in anorexia nervosa and ARFID; repetitive and abnormal regurgitation of food, as in rumination disorder; or binge eating, as in bulimia nervosa and BED. Some, but not all, of the disorders occur primarily in females and include disturbance of body image or overconcern with weight and shape. Most of the disorders have onset during childhood or adolescence, although adult onset can occur. Because of the nutritive impact of eating disorders, medical evaluations are important to assess for medical consequences and to ensure no other medical cause for the disordered eating. Additionally, the medical complications can be quite severe and, in some cases, lead to death. Suicide risk is also elevated in many eating disorders. Indeed, anorexia nervosa has the highest mortality rate of all psychiatric illnesses. Thus, prompt diagnosis and treatment are important.

ELEMENTS TO CONSIDER IN THE CULTURAL FORMULATION

- Feeding and eating behaviors are influenced by sociocultural contexts, cultural practices, religious beliefs, access to food, and family eating environments.
- Eating nonnutritive substances may be an important cultural, spiritual, or medicinal practice and therefore would not warrant a diagnosis of pica, unless the behavior occurs beyond what was socially normative.
- Despite similar prevalence across racial and ethnic groups for many eating disorders, treatment utilization is lower among marginalized ethnic groups.

DIAGNOSTIC PEARLS

- Although eating disorders are commonly thought to affect predominantly females, this predominance is true only of anorexia nervosa and bulimia nervosa. Binge-eating disorder (BED) is slightly more prevalent in females; pica, rumination disorder, and avoidant/restrictive food intake disorder (ARFID) are equally prevalent in both males and females.

- Anorexia nervosa and bulimia nervosa both include a disturbance in body image or overvaluation of shape and weight on self-evaluation. This disturbance is not present in ARFID and may or may not be present in other diagnoses.

- Age at onset for all feeding and eating disorders is generally before adulthood, although there are exceptions. Onset for bulimia nervosa and BED is typically in late adolescence and early adulthood. Onset for anorexia nervosa is early to late adolescence; and onset for pica, rumination disorder, and ARFID is often younger.

- Anorexia nervosa poses the highest mortality rate of all psychiatric illnesses. Thus, a diagnosis of anorexia nervosa supersedes diagnosis of other feeding and eating disorders to ensure adequate treatment.

- Adolescents are often secretive about their eating and may be poor reporters of their behaviors. Additionally, binge eating and compensatory behaviors may occur in secret, so parents and significant others may not be aware. It is important to get whatever collateral information is available and also attempt to remain nonjudgmental and compassionate during assessment to help reduce shame and guilt about behaviors.

- Toddlers and young children may narrow the range of foods they eat as part of normal developmental processes. This type of "picky eating" should not be diagnosed as ARFID unless severe nutritional deficits or significant psychosocial impairment occur.

- Feeding and eating disorders consist of a persistent disturbance in eating and eating-related behaviors with serious impacts to physical health and psychosocial functioning.

- Feeding and eating disorders affect individuals of all races, ethnicities, genders, sexual orientations, socioeconomic backgrounds, weight status, and cultures.

- Disordered eating and body image concerns are common even among individuals who do not meet criteria for an eating disorder diagnosis.

- Anorexia nervosa, bulimia nervosa, and BED are all mutually exclusive diagnoses.

- It is important to thoroughly evaluate for suicidal risk given high prevalence in this population.

SELF-ASSESSMENT

Key Concepts: Double-Check Your Knowledge

What is the relevance of the following concepts to the various feeding and eating disorders?

- Overvaluation of shape and weight
- Significantly low weight
- Fear of weight gain
- Restrictive eating behaviors
- Binge-eating episode
- Excessive exercise

Questions to Discuss With Colleagues and Mentors

1. What laboratory tests do you use when assessing medical complications in eating disorders?
2. How do you clarify the diagnosis when individuals refuse to disclose disordered eating behaviors although other sources suggest persistent food refusal?

Case-Based Questions

PART A

Jennifer is a 14-year-old Hispanic woman who reports restricting her food intake over the past few months because of discomfort in her stomach. She reports feeling so badly that she also makes herself throw up, hoping that it will alleviate the pain. Additionally, she sometimes feels severe hunger after periods of food restriction, which leads to loss of control in eating binges followed by self-induced vomiting to prevent abdominal pain. She has lost 20 pounds in the past 2 months, which puts her overall body weight in the 3rd percentile for her age, sex, and height. She is being hospitalized for bradycardia and requires enteral feeding because of her persistent food refusal.

Which diagnoses should be considered at this point?   At this point, Jennifer may meet criteria for avoidant/restrictive food intake disorder; anorexia nervosa, binge-eating/purging type; or a gastrointestinal problem. Additional information is needed to differentiate among these diagnoses.

PART B

Jennifer's medical doctors cannot find any clear medical basis for her abdominal pain. They believe that she has irritable bowel syndrome. Although the doctors offer recommendations for decreasing her discomfort, she continues to refuse food. Following release from the hospital after gaining weight (to the 10th percentile) through enteral feeding, she resumes her pattern of food restriction and occasional binge eating and purging.

Would she meet criteria for anorexia nervosa or bulimia nervosa?   On her release from the hospital, Jennifer no longer meets the low-weight criterion for a diagnosis of anorexia nervosa. Although she is engaging in binge eating and purging behavior, it is unclear that the frequency and duration would meet diagnostic criteria for bulimia nervosa. Additionally, and relevant for both anorexia and bulimia, there is no report of body image disturbance or emphasis on body image.

PART C

> After discharge from the hospital and cessation of the enteral feeding, Jennifer's weight drops again. She denies concern about shape and weight and reports that her eating patterns are entirely due to abdominal pain. However, the doctors report that most individuals with irritable bowel syndrome are able to eat normally, even if they report some discomfort.

Which diagnosis seems most appropriate? Because the persistent food restriction appears to exist beyond what would be reasonably expected given her medical condition, and she continues to require enteral feeding, Jennifer meets criteria for avoidant/restrictive food intake disorder.

Short Answer Questions

1. Which two of the feeding and eating disorders require body image disturbance or an overemphasis on weight and shape on self-evaluation?
2. What two characteristics are necessary for an eating episode to be considered binge eating?
3. What is the best way to differentiate anorexia nervosa from avoidant/restrictive food intake disorder?
4. Which feeding and eating disorder has the highest mortality rate?
5. Which feeding and eating disorder has onset from early to late adolescence and is often preceded by an overly anxious and harm-avoidant temperament?
6. Which of the feeding and eating disorders have greater prevalence in females?
7. What is the duration of time that symptoms must be present to meet diagnostic criteria for pica and rumination disorder?
8. Which of the feeding and eating disorders can be diagnosed in addition to the others within the category?
9. How is avoidant/restrictive food intake disorder different from a gastrointestinal problem?
10. When can both anorexia nervosa and OCD be diagnosed?

Answers

1. **Anorexia nervosa and bulimia nervosa require body image disturbance or an overemphasis on weight and shape on self-evaluation.**

2. **Binge eating involves consuming a large amount of food and feeling a loss of control over eating.**

3. **Individuals with anorexia nervosa also place undue emphasis on weight and shape and have disturbance in their body image.**

4. Anorexia nervosa has the highest mortality rate.

5. Anorexia nervosa has onset from early to late adolescence and is often preceded by an overly anxious and harm-avoidant temperament.

6. Anorexia nervosa, bulimia nervosa, and, to a lesser extent, binge-eating disorder are more prevalent in females.

7. Symptoms must be present for 1 month to meet diagnostic criteria for pica and rumination disorder.

8. Pica can be diagnosed in addition to other feeding and eating disorders.

9. Avoidant/restrictive food intake disorder can be diagnosed in the presence of a gastrointestinal disorder, but the disturbance of intake must be beyond what is directly accountable by the medical condition. Furthermore, some individuals may have lingering difficulties eating foods despite management of physical symptoms.

10. When diagnostic criteria for anorexia nervosa have been met but significant obsessions and compulsions not related to food or body image are also present, an additional diagnosis of OCD is considered.

RECOMMENDED READINGS

Agras WS, Robinson AH (eds): The Oxford Handbook of Eating Disorders, 2nd Edition. New York, Oxford University Press, 2018

Grilo CM, Mitchell JE (eds): The Treatment of Eating Disorders: A Clinical Handbook. New York, Guilford Press, 2011

Le Grange D, Lock J (eds): Eating Disorders in Children and Adolescents: A Clinical Handbook. New York, Guilford Press, 2011

Lock J (ed): Pocket Guide for the Assessment and Treatment of Eating Disorders. Washington, DC, American Psychiatric Association Publishing, 2019

Mitchell JE, Peterson CB (eds): Assessment of Eating Disorders. New York, Guilford Press, 2007

Walsh BT, Attia E, Glasofer D, et al (eds): Handbook of Assessment and Treatment of Eating Disorders. Washington, DC, American Psychiatric Association Publishing, 2016

REFERENCES

American Psychiatric Association: Diagnostic and Statistical Manual of Mental Disorders, 4th Edition. Washington, DC, American Psychiatric Association, 1994

American Psychiatric Association: Diagnostic and Statistical Manual of Mental Disorders, 5th Edition, Text Revision. Washington, DC, American Psychiatric Association, 2022

CHAPTER 15

Elimination Disorders

Jennifer Derenne, M.D.

"My daughter still wets the bed."

"My son messes his underpants at school."

- Enuresis
- Encopresis
- Other Specified Elimination Disorder
- Unspecified Elimination Disorder

Elimination disorders typically manifest in early childhood and are often associated with significant distress and frustration for the child and family. They are some of the most common pediatric concerns, yet parents often do not report symptoms because they believe that nothing can be done.

Enuresis, commonly referred to as "wetting," is uncontrollable leakage of urine that occurs after bladder continence would generally be expected. Symptoms may be *primary*, which means that toilet training is not successful in a child older than 5 years (or an equivalent developmental level); or *secondary*, which refers to new wetting episodes

Adapted from Derenne J, Fitzpatrick KK: "Elimination Disorders," in *Study Guide to DSM-5*. Edited by Roberts LW, Louie AK. Washington, DC, American Psychiatric Publishing, 2015, pp 251–266.

after a 6-month period of complete dryness. Urinary incontinence may be continuous or intermittent and may occur exclusively at night or during daytime hours as well.

Encopresis is voluntary or involuntary fecal soiling by a child who has previously attained (or would have been expected to attain) bowel continence. Similar to enuresis, a diagnosis of encopresis is made only after a period in which bowel continence would be expected, generally older than 4 years for a typically developing child, and can also be primary (failure to successfully toilet train) or secondary (developing after a period of continence). Bowel continence is expected to develop at a younger age than urinary continence, and a diagnosis is often made if the person is older than 4 years.

Both disorders involve the complex interplay of biological and psychological factors. Anatomical abnormalities such as posterior urethral valves or an ectopic ureter may impact continence. Physiological factors such as chronic constipation, bladder dysfunction, diabetes (mellitus or insipidus), ineffective colon motility (e.g., Hirschsprung's disease), and urinary tract infections must also be considered in the differential diagnosis. In cases with no obvious anatomical or physiological pathology, psychological factors such as stress, child maltreatment, depression, and anxiety must be considered. Symptoms can cause extreme distress to the child, who may be teased or bullied if peers or siblings are aware of the problem. Children with elimination disorders often avoid nighttime social activities such as sleepovers for fear of having an "accident" in front of friends.

The diagnostic criteria for enuresis and encopresis remain the same in DSM-5-TR (American Psychiatric Association 2022) as they were in DSM-5 (American Psychiatric Association 2013). They are included in the category of elimination disorders along with other specified elimination disorder and unspecified elimination disorder, which are used to describe symptoms characteristic of an elimination disorder that cause significant distress but do not fully meet diagnostic criteria for encopresis or enuresis. See Table 15–1 for key changes between DSM-5 and DSM-5-TR.

IN-DEPTH DIAGNOSIS: ENURESIS

Meera is an 8-year-old girl who is brought to her pediatrician's office for evaluation of nighttime wetting. She was very distressed about a recent overnight trip to visit relatives; her cousin noticed that she wet the bed and began teasing her. Meera began toilet training when she was 3 years old and seemed interested in wearing "big girl panties" featuring her favorite cartoon characters. She is dry during the day and can stay dry for a night or two but has wetting accidents most nights. There have been no consistent periods of nighttime dryness. Meera's parents try to be patient but admit that they are stressed with work and finances and sometimes yell when Meera has an accident. They deny corporal punishment. Disposable undergarments are expensive, and Meera's mom, who does most of the laundry, recently went back to work and does not have the time or energy to wash sheets every day. The parents do not limit fluids in the evening, and Meera likes to drink fruit juice. She is proud of drinking a big glass of milk at dinner, which is typically 2–3 hours before bed. They have tried sticker charts and point systems to reward dry nights but gave up after a few days because "it didn't seem to be working." Meera's physical examination yields normal results, as does her screening urinalysis.

Meera's presentation is typical—she is dry during the day and does have some dry nights. However, she is older than 5 years and has never been completely dry. There-

TABLE 15–1. Key changes between DSM-5 and DSM-5-TR

Prevalences have been updated.

Cultural-related diagnostic issues have been added.

fore, she has primary nocturnal enuresis. Nothing on examination indicates genitourinary, gastrointestinal, or neurological abnormalities. Her screening urinalysis does not reveal evidence of diabetes insipidus, diabetes mellitus, or a urinary tract infection. Her mom's return to work and the family's overall stress level are likely affecting Meera and making it difficult for her parents to be neutral, calm, and consistent with behavioral plans that would likely be effective if they gave them more time. It is important to assess whether the parents' frustration is leading to any sort of maltreatment, but it is very important to stress that most children with enuresis are not being abused.

Approach to the Diagnosis

The diagnosis of enuresis is made based on the child's history, physical examination, laboratory data, and imaging studies. A careful history will elicit the duration, timing, and severity of symptoms; exacerbating and ameliorating factors; and the presence of any extended periods of dryness. How many voids are there during the day? What is the child's bowel function like? It is important to determine whether the enuresis occurs solely at night or also occurs during the day, whether the incontinence is intermittent or continuous, and whether the child has any other genitourinary, gastrointestinal, or neurological symptoms. Is there any history of urinary tract infection or other medical illness? Does the child take any medications or have access to medications stored in the home, such as diuretics, lithium, or atypical antipsychotics? Caregivers should be questioned regarding their approach and attitude toward toilet training, their response to wetting accidents, and whether there have been any recent changes or stresses to the family. How is the child doing socially and academically? Are there any other developmental concerns (gross or fine motor skills, learning, speech, growth)? Providers should sensitively, yet directly, ask about any maltreatment or abuse.

Physical examination should generally be done by the pediatrician rather than by a psychiatrist and should focus on the genitourinary, gastrointestinal, and neurological systems. The back should be examined for birthmarks or tufts of hair that could indicate underlying pathology involving the spinal cord. The abdomen should be examined for presence of a distended bladder or excessive stool, which may indicate constipation and is frequently associated with enuresis.

In cases of primary nocturnal enuresis, a screening urinalysis is often the only diagnostic test necessary. If results are unremarkable, there is no need to request additional tests. However, the presence of a urinary tract infection in a male, a febrile urinary tract infection in a female, or repeated afebrile urinary tract infections would prompt renal and bladder ultrasonography. Abnormalities would indicate the need for further studies, such as a voiding cystourethrography.

Daytime wetting requires a bit more investigation to determine whether the underlying problem is one of storage or emptying. The clinician should request urinalysis and urine culture, as well as bladder ultrasonography to assess postvoid residual and uroflow testing to provide qualitative and quantitative assessment of the urinary stream. Certain features of the history and physical examination may signify the need for MRI, intravenous pyelography, or CT scan. For example, constant "dribbling" may suggest the presence of an ectopic ureter, whereas suspicious physical findings may indicate tethered cord syndrome.

Getting the History

A mother reports that her 10-year-old son, Luis, has daytime wetting episodes. The clinician starts with open-ended questions to determine the duration, frequency, and quality of symptoms: "Tell me what has been happening. How long has this wetting been an issue? Are there times when you stay dry? What happens when you have an accident?" The child or parent of a child with enuresis will typically report that the child never attained complete dryness or that the child is dry during the day but continues to have wetting episodes at night. The exact frequency of the wetting episodes can vary, but to meet DSM-5-TR criteria, they must occur at least twice per week for 3 consecutive months or cause significant distress or impairment in functioning across social, academic, and home domains.

The interviewer involves both Luis and his mother in the questioning in order to build rapport with the child and to get a more comprehensive sense of the issues involved. The interviewer asks, "How is Luis doing overall? Luis, how are things at school? How would Luis's teacher describe him? Tell me about your friends, Luis. What sorts of things do you like to do with your friends? Do you play sports? Do your friends ever have sleepovers? Do you go? How about at home? Do you have any arguments with your parents or siblings? Do you have any other areas of concern?" It is often helpful to conduct parts of the interview with both parent and child together as well as to meet with the child or parent alone, particularly if the conversation appears to be causing distress.

The interviewer will also need to ask specific questions about medical illnesses or medications that may cause urinary incontinence. "Does Luis have any medical illnesses? Any seizures? Diabetes? Spinal injuries? Luis, do you take any medications regularly?" The clinician should confirm with the parent that the child does not take (or have access to) diuretics, lithium, or antipsychotics.

The DSM-5-TR diagnosis of enuresis is relatively straightforward. The interviewer needs to determine whether the child is older than 5 years (or developmental equivalent) and must confirm that symptoms are present at least twice per week for 3 months *or* cause significant distress or functional impairment. Finally, the interviewer must confirm that there are no medical illnesses or exposures to substances that may better explain the symptoms of urinary incontinence. However, it is important to note that a child with an acute urinary tract infection or one who takes a diuretic may also be diagnosed with enuresis, providing those symptoms were present before the introduction of medication or presence of the illness.

Tips for Clarifying the Diagnosis

- Determine whether symptoms are primary or secondary, nocturnal or diurnal, and continuous or intermittent.

- Order a screening urinalysis for information about urine specific gravity, which would argue for or against diabetes insipidus; urine glucose, which may indicate diabetes mellitus; and the presence of bacteria, which would dictate need for a culture to rule out infection. Each of these conditions can be associated with enuresis.
- Remember that diurnal enuresis is less common than nocturnal enuresis, more common in females than in males, and more often associated with an underlying anatomical or physiological abnormality.
- Maintain a sensitive and empathetic approach to the family to obtain information that may be difficult to discuss but is important for the care of the patient. Take into consideration that it is important for the family to feel that the clinician is being complete and ruling out potential physical causes of enuresis rather than focusing solely on stress as a causative factor.

Consider the Case

Ivan is a 13-year-old boy with a history of well-controlled type 1, insulin-dependent diabetes mellitus and ADHD, with predominantly inattentive presentation, who presents to his pediatrician with concerns about new-onset nocturnal enuresis. He is too embarrassed to tell his parents why he wanted to see the doctor. He was previously completely dry but notes that he did have some difficulty with toilet training and was not completely dry until he was 10 years old. His parents used an alarm system, which worked after a couple months. The return of symptoms has caused him significant embarrassment, and he now goes to great lengths to hide his wetting episodes. He even bought another set of sheets and sometimes hides soiled sheets in his closet until his parents are not home and he can wash them in private. He actively tries to avoid fluids at night and voluntarily stopped drinking caffeinated diet soda because he recognized that it was increasing his need to urinate during the day. He reports that he is very stressed by his family's upcoming move to a new city. He describes himself as shy and interested in online gaming, and he worries about making friends in middle school. Otherwise, he feels well and denies recent weight loss, polyuria, polyphagia, or polydipsia. He reports complying with all doses of insulin, counting carbohydrates at every meal, and checking his blood sugar as he is supposed to. Physical examination results are unremarkable, and urinalysis results are within normal limits. His hemoglobin A1C is 6.5%.

Ivan's presentation is slightly atypical in that he is older than 8 years and has had a period of complete dryness, which indicates a diagnosis of secondary nocturnal enuresis. However, he did initially have primary nocturnal enuresis, which resolved with alarm therapy. Enuresis appears to be more common in children and adolescents with ADHD. The pediatrician is right to be more vigilant in Ivan's case because of his insulin-dependent diabetes mellitus. Adolescents with previously well-controlled blood glucose sometimes become nonadherent in the teen years as they become more independent and struggle with being "different" from their peers. Glucose spillage into the urine could present as polyuria, with difficulty at night. At this age, ethnicity and race are not likely to have much impact on diagnosis or presentation; however, in some cultures, children are expected to be toilet trained at an earlier age and may therefore present to a medical provider sooner than a child of a different background. Earlier toilet training is often related to concerns about cost or lack of readily available diapers. Developmentally, Ivan (appropriately) wants to be more independent with his activities of daily living. He may feel that his parents have high expectations for him, and he may not want to burden or embarrass them.

Differential Diagnosis

The differential diagnosis of enuresis centers on excluding the presence of medical conditions or substances that can cause urinary urgency or increased urine production, such as untreated diabetes insipidus or diabetes mellitus, an acute urinary tract infection, vaginal reflux, or neurogenic bladder related to spinal cord pathology (also lazy bladder syndrome, detrusor-sphincter dyssynergia, and Hinman syndrome). Exposure to medications such as atypical antipsychotics, lithium carbonate, and diuretics must also be excluded.

Children with enuresis may exhibit behavioral problems at a higher rate than other children. Developmental difficulties such as learning disabilities, speech delay, and fine and gross motor delays may be present. In children with other developmental delays, it is important to determine the child's developmental age rather than rely solely on chronological age to diagnose enuresis.

Enuresis is not diagnosed in the presence of a neurogenic bladder or a general medical condition that causes polyuria (increased urination) or urgency (e.g., untreated diabetes mellitus or diabetes insipidus), during an acute urinary tract infection, or during treatment with an antipsychotic medication. However, a diagnosis of enuresis is compatible with such conditions if urinary incontinence was regularly present before the development of the general medical condition or if it persists after the institution of appropriate treatment.

See DSM-5-TR for additional disorders to consider in the differential diagnosis. Also refer to the discussions of comorbidity and differential diagnosis in their respective sections of DSM-5-TR.

Summary

- The diagnosis of enuresis must be made in children older than 5 years (or developmental equivalent).
- Enuresis is not diagnosed in the presence of medical illness or use of medications that can result in polyuria or urge incontinence.
- Enuresis can lead to significant difficulty in the child's academic, social, and home functioning.

IN-DEPTH DIAGNOSIS: ENCOPRESIS

Milo is a 10-year-old boy who was referred from his local pediatric gastroenterologist because of a history of soiling in his underwear. The specialist has ruled out medical causes of these difficulties. Currently, voiding episodes of full, hard stools most often occur in the afternoon, after a day at school, approximately twice per week. Furthermore, he has frequent fecal overflow and soiling of his underwear. He describes being teased for being "smelly" and has attempted to avoid school for fear of soiling himself on the school bus or at the end of the school day. Milo met initial toilet training milestones within normal limits, achieving nocturnal bowel continence by 2.5 years of age and daytime bowel continence and urinary continence at 3 years of age. He has infrequent episodes of nocturnal enuresis approximately once per week.

Following a bout of severe stomach flu, Milo significantly restricted his food intake and subsequently developed constipation. Despite efforts to maintain Milo's regular stooling with laxatives and dietary maintenance (e.g., a high-fiber diet), Milo's mother describes him as appearing to deliberately retain his feces, evidenced by sphincter tightening and toe walking. She notes that at times he does not seem aware that he needs to use the bathroom and will often deny a need to defecate despite multiple reminders. Milo reports that he often does not feel the need "to go" until he experiences an intense urge or fecal overflow.

Medical evaluations have ruled out physical causes, but Milo continues to have high volumes of stool, evident on abdominal examination, and passes stools only twice per week. The family has worked to include regular fiber in their diet and through supplements but admit that they are inconsistent and that Milo resists the increased vegetable intake. They have otherwise attempted to avoid shaming or discussing these difficulties with Milo, expecting him to deposit his feces in the toilet and place his soiled underwear in a bag in the laundry area. Milo is described by his parents and teachers as a shy, somewhat withdrawn boy who avoids his peers and has a history of school avoidance, complaining of gastrointestinal symptoms. His mother reports he had difficulty separating when younger, but this resolved with his entry to elementary school. He does not have any history of disruptive or aggressive behaviors.

Milo's presentation is fairly typical, with a history of normal stooling followed by complications resulting from constipation. The establishment of normal bowel continence is important because it indicates that current symptoms are secondary to constipation and the reciprocal effects of withholding stool, followed by bowel impaction and fears of passing larger, more painful stools. The frequency of passing feces outside the toilet (more than once per month), coupled by the ability to engage in regular stooling at a younger age and exclusion of physical causes for these difficulties, clearly warrants a diagnosis of encopresis. Nothing on examination indicates anatomical, metabolic, endocrine, or neurological abnormalities, and Milo takes no medications associated with fecal incontinence. His history of shyness, separation fears, somatic complaints, and mild school refusal are consistent with higher levels of internalizing symptoms and attention to physical symptoms that exacerbate concerns around passing more painful stools. Developmental and familial challenges in maintaining a high-fiber diet and consistent routines around toileting often interfere with efforts to establish more typical stooling patterns and are likely applicable to Milo and his family.

A consultation with his pediatric gastroenterologist could help establish whether his current constipation might be managed with medications or warrants use of enemas for more thorough evacuation of stool. Evaluation of rectal distention could also be useful to establish whether more aggressive efforts, such as the use of anal biofeedback, would be useful to assist Milo in identifying the need to stool or whether these can be managed with laxative use. It is important to assess for the presence of maltreatment while keeping in mind that most children with incontinence are not experiencing abuse.

Approach to the Diagnosis

The diagnosis of encopresis is made clinically, based on history, physical examination, laboratory data, and occasionally imaging studies. A thorough evaluation to rule out physical causes of fecal incontinence is critical to this diagnosis and necessary to establish the diagnosis. Specialty medical evaluations are particularly important in cases where bowel regularity has never been established (primary encopresis). Encopresis can be associated with anatomical, metabolic, endocrine, and neurological causes, as well as substance use or abuse. The most important disorder to rule out is Hirschsprung's disease, in which the bowel lacks appropriate enervation and inhibits the ability both to identify the need to pass stool and to appropriately pass stools. In other cases, inflammatory bowel disorders may cause severe constipation. Effects may also be reciprocal, in that chronic and prolonged constipation can lead to bowel impaction that requires painful passage of stool. To prevent this pain, children may engage in retentive behaviors, most often tightening of the external anal sphincter muscles or tightening of the gluteal muscles or pelvic muscles to prevent stool passage. Ultimately, this retention slows total transit time in the colon, which exacerbates constipation. As the colon becomes impacted (megacolon), reflexive mechanisms for stool passage become impaired, which can prevent the child from identifying the need to pass stool. Many children with encopresis deny feeling an urge to defecate. The longer stool is retained in the colon, the more water is absorbed from the stool and the harder stools become, making passage more painful and potentiating further restriction. A diagnosis of encopresis is not made when physical causes for fecal incontinence are identified.

Other presenting issues often prompt the referral, and screening questions around toileting can uncover issues that require more evaluation. It is important to ask about the age at which regular toileting habits were established and the presence of any "accidents" or soiling. A careful history will elicit the duration, timing, and severity of symptoms; any exacerbating and ameliorating factors; and the presence of any extended periods of fecal continence (e.g., some children may avoid toileting at school but assume more regular bowel voiding during summer break). Further questions should evaluate the extent of symptoms of constipation. The specifiers of encopresis are "with constipation and overflow incontinence" and "without constipation and overflow incontinence." This can be assessed with physical examination and the following questions: Does your child pass large or very hard stools? Does your child appear to be holding in stool (retentive posture)? Does your child pass stools that are large enough to block the toilet? How frequently does your child pass stool into the toilet? How frequently does your child pass stool into other receptacles (most often underwear)?

It is important to determine the frequency of stool passage outside of appropriate receptacles and the timing of stooling when it occurs. Children and adolescents most often pass bowel movements in the late afternoon, after retaining stool for most of the day. Some experience the urge to pass stool during periods of more intense exercise, such as physical education classes or sports activities. It is also important to determine whether the fecal incontinence is intermittent or continuous and the conditions under which there is bowel regularity, if any, particularly in the context of constipation. Resolution of constipation itself is often an effective treatment for encopresis when efforts are maintained over 6–12 months. Important questions include the following: Other than the toilet, where does your child deposit bowel movements? How frequently does your child experience fecal soiling of the underwear (incontinence overflow)? Is there any evidence of nocturnal encopresis? Has your child ever been treated for constipation or other gastrointestinal difficulties? Has your child seen a gastroenterologist? If so, what is the maintenance routine for bowel regularity? How compliant is your child with these routines? How long have you maintained these routines? Have there been periods when your child was able to toilet regularly? How long have these periods lasted? Are there additional difficulties with enuresis (nocturnal or diurnal)?

Another important issue is whether the child takes any medications. In the absence of constipation, laxative use can cause encopretic behavior and may be associated with eating disorder behavior. Caregivers should be asked about their approach and attitude toward toilet training, their response to soiling, and whether there are any recent changes or stresses to the family. How is the child doing socially and academically? Are there any other developmental concerns (gross or fine motor skills, learning, speech, growth)? Are there concerns around neglect or failure to have appropriate toileting facilities available? Are there concerns around aggressive, violent, or regressive behaviors? Providers should sensitively, yet directly, ask about any maltreatment or abuse. Questions around general psychopathology are critical, given the wide range of comorbidity for this diagnosis. Specific questions should target anxiety, mood, and disruptive behavior disorders.

Getting the History

A mother reports that her 8-year-old daughter, Jasmyn, has daytime soiling episodes. The interviewer starts with open-ended questions to determine the duration, frequency, and quality of symptoms. The first questions are directed to the mother: "Tell me more about what you've been noticing. How long has this been an issue? Does Jasmyn pass stool outside the toilet, or does it just appear to be staining of the underwear? Is there a history of gastrointestinal difficulties, including stomach upset, vomiting, constipation, or diarrhea? How often does Jasmyn pass stools—daily or with less frequency? Are stools large or hard? Do they cause significant pain when passing?" The interviewer then directs questions to Jasmyn: "What is your understanding of what's happening? Do you think that it (constipation) is a problem now? How have you managed it? Have you changed what you eat or drink? Do you take any medicine to help you go to the bathroom? How often are stools passed in the toilet? Where else do they occur (such as underwear, somewhere in the bedroom)? Are there places you won't go to the bathroom (such as public places, at school, in certain restrooms)? Why or why not? What happens when you have an accident? Do you know that you need to use the bathroom, or does stooling just 'happen'?" The interviewer also asks the parent, "Does your child seem to know when she needs to use the bathroom?" The frequency of the soiling episodes can vary, but to meet DSM-5-TR criteria, they must occur at least once per month for 3 consecutive months.

The interviewer should also inquire about general functioning. It is important to include both Jasmyn and her mother in the questioning not only to build rapport with the child but also to get a more comprehensive sense of the issues involved. It is often helpful to do parts of the interview with the parent and child together and to meet alone with the child or parent, particularly if the conversation appears to be causing distress.

It is important to be nonjudgmental and empathetic because talking about soiling is very embarrassing to most children. Don't be afraid to use more child-friendly terminology to ease the discussion. The interviewer asks the parent, "How is Jasmyn doing overall? How are things at school? How would Jasmyn's teacher describe her? How are her grades?" The interviewer asks Jasmyn, "Do you have a best friend? What sorts of things do you like to do with your friends? Do they ever have sleepovers? Do you go? Do you play any sports? Which ones? How about at home—are there any arguments with your parents or siblings? Do you have any other areas of concern?"

As noted repeatedly in this section, ruling out physical causes is critical. Some important questions have already been captured here, but others include the following: "Has your daughter ever had any major medical illness or injury, such as a head or spinal injury? Does she take any medications or over-the-counter supplements? How much water does she drink?"

The DSM-5-TR diagnosis of encopresis is relatively straightforward, despite the need for ruling out physical causes of incontinence. The interviewer needs to determine whether the child is older than 4 years (or developmental equivalent) and must confirm the presence of symptoms at least once per month for 3 months. Unlike with enuresis, encopresis criteria do not specify frequency of symptoms or the presence of significant distress or functional impairment. Finally, the interviewer must confirm that there are not any medical illnesses or exposure to substances that may better explain the symptoms of fecal incontinence. The disorder is coded for the presence or absence of constipation because this specification directs treatment.

Tips for Clarifying the Diagnosis

- Refer the individual to their primary care provider and consider a consultation with gastroenterology to rule out physical causes of fecal incontinence.
- Assuming there is no physical cause of bowel incontinence, focus on determining the presence and extent of a history of constipation.
- Evaluate constipation and routines around maintenance of bowel regularity. Assess whether the family maintains appropriate fiber, water, and (where necessary) stool-softening regimens to reduce impaction. Advise them that in many cases, simply relieving constipation for a period of 6–12 months can resolve encopresis.
- In the absence of constipation, consider behavioral difficulties or environmental challenges to regular toileting, such as unclean or inadequate toileting facilities. Sensitively screen for current or historical abuse.
- Use a sensitive and empathetic approach to the family to obtain information that may be sensitive and difficult to discuss but is important for the care of the child. Most children, particularly older ones, experience significant shame around fecal incontinence.

Consider the Case

Adi is a 14-year-old boy with a history of oppositional defiant disorder and disruptive behaviors who presents to an outpatient child psychiatry clinic because of concerns around significant weight gain secondary to a trial of atypical antipsychotic medication. Following discontinuation of this medication, Adi has lost most of the excess weight but has experienced a return of more challenging disruptive behaviors and temper outbursts.

On evaluation, it is discovered that Adi has also never attained regular fecal or nocturnal urinary continence. He does not experience nocturnal fecal incontinence. His parents consulted a pediatric gastroenterology specialist 3 years before the current intake and are aware that Adi is outside of expected norms of toileting but have viewed his toileting difficulties as part of the larger scope of his "defiant" behaviors. He received a diagnosis of constipation at the time of the previous visit, but his parents were unclear if more significant testing was undertaken to rule out physical causes of incontinence. They were instructed to provide over-the-counter stool softeners to soften stools and did so for 1 month following their visit with the specialist. They expressed great frustration with Adi and have responded to toileting accidents with anger and privilege withdrawal, including having him wear soiled underwear as a punishment. This was discontinued when it resulted in a rash.

He has recently experienced increasing periods of dryness at night, with a recent stretch of nearly 10 dry nights, but these stretches are disrupted with any change in routine or structure. His parents tried using an alarm system, which they felt was unsuccessful in remediating his nocturnal enuresis. They have never engaged in any treatment to address fecal incontinence and noted that these symptoms had not been evaluated or discussed in his previous therapeutic relationship. On questioning, his parents note that at least one-third of the conflict at home stems from Adi's incontinence: either parental upset at these behaviors or Adi's response to punishments and privilege withdrawal.

On assessment, Adi presents as an active, inattentive young man who expresses great shame in describing himself, both behaviorally and in terms of toileting. He describes avoiding bathrooms at school because they are "disgusting" and other boys tease him if he enters a stall (e.g., throwing toilet paper over the door, knocking or hitting the door and calling him names). He also reports not always being aware of the need to stool, and his mother describes him as "zoning out" or "going into a trance" when he has a bowel movement. Otherwise, he feels well and denies nausea, vomiting, cramping, or painful stools. The family is instructed to take Adi for a physical examination, which reveals no presence of constipation or bowel impaction. They are also referred to follow up with a pediatric gastroenterologist for a thorough evaluation to rule out physical causes for his encopresis and nocturnal enuresis, which yields normal findings.

Adi's presentation is complicated, although not atypical, in that his symptoms were uncovered as part of a general psychiatric evaluation but not targeted in previous treatment. The failure to establish any regular history of either fecal or urinary continence is particularly concerning and warrants more in-depth evaluation to rule out physical causes for toileting difficulties, such as Hirschsprung's disease, inflammatory bowel disorders, and metabolic or absorption difficulties.

Differential Diagnosis

The differential diagnosis of encopresis centers on excluding the presence of medical conditions or substances that can cause fecal incontinence, including Hirschsprung's disease, inflammatory bowel disorders, a range of gastrointestinal difficulties, neurological impairment, spinal injuries that impair sensation in the bowel region or control over bowel evacuation, laxative abuse or overuse, and metabolic disorders. Exposure to medications can influence encopresis, most often by increasing constipation. As such, many medications may be implicated in exacerbating encopresis.

Children with encopresis may also exhibit medical and behavioral problems at a higher rate than children without the disorder. Specific learning disorder, anxiety disorders, depressive disorders, ADHD, and trauma- and stressor-related disorders all have high rates of comorbidity with encopresis. Encopresis should also be evaluated in children receiving treatment for other medical difficulties, particularly in hospital settings.

See DSM-5-TR for additional disorders to consider in the differential diagnosis. Also refer to the discussions of comorbidity and differential diagnosis in their respective sections of DSM-5-TR.

Summary

- The diagnosis of encopresis must be made in children older than 4 years (or developmental equivalent).
- Encopresis is not diagnosed in the presence of medical illness or medication use that can result in fecal incontinence.
- Encopresis has two specifiers that are important for directing treatment: "with constipation and overflow incontinence" and "without constipation and overflow incontinence."
- Encopresis can lead to significant difficulty in the child's academic, social, and home functioning.

SUMMARY: ELIMINATION DISORDERS

Enuresis and encopresis characteristically manifest in children and adolescents and can be extremely challenging to diagnose and treat. Because several medical conditions and medications can cause symptoms of bowel and bladder incontinence, it is essential that the mental health clinician work in concert with a medical provider to properly identify the biological, psychological, and social factors that contribute to the overall clinical picture. Children with elimination disorders are more likely to also have developmental delays, speech and language difficulties, learning disabilities, ADHD, and other behavioral problems.

ELEMENTS TO CONSIDER IN THE CULTURAL FORMULATION

- Enuresis and encopresis are seen in countries throughout the world.
- High rates of enuresis have been reported in orphanages and other residential institutions.

- Culture may impact the diagnosis and perceived etiology of enuresis and encopresis. Parents may be negatively impacted because of stigma or increased costs of childcare. They may be reluctant to seek treatment because of religious beliefs about the perceived impurity of urine and feces.
- Hot weather climates and differences in the intake of food and beverages in some settings may influence the development of constipation.
- Psychosocial adversity may lead to unexplained physical symptoms such as abdominal pain, which might trigger a cycle of withholding stool and constipation.

DIAGNOSTIC PEARLS

- Only a minority of elimination disorders can be traced to an underlying anatomical abnormality, malabsorption syndrome, endocrine issue, or neurological condition. Despite this, medical evaluation is a critical component of the evaluation.
- Bowel continence occurs before urinary continence, and children are expected to be consistently using the toilet for bowel voiding by 4 years of age (or developmental equivalent).
- Nocturnal encopresis is rare and is generally related to overflow incontinence from constipation; most cases occur during the day.
- Children with ADHD have about a 30% greater chance of experiencing enuresis. This increase is likely related to a neurochemical effect rather than to inattention or impulsivity.
- Nocturnal enuresis can be diagnosed based on history, physical examination, and a screening urinalysis. No additional testing is required in the absence of abnormalities, but additional testing may be required in cases of recurrent infection.
- Daytime incontinence or diurnal enuresis may be characterized as a problem of storage or emptying. In addition to a careful history and physical examination, children should also undergo urinalysis, urine culture, bladder ultrasonography, and uroflow testing.
- The diagnosis is largely based on clinical history, and extensive additional testing is often not necessary.
- Work with the child's primary care provider to ensure that a full physical examination has been completed. Obtain a screening urinalysis. Abdominal X-rays may be helpful in confirming the presence of constipation.
- Additional consultation with gastroenterology or urology can be requested in the event of diagnostic uncertainty or concerning findings.
- Always keep child maltreatment on your radar, but at the same time remember that most children with enuresis and encopresis are not being abused.

SELF-ASSESSMENT

Key Concepts: Double-Check Your Knowledge

What is the relevance of the following concepts to the various elimination disorders?

- Nocturnal versus diurnal enuresis
- Primary versus secondary enuresis
- Relationship between deep sleep and nocturnal enuresis
- Medical conditions and medications that may cause urinary incontinence
- Encopresis with and without constipation
- "Overflow" incontinence
- Relationship to comorbidity
- Physical causes of fecal incontinence
- Laxative use and contraindications for their use
- Behavioral training and biofeedback use

Questions to Discuss With Colleagues and Mentors

1. Do you screen all children and adolescents for elimination disorders, or do certain situations prompt you to take a more detailed history?
2. How do you make certain that families follow through on their child's medical prescriptions and adherence with bladder or bowel hygiene routines?
3. How do you overcome an individual's discomfort with talking about bladder and bowel habits?
4. Do you have an approach to working collaboratively with pediatricians and family practitioners to rule out medical causes of enuresis or encopresis before making a diagnosis?

Case-Based Questions

PART A

Delia is an 11-year-old girl who presents with her foster mother to her pediatrician with concerns about fecal smearing, as well as passage of bowel movements in a cabinet under the sink in the bathroom or into her underwear. Her early developmental history is generally unknown, but she was removed from her biological family because of concerns regarding neglect and physical abuse. Physical examinations have ruled out physical causes of fecal incontinence and are not suggestive of anal trauma. Since joining her foster family, she has never toileted appropriately with defecation and was initially enuretic, but she has responded to efforts to assist her with daytime dryness. She continues to wet several times per week. She is engaged in toilet training, and her foster parents are very patient with her. She passes regular stools and has fecal staining, which her foster mother relates to lack of wiping following bowel evacuation. The family has followed voiding schedules and incentive programs, with very limited success toward bowel continence. The family has not used stool softeners or laxatives, and currently Delia is not taking any prescription or over-the-counter medications. The doctor has ruled out constipation, and the family reports that at times Delia's bowel movements are appropriately soft and of sufficient bulk. They did not note blood in her stool but observed that some stools were soft and appeared to have a mucus-like texture or clear, foul-smelling discharge. Delia appears to know that she needs to have a bowel movement at times and will hide in the bathroom but will not use the toilet, preferring to evacuate her bowels under the sink instead.

Outside of toileting concerns, Delia has been defiant and aggressive in the home, occasionally engaging in head-banging and self-scratching behaviors. She has been found to be hoarding food in her room, although not eating it but allowing it to rot. She has learning difficulties, which may be related to inconsistent education in her early years because her family reportedly moved frequently. She has presented with some dissociative symptoms and flat affect at times, but she is responsive at other times. She can be difficult to establish rapport with, although her foster mother clearly has a caring and firm relationship with her. Delia has regressive behaviors with change, such as the foster family's older biological children returning home.

How should the pediatrician approach diagnosis in Delia's case?   Because Delia is older than 4 years and has no known history of constipation or physical causes for fecal incontinence, she receives a diagnosis of encopresis without constipation. Continued efforts at behavioral regulation, including a thorough diagnostic evaluation, are warranted. Additional evaluation by a pediatric gastrointestinal specialist is warranted to evaluate for physical causes of these difficulties.

PART B

Delia's physical examination results are significant for the presence of areas of inflammation of the bowel, consistent with ulcerative colitis. Furthermore, tracking of her bowel habits notes sensitivities to seasonings, including garlic and hot spices, despite her preference for these flavors. Use of steroid treatment significantly improves the consistency of her stools. However, challenges continue for voiding appropriately.

How should the pediatrician proceed?   The findings on examination are suggestive of physical causes for encopresis, but Delia's behaviors continued after resolution of these difficulties. The family has been consistent with behavioral interventions, and they do not react dramatically when soiling episodes occur. They implemented a clearer bowel regimen, including having Delia assist with cleanup. With time, Delia was able to note that she had a strong preference for quiet and privacy when voiding and was able to void at home, but she had continued difficulty transitioning to toileting outside the home, necessitating additional behavioral treatment to generalize these skills to toilets at school and in public.

Short-Answer Questions

1. By what age are children typically expected to be toilet trained and fully "dry"?
2. What tests must be ordered for children presenting with nocturnal enuresis?
3. List three medical conditions associated with urinary incontinence.
4. Name three psychiatric conditions that may be comorbid with enuresis.
5. By what age are children typically expected to no longer have daytime bowel incontinence?

6. Which specialists should be consulted for children presenting with encopresis?
7. Which medical disorder should be strongly considered as a rule-out, particularly for children who never achieve bowel continence?
8. Name at least three psychiatric conditions that may be comorbid with encopresis.

Answers

1. Children are typically expected to be toilet trained and fully "dry" by age 5 years (or developmental equivalent).

2. Screening urinalysis must be ordered for children presenting with nocturnal enuresis.

3. Medical conditions associated with urinary incontinence include diabetes insipidus, diabetes mellitus, acute urinary tract infection, and neurogenic bladder.

4. Psychiatric conditions that may be comorbid with enuresis include encopresis, ADHD, and sleep disorders.

5. Children typically are expected to no longer have daytime bowel incontinence by age 4 years.

6. Specialists in pediatric gastroenterology and possibly neurology and endocrinology may be consulted for children presenting with encopresis.

7. Hirschsprung's disease should be strongly considered as a rule-out, particularly for children who never achieved bowel continence.

8. Psychiatric conditions that may be comorbid with encopresis include specific learning disorder, anxiety disorders, depressive disorders, ADHD, and trauma- and stressor-related disorders.

REFERENCES

American Psychiatric Association: Diagnostic and Statistical Manual of Mental Disorders, 5th Edition. Arlington, VA, American Psychiatric Association, 2013
American Psychiatric Association: Diagnostic and Statistical Manual of Mental Disorders, 5th Edition, Text Revision. Washington, DC, American Psychiatric Association, 2022

CHAPTER 16

Sleep-Wake Disorders

Christina F. Chick, Ph.D.
Michelle Primeau, M.D.
Ruth O'Hara, Ph.D.

"I can't get to sleep."

"He snores so loud!"

- Insomnia Disorder
- Hypersomnolence Disorder
- Narcolepsy
- Breathing-Related Sleep Disorders
  - Obstructive Sleep Apnea Hypopnea
  - Central Sleep Apnea
  - Sleep-Related Hypoventilation
- Circadian Rhythm Sleep-Wake Disorders
- Parasomnias
  - Non–Rapid Eye Movement Sleep Arousal Disorders
  - Nightmare Disorder
  - Rapid Eye Movement Sleep Behavior Disorder
  - Restless Legs Syndrome
- Substance/Medication-Induced Sleep Disorder
- Other Specified Insomnia Disorder
- Unspecified Insomnia Disorder
- Other Specified Hypersomnolence Disorder

- Unspecified Hypersomnolence Disorder
- Other Specified Sleep-Wake Disorder
- Unspecified Sleep-Wake Disorder

Sleep disorders can manifest as a complaint of unsatisfactory sleep, impaired daytime function, or both. Several changes were implemented from DSM-IV (American Psychiatric Association 1994) in DSM-5 (American Psychiatric Association 2013) and DSM-5-TR (American Psychiatric Association 2022) chapters on sleep-wake disorders (Table 16–1). These changes were made to allow greater differentiation of the varied causes of sleep disruption and to help identify those who require referral to a sleep specialist.

- In the past, insomnia was at times considered an independent phenomenon (primary insomnia) or related to another condition (secondary insomnia). The distinction between primary and secondary insomnia was eliminated in DSM-5.
- The diagnosis of primary hypersomnia was replaced by hypersomnolence disorder, which includes greater specificity in the diagnostic criteria.
- Similarly, the diagnosis of narcolepsy requires not only subjective symptoms, such as sleep "attacks" or *cataplexy* (the loss of muscle tone with maintained consciousness triggered usually by a positive experience, such as hearing something funny), but also objective biological indicators, such as hypocretin and the occurrence of rapid eye movement (REM) sleep. Further specifiers cover other medical conditions associated with narcolepsy symptoms.
- In DSM-5 and DSM-5-TR, the DSM-IV diagnosis of breathing-related sleep disorder is separated into three disorders: obstructive sleep apnea hypopnea, central sleep apnea, and sleep-related hypoventilation.
- Circadian rhythm sleep-wake disorders include advanced sleep phase type, and the jet lag specifier has been removed.
- Disorders previously split as individual parasomnias, such as sleepwalking and sleep terrors, have been grouped into non–rapid eye movement (NREM) sleep arousal disorders to better reflect the clinical, etiological, and epidemiological characteristics. Nightmare disorder was modified to include specifiers to account for associated medical, psychiatric, and sleep disorders that may co-occur, as well as for duration and severity.
- Two new diagnoses were added to DSM-5 and DSM-5-TR: REM sleep behavior disorder (a parasomnia) and restless legs syndrome (RLS).
- Tobacco was added as a substance for substance/medication-induced sleep disorder in DSM-5 and DSM-5-TR.
- The category for sleep disorders related to another mental disorder was eliminated in DSM-5 and DSM-5-TR.
- Finally, for patients not meeting the full criteria for insomnia, hypersomnia, or another sleep-wake disorder, DSM-5 and DSM-5-TR contain other and unspecified diagnoses to apply to those experiencing clinically significant distress.

TABLE 16–1. Key changes between DSM-5 and DSM-5-TR

Narcolepsy, type 1 describes a diagnosis of narcolepsy with cataplexy or hypocretin deficiency, while narcolepsy, type 2 describes a diagnosis of narcolepsy without cataplexy and either without hypocretin deficiency or with hypocretin unmeasured.

Sleep complaints are common in everyday life. Most people have had the experience of being unable to sleep in the days leading up to a stressful event, such as a job interview. However, there are instances where disrupted sleep may reflect an underlying sleep disorder that leads to or exacerbates an existing psychiatric or other medical condition. Sleep disturbances can reflect very different sleep disorders, many of which have established treatments. Diagnosing and targeting co-occurring sleep disorders can help alleviate psychiatric symptoms.

Some sleep-wake disorders occur only during sleep; in fact, a person may be unaware that any unusual behavior is occurring. For example, children with NREM sleep arousal disorders, such as sleepwalking or sleep terrors, may not have any recollection of disruption the preceding night, even though their behavior may be quite unsettling to their parents.

Other sleep disorders are characterized by symptoms occurring during wakefulness. For example, RLS is characterized by a subjective discomfort in the legs with inactivity that is alleviated by movement.

Sleep disorders often co-occur with psychiatric conditions and can reduce an individual's quality of life. Given the important interactions between sleep-wake disorders and psychiatric illness, diagnosing co-occurring sleep disorders is important for effective long-term management of chronic, recurrent psychiatric illnesses.

IN-DEPTH DIAGNOSIS: INSOMNIA DISORDER

Ms. Albers, a 32-year-old woman, presents with a complaint of insomnia. She has experienced brief periods of insomnia in the past that were usually related to situational stressors or travel and relieved by a sleeping pill. However, she has had increasing difficulty with falling asleep over the past 6 months despite taking a sleeping pill nightly. Nine months ago, she started noticing that she would wake in the middle of the night and worry about work or her upcoming wedding, but more recently she has progressed to difficulties falling asleep at the beginning of the night. She finds that she is now worrying during the day about her inability to sleep and has come to dread the nights. She feels that her lack of sleep is causing her to be more irritable, have decreased concentration, and be ineffective at work. She has started canceling social outings and early morning meetings to accommodate her sleep. She has become so preoccupied with her sleep that her primary care physician prescribed a benzodiazepine to help with her anxiety, but she is reluctant to take it because "the only thing I'm worried about is my sleep."

Insomnia disorder occurs more frequently in females and tends to manifest in young adulthood. Often, individuals will report brief, prior episodes that resolved on their own. However, to meet the criteria for the diagnosis of insomnia disorder, the individual must experience an index episode where sleep disturbances occur at least 3 nights per week for a minimum duration of 3 months. The key component to note in Ms. Albers's case is the significant impact that she perceives the sleep disruption to have on her daytime function and her escalating preoccupation and concern over her sleep. It is common for individuals to awaken in the middle of the night, but becoming worried or stressed, striving to sleep, and being preoccupied with daytime impairments are indicators of insomnia. Mid–sleep period awakenings sometimes become so stressful that the individual worries about them to the point of having difficulty falling asleep at the beginning of the night. The fact that Ms. Albers presents as very anxious is evidence of the hyperarousal that is often seen in people with insomnia. Some individuals report that sleep is their only concern, even if they may have comorbid depression and anxiety. Finally, the use of sedative-hypnotic medications is common in patients with insomnia disorder.

Approach to the Diagnosis

Many people report problems with their sleep, but it is important to remember that not all sleep problems are insomnia. The first important consideration is whether the person is *complaining* about their sleep. For example, an individual may report a short sleep period but may not find that period to be distressing. It is important to identify exactly what the person's complaint is—difficulty falling asleep, difficulty maintaining sleep, early morning awakening, or some combination—because this information may indicate the presence of other sleep-wake disorders. Some people are able to identify discrete times at which they have some worsening of the complaint (e.g., "I have difficulty falling asleep every Sunday night, worrying about the coming week") or locations that affect their sleep (e.g., "I can only sleep well on vacation"), whereas others have sleeping trouble every day, no matter the situation.

Individuals with insomnia disorder frequently underestimate their actual sleep time and report more prolonged awakenings at night than are noted on objective studies of sleep. In general, the convention is to consider a sleep latency or wakefulness after sleep onset of more than 30 minutes to be outside of normal limits. Similarly, individuals with insomnia disorder report increased daytime symptoms, such as difficulty concentrating or performing complex, targeted tasks, but when tested, they frequently fall within normal limits. It is thought that the perceived difficulties may reflect the increased effort required to maintain the same outcomes.

Individuals with insomnia disorder are often described as "wired but tired," meaning that they report fatigue but are not overtly sleepy on subjective and objective measures of sleepiness, and they are unable to nap if given the chance. Individuals often report an inability to quiet their minds. Negative sleep-related cognitions often become prominent in individuals with insomnia disorder and can be used to assess the level of distress individuals are experiencing from their sleep complaints (e.g., "If I don't sleep well tonight, then I'm going to be horrible at my meeting tomorrow"). Individuals may become overly attentive to the effect that losing sleep has on performance and selectively attend to negative outcomes. The individual may make accommodations for their sleep difficulties. For example, individuals may cancel morning meetings so they can sleep later after a bad night or try to go to bed early to "catch up." In children, insomnia may manifest as bedtime resistance, calling parents back to the room multiple times, and requiring caregiver assistance in returning to sleep after night awakenings. Polysomnography is not essential to make the diagnosis of insomnia, unless other clinical correlates indicate a possible physiological sleep disorder, such as breathing-related sleep disorders, which are frequently comorbid with insomnia.

Getting the History

A 35-year-old patient presents with the chief complaint of "insomnia." The interviewer inquires about the duration of time that the symptoms have been present and asks the person about any identifiable trigger at onset. Specifics as to the nature of the problem are then obtained: Is it difficult falling asleep, staying asleep, or both? In a typical week, how often does this occur?

Often, to get an accurate picture of the problem, the interviewer asks questions that focus on sleep hygiene behaviors that may be targeted and guide the diagnosis. It is helpful to go through the night chronologically: "What time do you get into bed? What time do you turn off the television/lights/computer and allow for sleep? How long do you feel it takes to fall asleep? Once asleep, do you ever wake up during the night? How long does it take to return to sleep? At what time do you have your final awakening, and when do you get out of bed? Are those times different on weekends? What about taking naps (intentional) or dozing (unintentional)? Do your sleep patterns bother you? What is bothersome about your sleep?"

The answer to the following question can help point to circadian rhythm sleep-wake disorders: "Do you consider yourself a 'night owl' or a 'morning lark'?" Several questions can help rule out the potential contribution of substances such as caffeine, tobacco, or alcohol to the person's sleep: "Do you ever take medications for your sleep? If so, what do you take and at what time? Do you use any substances that may affect your sleep?" Some questions can help screen for obstructive sleep apnea hypopnea: "Do you snore? Has anyone ever told you that you appear to stop breathing while you are sleeping? Are you sleepy during the day?"

In insomnia evaluation, it is helpful to quantify the specifics of the sleep problem. Individuals with insomnia usually appreciate the interviewer's attention to detail in asking about all aspects of their night because they already have scrutinized all possible contributors to their impaired sleep and, being unable to identify a solution, are willing to discuss their sleep in minute detail. Identifying which part of the night is more impaired can help rule in or rule out other conditions. For example, difficulties initiating sleep may also be attributed to RLS or circadian rhythm sleep-wake disorder, delayed sleep phase type. It is important to consider these other sleep disorders because treatments are very different among them.

Tips for Clarifying the Diagnosis

- Evaluate the patient for co-occurring sleep and psychiatric conditions that may also be present.
- Understand whether the person has complaints about an impairment in some aspect of daytime function.
- Assess whether they are allowing adequate time for sleep.
- Determine whether they have cognitions about sleep, preoccupation with the negative impact of lack of sleep, or sleep-related anxiety.

Consider the Case

Mr. Hall, a 38-year-old Marine with a history of PTSD secondary to combat exposure, is being evaluated for residual sleep complaints. Mr. Hall was referred for sleep evaluation after he completed a research study on prolonged exposure therapy. Although his symptoms of PTSD have resolved almost completely, he still has difficulty initiating and maintaining sleep. He reports that he never had any sleep problems before his deployment; however, while deployed, he had to stand watch at night and sleep during the day, and he feels that his sleep patterns remain disorganized today. To compensate for his lack of sleep at night, he frequently naps and drinks coffee or smokes cigarettes to maintain alertness during the day. He worries about how his lack of sleep is affecting the way he relates to his children and is concerned that he will have difficulty reentering the workforce because of his sleep disruption.

Although insomnia is more frequently seen in females, it occurs often in males as well. People with psychiatric conditions also commonly have comorbid insomnia, and 40%–50% of people diagnosed with insomnia have a comorbid mental disorder. In the past, insomnia was often considered to be secondary to psychiatric conditions, but research indicates that considering the diagnoses to be co-occurring without prioritizing one diagnosis over another or attributing causality may be more accurate. Insomnia is the most frequently reported residual symptom in patients with major depressive disorder, and untreated sleep symptoms can precipitate another episode of depression. The symptom of insomnia is an independent risk factor for suicidal thoughts or behavior in both adolescents and adults.

Individuals with PTSD frequently have fragmented sleep, and Mr. Hall demonstrates inadequate sleep hygiene (e.g., frequent naps) and use of stimulating substances. Further elaboration of the history could help identify whether he has another sleep disorder, such as substance/medication-induced sleep disorder or circadian rhythm sleep-wake disorder, which might explain his disorganized sleep pattern. Insomnia is quite common in veteran populations.

Differential Diagnosis

The differential diagnosis of insomnia disorder includes normal sleep variations, such as those who physiologically require less sleep or those with age-related sleep changes. Situational/acute insomnia may be brief and precipitated by a change in life events. If an individual experiences sleep disturbances at least 3 nights per week and clinically significant impairment for a period less than 3 months, a diagnosis of other specified insomnia disorder may be made.

Circadian rhythm sleep-wake disorder is the primary diagnosis to consider when evaluating a person for insomnia disorder. Frequently, individuals with circadian rhythm sleep-wake disorder, delayed sleep phase type, are mistaken for having insomnia disorder because of their difficulty initiating sleep. These individuals tend to fall asleep and stay asleep later than is considered typical and in a way that interferes with their social or occupational functioning. Individuals whose circadian phase is advanced may describe excessive sleepiness in the evenings and early morning awakenings. However, when going to bed at a time better aligned with their natural rhythms, these individuals do not actually have difficulty initiating or maintaining sleep. Similarly, circadian rhythm sleep-wake disorder, advanced sleep phase type, may manifest in an older adult with early morning awakening. These individuals tend to fall asleep earlier in the evenings than intended, awaken earlier, and be unable to return to sleep. Circadian rhythm sleep-wake disorder, shift work type, differs from insomnia disorder by the recent history of shift work.

RLS can manifest as difficulty falling asleep or returning to sleep because of intrusive discomfort, usually in the legs. Individuals with insomnia disorder often report "tossing and turning," but people with RLS report an inability to sit still or feeling "tingling," "creepy crawly," or "as if my legs have to sneeze," which occurs around the same time of day or when being sedentary and improves with movement.

Other sleep-wake disorders to consider in the differential diagnosis of insomnia disorder include the following: Breathing-related sleep disorder is difficult to diagnose with history alone, but indicators of risk include being obese, snoring, witnessed apneas, and excessive daytime sleepiness. Individuals with narcolepsy sometimes may have comorbid insomnia, although the condition tends to be characterized by hypersomnia. Parasomnias are characterized specifically by events occurring while the person is asleep, and individuals usually are unaware of behaviors unless they awaken from them or are told about them by a witness. Substance/medication-induced sleep disorder may overlap with insomnia disorder but occurs in the context of acute intoxication or withdrawal from a substance or medication and is chronologically related to substance or medication use.

Insomnia disorder may co-occur with other sleep-wake disorders and psychiatric conditions, such as depression or anxiety, and the comorbid condition often may be seen as overlapping or contributing to the insomnia disorder.

See DSM-5-TR for additional disorders to consider in the differential diagnosis. Also refer to the discussions of comorbidity and differential diagnosis in their respective sections of DSM-5-TR.

Summary

- Insomnia is a common complaint, and the symptoms have an impact not only on the sleep period but also on daytime functioning.
- Insomnia is frequently comorbid with other medical and psychiatric conditions.
- A thorough history of the course of symptoms and how the insomnia manifests at night gives insight into the nature of the problem and can help direct future treatment.
- Diagnosis requires ruling out other sleep disorders, such as circadian rhythm sleep-wake disorder or breathing-related sleep disorder.

IN-DEPTH DIAGNOSIS: NARCOLEPSY

Annie, a 6-year-old girl without prior medical history, presents with her parents for evaluation of an acute change in her behavior. Her parents report that she had been her usual self until 3 months ago, when she acquired tonsillitis, and she has not been the

same since. They describe that she appears unable to stay awake during the day, frequently falling asleep at school and at home, even when engaged in an activity or conversation. Her nighttime sleep period has become disrupted as well, with apparent
vivid, terrifying dreams, some of which she physically reacts to, resulting in minor injuries from falling out of bed trying to run from whatever she was seeing. Her parents
also note that she appears "floppy"—with her mouth dropping open—or unable to
hold up her head. On one occasion, her father told a joke at dinner, and she laughed so
hard that her head fell into her spaghetti. There is no family history of anything similar,
and her siblings remain healthy.

Nocturnal polysomnography demonstrates an apnea hypopnea index (AHI) of
0.5 events per hour and REM sleep latency of 15 minutes. Next-day multiple sleep latency test (MSLT) had 5/5 sleep-onset REM periods with a sleep latency of 6 minutes.
Lumbar puncture was not done, given the classic presentation of symptoms, but human leukocyte antigen (HLA) typing demonstrated Annie to be a carrier of *HLA-
DQB1*06:02*.

Annie demonstrates the classic abrupt onset of narcolepsy. She has brief periods of
excessive sleepiness that she is unable to overcome by engaging in activity, as well as
classic cataplexy. Early in the condition, children often demonstrate hypotonia, with
parents describing them as "floppy," or have automatisms, such as tongue thrusting,
that are atypical for the child. As the condition progresses, cataplectic "attacks" may
be seen. These are triggered usually by a positive emotion, such as happiness or surprise, and can be dramatic, as in Annie's case, or even cause the individual to fall to
the ground. Not included in the diagnostic criteria of narcolepsy, but also suggestive,
is REM sleep behavior disorder, in which the person appears to be acting out terrifying imagery from a dream. It is also common for individuals with narcolepsy to have
sleep paralysis or hallucinations when falling asleep or when awakening, representing REM sleep intruding into wakefulness, which can be quite disturbing to them.

A nocturnal polysomnogram followed by an MSLT is used to confirm the narcolepsy diagnosis. Nocturnal polysomnography can rule out the presence of breathing-
related sleep disorders, which are more common than narcolepsy and may frequently
be comorbid with narcolepsy. The nocturnal polysomnography may indicate a short-
ened REM sleep latency (≤15 minutes, instead of the typical 90–120 minutes). The
daytime MSLT is considered positive if it shows two or more sleep-onset REM periods, with a mean sleep latency of 8 minutes or longer.

Of the individuals who have narcolepsy type 1 (NT1; narcolepsy with cataplexy
or hypocretin deficiency), 85%–95% are positive for *HLA-DQB1*06:02*. There are no
biomarkers for narcolepsy type 2 (NT2; narcolepsy without cataplexy and either
without hypocretin deficiency or with hypocretin unmeasured). Low or undetectable
hypocretin-1 levels are common among individuals with cataplexy.

Approach to the Diagnosis

Individuals who have narcolepsy are frequently misdiagnosed with other conditions,
such as major depressive disorder or obstructive sleep apnea hypopnea, before they
are correctly diagnosed and obtain adequate treatment. For a child with narcolepsy,
the parents may be able to provide a discrete onset of excessive sleepiness, often following an illness or vaccination, that is accompanied by other symptoms of visual

hallucinations, acting out terrifying dreams, sleep paralysis, and cataplexy. The child often sleeps through all or part of the history. Adults with narcolepsy may have more difficulty identifying the onset of symptoms, particularly if the symptoms have been present for many years. In adolescents or adults, the onset of symptoms may not be quite as dramatic as in young children. Excessive sleepiness and increased sleep are hallmarks of early narcolepsy, but over time it may be noted that the total daily hours of sleep are as expected, although the individual has difficulty maintaining sleep and wake states. Adults may describe having "sleep attacks" in which they do not even realize they were asleep until they awaken from a nap. Nighttime sleep becomes disrupted with insomnia or with vivid, disturbing dreams that the person may physically act out. Brief daytime naps are usually refreshing, but this is not necessarily specific to narcolepsy.

Cataplexy is present in NT1. Some individuals initially receiving a diagnosis of NT2 go on to develop cataplexy and are then reassigned to a diagnosis of NT1. If a person with cataplexy stops taking medications that suppress REM sleep, they can have a flurry of rebound cataplexy (status cataplecticus). Confirmation for the diagnosis of narcolepsy may be done in a sleep laboratory and by lumbar puncture. Overnight polysomnography may show a reduced REM sleep latency (≤15 minutes), or a daytime MSLT may be performed. The latter test should be performed after an overnight MSLT and while the person is not taking psychoactive medications. The person is then given the opportunity to take five naps over the course of the day, at 2-hour intervals, for up to 20 minutes each. Each nap is evaluated for the presence of sleep and a REM period. If the person goes into REM sleep within the 20-minute nap, that nap is considered a sleep-onset REM period. Two sleep-onset REM periods and a sleep latency of 8 minutes or shorter confirms the diagnosis of narcolepsy. Alternatively, a lumbar puncture may be performed to measure the level of hypocretin-1 present in the cerebrospinal fluid.

Getting the History

A 23-year-old man presents with a complaint of feeling "tired all the time." The interviewer clarifies whether the patient feels "sleepy" or "fatigued." The patient reports that he feels sleepy and has times when he feels an absolutely irrepressible need for sleep. The interviewer asks about automatic behaviors, such as writing notes without recollection and later realizing the notes made no sense, or losing time while driving. The interviewer then asks about symptoms of cataplexy: "Have you ever had times in which your muscles get weak or wobbly on you?" When the patient answers in the affirmative, the interviewer asks, "What seems to cause these symptoms?" If an emotional trigger occurs, it is important to note what type of emotion (i.e., positive or negative) and how long the symptoms last.

To elicit symptoms of sleep paralysis, the interviewer asks, "Do you ever wake up from sleep and feel that you are paralyzed? How often does that occur?" To elicit a history of hallucinations associated with falling asleep or awakening, the clinician asks, "Do you ever see things or hear things that others cannot see or hear? Do they occur at any particular time? Are they scary or disturbing to you?" Time course and perceived precipitants of symptoms are also elicited, as well as a thorough evaluation of sleep hours and medications. The patient is also screened for other sleep disorders that may cause excessive daytime sleepiness.

People often report feeling tired, but this symptom is very nonspecific. It is helpful to clarify whether a person feels overtly sleepy (e.g., eyes dry, eyelids heavy, yawning, on the verge of falling asleep) or fatigued (e.g., low energy, no "get-up-and-go"). Sleepiness is associated with sleep-disordered breathing, sleep deprivation, and narcolepsy; fatigue is associated more with insomnia or major depressive disorder. It also can be helpful to assess risk; individuals who are excessively sleepy may have "sleep attacks" even while driving, but those who have fatigue would be unlikely to fall asleep during an activity. Automatic behaviors may sometimes be seen as an individual inadvertently falls asleep but tries to continue the activities they were performing. With cataplexy, focused yet open-ended questions can be helpful. Individuals will often report that when they are very angry or anxious, they feel weak in the knees or unable to hold objects in their hands, but this symptom is not typical of cataplexy, which is generally elicited by positive emotions. Also, cataplectic attacks typically last a few seconds, so reports of persistent weakness over hours are also not typical of cataplexy. History regarding hallucinations is typically elicited; asking about the timing may indicate whether the hallucinations occur with falling asleep or waking up. However, it is important to remember that patients with narcolepsy have instability of sleep and wake periods, and therefore they may have hypnopompic or hypnagogic symptoms associated with daytime sleep episodes.

Tips for Clarifying the Diagnosis

- Determine whether the person is unable to maintain sleep and wakefulness.
- Assess whether they have brief periods of muscle weakness triggered by positive emotions. This weakness can be manifested by dropping head or drooping eyelids or more overtly by lower-extremity weakness that requires them to sit down.
- Ask how often these attacks occur and how long the sleep instability has been present.
- Confirm the diagnosis with the following tests: polysomnography with REM sleep latency of 15 minutes or less, MSLT with sleep latency of 8 minutes or less and two or more sleep-onset REM periods, or measurement of hypocretin-1 levels in cerebrospinal fluid.

Consider the Case

Mr. Pickell is a 35-year-old Black Marine referred to the sleep clinic by his psychiatrist for persistent excessive daytime sleepiness. Mr. Pickell has been working as a long-distance truck driver and was initially referred to a psychiatrist because he reported to his primary care physician that he was experiencing occasional perceptual distortions, such as seeing a person in the road or seeing the road as distorted. The psychiatrist also noted a restricted range of affect, disrupted nocturnal sleep, and daytime fatigue.

Mr. Pickell was prescribed a variety of antidepressants, with minimal improvement in daytime symptoms. Other medication at bedtime helped improve Mr. Pickell's sleep somewhat; but although he no longer reported visual hallucinations, he remained excessively sleepy. He was then referred for an evaluation of his sleep.

On evaluation, Mr. Pickell reports no history of snoring or witnessed apneas. Despite previously having short sleep hours while working, he has been on short-term disability for the past 3 months and has been sleeping at least 8 hours per night, and he reports frequently taking naps as well. He denies symptoms consistent with cataplexy, sleep paralysis, or parasomnias. He was tapered off his medications before obtaining polysomnography, which demonstrated an AHI of 7.8, with a REM sleep latency of 70 minutes. An MSLT the following day yielded positive results, with a mean sleep latency of 7 minutes and two sleep-onset REM periods occurring in the last two naps. Lumbar puncture was performed, and Mr. Pickell had a very low unmeasurable hypocretin level.

Mr. Pickell is an example of a patient with NT1. Safety is an important concern for this patient because of his work as a long-distance truck driver. Patients with narcolepsy are not only excessively sleepy but often may have automatic behaviors, in which they continue with an activity, even driving, while they are asleep. Once they are appropriately treated, most patients should be able to return to work, although Mr. Pickell may need to change to shorter local routes or some other form of employment. Some patients with narcolepsy are referred for psychiatric evaluation because of visual hallucinations; also, sometimes these patients are perceived to be depressed because of a restricted range of affect that may be acquired to help minimize cataplectic symptoms. When asked, however, this patient denied history of cataplexy, which is not uncommon. Some evidence indicates that individuals of African descent have less manifestation of cataplexy than do other populations; however, other explanations, such as duration of illness or presence of medications suppressing REM sleep, may also contribute to the presentation in this patient. Mr. Pickell's use of selective serotonin reuptake inhibitors and serotonin-norepinephrine reuptake inhibitors could also explain his lack of cataplectic symptoms. Because of the REM-suppressing effect of many psychiatric medications, it is important to coordinate care with other providers to ensure that an individual being assessed for narcolepsy with polysomnography and MSLTs is tapered off those medications if possible. Reduced REM sleep latency on polysomnography ($\leq$15 minutes) or on MSLT (in at least two naps) is required for the diagnosis, along with either cataplexy or hypocretin deficiency. Mr. Pickell had extremely low levels of hypocretin on lumbar puncture, confirming the diagnosis of NT1.

Differential Diagnosis

Narcolepsy must first be differentiated from hypersomnias. Individuals with these disorders may similarly complain of fatigue and sleepiness and may even have an MSLT with a short sleep latency and two or more sleep-onset REM periods. Individuals with hypersomnolence generally have longer, less disrupted nocturnal sleep, greater difficulty awakening, and persistent daytime sleepiness. Individuals with NT1 or NT2 may have "sleep attacks" during the day, and sleep-related hallucinations and sleep paralysis during sleep.

Sleep deprivation and insufficient nocturnal sleep are common reasons for excessive daytime sleepiness. Sometimes sleepiness may be caused by behavioral factors (e.g., parent busy with a full-time job, schoolwork, and children and "without enough hours in the day") or circadian misalignment (e.g., teenager with circadian phase delay who is unable to fall asleep until 2:00 A.M. and then must be up at 6:00 A.M. for school; shift worker who works nights and has difficulty sleeping during the day).

Breathing-related sleep disorders (i.e., sleep apnea syndromes) are far more common than narcolepsy and can cause sleep fragmentation leading to excessive daytime sleepiness. Individuals with major depressive disorder may experience hypersomnia and fatigue, but they are not typically sleepy and are not likely to have any of the other associated symptoms of cataplexy, sleep paralysis, or acting out of dreams. Individuals with functional neurological symptom disorder (conversion disorder) may present with prolonged, dramatic pseudocataplectic attacks, during which reflexes can be elicited. These patients also may insist that they slept on the MSLT, but such sleep is not evident on electroencephalography. In children, excessive sleepiness may be perceived as a behavioral issue or inattentiveness, although these children do not present with hyperactivity. Cataplexy, automatic behaviors, and sleep attacks could be interpreted as seizures, although when a person has a cataplectic attack, they are alert and conscious and less likely to become injured from the attack than is a person with seizure disorder; also, seizures are not triggered by emotional stimuli. Electroencephalography can help in ruling out seizure disorder. Chorea and pediatric autoimmune neuropsychiatric disorders associated with streptococcal infections (PANDAS) may be considered in children developing narcolepsy, particularly because narcolepsy may occur in the context of acute post–streptococcal infection. Schizophrenia may be considered in individuals with narcolepsy because of the presence of hallucinations and may be comorbid with narcolepsy, but persons with only narcolepsy will not demonstrate the thought disorder or negative symptoms characteristic of schizophrenia.

See DSM-5-TR for additional disorders to consider in the differential diagnosis. Also refer to the discussions of comorbidity and differential diagnosis in their respective sections of DSM-5-TR.

Summary

- Narcolepsy is characterized by inability to maintain sleep and wakefulness and can be difficult to diagnose because of the overlap of daytime sleepiness with other disorders.
- Cataplexy—a brief period of muscle weakness precipitated by a positive emotion—is a hallmark of NT1 but is not present in all individuals with narcolepsy.
- Overnight polysomnography demonstrating REM sleep latency of 15 minutes or less or a daytime MSLT with a mean sleep latency of 8 minutes or less and two or more sleep-onset REM periods can help make the diagnosis, but these results could be influenced by factors such as medications or sleep deprivation.

IN-DEPTH DIAGNOSIS: OBSTRUCTIVE SLEEP APNEA HYPOPNEA

Mr. Geri, a 52-year-old man with a history of obesity, hypertension, diabetes mellitus, gastroesophageal reflux disease, and erectile dysfunction, works in a building that contains a sleep laboratory. He decided to get evaluated for excessive daytime sleepiness.

He reports that he had always been a hard worker, dedicating long hours to his job, but over the past few years he had gained increased responsibility that he has been having difficulty maintaining because he frequently is falling asleep at his computer. He enjoys his work and does not feel bored but notes that he feels unable to maintain wakefulness when he is inactive during the day. Some days, he will even take a nap in his car before driving home because he is so tired that he fears he may fall asleep while driving. He has not had a bed partner in many years but has been told in the past that he snores and, on occasion, has "snorted" himself awake.

Physical examination demonstrates a blood pressure of 150/90 mm Hg, BMI of 37, neck circumference of 19 inches, and modified Mallampati score of 4. On overnight polysomnography, Mr. Geri had an AHI of 54 events per hour, with his longest apnea lasting 69 seconds and desaturating to 70%.

Mr. Geri represents a classic case of obstructive sleep apnea hypopnea. He is obese, which predisposes him to having this disorder, and he has multiple comorbidities that are associated with it. Hypertension can be seen in 60% of individuals with obstructive sleep apnea hypopnea, and there is evidence that the disorder can lead to impaired insulin resistance. Gastric reflux can be caused by the increased work of breathing while sleeping, and erectile dysfunction has been linked to obstructive sleep apnea hypopnea as well. Mr. Geri has excessive daytime sleepiness, as manifested by falling asleep when inactive, and individuals may also complain of cognitive dysfunction (e.g., poor concentration, attention, executive function). Individuals with obstructive sleep apnea hypopnea may report snoring, witnessed apneas, snorting themselves awake, and difficulty sleeping in certain positions (presumably because of positional airway collapse). If the person does not have a bed partner, obtaining history of nighttime symptoms may be difficult. Physical examination findings may be suggestive of obstructive sleep apnea hypopnea, as was the case for Mr. Geri. He demonstrates hypertension, obesity, a large neck circumference, and evidence of a crowded oral airway on the basis of his Mallampati score (which is used to assess for difficulty in intubation and risk for sleep apnea). Although the history and physical findings may suggest the diagnosis, ultimately it is confirmed by overnight polysomnography. Mr. Geri was found to have what is considered severe obstructive sleep apnea hypopnea (>30 events per hour), with significant oxygen desaturation. In an obese patient such as Mr. Geri, obesity hypoventilation syndrome should be considered, ideally with measurement of carbon dioxide levels.

Approach to the Diagnosis

Assessing a person for obstructive sleep apnea hypopnea requires a history and polysomnography. It is possible to make the diagnosis either by report of clinical symptoms with polysomnography demonstrating an AHI of at least 5 events per hour or by an AHI of 15 or more events per hour, regardless of symptoms. Symptoms to elicit in the history include both daytime symptoms and symptoms occurring during the sleep period. Individuals may report excessive sleepiness, fatigue, and cognitive symptoms such as diminished attention. A bed partner can be helpful in reporting symptoms occurring during sleep; for example, individuals may be unaware that they snore or have pauses in their breathing while they sleep unless another person tells them. Other symptoms that support the diagnosis but are not included in the diagnostic criteria are diaphoresis during sleep, sleep fragmentation, frequent nocturia, morning headaches, and dry mouth. Certain comorbid conditions, particularly hypertension, cardiovascular disease, gastroesophageal reflux, asthma, or allergies, also are suggestive of obstructive sleep apnea hypopnea. Family history of obstructive sleep apnea hypopnea may suggest its presence—there is likely a genetic basis to the syndrome as well as physical characteristics that predispose an individual to breathing-related sleep disorders. Physical examination characteristics are not included in the diagnostic criteria but may be suggestive, including obesity, hypertension, evidence of nasal obstruction (septal deviation, enlarged turbinates), tonsillar hypertrophy, Mallampati score of 3 or 4, and jaw structural abnormalities leading to a smaller oronasopharynx. Sex also is important to consider because males are at increased risk for obstructive sleep apnea hypopnea; however, when females go through menopause, the risk equalizes.

Polysomnography is required to make the diagnosis. It may be performed either in a hospital laboratory (usually considered an outpatient procedure) or at home by ambulatory monitoring. Polysomnography provides information on when the individual falls asleep, stages of sleep, and certain vital signs (e.g., heart rate and oxygen saturation), as well as whether there is any impairment in nasal or oral flow or in the work of breathing. Sleep and breathing events are scored according to criteria set by the American Academy of Sleep Medicine.

Getting the History

A 50-year-old patient presents with the chief complaint "I'm always tired!" First, the interviewer assesses if what the patient experiences is sleepiness (on the verge of falling asleep) or fatigue (low energy). The interviewer then asks about the duration and severity of the chief complaint. It can be helpful to have a bed partner provide collateral information, but if none is available, the interviewer asks the patient questions such as these: Has anyone ever told you that you snore? Has anyone ever told you that you seem to stop breathing in your sleep? Do you ever wake up gasping or choking or with a feeling of needing to catch your breath? Do you ever wake up with a dry mouth? Has anyone ever told you that you sleep with your mouth open? Do you have water at your bedside because you frequently need water in the middle of the night?

It can be helpful to review a typical night: What time do you go to bed? How long does it take you to fall asleep? Once asleep, do you usually wake up during the night? What is it that wakes you? How many times per night? How long does it take you to return to sleep? What time do you get up in the morning? When you wake up, do you feel refreshed or like you need to sleep longer? Do you wake with headaches? Do you ever take purposeful naps? Do you ever inadvertently doze off? Have you ever been so sleepy that you fell asleep while driving? Have you had any accidents or "close calls" because of being sleepy while driving? What do you do to prevent falling asleep while driving? For what medical illnesses do you regularly see a doctor? Do you have hypertension, coronary artery disease, gastroesophageal reflux, asthma, allergies, depression, or anxiety? Does anyone in your family have any problems with sleep?

Individuals with obstructive sleep apnea hypopnea may present as either sleepy or fatigued, but the tendency to use the vernacular "tired" is nonspecific and could indicate either symptom. Classically, people with this condition are thought to be sleepy more than fatigued, although certain populations (e.g., females) may more frequently report fatigue. As with any other complaint, the interviewer needs to assess duration, severity, and functional impact. It also is important to assess the person's level of sleepiness, particularly as it relates to driving, because driving while sleepy significantly increases the risk for motor vehicle crashes and is one area of particular concern for people with sleep disorders. As noted, a bed partner can be helpful in reporting symptoms observed during sleep, but even if a bed partner is not present, the person may have been told of symptoms in the past. Reviewing a typical night for the patient can be helpful both in ruling out other possible sleep disorders, such as insomnia or circadian rhythm sleep-wake disorders, and in providing additional information to support the diagnosis of obstructive sleep apnea hypopnea. For example, if a person awakens to use the bathroom five times per night and is able to return to sleep quickly, that pattern suggests obstructive sleep apnea hypopnea. Other supporting information would include medical conditions and family history.

Tips for Clarifying the Diagnosis

- Consider obstructive sleep apnea hypopnea in any person who is obese.
- Investigate sleep-disordered breathing as a potential cause of difficulties with sleep maintenance, as well as a cause of refractory sleepiness, fatigue, or concentration or cognitive problems.
- Assess for snoring or observed pauses in breathing while the person is sleeping, which are suggestive of obstructive sleep apnea hypopnea.
- Confirm the presence of obstructive sleep apnea hypopnea via polysomnography.

Consider the Case

Ricky is a 6-year-old boy who presents with his parents for evaluation for possible sleep apnea. They had researched online about ADHD and were wondering if sleep apnea could explain Ricky's current behavioral issues. He had been diagnosed with obstructive sleep apnea hypopnea when he was 3 years old, had his tonsils removed, and had subsequent significant improvement in his sleep, until about 6 months ago. His parents note that he has very restless sleep and moves around a great deal. He also gets very sweaty while sleeping. He does not snore but has loud, labored breathing and seems to breathe only through his mouth while sleeping. He was held back in kindergarten because of disruptive and inattentive behaviors in class, even though he had been successful in meeting other requirements for grade promotion.

On examination, Ricky's vital signs are in the normal range. He is excessively active, swinging between chairs in the exam room and climbing on the exam table and attempting to jump off. He requires significant intervention by his mother for redirection. He is observed to breathe through his mouth. His nasal examination reveals a midline septum with enlarged turbinates, and he has a high, arched palate, with a Mallampati score of 3. Overnight polysomnography demonstrates an AHI of 7.5, with desaturation to 92%.

Although obstructive sleep apnea hypopnea is less commonly recognized in children, it does occur in this population. Unlike adults, children usually present their sleepiness as hyperactivity rather than somnolence. Obtaining a clinical report of nighttime symptoms frequently is difficult, particularly for young children who have their own rooms; however, some parents do hear their children snore or have heavy, labored breathing. These children often move quite a bit in their sleep, sleep in unusual positions, and may become very sweaty while sleeping. They also are frequently behind their peers for height and may experience enuresis after having been dry. Identification of obstructive sleep apnea hypopnea and appropriate treatment can correct enuresis, lead to gains in height, and in some cases improve daytime behavioral issues. Ricky primarily breathes through his mouth, which indicates he may have nasal obstruction, either from his enlarged turbinates (likely secondary to allergies) or adenoid tissue hypertrophy. In some rare instances, a child may have regrowth of resected tonsillar tissue. The noted high, arched palate also suggests the presence of sleep-disordered breathing because it indicates a narrower space in which to contain soft tissue structures. In children, as in adults, polysomnography must be used to confirm the diagnosis. The relative severity in children differs from that in adults, with a lower threshold for diagnosis in the number of breathing events required to qualify for obstructive sleep apnea hypopnea (at least one event per hour).

Differential Diagnosis

Obstructive sleep apnea hypopnea should be differentiated from primary snoring and other sleep disorders. Ultimately, polysomnography will be most helpful in differentiating it from other disorders, but there are aspects of the history that may help in the consideration of other disorders. For example, a patient with a history of congestive heart failure may have obstructive sleep apnea hypopnea, but they may also have central sleep apnea (Cheyne-Stokes breathing). Similarly, a person who takes large doses of long-acting opioids would also be at risk for having central sleep apnea. Sleep-related hypoventilation should be considered in a person who is morbidly obese, takes sedative-hypnotics, or has neuromuscular or pulmonary conditions. Other sleep disorders that could cause excessive sleepiness should also be considered, such as narcolepsy, circadian rhythm sleep-wake disorders, or hypersomnolence disorder—although obstructive sleep apnea hypopnea may certainly be comorbid with these disorders.

Insomnia disorder is often seen with obstructive sleep apnea hypopnea; people with insomnia disorder typically complain more of fatigue and are not sleepy on objective measures of sleepiness. They also tend to demonstrate significant anxiety regarding sleep. Individuals with nocturnal panic attacks frequently report subjective symptoms that overlap quite a bit with obstructive sleep apnea hypopnea (e.g., gasping, choking, heart racing on awakening); however, these attacks usually are also seen in daytime panic attacks, occur less frequently, and would be less likely to be associated with excessive sleepiness. As in the case of Ricky described earlier, children may present with symptoms similar to ADHD (e.g., hyperactivity, inattentiveness, academic delays) that may improve with treatment of obstructive sleep apnea hypopnea. Substance/medication-induced symptoms may mimic obstructive sleep apnea hypopnea. For example, ingestion of alcohol before bed may cause greater muscle relaxation and airway collapse. Again, ultimately, polysomnography would be most helpful in differentiating these disorders.

See DSM-5-TR for additional disorders to consider in the differential diagnosis. Also refer to the discussions of comorbidity and differential diagnosis in their respective sections of DSM-5-TR.

Summary

- Obstructive sleep apnea hypopnea is characterized by snoring, witnessed apneas (pauses in breathing), snorting or gasping while sleeping, excessive daytime sleepiness, fatigue, or unrefreshing sleep.
- Polysomnography is required for the diagnosis.
- Individuals may be diagnosed with obstructive sleep apnea hypopnea if they have polysomnography demonstrating an AHI of at least 5 events per hour, with symptoms of snoring, pauses in breathing, excessive sleepiness, fatigue, or unrefreshing sleep; or an AHI of at least 15, regardless of symptoms.
- In persons with excessive sleepiness, it is important to screen for sleepiness while driving.

IN-DEPTH DIAGNOSIS: RESTLESS LEGS SYNDROME

Ms. Sanchez is a 67-year-old postmenopausal woman with a history of coronary artery disease, hypertension, severe obstructive sleep apnea hypopnea, and anxiety. She presents with a complaint of worsening insomnia. She notes that she was recently hospitalized for workup of a gastrointestinal bleed and that ever since her release from the hospital she has had difficulty falling asleep. She finds that each evening, while watching the television shows she normally enjoys, she has begun to feel restless and unsettled and "can't sit still." She has difficulty making it through an entire program without having to get up and walk around; she will usually feel fine for about 20 minutes after getting up, but then she begins to feel restless again. This feeling continues, even once she gets into bed, until she is so exhausted that she eventually falls asleep. She is unable to ignore the sensation, describing it as nonpainful but "uncomfortable, like my legs have to sneeze." She is worried because she had similar symptoms during her two pregnancies but to a much less severe degree. Aside from movement, she is unable to identify anything that improves or worsens the feelings. She is not aware of any family members with similar symptoms. Current medications include aspirin, an antidepressant, and a diuretic, and she has not had any lab levels checked since she was discharged from the hospital. Results of a neurological examination are normal, and sleep apnea remains well controlled with continuous positive airway pressure (CPAP).

RLS may be difficult to diagnose, and Ms. Sanchez's presentation highlights the importance of taking a thorough sleep history. Although she complains of "insomnia," greater detail demonstrates that she actually is experiencing RLS. This disorder occurs more frequently in females than in males, and that frequency is often attributed to increased prevalence in pregnancy. There is also an association with iron deficiency. This observation may explain the relationship with pregnancy, but in older adults presenting with new symptoms of RLS, a source of "occult" or unknown bleeding should be considered, as in Ms. Sanchez, who had a known gastrointestinal bleed. Individuals describe the symptoms in various ways, usually as a discomfort that is exacerbated by inactivity and relieved by movement. The symptoms do not have to occur daily; when they do occur, they tend to have a circadian rhythmicity. Family history may be positive (RLS has a known genetic component), but this history often is not recognized unless it is specifically solicited. Certain medications, such as selective serotonin reuptake inhibitors, may exacerbate the symptoms of RLS, but they would likely be less of a contributing factor in this case if Ms. Sanchez had been taking fluoxetine for some time preceding the gastrointestinal bleed.

Approach to the Diagnosis

The DSM-5-TR diagnosis of RLS is obtained solely from history, unlike some of the other sleep-wake disorders that entail laboratory testing to make a definitive diagnosis. Obtaining a history of RLS requires inquiry into a specific sensation of discomfort, usually in the legs, that the individual perceives as irrepressible. The discomfort should occur during periods of rest or inactivity, and movement must alleviate (at least partially) the sensation. The symptoms usually occur at a particular time of day and should occur at least three times per week. It is important to separate out whether the discomfort is caused by another medical condition. For example, an individual may feel excess soreness from an increase in physical activity, which tends to improve with additional increased physical activity, or a person who has peripheral neuropathy may experience lower-extremity discomfort that impairs sleep initiation, but the discomfort is constant. Also, the symptoms must cause some sort of distress or impairment in functioning. The symptoms of RLS can interrupt the ability to fall asleep or can even be significant enough to waken the person from sleep. Because of the sleep disruption, the individual may report sleepiness, fatigue, and impairment in cognition, mood, or behavior.

Information supporting the diagnosis, but not included in the DSM-5-TR criteria for RLS, is somewhat more concrete than the historical details required by DSM-5-TR. Family history indicates a likelihood of the diagnosis of RLS, and certain genetic markers (e.g., *MEIS1, BTBD9, MAP2K5/LBXCOR1*) have been associated with the diagnosis, although genetic typing is not currently clinically used for diagnosis. Iron deficiency, specifically a low ferritin level, in the context of a genetically vulnerable individual, may precipitate symptoms. For example, some people develop symptoms after severe anemia secondary to gynecological hemorrhage or, similarly, in pregnancy, which depletes iron stores. In other people, the symptoms of RLS may be a warning signal of otherwise unrecognized iron depletion. Although most labs consider a ferritin level of more than 20 µg/L to be within normal limits, a ferritin level in the range of 50–75 µg/L or more is preferable in a vulnerable individual. Also helpful in supporting the diagnosis is the presence of periodic leg movements on overnight polysomnography. Most people with RLS (70%) will also have periodic leg movements on polysomnography.

Getting the History

A 42-year-old woman presents with a history of "insomnia, tossing and turning each night." The interviewer inquires as to the specificity of symptoms: "Are you having difficulties with sleep initiation, maintenance, or both? How long has this been a problem? Have you ever had something like this before? What symptoms of daytime dysfunction are present?"

In attempting to solicit symptoms specific to RLS, the interviewer may find it helpful to preface the line of questioning with a qualifying statement such as, "Sleep disruption can come from a variety of different causes, so I'm going to ask some questions that may seem unrelated." Some people may have become preoccupied with the sleep disruption, so they minimize the symptoms of RLS. Asking the following questions in the context of unusual situations can be helpful: "Are you able to sit through an entire movie or long plane flight?" If the patient says no, the interviewer asks for further elaboration as to what causes her to get up, such as the need to use the restroom versus a need to move. More focused questioning may be required: "Some people describe a discomfort, a 'creepy crawly' feeling, or an itching or burning, deep within their legs. Do you ever get anything like that?" The patient answers in the affirmative, so the interviewer solicits occurrences in other situations, such as at home, and their frequency. The interviewer also elicits information about the circadian pattern: "Do the symptoms seem to happen at any particular time of day, or is there no pattern? Are they always there?" The interviewer assesses improvement in an open-ended manner: "Does anything seem to make the symptoms feel better or go away?" If the patient is unsure or gives a vague answer, a more direct question is important, such as, "Does it get better if you move?" With females, such as this patient, the interviewer may inquire whether they had similar symptoms when pregnant and, for any patient, whether anyone in the family has experienced anything similar. It may be helpful to inquire about health status, use of medications or other substances, and diet, as well as whether the patient has ever been diagnosed with anemia or has any evident blood loss.

People often have difficulty describing symptoms of RLS. They often identify a difficulty with sleep and require careful probing to identify symptoms of RLS as the cause. As with any other disorder, a description of the course of symptoms and impaired functioning should be elicited. Some individuals have become so distraught by their sleep disruption that they may present as people with insomnia disorder would—that is, with much anxiety and sleep-related worries. In this context, asking about the occurrence of symptoms during periods of rest or inactivity (i.e., not necessarily tied to sleep) can be helpful. Some people certainly will only note their symptoms in a circadian pattern. The discomfort is often difficult to describe, so giving descriptors such as "creepy crawly," "itching," or "like jumping beans" can sometimes resonate with them. Improvement with movement is also imperative, but sometimes people also describe elaborate rituals that they perform to ease the discomfort, such as a hot bath, massage, or even self-injurious behavior. Family history, health status, and use of medications or other substances also support the diagnosis.

In pediatric cases, inquiry as to "growing pains" at night may sometimes help identify the presence of RLS.

Tips for Clarifying the Diagnosis

- Question whether the person experiences discomfort or an unpleasant sensation in the legs, occurring typically around the same time of day.
- Clarify whether movement leads to *improvement* in the symptoms (i.e., there need not be *resolution* of the symptoms).
- Investigate whether the symptoms are exacerbated at night.
- Obtain supporting information (e.g., ferritin level <50 µg/L, presence of periodic leg movements, positive family history) that may help to clarify the diagnosis.

Consider the Case

Harvey is a 13-year-old nonverbal boy with a history of autism spectrum disorder whose parents brought him to the sleep clinic for evaluation of sleep disturbance. They note that he seems to fall asleep later than their older son did at the same age and are concerned that his sleep is causing him some anxiety. At night, they notice that he starts pacing around 9:00 P.M., and if they ask him to stay in bed, he performs automatisms of rubbing his legs, which he did not do previously. Once he does fall asleep, he occasionally wakes up and performs the same behaviors. They are concerned that he does not get enough sleep for school, and his teachers have noted some days at school in which he has greater behavioral disturbances, including tantrums and aggression.

Harvey has no other medical problems but recently started taking an atypical antipsychotic because of his behavioral issues at school and sleep problems. Family sleep history is positive for both insomnia disorder and RLS in his mother and obstructive sleep apnea hypopnea in his father.

On examination, Harvey is nonverbal and makes no eye contact. He responds to directions from his parents but resists physical examination. He is able to cooperate for polysomnography, which demonstrated sleep efficiency of 50%, an AHI of 0.7, and a periodic leg movement index of 25. His serum ferritin level was 18 µg/L.

Harvey presents an exceptionally difficult-to-identify case of RLS. Notably, the diagnosis of RLS requires a description of the symptoms in the person's own words; however, in some young children or individuals who are nonverbal, that narrative may be difficult to obtain, and other supporting information may point toward the diagnosis. In support of the RLS diagnosis are the circadian pattern of the symptoms, the family history of RLS in the mother, findings of periodic leg movements on the sleep study, and low serum ferritin. Children with autism spectrum disorder often are picky eaters, which may explain Harvey's low ferritin level. Also of note in this case is the exacerbation of daytime behaviors because of sleep disruption from the symptoms of RLS.

Differential Diagnosis

Differentiating RLS from other pain conditions, primarily in the extremities, is the first important separation. Positional discomfort would occur intermittently, without an obvious circadian pattern, and would likely completely resolve with repositioning. Leg cramps may also occur intermittently, and often patients can palpate a solid contraction of the muscle body while it is occurring. Movement can improve the cramp. Peripheral neuropathy would be suspected in a person with a history suggestive of peripheral neuropathy (e.g., a person who has diabetes mellitus or has used neurotoxic agents) and would be of a more chronic, constant nature. Neuroleptic-induced akathisia would not be expected to have circadian rhythmicity and would likely have a chronological relationship to medication initiation or increase. Other pain syndromes might be noted to worsen with inactivity but are not isolated to a certain time of day, and claudication would be precipitated by activity in an individual with peripheral vascular disease. Anxiety or insomnia may be tied to the perception of interference with sleep and can cause a feeling of restlessness that would not resolve with movement.

In pediatric cases, positional discomfort or injury should be considered in the process of arriving at the differential diagnosis. As with adults, these feelings would not likely occur with a circadian rhythmicity or awaken the child from sleep with regularity but would occur intermittently.

See DSM-5-TR for additional disorders to consider in the differential diagnosis. Also refer to the discussions of comorbidity and differential diagnosis in their respective sections of DSM-5-TR.

Summary

- RLS *requires* discomfort or urge to move the legs that worsens with inactivity, occurs with a circadian rhythmicity, and improves with movement.
- The symptoms cause some sort of impairment to sleep or daytime functioning.
- Certain details, such as family history, comorbid medical conditions, medications, ferritin level, and presence of periodic limb movements on polysomnography, help to support the diagnosis but are not included in the DSM-5-TR criteria.
- The symptoms should occur three times per week for at least 3 months.

SUMMARY: SLEEP-WAKE DISORDERS

Sleep-wake disorders can lead to, accompany, or exacerbate many psychiatric disorders. The diagnosis of sleep-wake disorders is important for the evaluation and treatment of such mental disorders as depression, PTSD, and anxiety. DSM-5-TR gives evidence of the importance of sleep-wake disorders to psychiatric phenotypes by elevating REM sleep behavior disorder and RLS to their own diagnostic categories. The state of the science is such that certain sleep disorders, such as obstructive sleep apnea hypopnea and narcolepsy, now have specialized testing. Increased clinical research has resulted in further refinement in DSM-5-TR of the subtypes of circadian rhythm sleep-wake disorders and breathing-related sleep disorders. In general, the approach to the patient with a sleep-wake complaint should include a thorough history of behaviors occurring in both sleep (e.g., snoring, sleepwalking) and wake (e.g., excessive sleepiness, substance use) states. Collateral information from a bed partner can also be helpful because many individuals are unaware of symptoms occurring while they sleep. Ultimately, certain sleep-wake disorders, such as obstructive sleep apnea hypopnea, require specialized tests or examinations, and these patients are best referred to a sleep medicine specialist. It is important for the mental health clinician to understand how sleep may be disordered, how sleep-wake disorders affect psychiatric and other medical conditions, and when it is important to refer someone to a sleep medicine specialist.

ELEMENTS TO CONSIDER IN THE CULTURAL FORMULATION

- Sleep disorders are universal.
- Individuals have unique sleep schedules and needs. "Early morning awakening," for example, may look different for different people.

DIAGNOSTIC PEARLS

- Many people complain of sleep-related problems, but they do not all have insomnia disorder. A variety of sleep-wake disorders should be considered.
- It is important to take a thorough sleep history and consider a full sleep evaluation by a specialist in sleep medicine to assess sleep complaints.
- Some individuals with primary sleep disorders present to mental health providers because of psychiatric-type symptoms. Daytime sleepiness, fatigue, poor concentration, irritability, anxiety, and hallucinations are just some of the symptoms that people with sleep disorders may report.
- Some sleep-related symptoms, including insomnia and nightmares, are risk factors for suicidal thoughts or behavior. Most individuals with suicidal thoughts or behavior have sleep problems, but only a subset of individuals with sleep problems have suicidal thoughts or behavior.
- In general, any person who is obese should be screened for breathing-related sleep disorders. Individuals with symptoms of snoring, gasping for breath, or stopping breathing while sleeping, as well as sleepiness or fatigue, should be referred for a full sleep evaluation.
- Individuals presenting with excessive daytime sleepiness of any etiology should be evaluated for safety while driving, and safeguards should be put in place if they are at risk of falling asleep while driving.

SELF-ASSESSMENT

Key Concepts: Double-Check Your Knowledge

What is the relevance of the following concepts to the various sleep-wake disorders?

- Sleepiness versus fatigue
- Impairment in daytime functioning
- Sleep-related anxiety

- Cataplexy
- Hypocretin deficiency
- Multiple sleep latency test
- Mean sleep latency
- Rapid eye movement (REM) sleep latency
- Sleep-onset REM periods
- Apnea
- Hypopnea
- Polysomnography
- Urge to move
- Circadian rhythm

Questions to Discuss With Colleagues and Mentors

1. Do you screen all patients for sleep-disordered breathing?
2. What questions do you use to help differentiate breathing-related sleep disorders from insomnia disorder or other sleep-wake disorders?
3. How do you assess for insomnia disorder versus circadian rhythm sleep-wake disorders?
4. How do you decide when to refer a patient to a specialist in sleep medicine?

Case-Based Questions

PART A

Mr. Xue, a 45-year-old man using stable-dose, daily methadone maintenance for opioid dependence, is referred to the sleep clinic for evaluation of sleep fragmentation and daytime sleepiness. He is referred for polysomnography because of concerns of central sleep apnea and sleep-related hypoventilation.

What is the differential diagnosis? Although obstructive sleep apnea hypopnea is the most common form of breathing-related sleep disorders, particularly in middle-aged males who may have other predisposing factors, it is important to evaluate for the presence of other types of breathing-related sleep disorders.

PART B

Polysomnography reveals that Mr. Xue has obstructive sleep apnea hypopnea and sleep-related hypoventilation, which are successfully managed with continuous positive airway pressure (CPAP). After being stable on CPAP for about 1 year, Mr. Xue decides to taper off methadone with the help of his physician. A few weeks after completion of his taper, he notes increasing difficulty falling asleep, which had not been a problem for him previously. He is concerned about the potential impact on his productivity at work.

What are the potential causes of his new difficulty falling asleep? Mr. Xue appears to have developed substance/medication-induced sleep disorder, insomnia type, in the context of opioid withdrawal. Perhaps he no longer has the sedating effect of the opioid medication or, because his breathing improved after the opioid was removed, the CPAP is interfering with his sleep. More history would be helpful in making the diagnosis.

PART C

> On further questioning, Mr. Xue reports that around the same time each night, he starts to get an uncomfortable feeling in his legs and cannot sit still, even when watching television. He will pace for a short period of time, which improves the symptoms, but they often return after about 20 minutes. This feeling keeps him from falling asleep.

Do these additional details change the differential diagnosis?   Mr. Xue now also appears to have restless legs syndrome (RLS), which has been unmasked. RLS can be treated with a variety of different classes of medications, one of which is opioids.

This case demonstrates the comorbidity that exists not only among sleep-wake disorders but also with other psychiatric conditions. It highlights the importance of digging into the history; treating Mr. Xue merely for insomnia disorder rather than RLS would not adequately address the symptoms and may impair his ability to remain off opiate medication.

Short-Answer Questions

1. Is it correct that an individual must have difficulty initiating sleep to be diagnosed with insomnia?
2. A teenager presents with difficulty falling asleep on school nights. Once asleep, he is able to remain asleep, but he is difficult to awaken, very tired during the day, and often falls asleep in class. What is the likely diagnosis?
3. What laboratory test can confirm the diagnosis of narcolepsy?
4. For a diagnosis of narcolepsy using polysomnography, what duration must the rapid eye movement (REM) sleep latency be?
5. Is it correct that snoring can indicate the presence of obstructive sleep apnea hypopnea?
6. What medical comorbidities have been linked with obstructive sleep apnea hypopnea?
7. What sleep-wake disorder may be seen in an individual with congestive heart failure?
8. A 72-year-old woman presents for a second opinion on a diagnosis of major depressive disorder. She started taking an antidepressant for early morning awakenings, but it has not helped to change her sleep or her mood, although she denies significant mood symptoms. What sleep-wake disorder likely explains her symptoms?
9. A 32-year-old Marine reports frequent, vivid nightmares impairing both his sleep and that of his bed partner. He awakens quickly from the dream but has difficulty returning to sleep. What sleep-wake disorder diagnosis should be considered?

10. A 62-year-old Vietnam War–era veteran presents with a complaint of "beating up my wife while sleeping." He reports that when this happens, he is often having combat-related dreams, and he feels badly that he has hurt his wife. What is the likely diagnosis?

Answers

1. No. Individuals with insomnia may have difficulty initiating sleep, difficulty maintaining sleep, early morning awakening, nonrestorative sleep, or some combination of those symptoms.

2. The likely diagnosis is circadian rhythm sleep-wake disorder, delayed sleep phase type.

3. Testing for hypocretin deficiency can confirm the diagnosis of narcolepsy.

4. For a diagnosis of narcolepsy using polysomnography, the REM sleep latency must be less than or equal to 15 minutes.

5. Snoring may indicate the presence of obstructive sleep apnea hypopnea, but only in combination with daytime symptoms (e.g., sleepiness, fatigue, unrefreshing sleep) and at least five obstructive apneas and/or hypopneas per hour of sleep.

6. Medical comorbidities that have been linked to obstructive sleep apnea hypopnea include hypertension, cardiovascular disease, cerebrovascular disease, diabetes mellitus, obesity, gastroesophageal reflux, and erectile dysfunction.

7. Central sleep apnea may be seen in an individual with congestive heart failure. Although a person with congestive heart failure may experience obstructive sleep apnea hypopnea, insomnia disorder, or any other sleep-wake disorder, it is also important to consider the possible presence of central sleep apnea.

8. The patient likely has circadian rhythm sleep disorder, advanced sleep phase type. Individuals with this disorder go to bed and wake up earlier than they desire. Sometimes, if individuals try to stay up to watch television or attend social activities, they may go to bed later but still wake up earlier, and so may become somewhat sleep deprived, with resultant daytime sleepiness and impaired functioning.

9. Nightmare disorder should be considered; however, PTSD is an obvious consideration in a veteran who is having nightmares.

10. This patient may be describing REM sleep behavior disorder, which typically consists of vocalizations or dream enactment behavior that may possibly hurt the individual or the bed partner. Symptoms occur during

REM sleep, when there typically is paralysis of voluntary muscles. REM sleep behavior disorder is associated with certain neurodegenerative conditions, such as Parkinson's disease, multiple system atrophy, or dementia with Lewy bodies, and neurological assessment may be indicated as well.

REFERENCES

American Psychiatric Association: Diagnostic and Statistical Manual of Mental Disorders, 4th Edition. Washington, DC, American Psychiatric Association, 1994

American Psychiatric Association: Diagnostic and Statistical Manual of Mental Disorders, 5th Edition. Arlington, VA, American Psychiatric Association, 2013

American Psychiatric Association: Diagnostic and Statistical Manual of Mental Disorders, 5th Edition, Text Revision. Washington, DC, American Psychiatric Association, 2022

CHAPTER 17

Sexual Dysfunctions

Richard Balon, M.D.

"He has never been interested in sex."

"I can't have sex—it hurts."

- Delayed Ejaculation
- Erectile Disorder
- Female Orgasmic Disorder
- Female Sexual Interest/Arousal Disorder
- Genito-Pelvic Pain/Penetration Disorder
- Male Hypoactive Sexual Desire Disorder
- Premature (Early) Ejaculation
- Substance/Medication-Induced Sexual Dysfunction
- Other Specified Sexual Dysfunction
- Unspecified Sexual Dysfunction

Sex is one of the three basic drives, in addition to eating and sleeping. Many mental and physical disorders and diseases affect the entire human body and all three basic drives. The impairment of sexual drive could thus occur within the context of another major mental disorder or physical illness (e.g., cardiovascular disease) or without any connection to another disorder or disease. The sexual dysfunctions discussed in this diagnostic class are those without any connection to other disorders. Sexual dysfunctions are characterized by a clinically significant inability to respond sexually and/or experience sexual pleasure (which could also be caused by pain in the case of genito-pelvic pain/penetration disorder). Sexual dysfunctions frequently coexist with each other, and one may be a consequence of another. In cases of more than one sexual dysfunction in a particular person, all diagnoses should be made.

The DSM-5-TR group of sexual dysfunctions includes the following (American Psychiatric Association 2022):

- Delayed ejaculation (delay in ejaculation or inability to ejaculate); erectile disorder (inability to attain and maintain erection)
- Female orgasmic disorder (delayed orgasm or anorgasmia)
- Female sexual interest/arousal disorder (lack of sexual interest/arousal)
- Genito-pelvic pain/penetration disorder (persistent difficulty or inability to have vaginal intercourse or penetration, marked vulvovaginal or pelvic pain during vaginal intercourse or penetration)
- Male hypoactive sexual desire disorder (lack of sexual fantasies and desire for sexual activity)
- Premature (early) ejaculation (ejaculation before the person desires, within approximately 1 minute after penetration)
- Substance/medication-induced sexual dysfunction (sexual dysfunction developing after introducing a substance, increasing the dosage, or discontinuing a substance of abuse or medication; the substance and the dysfunction should be specified)
- Other specified sexual dysfunction or unspecified sexual dysfunction (presentations in which symptoms characteristic of sexual dysfunction that cause clinically significant distress in the individual predominate but do not meet full criteria for any of the disorders in this diagnostic class)

For other specified sexual dysfunction, the clinician can note the specific reason the presentation does not meet the criteria for any specific sexual dysfunction—for example, "sexual aversion." For unspecified sexual dysfunction, the clinician chooses not to specify the reason that criteria are not met for a specific sexual dysfunction; this includes presentations for which there is insufficient information to make a more specific diagnosis.

DSM-5 (American Psychiatric Association 2013) introduced several significant, general changes from DSM-IV (American Psychiatric Association 1994) for making the diagnosis of sexual dysfunctions more specific, refined, and distinguished from transient sexual difficulties. These changes are maintained in DSM-5-TR. One change is the requirement of a specific duration of impairment of at least 6 months and, for most disorders, specification of frequency (i.e., symptoms experienced on approximately 75%–100% of occasions). Another change is the introduction of severity specifiers to rate distress as mild, moderate, or severe. DSM-5 and DSM-5-TR retain specifiers helpful in delineating the possible source or etiology of the sexual dysfunction, such as whether it is lifelong (i.e., present since the individual became sexually active) or acquired, and whether it is generalized (i.e., not limited to certain types of stimulation, situations, or partners) or situational (i.e., only occurring with certain

TABLE 17–1. Key changes between DSM-5 and DSM-5-TR

Diagnostic features updated for most sexual dysfunctions with the exception of male hypoactive sexual desire disorder.

Culture-related diagnostic issues have been updated to better reflect social determinants of health and sociocultural contexts and to reflect differences among cultures in prevalence of some sexual dysfunctions (e.g., in sexual desire).

Association with suicidal thoughts or behaviors has been added to some sexual dysfunctions, such as erectile disorder, female orgasmic disorder, female sexual interest/arousal disorder, and premature (early) ejaculation.

Prevalence has been updated for all sexual dysfunctions with the exception of female orgasmic disorder.

types of stimulation, situations, or partners). Some of the key changes between the DSM-5 and DSM-5-TR diagnostic criteria are summarized in Table 17–1.

Various factors may be helpful in determining the etiology and circumstances of sexual dysfunctions, such as partner factors (e.g., a partner's health status or sexual problem); relationship factors (e.g., poor communication, discrepancy in sexual desire); individual vulnerability factors (e.g., poor body image, psychiatric comorbidity such as depression, stressors such as job loss); cultural or religious factors; and medical factors (e.g., cardiovascular disease, surgery). It is also important to incorporate age-related changes into the diagnosis of sexual dysfunction because aging may be associated with a normative decrease of sexual desire and response. Sexual difficulties may also be related to a lack of sexual stimulation (when no diagnosis of sexual dysfunction should be made). Clinical judgment should be used in considering both age-related changes and possible lack of sexual stimulation.

DSM-5 also introduced two new diagnoses: female sexual interest/arousal disorder and genito-pelvic pain/penetration disorder. The first disorder was introduced because the distinction between phases of sexual response in females may be a bit artificial and not necessarily linear. The second disorder appears because the diagnoses of dyspareunia and vaginismus in prior versions of DSM were overlapping and thus difficult to distinguish in clinical practice. These two diagnoses are also included in DSM-5-TR. The diagnoses of sexual dysfunctions are all gender specific in DSM-5-TR.

Finally, DSM-5 removed sexual aversion disorder (a rare condition) as a separate diagnosis. It could be classified as other specified sexual dysfunction.

Discussing sexual functioning could be difficult for many, if not all, people in any situation or context, including the clinical setting. The interviewing clinician should be sensitive to the fact that people may hesitate to acknowledge that they are having sexual difficulties. For some, confidentiality is a concern; for others, barriers to disclosure relate to self-esteem, fears, culture, and religion. The careful interviewer will not be satisfied with vague answers to general or specific questions. Confidentiality of the interview should always be emphasized. Questions should progress from general to specific and should consider the sensitivity and intimacy of discussing sexuality. Sexual dysfunctions have a broader impact than clinicians usually realize—they affect the individual and their partner. Thus, the clinician may consider interviewing (and educating) the patient's partner in addition if the patient agrees. The interviewing clinician should also remember that sexual functioning is intertwined and affected by various mental and physical disorders and illnesses and therefore should ask about these conditions in connection with sexual functioning.

IN-DEPTH DIAGNOSIS: FEMALE ORGASMIC DISORDER

> Ms. Mitchell, a 27-year-old physically healthy married woman, complains of inability to reach orgasm. She states that she has never experienced orgasm. She became sexually active around age 20 and had three sexual partners before she got married. She describes those sexual partners as "typical student sexual partners; we dated and had sex occasionally. I was not really invested in the relationships and having orgasms with these guys was not that important to me." She was interested in having sex and had het-erosexual fantasies. She hoped that orgasms "would come in a real relationship." She got married 2 years ago to "a great guy. I have been and still am really sexually attracted to him." They have been having sex several times a week. She states, "I love having sex with my husband. He is caring, a great lover, and he has been trying very hard to satisfy me." She hoped that she would start to have orgasms, but "it did not happen." They have tried various things, such as oral stimulation, masturbation during intercourse, and using a vibrator. "Nothing helps." Her husband started to question his abilities and then whether anything was wrong with her. The absence of orgasm has become a "sore point in our relationship." She has been afraid that "he may start to look somewhere else." She has tried to masturbate and use a vibrator on her own, "but I cannot come, no matter what." She denies substance abuse and does not take any medication.

Ms. Mitchell meets criteria for female orgasmic disorder. She has never experienced orgasm (i.e., meeting the duration criterion that the difficulty has been present for more than 6 months, and the specifier of not having an orgasm under any situation). She has tried various ways of stimulation without any success. She has had sexual fantasies and becomes aroused when with her husband and with her previous sexual partners. She does not describe any other sexual problem; she does not mention any pain during sexual intercourse. She is healthy, does not take any medication, and does not use any substances. She is happily married, and her husband is caring, trying to satisfy her; their relationship has been good. She has been sexually satisfied and has had sex several times a week yet has not been able to reach orgasm. She started to be distressed by her inability to reach orgasm and by the fact that it has become an issue, a "sore point," in her relationship with her husband.

Ms. Mitchell has never been able to reach orgasm; thus, her dysfunction started early in her life. Her orgasmic disorder should be subclassified as lifelong and generalized because she has never experienced an orgasm under any situation (also a DSM-5-TR specifier), and probably of moderate severity.

Approach to the Diagnosis

For diagnosis of this disorder, a woman must be distressed over her inability to reach orgasm, or significant interpersonal difficulties should result from this sexual difficulty (e.g., her partner may be upset, she may feel inadequate, her partner may cease having sex with her and look for satisfaction elsewhere). Not all women are distressed by an inability to reach orgasm. On the other hand, some women may not report their inability to reach orgasm, even though they are distressed about it, possibly because of being otherwise satisfied or not wanting to upset their sexual partner. They may have difficulties discussing sexual issues. It is thus very important to inquire directly about a patient's ability to reach orgasm, without relying on spontaneous reporting. In a woman who can reach orgasm, orgasmic sensation should be consistent, occurring on most (at least 75%) occasions of sexual activity; therefore, individuals with female orgasmic disorder may experience orgasm up to about 25% of the time. An important factor to consider in making the diagnosis of orgasmic disorder is adequate stimulation. Not all women experience orgasm during penile-vaginal intercourse all the time. Many women may require more stimulation, such as by masturbation or a vibrator (women's rates of orgasmic consistency are higher during masturbation than during partnered sexual activity). The woman's and her partner's orgasms also do not usually occur at the same time, and the woman may require more stimulation after her partner reaches orgasm to reach her own orgasm. Female orgasmic disorder may develop at any age, from the prepubertal period to late adulthood.

The inability to experience orgasm (or having a significantly delayed orgasm) should be evaluated in a wide context of numerous issues. The clinician needs to consider whether the absence of orgasm could be explained within the frame of another mental disorder (e.g., depression); if so, a diagnosis of female orgasmic disorder would not be made. However, the presence of another sexual dysfunction (e.g., female sexual interest/arousal disorder) does not exclude the diagnosis of female orgasmic disorder.

DSM-5-TR provides specifiers that should help to refine the diagnosis of female orgasmic disorder and make treatment planning more precise. The diagnosis should specify whether the individual has never experienced an orgasm under any situation, whether the orgasmic disorder is lifelong or acquired (i.e., it started after a period of having orgasms or of not having any orgasmic difficulties such as delay or decreased intensity), and whether the absence or impairment of orgasm is generalized (i.e., occurring basically in all situations and with all partners, if there were more than one) or situational (i.e., occurring with certain stimulation, situations, or partners). The clinician should also specify whether the associated distress is mild, moderate, or severe.

Relying on their judgment, the clinician should evaluate and discuss the following topics, even though they are not included among the DSM-5-TR specifiers:

- Relationship factors (e.g., discrepancies in desire for sexual activity, poor communication).
- Partner factors (e.g., partner's health, partner's interest in the patient's ability to achieve orgasm, partner providing adequate stimulation).
- Individual vulnerability (e.g., the loss of a job or other stresses that may be associated with inability to achieve orgasm; a change in living arrangements, such as living in a crowded space or sleeping with a baby in the room; history of sexual or emotional abuse).

- Medical factors relevant to prognosis, course, or treatment (e.g., hypothyroidism, arthritis).
- Cultural or religious factors (e.g., sex being designated for reproductive purposes only, negative attitude toward sexuality in general).

Getting the History

A 25-year-old woman reports having "sexual problems. I am unable to come." The interviewer should evaluate thoroughly all aspects of her sexual functioning and then focus on her ability to reach orgasm by asking a set of questions, gradually increasing the specificity, as follows: "Do you always have difficulties reaching orgasm? Do you reach orgasm at all? Have you ever been able to reach orgasm, or have you never been able to reach it?" Once the difficulty in experiencing orgasm is established, the interviewer should ask additional questions: "How long have you had problems reaching orgasm? Do you feel upset that you cannot? Is your partner upset with you because of this problem? Do you think that you may need more stimulation to reach orgasm? Have you ever tried to masturbate to reach orgasm? Do you and your partner use a vibrator?" It is important to establish possible partner factors: "Have you asked your partner to help you by stimulating you more? Does your partner reach orgasm too quickly? Is your partner demanding that you reach orgasm at the same time? Is your partner healthy?"

The following questioning focuses on more specific issues (to establish the specifiers): "Have you always had difficulties reaching orgasm? Let me clarify—have you never reached orgasm in your life? Are you unable to have an orgasm in any situation? Have you been unable to reach orgasm with other partners too? How much does this stress you out?"

Further questions may help clarify the diagnosis and the entire problem: "Did anything happen around the time you started to have difficulties reaching orgasm? For instance, have you started taking any new medications (e.g., selective serotonin reuptake inhibitors), or were any of your prescription dosages increased? Have you been using any illicit substances? When was your most recent gynecological or physical examination? Do you have any pain during intercourse? Are you happy in your relationship? Do you and your partner have any problems? Have there been any problems at home or at work? Do you feel stressed? Do you feel depressed? Are you anxious? Do you have other sexual problems?"

It is always important to establish whether the patient experiences female orgasmic disorder by asking whether she is able to reach orgasm, whether her current situation constitutes a change from her previous ability to reach orgasm, or whether she has been unable to reach orgasm from her first sexual encounter. Furthermore, the interviewer needs to ascertain that the inability to reach orgasm is not caused by a lack of stimulation; thus, questions need to be asked about the adequacy of stimulation, use of vibrators, and masturbation. Once the inability to reach orgasm is firmly established and the inadequacy of stimulation is ruled out, the length of the disturbance (e.g., 6 months vs. transient, short disturbance) and distress (e.g., being upset about inability to reach orgasm, feeling inadequate, partner complaints) should be established. Focusing on specific partner issues may be helpful in treatment planning; thus, the interviewer should ask about the partner's premature ejaculation, communication problems, and difference in demands of sexual activity. Inability to reach orgasm may occur within the context of mental and physical illness or as a side effect of a medication or a consequence of substance abuse. Because many women have difficulties communicating their sexual problems, the interviewer's questions need to be sensitive yet very specific.

Tips for Clarifying the Diagnosis

- Address whether the patient has ever experienced orgasm.
- Question whether the patient has been adequately stimulated and whether she has attempted to reach orgasm through masturbation.
- Clarify whether she feels distressed about her inability to experience orgasm, how much distress she feels, and whether she has been sexually satisfied.
- Ask whether she has discussed her inability to reach orgasm with her partner and whether she is able to discuss sexual issues with her partner and her physician.
- Investigate whether lack of orgasm has been consistent for at least 6 months, or whether the problem is temporary or transient.
- Investigate whether the patient is healthy and is taking any medication.

Consider the Case

> Ms. Cook, a 51-year-old woman, complains of a gradual decrease in her ability to reach orgasm over the past 1–2 years. "Most of the time I don't have any orgasm. I may have one every month or two, no matter how excited I get, no matter how wet I get," she says. "We are having sex twice a week." She has been with her partner for 3 years. They got together 2 years after her husband died. "My partner is trying, but I am also not what I used to be. I may not have the drive I used to have." She claims that her partner does "whatever I want, and at times we tried to get me excited for hours, even masturbating, and nothing happens." Ms. Cook is physically healthy. She admits being mildly depressed for the past 3 months after she was demoted at work for performance problems. She emphasizes that her orgasmic difficulties started before her work problems, although "it has been even more difficult in bed since I started to have problems at my job."
>
> Ms. Cook is upset about her inability to reach orgasm: "I love to have one, but once in a blue moon after a whole night of hard work for it is not really any pleasure." She denies any substance abuse. She takes multivitamins and occasionally zolpidem (a non-benzodiazepine hypnotic) for sleep. Her menstrual periods ceased when she was 42 years old. She tried "hormones" for her orgasmic problems in the past, "but it did not help."

Ms. Cook's ability to reach orgasm gradually ceased around age 50. Women usually learn to experience orgasm as they learn more about their bodies and have more experience with various stimulations. Ms. Cook is still able to achieve orgasm, but very rarely and after a lot of stimulation. She experiences anorgasmia on almost all occasions of sexual activity, about 90% of the time. She has been anorgasmic for about 1–2 years. She is mildly depressed—anorgasmia may occur within the context of depression and other mental disorders—however, her depression developed much later than her inability to reach orgasm. She is in menopause, but menopausal status is not consistently associated with difficulties in reaching orgasm. Also, she had reached menopause before the onset of her sexual difficulties. She takes zolpidem occasionally, but this medication is not known to be associated with impaired ability to reach orgasm. She is unhappy about not having orgasms. Her presentation is a bit atypical because of the fairly late development of her inability to have orgasm and some symptomatology such as depression. Her sexual drive may be decreased, but it does not seem to reach criteria of another sexual dysfunction.

Differential Diagnosis

The differential diagnosis of female orgasmic disorder includes nonsexual mental disorders and symptoms, such as major depressive disorder, severe anxiety disorder, psychosis, or substance use disorder. However, if a patient with anorgasmia has a history of depression or another major mental disorder that does not include inability to reach orgasm in its symptomatology, then the diagnosis of both the major mental disorder (e.g., major depressive disorder) and female orgasmic disorder should be made. Similarly, if the inability to reach orgasm precedes the development of symptomatology of major mental disorder (e.g., the patient has a lifelong history of inability to reach orgasm and recently became depressed), the clinician should diagnose both female orgasmic disorder and the major mental disorder. Female orgasmic disorder may co-occur with other sexual dysfunctions (e.g., female sexual interest/arousal disorder); thus, existence of another sexual disorder does not rule out female orgasmic disorder. The differential diagnosis of female orgasmic disorder also includes another medical condition (e.g., multiple sclerosis, spinal cord injury, fibromyalgia, endocrine disease) and interpersonal factors (e.g., intimate partner violence, severe relationship distress). The impact of using illicit substances (e.g., opioids) and medications (e.g., antidepressants, antipsychotics) should be evaluated in the differential diagnosis. The clinician should consider that even an increase in prescription medication dosage might impede the ability to reach orgasm.

Women with female orgasmic disorder may develop various associated symptomatology. They may subsequently be less interested in engaging in sexual activity. Failing to reach orgasm and subsequent possible interpersonal difficulties surrounding this failure may lead to anxiety regarding sexual activity and depression about their inability to have orgasm. Other factors, such as their partner's demands despite their difficulties in reaching orgasm or their partner reaching orgasm too quickly, may affect their associated symptomatology. If a woman is distressed about her inability to reach orgasm, she may become more anxious and then less interested in sex and less aroused. In a vicious circle, this could lead to more sexual difficulties and less ability to reach orgasm (if there was any before) and even associated pain during intercourse. It is important to note that many patients report high levels of sexual satisfaction despite rarely or never reaching orgasm.

See DSM-5-TR for additional disorders to consider in the differential diagnosis. Also refer to the discussions of comorbidity and differential diagnosis in their respective sections of DSM-5-TR.

Summary

- The core symptom of female orgasmic disorder is a marked delay in, decreased frequency of, or inability to reach orgasm or a marked decrease in orgasmic intensity on at least 75% of occasions of sexual activity, including masturbation.
- The impairment should last at least 6 months.
- A patient must demonstrate significant distress or impairment (e.g., interpersonal difficulties, feelings of inadequacy).
- The adequacy of sexual stimulation should always be carefully probed.
- Individuals may feel sexually satisfied yet still have orgasmic difficulties or be unable to reach orgasm.
- Other mental disorders (e.g., those involving depression, psychosis, anxiety, substance abuse) and side effects of medications should be ruled out as possible causes of female orgasmic disorder.
- Female orgasmic disorder may be diagnosed in the presence of other sexual dysfunctions.

IN-DEPTH DIAGNOSIS: DELAYED EJACULATION

Mr. Jones, a 21-year-old physically healthy man, complains of problems being sexually satisfied during intercourse. He says he takes a very long time to ejaculate: "at least half an hour of hard work." At times, he is unable to ejaculate at all because he is exhausted by his efforts to reach ejaculation. His girlfriend has been complaining that he reaches ejaculation a long time after she achieves orgasm. She is hesitant to have sex with him because "it is not comfortable or enjoyable at times; it is just an exhausting exercise." They tried various things, such as foreplay with "a lot of oral sex," mutual masturbation, and watching erotic movies together, but "nothing helps."

The patient states that he wants to have sex often, he thinks about it frequently, but he is becoming really discouraged about the difficulties. "I hope I will be able to have children." He has no problems getting an erection. He says that he has been having difficulties with ejaculating "for as long as I can remember, even the first time I masturbated, but I believed that it would get better with some training."

He denies any depression or other symptoms of mental illness except for getting anxious about being able to ejaculate. He does not take any medication and denies using any drugs: "It is not in my repertoire."

Mr. Jones demonstrates typical features of early onset delayed ejaculation. He has difficulty achieving ejaculation, and the time to ejaculation is very long. At times, he cannot ejaculate at all. He has always had this difficulty (i.e., for more than 6 months). At times, his efforts to achieve ejaculation have led to exhaustion. He has tried to ease his difficulty (e.g., implementing mutual masturbation with his girlfriend), but nothing has helped. His delayed ejaculation and inability to reach ejaculation have become distressing for him—he feels anxious and even doubts he will be able to have children. His dysfunction has also caused interpersonal difficulties with his girlfriend (e.g., she has been hesitant to have sex with him). The man's delayed ejaculation could not be explained in terms of any physical illness, mental disorder, or use of any substance.

Approach to the Diagnosis

Delayed ejaculation is the least frequent sexual dysfunction in men (<1% of men complain of problems with ejaculation that last more than 6 months; the prevalence of delayed ejaculation in the United States is estimated at 1%–5%). It could develop at any age; however, the prevalence of delayed ejaculation remains relatively constant until around age 50, when it begins to increase significantly. Taking the sexual history should always include detailed questioning about the ability to ejaculate and any delayed ejaculation. Males, especially older males, may attempt to explain their difficulty in terms of erectile dysfunction; erectile disorder and delayed ejaculation could coexist and should be diagnosed separately if a man meets the diagnostic criteria for both. Careful attention should be paid to a patient's description of ejaculatory dysfunction. At times, men may be able to ejaculate but not describe orgasmic pleasure (which has been described as anhedonic ejaculation). Ejaculation itself is a "peripheral" or genital phenomenon, whereas the experience of orgasm is a "cerebral" subjective phenomenon. Thus, these two events, although usually occurring together, can occur separately. In such a case, the diagnosis is not delayed ejaculation, but rather sexual dysfunction not otherwise specified (because ejaculation occurred and was not delayed).

The absence of ejaculation in the presence of adequate desire, arousal, and stimulation makes the diagnosis of delayed ejaculation clear. However, there is no definite agreement about what "delayed" ejaculation means, and in cases of delayed but present ejaculation, diagnosis of delayed ejaculation is a matter of clinical judgment. The delay in ejaculation should be present consistently over a period of at least 6 months, reported by the patient and probably his sexual partner (although the DSM-5-TR criteria do not require the partner's report), and distressing to the patient and/or his partner, or it could cause some impairment in the form of interpersonal difficulties, avoidance of having intercourse, or inability to conceive. Partners may feel inadequate or unattractive and may blame themselves for the man's inability to ejaculate.

Explanation in terms of other sexual dysfunction (e.g., lack of sexual desire or ability to achieve erection), comorbid mental disorder (e.g., severe major depressive disorder), physical illness (e.g., interruption of innervation of sexual organs during surgery, neurological disease such as multiple sclerosis, consequence of an illness such as diabetic neuropathy), and use of various medications (e.g., serotonergic antidepressants, antihypertensives, tamsulosin) and substances of abuse (e.g., opioids) should be considered, especially in cases of late-onset delayed ejaculation.

The approach to the diagnosis of delayed ejaculation should thus progress from 1) establishing delayed or missing ejaculation and the psychological experience of orgasm for at least 6 months in the evaluator's clinical judgment, to 2) determining the existence of distress or impairment in terms of the patient's and his partner's experience. This approach could be followed by questions about the possible etiology using the framework of the DSM-5-TR specifiers.

Getting the History

A 30-year-old man complains that it "takes me forever to ejaculate." The interviewer should ask about all aspects of the patient's sexual functioning and sex life, and thus they should start with general inquiries as follows: "Please tell me whether you are satisfied with your sex life. If not, why not? How often do you have sex? Is your partner satisfied with the frequency and quality of your sexual encounters?" Questioning should then become more specific, focusing on particular aspects. For example, after asking about sexual desire (e.g., "Do you feel like having sex often?"), erectile disorder (e.g., "Are you getting hard enough when you have sex? Have there been any changes in your ability to get an erection?"), and ejaculation ("Have you had any problems reaching orgasm or ejaculating?"), it may become clearer that the prevailing sexual problem is delayed ejaculation or inability to ejaculate. The questions should then become even more specific, as follows: "Do you ejaculate at all? Does it take you more time to come or to ejaculate lately? Have you tried any additional stimulation to reach orgasm? Are you able to ejaculate when masturbating? Can you ejaculate when having sex with someone else? What sexual fantasies do you have while having sex and while masturbating? Are you upset that it takes you a long time to ejaculate or that you cannot ejaculate? Is your partner also upset? Are you taking any medication? Which one(s)? Do you use any substances? Do you feel depressed? Are you healthy? Have you had any recent medical problems?"

Once the patient opens up about his sexual problem, establishing the descriptive diagnosis of delayed, less frequent, or nonexistent ejaculation may be relatively simple. The patient has to believe that the information they share is confidential and being considered seriously because the inability to ejaculate may be damaging to feelings about male function and ability to conceive (especially among younger males with early-onset delayed ejaculation, or in those with lifelong delayed or absent ejaculation). It is important to determine that the impairment is continuous (i.e., almost all occasions), lasting (i.e., 6 months or longer), and not temporary (e.g., because of interpersonal difficulties). Delayed ejaculation or an inability to ejaculate should also cause distress (e.g., anxiety, self-doubt) or interpersonal difficulties (e.g., partner's unhappiness, arguments) in order to meet the DSM-5-TR criteria for delayed ejaculation. The judgment about the delay in ejaculation is clinical and should be considered within a wide context because there is no consensus regarding what constitutes a reasonable and generally acceptable time to reach orgasm. The DSM-5-TR specifiers (lifelong vs. acquired; generalized vs. situational) should be utilized as a framework for more specific questioning that may help to clarify the possible cause or any contributing factors.

Tips for Clarifying the Diagnosis

- Ask whether the patient has ever had an orgasm in terms of ejaculation and experiencing orgasm at the same time.
- Question whether the ejaculation is markedly delayed or significantly less frequent in spite of adequate desire, arousal, and stimulation.
- Verify that this dysfunction has been ongoing for at least 6 months.

- Assess whether the delay in ejaculation, decreased frequency, or inability to ejaculate is causing distress or personal difficulty.
- Ask the patient whether he is taking any substances that could delay ejaculation.
- Investigate whether he experiences other sexual dysfunctions, such as male hypoactive sexual desire disorder or erectile disorder.

Consider the Case

Mr. Wong, a 55-year-old man of Chinese origin, is brought in by his wife, who complains that "lately, at least a year or two, he is demanding to have sex that lasts forever.. I am not able to satisfy him." He admits that as he is getting older, he has been having "more difficulties ejaculating, and my erections are getting weaker."

Mr. Wong says that he has always been proud of being able to satisfy his sexual partners, although "they usually came much earlier than I did, but they liked the fact that they always came." His time to reach ejaculation was longer, but he was able to ejaculate on all occasions. However, during the past several years, his ejaculations have been significantly delayed. At times, at least once or twice a month, he is unable to ejaculate at all. His mild erectile difficulties usually happen in the context of trying to achieve ejaculation "at the end of my effort to satisfy my wife or at the end of my trying to ejaculate while masturbating." He is upset about his wife's complaint. They have argued a lot because she has been refusing to have sex with him lately. He is fairly healthy and has been taking medication for lowering cholesterol for about 10 years and "some pills for heartburn occasionally." He has never used any illicit substances. He drinks a glass or two of wine over the weekend.

Mr. Wong gradually developed delayed ejaculation and, at times, inability to ejaculate during his early fifties. In addition to his age, he has some predisposition for developing delayed ejaculation: he is of East Asian origin (more males of East and Southeast Asian origin report delayed ejaculation), and he has always taken a longer time to reach ejaculation. However, he was not distressed about his somewhat delayed ejaculation in his earlier years, and it did not cause him reportable interpersonal difficulties. He is, however, distressed by the development of more delayed ejaculation to the point of inability to ejaculate in the past several years, and his sexual dysfunction has caused interpersonal difficulties (e.g., he and his wife argue about it). He has some associated mild erectile disorder but is fairly healthy, and his medications or consumption of wine cannot explain his sexual dysfunction, which clearly meets the delayed ejaculation diagnostic criteria. His disorder could be specified as acquired and probably generalized. He seems at least moderately distressed.

Differential Diagnosis

Differential diagnosis of delayed ejaculation includes numerous factors, especially in cases of acquired delayed ejaculation. In a young healthy male, the differential diagnosis includes mainly use of medications (e.g., selective serotonin reuptake inhibitors), substances of abuse, and psychological factors (e.g., inability to ejaculate with one partner while being able to ejaculate with others; paraphilic interests; and even a consequence of prolonged infertility treatment with pressure on "performing"—i.e., ejaculating at certain times and circumstances). Differential diagnosis could also include the disjunction between ejaculation and orgasmic experience (anhedonic ejaculation).

Differential diagnosis of late-onset delayed ejaculation is probably wider and includes various medical illnesses (e.g., impaired innervation of genitals in disorders such as multiple sclerosis, diabetes mellitus, and alcoholic neuropathy; intentional or unintentional injury of innervation during surgery); use of medications (e.g., antihypertensives, antipsychotics, selective serotonin reuptake inhibitors, painkillers [opioids]) or drugs of abuse (opioids); psychological factors (e.g., ability to ejaculate with one partner but not another of the same sex, paraphilias, other sexual dysfunctions, major depression); and anhedonic ejaculation (or other dysfunction with orgasm, such as painful ejaculation associated with some medications).

Factors that may affect the clinical presentation of delayed ejaculation include

- Associated depression or anxiety
- Other sexual dysfunction that may either precede or develop as a consequence of delayed ejaculation (e.g., lack of desire to have sex anymore, erectile dysfunction)
- Distress caused by inability or fear of inability to conceive; history of sexual abuse
- Poor body image
- Cultural and religious influences (e.g., religious belief that man should ejaculate just for the purpose of conception and that masturbation is a sin)
- Partner demands (e.g., more sex, no sex) and complaints (e.g., that it takes too long to get sex [which could perpetuate the difficulty because of performance anxiety], that the sex is painful or exhausting)
- The man's own exhaustion during the long attempts to achieve ejaculation while not being particularly physically fit

See DSM-5-TR for additional disorders to consider in the differential diagnosis. Also refer to the discussions of comorbidity and differential diagnosis in their respective sections of DSM-5-TR.

Summary

- Delayed ejaculation is the least frequent male sexual dysfunction.
- To establish the diagnosis of delayed ejaculation, the clinician should inquire about markedly delayed ejaculation or marked decrease in frequency of ejaculation or inability to ejaculate.
- The dysfunction should be continuous, occurring in almost all or all attempts to have intercourse or masturbation, and should last at least 6 months.
- The decision about the delay of ejaculation is clinical. There is no clear consensus about what constitutes delayed ejaculation in terms of time or frequency.
- The dysfunction should cause distress or impairment (especially in the man's relationship with his partner).
- Various factors that could explain or modify the clinical picture of delayed ejaculation include those related to the patient, his partner, physical illness, medical illness, and medications or substances of abuse.

IN-DEPTH DIAGNOSIS: FEMALE SEXUAL INTEREST/AROUSAL DISORDER AND MALE HYPOACTIVE SEXUAL DESIRE DISORDER

Female Sexual Interest/Arousal Disorder

Ms. Parker is a 23-year-old healthy woman who states that she has not been interested in having sex for as long as she can remember. She is attracted to men in general and has had partners, but only as "companions. I have never thought of men in sexual terms very much, and I don't have any sexual fantasies." She is not receptive to her boyfriend's attempts to start sex, although "I give up at times, to make him happy." She may get aroused ultimately, but "I don't feel much when having sex, and it is the same when I tried to masturbate per someone's suggestion." Once aroused, she has no problem reaching orgasm. She has been having arguments with her boyfriend about her lack of interest in sex. "He thinks I don't love him. He is a great, caring guy, and I do love him, but I don't care about sex." She is upset about their arguments and worried that "he may run away." She denies taking any medication or using any drugs.

Ms. Parker meets the DSM-5-TR criteria for female sexual interest/arousal disorder, lifelong and generalized, because she has lacked sexual desire since her first sexual encounter. She does not have any sexual fantasies and is not receptive to her boyfriend's attempts to have sex. She also reports decreased intensity of sexual sensations during sex. Thus, she clearly presents with a mixture of lack of sexual desire and some impairment of arousal. She can get aroused occasionally and reach orgasm. She loves her boyfriend and is attracted to him, but not sexually. Her sexual dysfunction is persistent and has lasted more than 6 months. She has been having arguments because of her "sexual problems" and is worried about losing her partner, thus meeting the distress criterion (probably at a moderate level). She is healthy and denies any problems or substance abuse and does not take any medications.

Male Hypoactive Sexual Desire Disorder

Mr. Carr, a 30-year-old married man, tells his doctor that his wife is complaining of his "total lack of interest in her and in having sex with her." They have been married for 3 years and have had sex "less than a dozen" times during their marriage. His wife says that she would be happy to have sex once every month or two, but "he is not interested." He denies any extramarital affair and reveals that he has never been interested in sex, and "I really never think about it." His wife bought him some testosterone gel, and he applied it a few times, without any change in his desire. He has been able to have an erection after a "lot of stimulation by my wife, and after that, ejaculation is not a problem." He is healthy, uses no substances or prescribed medications, does not drink alcohol, and denies any depression. He is getting anxious because his wife is threatening to divorce him, saying that his lack of sexual interest "shows" he does not love her.

Mr. Carr has not had interest in sex for most of his life, and he meets the criteria for male hypoactive sexual desire disorder (lifelong, probably generalized). He and his wife are having sex very infrequently for their age group, and his wife would clearly like to have sex more frequently, although her demands are not excessive. Mr. Carr has had no sexual fantasies, and his lack of interest in sex does not seem to be related to the lack of testosterone (application of testosterone gel did not make any difference in his lack of sexual desire). He is able to get an erection and ejaculate during sex. His sexual dysfunction is causing some interpersonal difficulties (mild). He is healthy, and his lack of sexual desire does not seem to be explainable in terms of other physical or mental illness or use of substances or medications.

Approach to the Diagnosis

FEMALE SEXUAL INTEREST/AROUSAL DISORDER

Female sexual interest/arousal disorder became a new diagnosis in DSM-5 (and is included in DSM-5-TR), requiring at least three symptoms that have persisted for at least 6 months. Because this disorder in a way combines the symptoms of low or nonexistent sexual desire and lack of arousal, both of these sets of symptoms must be carefully explored. Various combinations of symptoms are possible. In assessing the sexual interest of a female, the clinician must consider a possible discrepancy in sexual desire between the patient and her partner; the clinician may not include the alleged lack of sexual desire, which could be accounted for by "desire discrepancy" in symptoms counted toward the diagnosis of this disorder. The normative decline in sexual desire with age should also be considered in determining the lack of sexual desire. The lack of sexual receptivity to a partner's attempt to initiate sex should be carefully evaluated with consideration of the patient's and her partner's beliefs and preferences for initiation of sex. Wide variety in expression of sexual fantasies occurs in women, and individual patterns need to be taken into account in diagnosing female sexual interest/arousal disorder because specifications for sexual fantasies, desire, and feelings are neither known nor established. For the diagnosis, the presence of three or more symptoms of impaired sexual interest/arousal must cause significant distress or impairment. Finally, clinicians should consider physical or mental illness and substance or medication use as possible causes of female sexual interest/arousal disorder. Further considerations include partner factors (e.g., poor health, lack of interest in proper stimulation), interpersonal problems (e.g., discrepancy in sexual desire, poor communication about sex, intimate partner violence), individual vulnerability (e.g., depression, anxiety, poor body image, stress over job loss), medical factors, and cultural or religious factors (e.g., religious prohibition of sex before marriage).

MALE HYPOACTIVE SEXUAL DESIRE DISORDER

When making the diagnosis of male hypoactive sexual desire disorder, the clinician must establish that the lack of sexual desire and the absence of sexual thoughts or fantasies are persistent and have lasted at least 6 months. An adaptive response to an adverse life condition (e.g., partner's pregnancy, intention to terminate relationship) should also be considered. In addition, questions about a possible discrepancy in sexual desire between partners should be asked (not all men claiming low sexual desire have low sexual desire). Increased age is a significant risk factor for decreased sexual desire. Although decrease in testosterone levels is not always associated with decrease in sexual desire, a clear-cut hypogonadism is associated with low sexual desire and should be ruled out as an underlying cause of this disorder. For the diagnosis of male hypoactive sexual desire disorder to be made, low or nonexistent sexual desire must be associated with significant distress (e.g., "not being a man") or impairment (e.g., dissolution of a relationship).

A wide spectrum of risk factors for developing low sexual desire needs to be considered in diagnosing this disorder, including depression, hyperprolactinemia, alcohol use, the patient's feeling about his masculinity, religiosity, paraphilic tendencies, marital alienation, extramarital affairs, intrafamilial sexual abuse, pornography addiction, poor sexual education, and early life trauma. It is important to realize that male hypoactive sexual desire disorder is rarely the sole sexual diagnosis in men and that comorbidity with other sexual dysfunctions, depression, and endocrinological factors is common. Thus, the diagnostic process should be a very careful exploration of multiple areas of sexual and psychological functioning and personal history.

Getting the History

FEMALE SEXUAL INTEREST/AROUSAL DISORDER

A 35-year-old female presents with a vague complaint of not satisfying her sexual partner. The interviewer begins by asking about the nature of the patient's sexual activity and sexual satisfaction: "Are you satisfied with your sexual functioning? Why not? How often do you have sex? Has there been any change in how often you have sex lately? Is your partner satisfied with your sexual encounters? Is your partner demanding more sex lately?" Once the impairment of sexual functioning is generally established, questions should focus on various aspects of sexual interest/arousal: "Do you feel like having sex often? Do you think about sex often? Why not? Do you fantasize about having sex? If not, why not? Has there been any change in your sexual fantasies and thoughts? Who initiates sex, you, or your partner? How do you respond when your partner initiates sex? Does your sexual desire appear or increase when your partner tries to initiate sex? Does your partner arouse you? Do you get wet easily, or have you had problems with lubrication lately? Have you needed more sexual stimulation to get aroused lately? What about the feelings in your genitals and vagina during intercourse? Any change? Less intense? Any pain?" The interviewer then asks, "How long has this been going on? Has there been anything that may have triggered these problems? Are you upset about your sexual problems? Why? Do you feel stressed out about the problem? Any related problems with your partner?" The interviewer also asks questions about health and substance use, such as, "What about your health? What about your menstrual periods—any changes, any difficulties? Are you taking any medication? Are you drinking? Are you using any illicit substances?"

The diagnosis of female sexual interest/arousal disorder is the most symptom-specific (i.e., Criterion A requires a specific number of symptoms to be present) among the sexual dysfunction diagnoses and basically combines the symptoms of sexual desire/interest and arousal. Therefore, all symptoms of possibly impaired sexual desire/interest and possibly impaired sexual arousal should be carefully evaluated. Symptoms should be evaluated in relation to the patient (e.g., sexual thoughts, fantasies), the dyad (e.g., the initiator of sex, the response of the partner, discrepancy in sexual desire or demands), and subjective feelings and physiological response (e.g., genital feelings, psychological excitement, lubrication, vasocongestion). Once the symptom configuration is established, their persistence and duration need to be ascertained (brief decreases in sexual desire and arousal may occur in various situations and may resolve). Occurrence of other sexual problems (e.g., lack of orgasm, sexual pain) should also be explored because these problems may develop as a consequence or contribute to the development of female sexual interest/desire disorder.

MALE HYPOACTIVE SEXUAL DESIRE DISORDER

A 23-year-old male states that "my partner says I am not interested in sex." As in cases of any sexual dysfunction, the interviewer first elicits responses about sexual functioning in general, by asking, "Can you tell me whether you are satisfied with your sexual functioning? If not, why not? How often do you have sex? Do you masturbate in addition to having sex with your partner? Is your partner satisfied with your sexual encounters? Is your partner more demanding, or has there been any change in your partner's demands of sex?" Then the interviewer asks more specific questions, such as, "Do you feel like having sex often? Do you think about sex often? No? Why not? Have you always had low interest or no interest in sex? Has there been any change in your interest in sex or desire to have sex? How long has it been going on? Do you have any other sexual problems? Can you get an erection? What about ejaculation? Can you ejaculate? Do you have any problems with ejaculation?" If necessary, further questioning should establish whether the lack of sexual desire is the primary sexual dysfunction: "Which of your sexual problems appeared first: lack of libido, problems with erection, or problems with ejaculation?" These questions should be followed by queries about the distress: "Are you upset about your lack of desire? Why? How much? Has it caused any problems between you and your partner?" Finally, the interviewer asks about possible contributing factors: "Have you been depressed or anxious? How has your physical health been? Are you taking any medications? How much do you drink? Do you use any other substances? Have you been sexually involved with anybody else? Did you have similar problems in that relationship?"

The diagnostic questioning for male hypoactive sexual desire disorder focuses first on establishing the existence of sexual dysfunction and then on determining what dysfunction it is by asking about all aspects of the patient's sexual functioning (e.g., desire, arousal [erection], and orgasm [ejaculation]) and questioning whether lack of desire is the primary problem. Lack of sexual desire could possibly develop as a reaction to inability to attain erection or delayed ejaculation. It is also important to establish the existence of distress; a minority of men may not be distressed about their lack of sexual desire and may not be interested in sexual or other relationships (if the low or nonexistent desire is explained by self-identification as asexual, then a diagnosis of male hypoactive sexual desire disorder should not be made). Finally, questions about possible psychological factors (e.g., depression, marital problems, emotional connection with his partner, extramarital affairs, even frequent compulsive watching of pornography) and "environmental" factors (alcohol and other substance abuse, medication, religious or cultural issues) are also very important. Contrary to many beliefs, hypogonadism and "idiopathic" male hypoactive sexual desire disorder are not the only causes of low desire in many males. Using the framework of DSM-5-TR, specifiers and risk factors may help elucidate and specify the diagnosis further.

Tips for Clarifying the Diagnosis

FEMALE SEXUAL INTEREST/AROUSAL DISORDER

To investigate whether a patient has female sexual interest/arousal disorder, explore the following questions:

- Does the patient have low sexual desire in the form of absent or reduced interest in sexual activity? What about sexual fantasies? Does she become interested or aroused while talking about sex with her partner or watching a sexually explicit movie? Does she attempt to masturbate? Is she adequately stimulated during the partnered sexual activity?
- Who initiates sexual activity in the couple? How is initiation of sexual activity accepted by the patient? Any resistance?
- Does she experience any pleasure during sexual intercourse?
- Does she become aroused during intercourse? Is there adequate lubrication? Do her genital feelings change during intercourse?
- Is the patient distressed about her lack of sexual interest/arousal? How much and what is the nature of her distress or impairment?
- Is the patient healthy? Does she have any signs of depression, anxiety, or substance abuse? Any medical condition (e.g., diabetes mellitus, thyroid disease)?

MALE HYPOACTIVE SEXUAL DESIRE DISORDER

To investigate whether a patient has male hypoactive sexual desire disorder, explore the following questions:

- Does the patient report any change in sexual desire/interest? Does he have any sexual fantasies? Is this situation different than before or has this lack of sexual desire/interest been a lifelong pattern? Is the lack of desire persistent?
- How long has sexual desire/interest been absent?
- Is he upset or distressed about his lack of sexual desire? Has it caused any problems for him?
- Is the lack of sexual desire specific for a particular person (partner) or situation, or does it occur for any sexual partner or situation?
- Is he depressed or anxious, or concerned about his body image or sexual performance? Any other sexual dysfunction?
- Does he have any physical signs of hypogonadism or low testosterone level?

Consider the Case

FEMALE SEXUAL INTEREST/AROUSAL DISORDER

> Ms. Stone, a 45-year-old married woman, states that her husband has been complaining about her lack of interest in having sex with him. "I realize that he is right. The problem is that I have not been feeling much during intercourse except for a bit of pain occasionally because I don't get wet. I just do not feel excited, no matter what we try—looking at movies, oral sex, vibrator. Sex is just not pleasurable for me anymore. I don't know

how it happened and when; it has been a while, many months. I'm not interested in sex anymore. It's not my husband; he is okay. It's sex that I'm not interested in. It's sad—I used to love sex." Ms. Stone is nervous because her husband's behavior "has changed lately. He is not home frequently. I am afraid he found someone to have sex with." She denies any depression. She is fairly healthy, and her periods are regular, without any changes. She takes a sleeping pill occasionally and multivitamins daily. She admits smoking a small amount of cannabis weekly "since I was in college."

Ms. Stone developed sexual dysfunction several months ago after functioning sexually fairly well. She has difficulties in getting aroused and feeling any pleasure and has also lost interest in sex. She meets symptom criteria for female sexual interest/arousal disorder (at least four symptoms). She has been suspicious that her husband may be having an affair because of her lack of interest in having sex with him, and she feels distressed about it. She has not reached menopause yet. Ms. Stone is healthy and does not take any medication that would affect her sexual functioning. She has been smoking small amounts of cannabis for years, so that activity could not explain her change in sexual functioning several months ago. The duration of her sexual functioning is not clear ("several months"); however, her impairment of sexual functioning has been persistent (if the duration of dysfunction is not precisely clear, the persistence of symptomatology may ascertain the diagnosis of female sexual interest/arousal disorder). Ms. Stone's disorder could be subtyped as acquired and probably generalized and specified as severe because she is significantly distressed.

MALE HYPOACTIVE SEXUAL DESIRE DISORDER

Mr. Carpenter, a 52-year-old married man, reports that he has been having occasional problems with erection and that his sexual desire has been "fading away lately." He can still have full erections occasionally, "but I am not really interested that much." The frequency of intercourse with his wife gradually decreased to once every several months, "after we used to have sex two to three times a week less than 2 years ago." He admits that he stopped thinking about sex, and "my fantasies about other women disappeared. I don't masturbate anymore." His testosterone level is lower than before but still within normal limits. A testosterone patch did not help, and the "little blue pill" did not help either. Mr. Carpenter is very upset about his lack of sexual interest and declining performance because his friends have been constantly teasing him after he mentioned it to them a while ago. "I don't feel as if I am a man anymore." He exercises regularly and is in good shape. He denies any depression. He was diagnosed with hypothyroidism several years ago and takes thyroid hormone supplement daily (his thyroid-stimulating hormone and free thyroxine levels are within normal limits). He has been drinking a beer or two with friends occasionally for years but does not use any illicit substances.

Mr. Carpenter developed a lack of sexual desire relatively late in his life. His decline in sexual desire is associated with some erectile dysfunction (associated sexual dysfunction), but his erectile dysfunction does not explain his total lack of desire or interest in sex after a long period of good sexual functioning. His testosterone level is a bit low but not abnormally low, and because testosterone patches were not helpful, low testosterone does not seem to be the underlying cause of his lack of desire (hypogonadism should be ruled out in all cases of low sexual desire). His sexual activity has almost completely ceased, and he feels distressed about it. Alcohol use may increase the occurrence of male hypoactive sexual desire disorder. He drinks beer occasionally, but has done so for a long time, so his drinking could not explain his recent decrease in sexual desire. Mr. Carpenter has two risk factors for developing male hypoactive sexual desire disorder: he is older than 50 and has physical illness. He has hypothyroidism, which, if not properly treated, could explain the decrease in his sexual desire. However, in this case, the laboratory evaluation of thyroid functioning shows that it is within normal limits.

Differential Diagnosis

FEMALE SEXUAL INTEREST/AROUSAL DISORDER

The differential diagnosis of female sexual interest/arousal disorder is fairly broad because the symptomatology of this sexual dysfunction covers the areas of desire and arousal. As in other sexual dysfunctions, a broad variety of mental and physical illnesses may affect sexual desire and arousal.

Nonsexual mental disorders need to be considered. For example, major depressive disorder (one of the symptoms is markedly diminished interest or pleasure in all, or almost all, activities) and persistent depressive disorder (dysthymia; symptoms include low energy, fatigue, low self-esteem) may account for the lack of sexual interest/arousal or its decrease. Some anxiety disorders and trauma- and stressor-related disorders (e.g., PTSD) as well as OCD should also be ruled out as a possible cause of low sexual interest/arousal. Major psychotic disorders and some personality disorders may also be associated with lack of or reduction in sexual interest/arousal. Similarly, substance use (e.g., opioids), not only during the episode of acute intoxication, and some medications (e.g., antihypertensives, antipsychotics, antidepressants, chemotherapeutics, hormones) may account for the lack of sexual interest/arousal.

Medical illnesses or conditions associated with the lack of or diminished sexual interest/arousal include, for instance, diabetes mellitus, thyroid disease, multiple sclerosis and other neurological diseases, and cardiovascular diseases (e.g., endothelial disease).

Clinicians should also consider other sexual dysfunctions (e.g., chronic genital pain; genito-pelvic pain/penetration disorder) as an explanation of female sexual interest/arousal disorder symptomatology. Other sexual dysfunctions (e.g., female orgasmic disorder) may also coexist with this disorder.

Sexual arousal and, in some women, sexual desire may develop in response to the partner's initiation and stimulation. The discussion of presence and adequacy of sexual stimulation should be part of the patient interview. If inadequate or absent sexual stimulation is part of the clinical picture, diagnosis of a sexual dysfunction should not be made.

Finally, interpersonal factors such as interpersonal distress, intimate partner violence, partner poor health, and stresses (e.g., job loss) may also play a role in the lack of or diminished sexual interest/arousal. Some of these factors may be transient and could be a secondary adaptive alteration in sexual functioning.

The differential diagnosis of female sexual interest/arousal disorder may be complicated by development of associated factors or complications, such as another sexual dysfunction (e.g., female orgasmic disorder)—in which case it is important to establish which dysfunction is the primary one—and various psychological reactions to the lack of or diminished sexual interest/arousal, such as anxiety, depression, and interpersonal difficulties (e.g., the lack of receptive response may lead to arguments, which may further reduce the lack of interest).

See DSM-5-TR for additional disorders to consider in the differential diagnosis. Also refer to the discussions of comorbidity and differential diagnosis in their respective sections of DSM-5-TR.

MALE HYPOACTIVE SEXUAL DESIRE DISORDER

The differential diagnosis of male hypoactive sexual desire disorder includes a broad variety of mental and physical illnesses that may affect sexual desire. Using the framework of subtypes (i.e., lifelong, acquired) and specifiers (i.e., situational, generalized) may be helpful in considering the differential diagnosis.

Nonsexual mental disorders need to be considered. For example, major depressive disorder (for which one of the symptoms is markedly diminished interest or pleasure in all, or almost all, activities) and persistent depressive disorder (dysthymia; symptoms include low energy, fatigue, low self-esteem) may account for the lack of sexual interest or its decrease. Some anxiety disorders and trauma- and stressor-related disorders (e.g., PTSD) may also affect sexual desire. Major psychotic disorders and some personality disorders (e.g., schizoid personality disorder) may also be associated with lack of or reduction in sexual interest.

Substance use (e.g., chronic alcohol use, use of cannabis or opioids), not only during the episode of acute intoxication, and some medications (e.g., anticonvulsants, antihypertensives, antipsychotics, antidepressants, chemotherapeutics, and medications used in urological diseases) may also account for the lack of sexual desire.

Various medical conditions, such as hypogonadism (verified by low testosterone level), hypothyroidism, diabetes mellitus, cardiovascular diseases, epilepsy, chronic renal failure, chronic liver disease, and testicular disease (e.g., cancer, undescended testes, mumps orchitis), are often associated with low or nonexistent sexual interest.

Various stressors (e.g., job loss), interpersonal factors (e.g., arguments with partner, extramarital affair, partner's pregnancy, violence), and individual factors (e.g., poor body image, history of sexual trauma) need to be ruled out as possible causes for the deficient or absent sexual desire.

Some men (1%–2%) may identify themselves as asexual. For them, male hypoactive sexual desire disorder should not be diagnosed.

The differential diagnosis of male hypoactive sexual desire disorder may be complicated by the development of associated factors or complications, such as another sexual dysfunction (e.g., erectile disorder, delayed ejaculation). Many men (up to one-half) with male hypoactive sexual desire disorder may have other sexual dysfunction(s) that play a role in the lack of or diminished sexual interest. These dysfunctions do not necessarily rule out the diagnosis of male hypoactive sexual desire disorder. In such cases, it is important to establish which dysfunction is primary and to identify the various psychological reactions to the lack of or diminished sexual interest or arousal, such as anxiety, depression, and interpersonal difficulties.

See DSM-5-TR for additional disorders to consider in the differential diagnosis. Also refer to the discussions of comorbidity and differential diagnosis in their respective sections of DSM-5-TR.

Summary

FEMALE SEXUAL INTEREST/AROUSAL DISORDER

- Female sexual interest/arousal disorder is a relatively new diagnosis in the DSM system that basically combines the symptomatology of diminished or absent sexual interest and diminished or absent sexual arousal.
- The symptoms of impaired sexual interest or arousal must have persisted for at least 6 months.
- The patient must be distressed about her level of sexual interest/arousal or experience impairment in her psychological well-being or interpersonal difficulties as a consequence of it.
- Various mental disorders (particularly major depressive disorder), other medical conditions, substance/medication use, and interpersonal and individual factors should be considered in the differential diagnosis.

MALE HYPOACTIVE SEXUAL DESIRE DISORDER

- The lack of sexual or erotic thoughts and fantasies and lack of desire to have sex (including masturbation) is the hallmark of this disorder. This lack of interest is based on clinical judgment.
- The absence or diminishment of sexual desire/interest must have persisted for at least 6 months.
- The absent or deficient sexual desire/interest should cause clinically significant distress.
- The differential diagnosis of this disorder includes various mental disorders (e.g., depression), physical conditions (e.g., endocrine disease such as hypogonadism or thyroid disease), substance/medication use, and individual and interpersonal factors.
- Male hypoactive sexual desire disorder may be associated with other sexual dysfunctions (e.g., erectile disorder, delayed ejaculation). These dysfunctions may either precede it (in which case the diagnosis of male hypoactive sexual desire disorder should not be made) or develop as its consequence.
- The framework of subtypes and specifiers (i.e., acquired vs. lifelong, situational vs. generalized) will be useful in considering the differential diagnosis of this disorder.

SUMMARY: SEXUAL DYSFUNCTIONS

Sexual dysfunctions are fairly prevalent impairments of sexual functioning. Prevalence of sexual dysfunctions may vary among different cultures and world regions—

the highest prevalence of various sexual dysfunctions was found in East and Southeast Asia.

In an effort to make diagnosis of sexual dysfunctions more precise and to decrease the likelihood of overdiagnosis, DSM-5-TR criteria require a minimum duration of dysfunction of at least 6 months and include more precise severity specifiers (i.e., distress being mild, moderate, or severe) and more detailed subtypes (i.e., lifelong vs. acquired) and specifiers (i.e., situational vs. generalized). Clinicians may also examine interpersonal, partner, relationship, cultural, religious, and individual vulnerability factors in considering the diagnoses and the differential diagnoses of these disorders. These specifications make it easier to distinguish the true sexual dysfunctions from transient impairment of sexual functioning that possibly relates to various interpersonal problems and stresses. For the diagnosis of a sexual dysfunction, impairment of sexual functioning must also cause distress in interpersonal relationships and possibly in other functioning. All of the diagnostic criteria rely on the clinician's judgment. The diagnosis of sexual dysfunctions is no longer anchored solely in the so-called sexual response cycle and now is gender specific. Sexual dysfunctions should always be evaluated and diagnosed in the wider context of other mental disorders, substance abuse, physical illnesses, medications taken by individuals with sexual dysfunctions, individual vulnerability, partner issues, stress, religious and cultural issues, and interpersonal factors. Inadequate stimulation and discrepancy in sexual demands between partners should always be considered in clarifying the diagnosis.

DSM-5 introduced two new diagnoses—female sexual interest/arousal disorder and genito-pelvic pain/penetration disorder—and no longer includes the diagnosis of sexual aversion disorder as an individual diagnosis. These changes are maintained in DSM-5-TR.

ELEMENTS TO CONSIDER IN THE CULTURAL FORMULATION

- Culturally determined views, expectations, and practices concerning marital relationships, sexual performance, fertility, and gender roles can influence anxiety and other symptoms that may affect sexual dysfunction.
- In some cultures, women's sexual satisfaction may be undervalued or devaluated, and marital sex may be viewed as a duty for women rather than a pleasurable activity.
- Women's help-seeking behavior may be lower than men's.
- Sexual desire varies across cultures.
- The population of gender-diverse persons, including transgender, nonbinary, and agender, may not identify with or appear to fit the existing sex- and gender-based diagnostic categories. Despite the names given to male hypoactive sexual desire disorder and female sexual interest/arousal disorder, the diagnostic criteria describe symptoms and experiences that are not dependent on the person's specific sex or gender. Thus, either diagnosis can be applied to gender-diverse individuals.

- For diagnoses linked to reproductive anatomy, diagnoses of sexual dysfunction should be based on the individual's current anatomy and not on the individual's sex assigned at birth.

DIAGNOSTIC PEARLS

- Sexual dysfunctions need to be distinguished from transient impairment of sexual functioning; therefore, the duration of impairment should be at least 6 months.
- Sexual difficulties, especially in women, could result from inadequate sexual stimulation. In such cases, sexual dysfunction should not be diagnosed.
- Sexual functioning may decline with aging; therefore, age-related changes should be considered when diagnosing sexual dysfunction.
- Sexual dysfunctions are gender specific.
- Impairment of sexual functioning could be associated with various mental disorders (e.g., depression) and physical illnesses (e.g., diabetes mellitus, neurological diseases).
- Impairment of sexual functioning could result from various substances of abuse (e.g., alcohol, nicotine, opioids) and numerous psychotropic (e.g., antidepressants, antipsychotics) and nonpsychotropic (e.g., antacids, antihypertensives, beta-blockers) medications.
- Cultural, interpersonal, and religious factors may play important roles in impairment of sexual functioning and should be considered when making the diagnosis.
- Several sexual dysfunctions may occur or overlap in one person.
- The etiology of sexual dysfunctions is usually unknown; impairment of sexual functioning is frequently a result of a complex interplay of biological, psychological, and sociocultural factors.
- Individuals should be evaluated in the context of their cultural milieu.
- Sexual dysfunctions should be differentiated from transient sexual difficulties caused by various interpersonal, social, cultural, and other demands.

SELF-ASSESSMENT

Key Concepts: Double-Check Your Knowledge

What is the relevance of the following concepts to the various sexual dysfunctions?

- Low sexual desire
- Impaired interest or arousal
- Erectile dysfunction
- Delayed orgasm

- Anorgasmia
- Genital pain
- Sexual fantasies
- Premature (early) ejaculation
- Impaired sexual functioning due to medical illness or medications
- Impaired sexual functioning due to substance abuse

Questions to Discuss With Colleagues and Mentors

1. Do you routinely discuss sexual functioning and sexual practices, behaviors, and preferences with your patients?
2. Do you feel comfortable asking your patients about their sexuality or sexual habits, preferences, and practices? If not, why not? Do you avoid certain questions about patients' preferences and practices?
3. What questions do you ask your patients about their sexual functioning?
4. How do you conceptualize sexual functioning and its impairment? What do you think about the DSM-5 and DSM-5-TR changes in that the diagnoses are now gender specific?
5. Once you establish a diagnosis of sexual dysfunction in your patient, do you explore other aspects of your patient's sexual functioning to find out whether other sexual dysfunctions are present?
6. What do you know about the impact of other mental disorders, physical conditions, medication use, and substances of abuse on sexual functioning?

Case-Based Questions

PART A

> Ms. Gonzalez, a 35-year-old woman, states that she does not enjoy sex anymore. "Actually, I haven't had sex in a long time, and we used to have sex almost daily when we got married 3 years ago. I used to think about sex on my way home from work, but that is gone. I don't think about it. My husband has been trying to get me into the mood, but I usually turn around and go to sleep. Part of the problem is that I don't feel anything anymore down there. I used to have very pleasurable feelings when penetrated. We tried a vibrator to get back to those feelings, but it did not help." She admits worrying about her recent lack of orgasm because "that is necessary to get pregnant and we planned to have a kid or two." She states that she and her husband have been stressed by the fact that they may lose their house. "He lost his job. He got a new one, but it does not pay enough to cover the mortgage payments or the rest of our bills. We have argued about this a lot." She denies any physical illness or problems. She does not take any medication. She drinks wine occasionally, one or two glasses with dinner. She has smoked cigarettes, a pack per day, since her early twenties. She denies using any illicit substances.

What diagnosis would you consider at this point? Could substance use have an impact on her sexual functioning? Ms. Gonzalez meets the diagnostic criteria for female sexual interest/arousal disorder: she has lost her interest in sex, does not respond to her husband's sexual advances, and has lost genital feelings during intercourse. The exact duration of her dysfunction is not known, but it has been persistent. She has probably also developed female orgasmic disorder lately, possibly as a consequence of her lack of sexual interest/arousal. She is fairly healthy and does not use any illicit substances or medications. Her occasional glass or two of wine would not explain her sexual problems, and her smoking long preceded the development of her sexual dysfunctions. The stress related to her husband's loss of job, possibility of losing their house, and frequent arguments probably contributes to her loss of sexual desire, but probably not to the loss of her sexual feelings.

PART B

> Ms. Gonzalez admits that she became depressed within the past month or so, "because it's really upsetting to me that I do not enjoy sex and am not intimate with my husband. I used to enjoy sex so much." She also admits feeling some pain on her husband's attempts to have sex with her.

Is there any diagnosis of sexual dysfunction to add to the diagnostic consideration on the basis of the presence of pain during intercourse? In addition to this patient's already complex sexual problems, she may be developing sexual pain (genito-pelvic pain/penetration disorder) and has become depressed. Her case demonstrates that several sexual dysfunctions may co-occur or may develop as a consequence of another dysfunction. It also demonstrates the possible role of psychological factors in the development of sexual dysfunctions and the development of psychiatric symptoms (e.g., depression) as a possible consequence of impaired sexual functioning.

Short-Answer Questions

1. How long must any symptoms of impaired sexual function last to meet the diagnostic criteria for sexual dysfunction?
2. Should a diagnosis of sexual dysfunction be made if there is inadequate stimulation during intercourse?
3. What happens to sexual functioning with aging?
4. What are some risk factors for female orgasmic disorder?
5. How soon after vaginal penetration must ejaculation occur to meet the diagnostic criterion of premature (early) ejaculation?
6. Which major psychiatric disorder is probably most frequently associated with diminished or absent sexual interest/desire?
7. Which class of psychotropic medications is most frequently implicated in delayed ejaculation?
8. What are the differences between the previous classification of sexual dysfunctions and the DSM-5 and DSM-5-TR classification regarding gender specificity and the role of the sexual response cycle?
9. True or False: Distress is a necessary criterion for making the diagnosis of sexual dysfunction.

10. What are the new diagnoses of sexual dysfunctions included in DSM-5 and DSM-5-TR?

Answers

1. Any symptoms of impaired sexual function must last 6 months to meet the diagnostic criteria for sexual dysfunction.

2. Sexual dysfunction should not be diagnosed if there is inadequate stimulation during intercourse.

3. With aging, sexual function usually declines, and frequency of sexual impairment increases.

4. Poor physical health, anxiety, depression, and relationship factors are risk factors for female orgasmic disorder.

5. Ejaculation must occur within approximately 1 minute after vaginal penetration to meet the diagnostic criterion of premature (early) ejaculation.

6. Major depressive disorder is probably the most frequent major psychiatric disorder associated with diminished or absent sexual interest/desire.

7. Serotonergic antidepressants are most frequently implicated in delayed ejaculation.

8. The DSM-5 and DSM-5-TR classification is gender specific, and the diagnoses no longer relate to the so-called sexual response cycle.

9. True. Distress is a necessary criterion for diagnosing sexual dysfunction.

10. The diagnoses of female sexual interest/arousal disorder and genito-pelvic pain/penetration disorder are new in DSM-5 and DSM-5-TR.

REFERENCES

American Psychiatric Association: Diagnostic and Statistical Manual of Mental Disorders, 4th Edition. Washington, DC, American Psychiatric Association, 1994

American Psychiatric Association: Diagnostic and Statistical Manual of Mental Disorders, 5th Edition. Arlington, VA, American Psychiatric Association, 2013

American Psychiatric Association: Diagnostic and Statistical Manual of Mental Disorders, 5th Edition, Text Revision. Washington, DC, American Psychiatric Association, 2022

CHAPTER 18

Gender Dysphoria

Daryn Reicherter, M.D.

"I'm transgender."

"I always knew I was really a girl."

"I can't be who I am."

- Gender Dysphoria
  - Gender Dysphoria in Children
  - Gender Dysphoria in Adolescents and Adults
- Other Specified Gender Dysphoria
- Unspecified Gender Dysphoria

Gender is used to describe one's public, sociocultural, lived role as a man, a woman, or another gender. *Gender dysphoria* describes the distress that may accompany an incongruence between the gender assigned at birth and one's experienced gender. The

Adapted from Greaves CC, Reicherter D: "Gender Dysphoria," in *Study Guide to DSM-5*. Edited by Roberts LW, Louie AK. Washington, DC, American Psychiatric Publishing, 2015, pp 317–334.

individual with gender dysphoria has a strong identification with and desire to be part of the social world of the experienced gender. A significant conceptual shift occurred in the diagnostic category of "gender identity disorder" in DSM-IV (American Psychiatric Association 1994) and "gender dysphoria" in DSM-5 (American Psychiatric Association 2013), with DSM-5 emphasizing the symptomatic response as opposed to pathologizing the condition itself, as in DSM-IV. The terminology used in DSM-5-TR (American Psychiatric Association 2022) for gender dysphoria has been updated based on the literature; for example, "natal male"/"natal female" is now "individual assigned male/female at birth" and "desired gender" is now "experienced gender." *Transgender* is not a diagnostic term and simply refers to any individual whose gender is different from the gender assigned at birth. *Cisgender* refers to individuals whose gender aligns with the gender assigned at birth.

The diagnosis of gender dysphoria does not refer to distress related to stigma, although this may be significant. Gender dysphoria and stigma related to gender dysphoria may deeply affect self-concept, identity, family structure, and social adaptation. A great deal of distress, including anxiety, tension, and questions about what is real and who to believe (self or others) can develop around family dynamics, the school environment, interpersonal relationships, and the capacity for intimacy. Not all individuals who experience incongruence between their gender assigned at birth and their experienced gender will be distressed. The inability to access desired gender-affirming medical treatments, such as hormones or surgery, that would align one's physical characteristics with one's experienced gender, may be very distressing, however.

Gender dysphoria tends to manifest differently in different age groups and in the different genders. Prepubertal individuals assigned female at birth who have gender dysphoria characteristically express the wish to be a boy and assert that they are male or that they will grow up to be a man. They may prefer traditional boys' clothing or hairstyles and engage in rough-and-tumble play. They may have very negative reactions to parental attempts to have them wear dresses or to have the physical appearance of a girl. Role-play, dreams, and fantasies are often more consistent with typical male themes. They may express serious concern or disgust with the prospect of developing into mature women. Prepubertal individuals assigned male at birth with gender dysphoria may express the wish to be a girl and assert that they are female or will grow up to be a woman. They may dress in girls' or women's clothes or may improvise feminine clothing. They may role-play as women and may have an intense interest in women fantasy characters. They may prefer traditional girls' toys and games and may be uninterested in or resentful toward traditional boys' toys and games.

In children, the gender dysphoria diagnosis requires that the child have a strong desire to be another gender (what is felt as "natural to who I really am") from the gender assigned at birth—or insistence that they are of another gender. This desire may also occur in adolescents and adults with gender dysphoria but is not required for the diagnosis as it is for children. In addition, the dysphoria is based on clinically significant distress or impairment in social, school, or other important areas of functioning. Distress or impairment can result from pretending to live as a member of the gender assigned at birth, or it may come from the pervasive need to convince other people (e.g., parents, siblings, friends) of the experienced gender—and from dealing with the serious social consequences of rejection, teasing, ridicule, opprobrium, ostracism, contempt, threats, and violence.

In young adolescents with gender dysphoria, clinical features are similar to those of children or adults, usually depending on developmental level. In adolescence, a time of an acute need for peer approval, the awareness of being different is accompanied by substantial alienation, hiding, shame, and/or impairment of identity formation. Younger adolescents may be very distressed by the imminent physical changes of puberty. Older adolescents and adults often, but not always, express a desire to acquire physical attributes associated with their experienced gender and a desire to be rid of physical attributes associated with their gender assigned at birth.

Adults with gender dysphoria may wish to change their physical characteristics to better align their body with their gender and to be viewed by society as their experienced gender. For these individuals, gender-affirming care may include hormonal treatments, hair removal or implantation, facial bone realignment surgeries, and genital, breast, or other plastic surgeries. Older adolescents and adults may, to varying degrees, dress, behave, and act as members of their experienced gender, with or without seeking medical treatment. Individuals may live fully or partially within their experienced gender role or within a neither conventionally male nor conventionally female role.

DSM-5-TR identifies two specific states of gender dysphoria: gender dysphoria in children and gender dysphoria in adolescents and adults. Both diagnoses begin with "a marked incongruence between one's experienced/expressed gender and assigned gender, of at least 6 months' duration." The child and adult variants have different specific criteria but share the common themes of strong identification with the experienced gender, desire to be recognized as the experienced gender, and desire for primary and/or secondary sex characteristics that match one's experienced gender.

Both diagnoses ask for a specification of whether the condition is tied to a physical syndrome (e.g., androgen insensitivity syndrome). DSM-5-TR has changed the wording for this specification to "a disorder/difference of sex development."

DSM-5-TR also identifies two nonspecific diagnostic categories: other specified gender dysphoria and unspecified gender dysphoria. These diagnoses are used when the full diagnostic criteria are not met for the specific disorders, but the major clinical concern is related to the themes contained in the specific diagnoses. See Table 18–1 for key changes between DSM-5 and DSM-5-TR.

The gender dysphoria diagnoses should not be confused with the diagnoses in the DSM-5-TR chapter on paraphilic disorders. For instance, the DSM-5-TR diagnosis of transvestic disorder may be within the differential diagnosis of a gender dysphoria diagnosis; however, transvestic disorder should be easily distinguished diagnostically from any gender dysphoria diagnosis.

The prevalence of gender dysphoria is not known but is estimated to be low (<0.1%).

DSM-IV contained diagnoses very similar to gender dysphoria in the diagnostic class of sexual and gender identity disorders. A specific diagnostic class in DSM-5 and DSM-5-TR is dedicated to gender dysphoria. The gender identity disorders characterized in DSM-IV have very similar features to the gender dysphoria in DSM-5 and DSM-5-TR.

TABLE 18–1. Key changes between DSM-5 and DSM-5-TR

Substantial updates have been made to paragraphs in the "Introduction," "Diagnostic Features," "Associated Features," and "Development and Course" sections.

Additional updates have been made to the "Prevalence," "Risk and Prognostic Factors," and "Culture-Related Diagnostic Issues" sections and the second paragraph of the "Functional Consequences of Gender Dysphoria" section.

"Sex- and Gender-Related Diagnostic Issues," "Diagnostic Markers," and "Association With Suicidal Thoughts or Behaviors" sections have been added.

IN-DEPTH DIAGNOSIS: GENDER DYSPHORIA IN CHILDREN

Jill is a 16-year-old adolescent. Her parents brought her to consultation because they have despaired for several years at her insistence that she is a boy. What they thought would be a passing whim over the years, they now realize is a deeply set conviction. Jill would like to start dressing in boy's attire, begin using a masculine name and pronouns, and pursue masculinizing hormone treatments.

The history reveals that at approximately age 3, Jill began showing a greater interest in playing with her brother's toys rather than girl-typical toys, such as dolls. At age 4 she declared that she was a boy; any attempt of telling her otherwise was met by crying protests. In kindergarten, at age 5, Jill preferred the company of boys, with whom she would engage in competitive body-contact games. At girls' social gatherings, she kept apart, choosing aloneness rather than joining in games and other activities. For school, she insisted on wearing boyish clothes. At around age 7, her favorite movies and television shows involved a young male hero, a boy-centered story, or a medieval knight with whom she would identify.

Jill enjoyed soccer and other sports during late childhood but would feel deeply hurt when a group of boys rejected her as a member of their team on account of her being a girl. By this point she had learned not to overtly declare being a boy, given the experiences of teasing and ridicule that her assertion elicited.

As Jill entered puberty, she found herself isolating more and more. She felt that she did not fit in anywhere, and she was often teased for being "weird." She was distraught at the emergence of her breasts. When her menarche occurred at age 13, she "cried for days," experiencing, for the first time, a 3-month-long depressive episode.

Jill has shown from early life an awareness and conviction that she does not belong to the gender she was assigned at birth. She has consistently preferred to look like and play like a boy and feels very comfortable in typically male roles over female gender roles. She is uncomfortable with her secondary sex characteristics and has become withdrawn and depressed. Jill reports that she is ready to socially and medically transition, but her parents remain concerned.

Approach to the Diagnosis

The diagnosis of gender dysphoria in children should be considered when the clinician is presented with a child patient, usually brought to clinical attention by their parents, who since early age has been experiencing significant distress because of doubts or confusion about the nature of their gender or who carries the unshakable conviction that they belong to a gender other than the one assigned at birth. This doubt or conviction, per se a source of distress, may have in turn brought about alienation within the family structure, affected acceptance among playmates, and disrupted school activities and performance.

Parents and others may perceive this child as "odd," "weird," "strange," "different," "not fitting," and so on, and in reacting to this peculiarity, they may reject, tease, disparage with put-downs, humiliate, or—not infrequently—be violent toward the child. In consequence, the child feels different or alien, developing a concept of the self as deviant, bizarre, damaged, and undesirable. The individual's initial perplexity at others not seeing what is obvious—that a "mistake" was made in the assignation of gender at birth—gives way to despair at the realization that, biologically, they were born with anatomy that does not correspond to their psychological gender construct, deep conviction, and actual subjective experience of their "true" gender identity.

Some individuals are able to disguise this predicament, developing an elaborate "false self" that consumes a great deal of attention and vital energy, while the hidden "real self" is further separated from the outside world. Individuals in this circumstance feel tremendous distress.

It is important to emphasize the shift from the diagnosis of gender identity disorder in DSM-IV to the one of gender dysphoria in DSM-5 and DSM-5-TR. The psychiatric diagnosis is not based solely on the presence of a different gender identity or the wish to be a certain gender but includes the personal distress, the disruption of family life, and the difficulties experienced in the social realm that this particular human variance has brought about to the individual. If, even in the context of a fully accepting environment, the individual still struggles with the paradoxical nature of their existence, the diagnosis of gender dysphoria is made.

The clinician, therefore, needs to focus on the disruptions of identity formation, adaptation to the outside world, successful coping mechanisms or lack thereof, problems of integration into the social milieu, and negative introjects the individual has embraced that would generate self-hatred, depression, anxiety, and poor performance in academic and interpersonal realms.

Getting the History

The following set of questions for parents can help elicit the diagnosis: You are concerned for your child. What have you noticed that is troubling you? For how long has this been going on? What is the first thing you noticed? What sort of clothing does your child prefer to wear? What games, activities, and toys does your child prefer? What happens if you deny the preferred ones and insist on others? Who does your child like to be with for play and companionship? Do you have a sense of the sort of fantasy play in which your child engages? Has your child expressed dislike for their body or genitals? Has your child expressed a desire to be of another gender, or has your child expressed the conviction of belonging to another gender? How troublesome is this for your child? Have you noticed sadness, isolation, nervousness, or any other signs that your child is troubled? How is your child doing at school? Do you have any pertinent information from teachers or other parents? Does your child have friends? What sort of friends? Has there been a change in the way you relate to your child? Has this condition changed the way you think about your child or the degree of closeness you experience?

In eliciting the diagnosis of gender dysphoria in children, the interviewer will be using at least two sources: the parents and child. In examining the young person, besides observing constitution, presentation, mannerisms, ways of expression, movements, speech, and so on, the interviewer can adapt these questions for the young person depending on their age and developmental stage.

The parents will most likely be tense, worried, and fearful about the results of the consultation. They may have postponed arranging the appointment for months, sometimes years, in the hope that the gender-atypical behaviors they have observed—the "tomboyness" or "sissiness," for example—are a "passing phase" or "something our child will outgrow." Only when these behaviors remain consistent over time and are accompanied by the young person's assertions of other-gender wishes do parents become alarmed and seek consultation. Parents may confuse sexual orientation variances with gender variances, which delays consultation and diagnosis.

Information from siblings and peers, as well as from teachers and extended family members, can help clarify the relevance of the diagnosis of gender dysphoria in children. In a diagnosis of such sensitivity as this, the clinician needs to muster as much objectivity, nonjudgmental attitude, understanding, support, and compassion as possible.

Tips for Clarifying the Diagnosis

Consider the diagnosis of gender dysphoria in children:

- The hallmark theme of gender dysphoria in children is a "marked incongruence between one's experienced/expressed gender and assigned gender" that causes distress of dysfunction. This phenomenon must be present for the diagnosis.
- The general description and six of the eight DSM-5-TR criteria must be met to make the diagnosis.
- Diagnostic criteria must be present for at least 6 months.
- Many of the diagnostic criteria involve the strong dislike of the physical attributes of the individual's assigned gender, as well as preferences to behave as members of a different gender.
- Differential diagnostic concepts must be ruled out as better explanations of the observed phenomena. Other variants of nonconformity to gender roles must be considered and ruled out to complete the diagnosis.

Consider the Case

John, the child of Chinese immigrants, is referred at age 14. He felt and exhibited signs of depression for 2 years before consultation. Other than that, his parents describe their young son as "quiet, gentle, and obedient," and they have not observed anything atypical about him. When John entered school at 6 years of age, his teachers noticed his avoidance of the playground and preference for being on his own. While by himself, in school or at home, John would sing to himself, at times dancing, according to his mother. He began to explore his mother's wardrobe around this time, trying out garments and looking at himself in the mirror, or experimenting with her lipstick and other cosmetics.

Any attempts at dissuading him from these behaviors were met with a passive, downcast, deflated attitude, followed by a sullenness lasting a few days. If allowed to do these things, John would be "animated, talkative, and happy." He was not interested in boys' games and toys, but he also was not particularly interested in girls' toys. He liked "colorful fabric, pretty buttons, a needle and scissors, and colorful thread," which he would use to create unique items of clothing. Again, when denied these, he would "go into a funk" that lasted until he got what he wanted.

John reveals to the examiner that he had always doubted whether he was a girl or a boy or something else, "maybe nonbinary," a feeling that he had never revealed to anyone. Now that it is clear to him that he was born as a boy, he wants to be a girl because "I feel like a girl inside. I love girly things. I always imagined myself growing up a girl and maybe dating boys." John is sad that he can never give birth to children. He describes his genitals as "all wrong." For as long as John can remember, he has felt "different," unable to relate to either boys or girls, choosing aloneness rather than risking scorn and rejection.

John's only close friend is another boy who is also questioning his own gender. John has given himself a girl's name that only he knows. John has experienced chronic depression for 2 years, that being the reason he gave his mother to bring him for a psychiatric consultation; he knew that his mother would dismiss his gender issues as "stupid and irrelevant."

John lacks certainty as to his gender: "Am I a boy or a girl? Am I nonbinary?" He leans toward identifying as a girl, and he has given himself a secret girl's name. These deep doubts have been ongoing for several years. John avoids social interaction with peers because he feels he does not fit in and also wants to avoid the hassles that would descend on him were he to show his "real girl self." He experiences a pervasive desire to take on the social roles and external presentation of his desired girl identity; his inability to do so is a source of distress and low mood. John feels that he has a great deal of disconnect and conflict with his parents. He worries that his gender dysphoria would be misconstrued by them somehow as the bad influence of American culture.

Differential Diagnosis

DSM-5-TR describes a typical list of behavioral and diagnostic concepts that should be considered in the differential diagnosis of gender dysphoria. A young person who is nonconforming to stereotypical gender role behavior may reject gender-typical activities and play but have no doubt that their gender matches the one assigned at birth. Their nonconformity will tend to be transitory, shifting as the individual matures or is influenced by peers. Disorders of sex development may or may not be associated with gender dysphoria and need to be ruled out.

An individual with body dysmorphic disorder focuses on the alteration or removal of a specific body part because it is perceived as abnormally formed, not because of any gender-related issue.

Other symptomatology, such as hallucinations, paranoid delusions, and course of illness, would differentiate a patient with schizophrenia or other psychosis—which could include delusions related to gender—from a child with gender dysphoria. In the absence of psychotic symptoms, a child with gender dysphoria is not considered delusional.

DSM-5-TR also includes autism spectrum disorder in the differential diagnosis. Rigid, concrete thoughts around gender roles or poor comprehension of usual social and gender relationships should be differentiated from gender dysphoria. Children may be diagnosed with an autism spectrum disorder and gender dysphoria if criteria for both are met.

See DSM-5-TR for additional disorders to consider in the differential diagnosis. Also refer to the discussions of comorbidity and differential diagnosis in their respective sections of DSM-5-TR.

Summary

- Gender dysphoria is considered as a diagnosis if for at least 6 months a child has had serious doubts about their gender or is convinced and insists that they belong to another gender, resulting in tension, confusion, and general distress.
- A child with gender dysphoria prefers to play, dress, fantasize, seek companionship, and assume roles that are typical for the experienced gender rather than the gender assigned at birth.
- A child with gender dysphoria dislikes their anatomy, particularly their genitals; dreads the emergence of secondary sexual characteristics; and/or wishes for a different body configuration—one that matches the experienced gender.
- Over time, the condition has disrupted the individual's development within the family dynamics, interpersonally, and in the general social world.
- The hallmark theme of gender dysphoria in children is a "marked incongruence between one's experienced/expressed gender and assigned gender" that causes distress or dysfunction.
- Six of the eight criteria must be met to make the diagnosis.
- Many of the diagnostic criteria involve strong preferences to behave as a member of the experienced gender.
- There are significant differences (aside from age) in the typical presentations between gender dysphoria in children and gender dysphoria in adolescents and adults.
- The differential diagnosis must be considered before ruling in gender dysphoria in children.

IN-DEPTH DIAGNOSIS: GENDER DYSPHORIA IN ADOLESCENTS AND ADULTS

Sally is a 38-year-old transgender woman who began hormone replacement therapy a few months before consultation. Sally is the only child of a rural Midwestern, White family. She was assigned male at birth. Until mid-adolescence, other than a distinct yet vague feeling that she was "different," her childhood developed along the lines expected for boys. She was not enthusiastic about sports, preferring intellectual activities and discussions. When she was about 15 years old, an increasing sense of alienation from her body developed, particularly regarding body hair, genitals, voice, and facial features, with a concomitant desire for female attributes.

Sally denied all of this to herself at the time: "I put it aside; it was too much and too complex to deal with. In my neck of the woods, I would have been kicked out of my home, thrashed by others, maybe killed." Sally felt attracted to women. After a couple of short-lived affairs with girlfriends, she fell in love with a college friend, marrying her just after graduation. Sally and her wife have three children, a boy and two girls. Sally completed a master's degree in business and got a good job. When alone at home, she wears her wife's clothing and cosmetics. Sally imagines herself as a woman, feeling a "huge relief" from the permanent tension she experiences at the growing realization that she is "authentically, a woman." Sally feels that in denying her early sense of being female, she deeply betrayed herself and her "true nature."

Although professionally successful and happy to be a parent, Sally is otherwise quite dysphoric, feeling constant tension, depressive feelings, serious anxiety, increasing difficulty with sexual performance, and despairing as to what to do. Soon after the birth of their third child, Sally had announced to her wife, who by now knew about her dysphoria and its origin, that she intended to socially and medically transition to the female gender. "I just could not handle it any longer; when suicidal thoughts entered my mind, I knew it was time to act."

Sally's awareness of being alienated from her assigned gender emerged after puberty and manifested at first by dislike for her male physical attributes; later by the desire to dress up, use cosmetics, and be a woman in private; and eventually, by a desire to medically transition. She is married and subjectively experiences herself not as her wife's male counterpart but as a kindred entity, physically, emotionally, and spiritually. Her children have known her as "Dad," but she has explained to them that she "always felt like a girl inside and is now becoming a girl outside too," and they seem enthusiastic about the prospect of having two moms.

Sally is happy that she is pursuing her "true gender" but remains worried about the implications that her transition will have on her marriage, parenthood, family of origin, friendships, and social and work environments. She knows that she is making the right decision because her suicidal ideation and depressive symptoms have been greatly reduced.

Approach to the Diagnosis

With an adolescent or young adult, usually the parents seek consultation. They may be concerned about the recent (or longer) development of symptoms of unease, withdrawal, depression, isolation, tension, and stress in their adolescent or young adult, or they may complain about acting-out behaviors, with the possible use of alcohol or illicit drugs. The parents may have noticed disruptions in their child's socializing with friends, excessive use of the computer, sullenness, and poor communication, with angry responses or evasion.

The adolescent may or may not have revealed that they are questioning their gender. A parent may have discovered internet searches on a computer or found clothing, books, magazines, and so on that tip them off that there is something "different" concerning their child's gender. The adolescent or young adult, once they are able to trust the clinician, may request that what is disclosed be kept confidential from their parents.

The adolescent will likely disclose a deeply felt dislike for their anatomy, secondary sex characteristics, and the roles and social expectations associated with the assigned gender at birth; they may hold the conviction that they must express their experienced gender. Some adolescents may vehemently insist that they must begin living as their experienced gender and/or begin pursuing gender-affirming medical care so as to avoid further traits, physical and social, of belonging to the assigned gender. They may greatly worry about what seems an impossibly difficult and costly process, which without parental support will be unattainable for "who knows how many years!"

Adults are typically self-referred. After explaining their gender dysphoria, the duration, the development, and their difficulties with their experience, some will ask for counsel on how to proceed with the transition process; for support for the completion of a course of action they have already decided on; or for help in dealing with how to adapt to and process the posttransition realities. Some may be uninterested in either supportive or insight-oriented psychotherapy and instead ask for a formal diagnosis in order to meet criteria for gender-affirming medical care.

As stated in DSM-5-TR, "Prior to receiving gender-affirming treatment and legal gender reassignment, adolescents and adults with gender dysphoria are at increased risk for suicidal thoughts and suicide attempts" (p. 518). Risk factors for suicidality also include a history of mistreatment or gender victimization, depression, substance use, and younger age.

Getting the History

> Sam, a 30-year-old man, presents for evaluation of "some mild depression." He is dressed in baggy men's clothing. The name on his medical chart is listed as Sarah. He quickly clarifies that he is transgender and is in the process of legally changing his name and gender marker. He reports that he is also awaiting "top surgery" to remove his breasts and masculinize his chest.
>
> Although the stated purpose of the visit is depression, he begins by explaining the gender issue that seems to be the context around his mood symptoms. He describes a long history of incongruence between his experienced gender and his assigned gender, beginning in childhood. He clearly describes distress as a result throughout his life. These gender issues have led to significant interpersonal stressors. He reports having grown up in a strictly religious family in which his gender issue was ignored or met with disdain.
>
> The interviewer asks about his transition: "How do you like to be addressed? Your stated name is different from the name in your medical (legal) chart." Sam laughs at the question, initially. Then he responds, "I have been living as a man for years now. I am in the process of getting all this worked out 'technically.' Once I legally change my name to Sam and have surgery, hopefully there won't be any more confusion. Please call me Sam."

This case clearly fits the themes in the diagnosis of gender dysphoria in adolescents and adults. The key features are clear. Sam meets at least two of the six criteria and has for 6 months or more. Social dysfunction and distress have been present for Sam for many years.

This case not only meets criteria for the diagnosis but also meets the stated criteria for the specifier "posttransition." Sam is preparing to undergo a gender-affirming medical procedure and has lived as a man for years, per the history.

With adults, a cohesive, processed, and integrated picture will most likely be offered without much questioning. Once the individual's gender-related issues are revealed and the concomitant dysphoria elucidated, the examiner ought to address the differential diagnosis and refine an understanding of the peculiarities and uniqueness of this person's experience and situation.

Getting the history from an adolescent may require more finesse. The following are examples of helpful comments: "I am here to understand and help you, not to judge you"; "Whoever you are or want to be is fine, as long as you don't hurt yourself or others"; "I realize you have been going through a great deal; let us work together to understand what is happening to you and to alleviate your distress." Questions about the actual phenomena the youth is experiencing internally and externally are important: "What is it that you feel you are? For how long has this been so? What are the things you'd like to do if you were free to do as you wish? How would you like to dress? What kind of person would you like others to see you as, and how do you want to come across to others? How do you feel about your body?"

Once answers to these and similar questions have been ascertained, a more in-depth set of questions involving the youth's hoped-for world can provide valuable diagnostic information: "How do you imagine yourself to be? What sort of images of yourself seem right and fitting for you? How are you pictured in your dreams? How would you like to be, say, 5 or 10 years from now? Describe for me the type of body you would like to have. How do you imagine your life would be if you were to change your gender? What do you imagine the reaction would be to that change from your family, your friends, and society? How does all of this make you feel: good, bad, happy, sad, scared, frustrated, angry, anxious? Have you entertained suicidal thoughts? What is going on now between you and your friends? How does your situation fit with your values, religious teachings, principles, and ideal vision of yourself? What name would you like me to call you? Is there anything I have not asked you about that is important to you?"

Tips for Clarifying the Diagnosis

For a diagnosis of gender dysphoria in adolescents and adults, the individual must

- Have a consistent, persevering conviction of belonging to the experienced gender.
- Dislike or be averse to the external identifiers of their assigned gender, which may or may not include a wish for a change in genital anatomy.
- Wish for the social role of the experienced gender and wish to be seen, thought of, and reacted to as a member of the experienced gender.
- Experiment with clothing and accessories generally attributed to the experienced gender.
- Experience significant stress, tension, anxiety, depression, or anger and disturbances of family, intimate, and social relationships. Their academic or work performance may or may not be affected.

Consider the Case

Ron was 60 years old when they came for consultation. They remember their mother saying to them at some point in early childhood that she wished they had been a girl. Ron thought of themself as having been a "sissy boy" who later, in adolescence, was able to "man up": "my older brothers taught me to be tough." The softer, more sensitive inner self of their childhood was masked, finding expression in poetry and music. Ron went through high school and college feeling, acting, and being accepted as any other young man on campus.

Ron began experimenting with gender in their forties: "exploring the woman in me; caring for my hair and nails; paying attention to the detail of my clothing; dressing as a woman for Halloween parties and, in regular parties, hanging out with women's groups, cooking, arranging flowers."

Soon after, gender dysphoria began to bother them. They began dressing up from time to time, using makeup, wearing wigs, and "acting like Bette Davis or Marilyn Monroe." They state that "gender has always been a great performance" and that masculinity and femininity feel equally "theatrical" to them.

They found their partner through internet dating, a 65-year-old cisgender woman who prefers to wear men's attire. "We are a good match because we have a great appreciation for one another's style and flair."

For Ron, the revelation of gender nonconformity occurred at a mature age. Their sense of femininity overwhelmed their previous male identification, at which point they began to experience gender dysphoria. This late onset of gender dysphoria is uncommon. Ron identifies as nonbinary and as having a more "fluid" gender, but they are interested in discussing gender-affirming medical care and whether this might be helpful for them and their experience of gender dysphoria.

Ron does not meet the criteria for transvestic disorder because they do not use cross-dressing for sexual excitement and their sexual arousal does not depend on certain clothing.

Differential Diagnosis

For adolescents and adults, several possibilities on the differential diagnosis should be considered and ruled out before diagnosing gender dysphoria. A gender nonconforming individual may feel disturbed, angry, contemptuous, disaffected, and critical of the roles culture and society impose on either gender, but have no desire to be a different gender from the one assigned at birth and feel no alienation from their anatomy or current external gender traits.

Transvestic disorder describes a distressing or impairing pattern of cross-dressing for the sake of sexual arousal among individuals who are otherwise perfectly content with their gender and anatomy.

Body dysmorphic disorder is characterized by an individual's focus on the alteration or removal of a specific body part because it is perceived as abnormally formed, not because it represents a particular gender.

Schizophrenia and other psychotic disorders, as well as OCD, are considered part of the differential diagnosis. Some personality disorders can manifest with gender themes but should be distinguishable from gender dysphoria.

Some deeply homophobic individuals may entertain the idea of changing genders in order to avoid rejection or shame associated with being gay or lesbian. Changing genders could provide sanction from family or religion for the now heterosexual orientation. This wish does not reflect a pervasive sense or conviction of belonging to a gender that is different from the one assigned at birth.

Autism spectrum disorder may be associated with rigid, concrete thoughts regarding gender roles or poor understanding of social relationships.

Some adults enjoy cross-dressing and assuming the roles of another gender for the purposes of entertainment, leisure, or plain fun (e.g., "drag queens and kings") without any desire to change the gender assigned at birth.

Other clinical presentations include, for example, males who seek castration or penectomy for aesthetic reasons or to remove the psychological effects of androgens, without changing male identity or gender; these presentations do not meet criteria for gender dysphoria.

See DSM-5-TR for additional disorders to consider in the differential diagnosis. Also refer to the discussions of comorbidity and differential diagnosis in their respective sections of DSM-5-TR.

Summary

- The hallmark theme of gender dysphoria in adolescents and adults is a "marked incongruence between one's experienced/expressed gender and assigned gender" that causes distress or dysfunction.
- An adolescent or adult with gender dysphoria consistently experiences the certainty of belonging to a gender other than the one assigned at birth.
- This desire is accompanied by dislike of or aversion to one's own body, with a desire to have the body and attributes of the experienced gender, including or not including genital anatomy.
- There is an attraction for and desire to experience life as a member of the experienced gender, to be seen and acknowledged as such, and to be treated accordingly.
- The gender dysphoria results in great pressure, tension, mood changes, anxiety, discomfort, and alterations in the interpersonal sphere of the person.
- A great deal of time and energy is spent in fantasizing how life would be if lived as the experienced gender, bringing a sense of completion and fulfillment to the person.

SUMMARY: GENDER DYSPHORIA

The diagnosis of gender dysphoria is applicable when an individual has clinically relevant distress as the result of a pervasive sense or conviction that they are the member of a gender that is different from the one assigned at birth. As a result, the person must have been experiencing, for at least 6 months, a few or several of the following symptoms: distress, anxiety, tension, affective disturbances, alteration in family dynamics, personal doubts and confusion, alienation from others, and disruptions in school, work, or social settings in general.

These individuals may have a subjective certainty that something went amiss in their biological development, resulting in their being born in a body that does not fit the gender to which they know they belong. This predicament creates, in an individual, an intense desire to "fix what is wrong"—thus, in children, to play, dress, and be with those of their desired gender; in adolescents and adults, to get rid of any observable traits that would identify them, to themselves and others, as belonging to the gender assigned at birth, and to live, work, socialize, be intimate, and find fulfillment in life as a member of the experienced gender later in adulthood.

Transgender individuals inevitably face obstacles in life, not necessarily because of their identity, per se, but because of stigma, ignorance, and interpersonal violence within society. In childhood, obstacles may include difficulties surrounding naturally chosen play, companionship, and dress. Later, in adolescence and adulthood, obstacles may include redefinitions of self-concept, bodily configuration, and family and peer structures; having to master social expectations; building compensations for the shame of disapproval, hostility, or rejection; and creating an effective masking to achieve survival.

Parents, family, friends, and acquaintances may experience a symptomatic response to witnessing their loved one transition, either because of empathy, sympathy, compassion, opposition, fear, rejection, confusion, violence, ignorance, or anticipated financial challenges.

ELEMENTS TO CONSIDER IN THE CULTURAL FORMULATION

- Transgender persons are observed in many different cultures the world over. The cultural reaction to transgender people can widely vary.
- Some cultures approach gender diversity with stigma and shame, whereas others may have less of a negative reaction.
- Some cultures sanction gender nonconformity—and it is unclear whether the diagnosis of gender dysphoria would have meaning in this context.
- It is unclear whether the diagnosis of gender dysphoria exists at all or at a different prevalence rate in cultures that have less negative stigma toward transgender people.

DIAGNOSTIC PEARLS

- Gender dysphoria is the distress from an experienced disconnect between an individual's assigned gender at birth and experienced gender.
- Gender dysphoria is not a sexual dysfunction or paraphilic disorder.

- The key characteristics of gender dysphoria center around the distress caused by the incongruence between the person's experienced/expressed gender and their assigned gender.
- Because features may manifest differently in various stages of development, DSM-5-TR has two distinct diagnostic criteria sets: gender dysphoria in children and gender dysphoria in adolescents and adults.
- Gender dysphoria must be present for more than 6 months, but in most cases this time criterion will be easily met because the experience tends to be chronic.
- Gender dysphoria diagnoses have qualifiers that inform whether a physical or medical issue is related to the diagnosis. DSM-5-TR asks clinicians to clarify whether the gender dysphoria is associated with "a disorder/difference of sex development." This specifier may be important in the formulation of an individual overall.
- The hallmark theme of gender dysphoria in children is a "marked incongruence between one's experienced/expressed gender and assigned gender" that causes distress or dysfunction. This phenomenon must be present for the diagnosis.
- Many of the diagnostic criteria for children involve the strong dislike of the physical attributes of the child's assigned gender, as well as preferences to behave as members of a gender that is not the assigned gender.
- Gender dysphoria in adults generally involves a consistent conviction of belonging to the experienced gender; a dislike or aversion to the external identifiers of the assigned gender (which may or may not include anatomy); a wish for the social role of the experienced gender; and a wish to be perceived, thought of, and reacted to as a member of the experienced gender.
- Gender dysphoria may result in significant stress, tension, anxiety, depression, or anger, as well as disturbances of family, intimate, or social relationships.
- Other variants of nonconformity to gender roles must be considered and ruled out.

SELF-ASSESSMENT

Key Concepts: Double-Check Your Knowledge

What is the relevance of the following concepts to gender dysphoria?

- Distress caused by experienced gender incongruence
- Difference between assigned gender and experienced gender
- Lack of relationship to sexual dysfunctions or paraphilic disorders
- Different presentation in various stages of development
- Distinct diagnostic criteria sets for children and for adolescents and adults
- Duration of at least 6 months
- Medical specifier in the overall formulation

Questions to Discuss With Colleagues and Mentors

1. What is the relationship of societal views regarding gender identity to the manifestations of gender dysphoria? Would there be such a thing as gender dysphoria if society ascribed equal value to all forms of gender expression?
2. How do we understand the fact that there are many forms of gender expression?
3. Can there be gender dysphoria in individuals who do not question the gender they were assigned at birth? Do other forms of dysphoria relate to gender?
4. If a child clearly has an atypical gender identity and is nonconformist regarding their gender role, what factors should the clinician consider before diagnosing gender dysphoria in the child?
5. How should gender be defined and referred to in a person with a diagnosis of gender dysphoria?
6. Why is it important to consider suicidality when working with gender dysphoria? Especially early in a patient's gender transition?
7. Should the presence of a "disorder/difference of sex development" influence the way in which a case of gender dysphoria is handled clinically? If yes, why? If no, why not?

Case-Based Questions

PART A

Maria was assigned the female gender at birth; she is the third child of a West Coast, upper-middle-class family. Her father, an engineer, came from the Midwest; her mother's family, originally from Mexico, has been in the United States for four generations. Neither family was religiously inclined. At the time of her birth, Maria's two older sisters were ages 5 and 7, her father was 45, and her mother was 39. Postpartum complications and age made her mother unable to bear any more children.

Since her earliest recollections Maria thought of herself as different from other children and her sisters. She was active, curious, and willful, whereas her sisters were more easygoing. In kindergarten she preferred to play "boy games" with the boys, rejecting the company and play toys of the girls. At home she was given the toys she preferred: cars, trains, and cowboy hats and boots. Wishing to differentiate herself from her sisters, Maria favored masculine attire, which her parents indulged because they found it "cute and different."

On the basis of the information given so far, can the diagnosis of gender dysphoria be made?   No. Although some information is consistent with a theme of gender dysphoria, full criteria have not been met in the information given.

PART B

In later childhood, Maria engaged in rough play with boys in her neighborhood and at school, and she began to assert with increasing vehemence that she was a boy. These assertions were met with dismissive smiles from her parents and close family members, but at school she was ridiculed. During puberty and early adolescence, at her insistence, Maria was allowed to dress as a boy at home and began to use a boy's name, Marcus, which became her "nickname" among intimates. She also began to wear boyish clothing to school. She dreaded and eventually hated her breasts, using compression garments to hide them; her menarche was a great disappointment.

She learned about transgender identities and gender-affirming treatments through the internet, and she began to correspond with other youths experiencing similar predicaments. She expressed the desire to medically transition and was eager for the secondary sex characteristics of maleness. Her parents did not oppose this wish but asked her to wait "so that you are sure this is really what you want."

At age 16, Marcus insisted everyone call him by his male name and male pronouns, and, with parental sanction, began androgenic hormone treatments. At age 17, he underwent surgical breast reduction. He began developing facial and body hair, and his voice deepened considerably.

Marcus had fully transitioned to the male gender by the time he went to college. There he played sports on the men's teams. He avoided locker rooms but used men's bathrooms, adducing "pee shyness" to justify his avoidance of urinals. Academic difficulties led Marcus to drop out of college; his parents helped him financially through a few years of various jobs. At age 24, he applied to and was accepted into the fire department of a major West Coast city. By the time of consultation, at age 32, Marcus had been a firefighter for 8 years.

After Marcus became comfortable with his life as a man, did he meet criteria for gender dysphoria? No. Marcus is living happily (without distress or dysfunction) as a transgender individual.

SHORT-ANSWER QUESTIONS

1. What is gender dysphoria?
2. What are the separate criteria sets of gender dysphoria?
3. What are the key features of gender dysphoria in children?
4. What are the key features of gender dysphoria in adolescents and adults?
5. What is meant by "hormone treatments" in this context?
6. What is the minimum necessary duration of symptoms for the diagnosis of gender dysphoria?
7. What are important attitudes in the examiner?
8. If a child assigned male at birth identifies as a girl but does not experience any dysfunction or distress, should gender dysphoria be diagnosed?
9. What is the prevalence of gender dysphoria?
10. What is the differential diagnosis for gender dysphoria in adolescents and adults?

ANSWERS

1. *Gender dysphoria* refers to a complex set of symptoms that result when an individual experiences their gender identity to be at odds with the gender assigned at birth.

2. The separate criteria sets of gender dysphoria are gender dysphoria in children and gender dysphoria in adolescents and adults.

3. Key features of gender dysphoria in children are a consistent pattern of preferring the play toys, attire, company, games, make-believe fantasies, and activities that are typical of a gender other than the one assigned at birth. The sense of belonging to another gender, the feeling of being in the wrong body, the dreading of the external bodily attributes of the assigned gender, and the wish for the primary and/or secondary sex characteristics of the desired gender bring about gender dysphoria symptoms.

4. Key features of gender dysphoria in adolescents and adults include a pervasive conviction that they are a member of another gender from the one assigned at birth; a strong desire to get rid of the primary and/or secondary sex characteristics of the birth gender; a strong desire to possess the primary and/or secondary sex characteristics of the desired gender; a subjective sense that their thoughts and feelings are similar to those of the desired gender; and a wish to be seen and treated as typically expected for a member of the desired gender.

5. Hormone treatments involve the administration of either estrogenic or androgenic hormones to achieve a feminization or masculinization of the individual.

6. Six months is the minimum necessary duration of symptoms for the diagnosis of gender dysphoria.

7. The examiner adapts to the age of the patient and exudes attitudes of warmth, understanding, acceptance, empathy, lack of judgment, openness, support, and encouragement.

8. No. Gender dysphoria should not be diagnosed in a child who does not experience any dysfunction or distress.

9. The prevalence of gender dysphoria is less than 0.1%.

10. The differential diagnosis for gender dysphoria in adolescents and adults includes nonconformity to gender roles, transvestic disorder, body dysmorphic disorder, schizophrenia and other psychotic disorders, autism spectrum disorder, and other clinical presentations.

REFERENCES

American Psychiatric Association: Diagnostic and Statistical Manual of Mental Disorders, 4th Edition. Washington, DC, American Psychiatric Association, 1994

American Psychiatric Association: Diagnostic and Statistical Manual of Mental Disorders, 5th Edition. Arlington, VA, American Psychiatric Association, 2013

American Psychiatric Association: Diagnostic and Statistical Manual of Mental Disorders, 5th Edition, Text Revision. Washington, DC, American Psychiatric Association, 2022

CHAPTER 19

Disruptive, Impulse-Control, and Conduct Disorders

Whitney Daniels, M.D.

"He just explodes."

"It seems he always has to do exactly the opposite of what I tell him."

- Oppositional Defiant Disorder
- Intermittent Explosive Disorder
- Conduct Disorder
- Antisocial Personality Disorder
- Pyromania
- Kleptomania
- Other Specified Disruptive, Impulse-Control, and Conduct Disorder
- Unspecified Disruptive, Impulse-Control, and Conduct Disorder

Adapted from Daniels W, Steiner H: "Disruptive, Impulse-Control, and Conduct Disorders," in *Study Guide to DSM-5*. Edited by Roberts LW, Louie AK. Washington, DC, American Psychiatric Publishing, 2015, pp 335–348.

The disruptive, impulse-control, and conduct disorders are grouped together in DSM-5-TR (American Psychiatric Association 2022) and include the following: oppositional defiant disorder (ODD); intermittent explosive disorder (IED); conduct disorder; antisocial personality disorder; pyromania; kleptomania; other specified disruptive, impulse-control, and conduct disorder; and unspecified disruptive, impulse-control, and conduct disorder. The core feature of these conditions is persistent dissocial patterns of behavior apparent across a variety of developmental stages. The diagnostic criteria for these disorders have undergone only relatively minor changes with regard to time and age requirements of certain diagnoses.

In assessing individuals to clarify the presence of a diagnosis, a thorough history, including details about symptoms, timing, and age, is highly important. In addition, collateral historical information is imperative to fully grasp the nature of the symptoms, their presentation, and the contribution of the symptoms to the level of dysfunction for the individual.

DSM-5 (American Psychiatric Association 2013) made great strides to group these disorders under one classification, with great considerations for shared domains of several specific disorders. Some explicit purposes of DSM-5-TR were to specify, through text revisions, additional research evidence to support diagnoses, as well as to identify and highlight racial, ethnic, and cultural considerations in relation to a variety of diagnoses (see Table 19–1). Within this classification of DSM-5-TR, much of the evidence has remained unchanged since DSM-5's publication.

This chapter focuses in-depth on the disorders ODD and IED:

- ODD involves a persistent pattern of aggression, irritability, and anger, coupled with defiant and vindictive behaviors. This disorder typically manifests before adolescence but in some cases can manifest later. One of the keys to this disorder is the presence of symptoms that exceed what is normative for the age range. In the approach to a possible diagnosis of ODD, taking a thorough history—including gathering of collateral information—is of uppermost importance. Clinicians assessing for this diagnosis should inquire about symptoms that are pervasive across multiple settings and environments, although symptoms need only occur in one setting to meet criteria for the diagnosis.
- IED is characterized by recurrent behavioral outbursts during which the individual does not control their aggressive impulses. These recurrent behavioral outbursts are beyond what might be expected for the stimulus.

IN-DEPTH DIAGNOSIS: OPPOSITIONAL DEFIANT DISORDER

The mother of Adam, a 7-year-old boy, brings him to a suburban outpatient clinic for evaluation and possible treatment because of disruptive behavior at school. Adam's mother is a single mother of four children (ages 2–15 years), works full-time outside the home, and reports that she is seeking help because she feels as though Adam's behavior has become unmanageable at home and is beginning to manifest at school. His mother reports excessive arguments at home between Adam and his siblings, both younger

TABLE 19–1. Key changes between DSM-5 and DSM-5-TR

Adjustment disorder and PTSD have both been added to the list of differential diagnoses for oppositional defiant disorder.

Relevant statistics have been added for intermittent explosive disorder's racial, ethnic, and cultural prevalence.

and older; Adam often talks back and does not follow rules at home or school. His mother recalls that he has been the most challenging to manage of her children, starting when he was between ages 3 years and 4 years. She felt the immediate need to seek assistance when the school notified her because security guards had been called for the second time in 3 weeks in response to Adam's behavior. The most recent incident involved Adam climbing onto the roof of one of the school buildings and taunting the teachers and security guard as they tried to get him to come down safely. He reports that he climbed up there because he thought hiding from his teacher was fun, and because she deserved it and he did not care if he got in trouble.

Adam's case is a very common presentation of ODD: a young child with long-standing behavioral concerns noted across multiple settings. It is most typical that the child's behavior is tolerated by the parent(s) at home from a very young age and is met with discord when the child attends school and has difficulty with peers, figures of authority, and following the rules. In addition to better understanding Adam's home environment, it is important to screen for any other disorders that may have a similar presentation or a high risk of comorbidity, such as mood disorders or ADHD.

Approach to the Diagnosis

When approaching the diagnosis of ODD, the clinician needs to consider the criteria for this and other disorders very carefully. As just mentioned, one of the most critical parts of the ODD diagnosis is ruling out other diagnoses such as a mood disorder or ADHD. A clinician should understand the age of the child and their current developmental stage, consider the complaint from the parents, and corroborate the information in a collaborative approach, working with the parents to contact other caregivers, teachers, and school officials if possible. Outside information may provide insight into recent environmental or relationship changes for the child.

Once the child's context is clearly understood, the clinician can begin to align confirmed symptoms with assigned criteria to determine if they corroborate the diagnosis. Isolating the single diagnosis of ODD can be difficult, given that this diagnosis is often accompanied by what are referred to as "internalizing" and "externalizing" symptoms. DSM-5-TR has attempted to address this difficulty by outlining categories under Criterion A to guide clinicians in assessing the presence of angry/irritable mood, argumentative/defiant behavior, and level of vindictiveness, if appropriate.

The DSM-5-TR criteria are specific in that the pattern of behavior needs to be persistent and have a particular frequency, based on whether the child is younger than 5, or age 5 or older. If the child is younger than 5, the behavior is required to be persistent on "most days" for at least 6 months. If the child is age 5 or older, the behavior must occur at least once per week for at least 6 months. Thorough understanding of the nature and number of settings where the behavior is observed will provide severity classification of the disorder as mild, moderate, or severe.

As stated in DSM-5-TR, "oppositional defiant disorder has been associated with increased risk for suicide attempts, even after comorbid disorders are controlled for" (p. 524).

Getting the History

> A mother comes to the clinic with Michael, her 9-year-old son, just before the New Year's holiday, concerned that he will not behave well and "will ruin everybody's vacation by being bad." She goes on to report that she has done some of her own research online at home, and she found some websites about children who have ODD who "sound exactly like him." The interviewer then asks the mother to share more about what she has read that fits what she has experienced with her son. The mother reports that since his third birthday, Michael "has broken every rule possible." She describes symptoms such as irritability, teasing others ("to the point where it really is awful and he won't stop!"), blaming his sister "for everything," being "cranky all the time," and not going to bed in the evenings even when reminded several times.
>
> The interviewer then attempts to obtain an accurate time frame of the symptoms: "You mentioned that you feel as if this difficulty started around his third birthday. Do you feel as if these symptoms that you just mentioned have happened since before the start of this school year, perhaps in the summer?" The mother replies, "Absolutely!" The interviewer then asks for data regarding frequency: "How often does he get in trouble because of not following the rules? Is it every day after school? Is it mostly on the weekends? What do you think?" The mother replies, "I feel as if I'm taking his video games away almost every day now." The examiner continues, "How often do you hear feedback from the teacher?" The mother responds, "Well, now the teacher has taken to sending me a weekly email about Michael's behavior because it is so frequent that he is arguing with one of his friends or getting a referral to the principal's office."
>
> The interviewer continues to determine if any recent environmental or social changes have occurred for Michael and also elicits his academic and medical history.

Michael's case represents a very typical presentation of ODD, when the parent has observed a child's defiant behaviors from a very young age and is prompted to seek assistance when the child's academic and social function have become impaired. It is very common for a parent to present having previously "diagnosed" the child via websites. It is the interviewer's responsibility to clarify the symptoms and take a thorough history. The interviewer first determines that Michael has more than the required number (four) from Criterion A. The interviewer then verifies the temporal pattern. Parents often feel as though their child has "always been like this" and have difficulty specifying exact time intervals. Typically, providing a time frame for parents or children as benchmarks in their memory can help elicit a more distinctive temporal history. To further understand the frequency, the interviewer asks about the number of times the child has been disciplined not only at home but also at school. This line of inquiry provides salient information, covering more than just frequency. Additional information to acquire is whether this behavior is observed by others at school, affects the child socially, and ultimately occurs at least once weekly. As always, the context of the child should be examined, and any medical diagnosis that may be contributing to the child's presentation should be ruled out.

Tips for Clarifying the Diagnosis

- Clarify that the child has at least four symptoms from these three categories: angry/irritable mood, argumentative/defiant behavior, and vindictiveness.
- Be very clear on the persistence and frequency based on the age of the child (i.e., younger than 5, or 5 or older).
- Understand the level of dysfunction and disruption for the child that is causing impairment.
- Consider whether the behavior may be accounted for by any other disorder, and verify that it does not occur exclusively during the course of another disorder.

Consider the Case

Tina is a 5-year-old girl whose parents have brought her to the clinic for assistance with her behavior at home. Her mother, father, and stepfather report that they have recently caught her lying more, cheating at family board games, and fighting and arguing with her older sister. Her teachers have sent reports home about similar behavior happening at school and during her after-school program. Tina has a few friends at school, but her parents have witnessed her threatening and bullying her friends when they do not play games she wants to play or play according to her rules. Her mother recalls noticing this behavior worsening since Tina was 3 years old, when Tina had difficulty following directions. She recently has become more irritable. She has always been known to be fidgety and has never been known to remain seated to complete homework or leisure activities at home. Tina refuses to do her homework, among other tasks that she is asked to complete both at home and at school, and feels as though she is always getting in trouble for situations that are not her fault.

Tina's parents are bringing her in for care at a younger age than would typically be expected. Tina is apparently experiencing complex symptoms that relate to two diagnoses, ODD and ADHD. At times, children who have difficulty following instructions or seem as though they are not listening may appear to be defiant. In Tina's case, she has displayed symptoms across diverse settings—that is, at home, at school, and in after-school care. Tina has been defiant despite identifying that she has heard and understands instructions, and she frequently blames her behavior on others. In addition, she has had difficulties with friendships, not only blaming her friends for her argumentative behavior but also forcing them to play in certain ways, cheating on games, and planning schemes with ill outcomes toward her friends and sister. Tina's history is also suggestive of ADHD, given that she is described as fidgety, having difficulty sitting still, impulsive, and appearing to not listen at times. Questions that might confirm a comorbid diagnosis of ADHD include whether Tina frequently loses things, forgets instructions and activities, or has difficulty waiting for her turn.

Differential Diagnosis

The differential diagnosis for ODD includes conditions such as conduct disorder, ADHD, depressive and bipolar disorders, IED, disruptive mood dysregulation disorder, language disorder, intellectual developmental disorder (intellectual disability), or social anxiety disorder. ODD and ADHD often co-occur. Clinicians should rely on the characterization of symptoms, including the timing and setting, to establish whether criteria have been met. It is important to define the age at onset, contextual presence, and temporal relationship of symptoms, including examination of a continual nature versus intermittent. Disruptive behavior noted with ADHD is a result of the inattention and impulsivity of the disorder and thus should not be considered a diagnosis of co-occurring ODD unless it is clear that the criteria for both diagnoses have been met. Furthermore, if an individual resists completing tasks, it should be made clear that the tasks do not demand sustained attention and effort, which would be more indicative of an ADHD diagnosis.

ODD is best differentiated from conduct disorder by the impulsivity of mood and irritability that is characteristic of ODD. Conduct disorder is more severe in that it also includes the criteria of aggression toward people or animals, destruction of property, or a pattern of theft or deceit. It is also possible to observe the manifestation of aggression or irritability in the context of a depressive disorder or episode. The time frame of disruptive behavior may help in discerning the correct diagnosis or diagnoses. Furthermore, the irritability manifested in ODD is characterized by defiant behavior and possible vindictive behavior. To further identify the presence of a distinct mood episode or mood disorder, a clinician would rely on the required neurovegetative criteria met for a mood episode, in addition to the differences in required time intervals.

See DSM-5-TR for additional disorders to consider in the differential diagnosis. Also refer to the discussions of comorbidity and differential diagnosis in their respective sections of DSM-5-TR.

Summary

- ODD is characterized by the presence of persistent, nonepisodic patterns of angry/irritable mood, defiant behavior, or vindictiveness for at least 6 months.
- The presence of oppositional behavior creates a significant disruption in a variety of settings, such as school and home.
- The severity of ODD can be specified as mild, moderate, or severe, depending on the number of settings in which behaviors occur.
- The diagnosis of ODD requires that other diagnoses in this class be ruled out, as well as medical and neurodevelopmental disorders.

IN-DEPTH DIAGNOSIS: INTERMITTENT EXPLOSIVE DISORDER

Mr. Peters is a 28-year-old software engineer who presents at the request of a recent court order for mandatory anger management treatment. He reports that he was charged with domestic violence after a physical altercation with his wife of 2 years. He endorses a distant history of school expulsion on two separate occasions in middle school and high school, each for a physical fight. He reports that as a young boy he witnessed a significant degree of domestic violence between his parents, who both had alcoholism. He feels that over the years he has been able to control his anger and his rage, except every now and then when it has become more difficult and resulted in mild to moderate destruction of his own property. On further examination, Mr. Peters expresses an overwhelming amount of guilt and shame about his outbursts, reporting that he knows his anger is often not warranted. He says he loves his wife more than himself, and he recognizes that the punishment he inflicts on her does not fit the "crime." He is now fearful of the dissolution of his marriage and the loss of his job and benefits.

IED is characterized by repeated serious outbursts and aggressiveness that are grossly out of proportion to the situation or to known precipitants. The outbursts are impulsive and not calculating or premeditated. They are very upsetting to the individual and to others who are affected or who witness them. IED is not caused by another disorder or condition, for example, the expansiveness or irritability seen in bipolar disorder or the behavioral dysregulation after a head injury.

It is not uncommon for an individual with IED to present for treatment long after symptoms have started and as the consequences of behavioral problems have accumulated. IED often is most evident at a stage in life when social, vocational, or occupational demands are placed on an individual. For Mr. Peters, the disorder manifested itself most distinctly and jarringly in the threat of dissolution of his marriage and occupation. Mr. Peters's report regarding his childhood is relevant to the diagnosis. He recalls school expulsion on more than one occasion spanning between middle and high school, indicating a likely adolescent onset. He identifies that his symptoms have been a chronic problem for him, resulting in physical damage to objects and people and, ultimately, causing extreme dysfunction in a variety of areas. Most important, he is able to identify that his reactions to certain minor provocations are also greater than what others might expect. As with all disruptive, impulse-control, and conduct disorders, it is important to understand the temporal relationship of his symptoms and to rule out any episodic nature to them that might be more indicative of a mood disorder diagnosis. IED can be diagnosed in children older than 6 years and in adolescents, as well as adults.

Approach to the Diagnosis

Making the diagnosis of IED can be difficult, given the strict criteria outlined and the symptoms of other disorders that may appear to manifest as IED. A thorough history will reveal whether the specific time requirements for the diagnosis have been met. In addition, the quality of the outbursts must be accurately assessed to determine whether criteria are met. Parents and families will often present clear descriptions of a specific tantrum or outburst. It is important to determine whether the outburst is outside the realm of what might be a typical or expected response to an environmental provocation.

One key indication that an outburst response is out of proportion to the stimulus is destruction of property. If the nature of the outbursts tends to include destruction of property, investigating the frequency of outbursts is appropriate, determining whether there has been one in the past 3 months and how many have occurred in the past 12 months. The quality of the outburst can be more difficult to assess when it consists of verbal altercation or assault, without destruction of property or physical assault. Even in this case, it is appropriate to screen for additional qualifiers, such as cruelty toward an animal or another human being or physical aggression.

Age at onset is critical to the diagnosis of IED. Symptoms can begin at any time throughout the life span, with onset often found to be within childhood (age 6 or older) or adolescence, but rarely if older than 40. Once the age at onset is known, it is important to understand that the course of symptoms may be episodic in nature, following a chronic and persistent course.

IED outbursts can be triggered by what appear to be very small matters, producing unexpected results. Regardless of the provocation, the outbursts are generally frequent, with rapid onset, lasting less than 30 minutes. The character of the outbursts may be either in the form of low-intensity verbal or physical aggression without resulting damage or destruction, averaging twice weekly for 3 months, or in the form of high-intensity physical aggression with physical injury or destruction of property three times within 1 year.

Care should be taken during historical and diagnostic interview to clarify and confirm the presence or absence of a major mood disorder, episode of psychosis, direct physiological effects of a substance, or a general medical condition. In the context of these disorders, the diagnosis of IED should not be made. The presence of a childhood history of a disruptive behavior disorder of childhood is not uncommon (i.e., ADHD, ODD, conduct disorder).

Getting the History

Mr. Fields, age 42, presents to a clinician's office reporting that he needs help with anger management. The clinician proceeds by asking about his most recent complaints and why he feels he needs to manage his anger. Mr. Fields reports a story from the previous week, when he became enraged at his coworker who interrupted him in a meeting, which prompted Mr. Fields to abruptly end the meeting by yelling and storming out. The clinician asks Mr. Fields to consider how many times these "enraged" moments happen to him in a given week. Mr. Fields replies that some weeks it does not happen, but other weeks it may happen nearly every day, so "on average three to four times each week." The interviewer then investigates the quality of the outbursts: "Does that enraged feeling you get ever become so great that you end up physically throwing things, damaging property, or hurting others?" Mr. Fields reports that although he feels as if the outbursts could get to that point, he somehow has been able to refrain from hurting anyone and breaking things.

The interviewer then asks, "Do you remember when you first started noticing feeling like your anger was out of control?" In an effort to clarify the amount of functional impairment the patient currently experiences, the interviewer asks, "How long have you been at your current job?" Mr. Fields reports that he started at his current company 3 months ago, after having been terminated from his previous company the year prior. He continues on to say that this is his third job in 3 years, with the common feedback that he is "difficult to work with." Mr. Fields recalls that he felt "these anger impulses" during college. He stopped drinking and started "working out" more and going to church regularly. He felt that these efforts helped, and he has continued these "good habits" to help him manage his outbursts—"but it's still such a problem for me!" The clinician is prompted to delve further into the patient's childhood history, asking, "Did either of your parents or anyone in your family ever complain about your anger when you were in, say, middle school or high school?" Mr. Fields reports that he rarely got in trouble during his school years and often made the honor roll.

The interviewer allows Mr. Fields to lead with his initial broad complaint before targeting specifics of the described symptoms. The interviewer makes sure to elicit the time of onset of symptoms, investigates whether the symptoms occurred earlier in childhood, and seeks to determine the presence of other disorders during childhood. The interviewer further investigates the quality of Mr. Fields's outbursts by highlighting the presence or absence of property destruction and the frequency of the outbursts. To qualify for the diagnosis of IED, verbal aggression should occur approximately twice per week, on average, for at least 3 months. The interviewer would also want to investigate carefully the presence of other disorders, such as major mood or psychotic disorders, a general medical condition, or substance intoxication or withdrawal.

Tips for Clarifying the Diagnosis

- Question when the symptoms began.
- Determine the time course of the symptoms.
- Establish the intensity of symptoms. Learn whether there is damage or destruction to people or property.
- Find out whether the outbursts are provoked and in what situation(s).
- Determine whether it is possible to predict when an outburst is going to occur.

Consider the Case

Gary is a 15-year-old boy whose grandmother is concerned about his behavior at home and school. She reports that he recently spent one night at the juvenile detention center after the police were called to his school for verbal threats he was making toward his teacher. Gary and his grandmother report that his outbursts have been an increasing problem since he was in first grade; however, this is the first time the police have been called to a public place for his behavior. Gary migrated to the United States with his father and grandparents approximately 6 months ago. Gary's grandmother reports that since he was 6 years old, Gary has had extreme temper tantrums on numerous occasions, throwing his toys and often destroying his small handheld electronics. Recently, he has begun breaking objects in his room, such as a lamp and his dresser drawer. Once he punched a hole in his wall. She recalls that since Gary was 12 years old, not a month has gone by when she hasn't seen a serious tantrum resulting in property destruction in some way.

Gary's case shows an onset of symptoms dating back to at least age 6, as documented by his grandmother's history. To qualify for the diagnosis of IED, an individual must be 6 years of age or older. Gary meets criteria on the basis of the degree of his symptoms and their frequency, in that his grandmother notes a history of property destruction during his tantrums, occurring on a monthly basis over several years.

Most recently, his outburst occurred at school and resulted in verbal assault of his teacher and the involvement of law enforcement. His symptoms demonstrate reactions that are outside of the expected social norm, with excessive consequence severity. Given the timing of Gary's presentation for care, not long after coming to a new country, an element of adjustment may be playing a role. Because Gary is now presenting 6 months after his immigration, the diagnosis of IED is appropriate. In addition, he has a history of symptoms documented back to an early age, supporting the diagnosis.

Differential Diagnosis

Because of the low prevalence of IED, the clinician should consider the presence of another mental disorder during assessment. Irritable and aggressive behavior that is thought to be related to IED may, in fact, be a manifestation of a general medical condition, substance abuse or intoxication, mood disorder, personality disorder, or psychotic disorder, among other possibilities. It is important to understand the temporal relationship of symptoms and to rule out any episodic quality to them that may be more characteristic of a mood disorder, as well as the presence of a substance or medication or withdrawal from a substance that may be having a direct psychological effect on the individual. This evaluation occurs by a thorough clinical interview and examination, as well as, when indicated, a blood or urine toxicology screen. The presence of a general medical condition precludes the diagnosis of IED. Ruling out other mental disorders or general medical conditions is best accomplished by a thorough psychiatric and neurological examination.

Aggression that is well thought out, motivated, or vindictive in nature does not meet criteria for IED. The presence of a personality disorder, such as borderline personality disorder or antisocial personality disorder, does not rule out the presence of IED. The disorders each should be carefully considered, including their symptom and temporal patterns, and both diagnoses may be made if criteria are met. Most often, the personality disorder is an established diagnosis, with a new persistent change in the quality of intermittent impulsive aggression.

See DSM-5-TR for additional disorders to consider in the differential diagnosis. Also refer to the discussions of comorbidity and differential diagnosis in their respective sections of DSM-5-TR.

Summary

- IED may be considered when clinically significant aggression is present.
- Before making the diagnosis of IED, it is important for the clinician to rule out a general medical condition, substance intoxication or withdrawal, or another mental disorder that may account for the symptoms.
- A thorough clinical and neurological examination should be completed as part of the symptom assessment.
- Symptom severity should be assessed on the basis of the functional impairment that the symptoms are causing.

SUMMARY: DISRUPTIVE, IMPULSE-CONTROL, AND CONDUCT DISORDERS

The disruptive, impulse-control, and conduct disorders are among the most frequent disorders seen by child and adolescent mental health professionals. The underlying symptom that brings all of these disorders together under one diagnostic umbrella is the nature of self and interpersonal dysfunction that occurs. ODD initially manifests within the family, disrupting those relationships, and is most often brought to clinical attention once the child reaches school age and is beginning to demonstrate difficulties at school with peers and authority figures. IED often begins in adolescence but is most likely to present to clinical attention when dysfunction affects a young adult's peer relationships and occupational endeavors.

Behavioral dysregulation is an underlying commonality in this diagnostic class. Nevertheless, each diagnosis is distinct and has specific diagnostic criteria. It is important to understand the temporal relationship of symptoms, in addition to understanding when they may have first manifested in the individual's history and how consistent or persistent they have remained. With IED, for example, the timing of explosive behaviors, including the duration and frequency, is imperative information to glean in arriving at the correct diagnosis or diagnoses. As always, for each of these disorders, keeping the individual's appropriate expected developmental stage at the forefront is essential for clarity in understanding the diagnosis.

ELEMENTS TO CONSIDER IN THE CULTURAL FORMULATION

- Male prevalence of ODD should be considered in accordance with social norms of a particular geographical location or culture (Canino et al. 2010; Demmer et al. 2017; Wiesner et al. 2015).
- Some evidence demonstrates that first-generation migrants and refugees may be at decreased risk of ODD symptom development (Atherton et al. 2018; Betancourt et al. 2017).
- Cultural factors in some countries may contribute to a lower prevalence of IED because of the way clinical questions are presented or understood.

DIAGNOSTIC PEARLS

- Across this diagnostic class, all disorders involve the violation of some aspect of social norms and individual rights, and most demonstrate an increased rate of anger.
- The disruptive, impulse-control, and conduct disorders create clinically significant disturbance and impairment in social, educational, and vocational activities, as well as in interpersonal and intrapersonal relationships.

- Although high rates of aggression are common across all diagnoses in this class (except kleptomania), the types of aggression are distinctly different, specifically regarding premeditated aggression for secondary gain versus impulsive aggression.
- Imagine the everyday life of your patient, and have them and their caretaker walk you through a typical day from sun up to sun down; certain contexts may make the presentation normative.
- Language matters! Be certain of the language of your patient *and* all of the caretakers involved in your clinical interview and diagnostic process.
- Clinicians should begin each interview with their own brief self-assessment of potential bias pitfalls.

SELF-ASSESSMENT

Key Concepts: Double-Check Your Knowledge

What is the relevance of the following concepts to the various disruptive, impulse-control, and conduct disorders?

- Social norms
- Sequelae of behavioral disruption
- Consequence severity
- Interpersonal functioning
- Expected developmental stage
- Irritability
- Comorbid diagnoses
- Severity of aggression

Questions to Discuss With Colleagues and Mentors

1. How much do you, or can you, rely on the collateral data from sources such as teachers, parents, employers, and spouse to inform your diagnostic approach when you are evaluating a new patient with a disruptive, impulse-control, or conduct disorder?
2. Given the common co-occurrence of other disorders, how do you clarify the diagnoses in this diagnostic class?
3. How do you approach gender and cultural considerations in this diagnostic class?

Case-Based Questions

PART A

Mr. Hill is a 42-year-old man who reports a history of being "moody" since he was in college. He reports that he has been so moody at times in the past that he has lost a few friends and been divorced three times. His occupational history has been one of instability, and he wonders if he will ever be able to hold a job longer than a year. He reports that when he was about 35 years old, alcohol helped him calm down in the evenings when he was afraid he would just absolutely explode on somebody. He denies any other substance use or abuse, and the results of his medical workup are negative.

What is the most striking aspect of Mr. Hill's history with which a clinician should be first concerned? Mr. Hill is describing significantly impaired self-control and interpersonal functioning, a hallmark for disruptive, impulse-control, and conduct disorders.

PART B

Mr. Hill mentions that most days he is "fine" and can remain calm, but he has always lived in fear that he is going to explode on anyone at any moment. He says he never has a stretch of days when he is "moody" or "down," but rather that "it is just kind of unpredictable, and so random. Things that should only make me a little upset or cranky make me lose my mind it seems!"

Could Mr. Hill possibly have a mood disorder? Given that Mr. Hill says his symptoms are random, not episodic, and do not last for a significant period of time, a mood disorder diagnosis is less likely.

PART C

Given the opportunity to talk about his childhood, Mr. Hill reports, that in retrospect, "I wasn't necessarily moody as a kid, but I had a couple of times when I got in trouble at school and got in a few fights in middle school."

Which diagnosis should most likely remain at the top of the differential for Mr. Hill? Mr. Hill is describing symptoms that are most consistent with intermittent explosive disorder, with a slight history of disruptive behavior dating back to childhood. The level of dysfunction is concerning, especially because it has persisted for quite some time, in that he has been through three marriages and multiple jobs.

Short-Answer Questions

1. For a child younger than 5 to be diagnosed with oppositional defiant disorder (ODD), how often must the symptoms occur?
2. For a child age 5 or older to be diagnosed with ODD, how often must the symptoms occur?
3. What are the key categorical components of ODD behavior that must be evidenced for diagnostic qualification?
4. How often must vindictive or spiteful behavior occur for ODD?
5. What is the required time criterion for an individual to manifest aggressive impulses for the diagnosis of intermittent explosive disorder (IED)?
6. What is the youngest age at which IED may be diagnosed?
7. What is the typical age at onset for IED?

Answers

1. Generally, symptoms must occur on most days for a period of at least 6 months for a child younger than 5 to be diagnosed with ODD.

2. Generally, symptoms must occur at least once per week for at least 6 months for a child age 5 or older to be diagnosed with ODD.

3. The key categorical components of ODD behavior that must be evidenced for diagnostic qualification are angry/irritable mood, argumentative/defiant behavior, and vindictiveness.

4. Vindictive or spiteful behavior must occur at least twice within the past 6 months for ODD.

5. For the diagnosis of IED, the individual must manifest verbal or physical aggression twice weekly, on average, for the past 3 months (without damage or destruction to property or physical injury to animals or other individuals), or three behavioral outbursts involving damage or destruction of property and/or physical assault involving physical injury to animals or other individuals within a 12-month period.

6. The youngest chronological age for which IED may be diagnosed is 6 years (or equivalent developmental level).

7. The typical age at onset for IED is childhood or adolescence.

REFERENCES

American Psychiatric Association: Diagnostic and Statistical Manual of Mental Disorders, 5th Edition. Arlington, VA, American Psychiatric Association, 2013

American Psychiatric Association: Diagnostic and Statistical Manual of Mental Disorders, 5th Edition, Text Revision. Washington, DC, American Psychiatric Association, 2022

Atherton OE, Ferrer E, Robins RW: The development of externalizing symptoms from late childhood through adolescence: a longitudinal study of Mexican-origin youth. Dev Psychol 54(6):1135, 2018

Betancourt TS, Newnham EA, Birman D, et al: Comparing trauma exposure, mental health needs, and service utilization across clinical samples of refugee, immigrant, and US-origin children. J Trauma Stress 30(3):209–218, 2017

Canino G, Polanczyk G, Bauermeister JJ, et al: Does the prevalence of CD and ODD vary across cultures? Soc Psychiatry Psychiatr Epidemiol 45:695–704, 2010

Demmer DH, Hooley M, Sheen J, et al: Sex differences in the prevalence of oppositional defiant disorder during middle childhood: a meta-analysis. J Abnorm Child Psychol 45:313–325, 2017

Wiesner M, Elliott MN, McLaughlin KA, et al: Common versus specific correlates of fifth-grade conduct disorder and oppositional defiant disorder symptoms: comparison of three racial/ethnic groups. J Abnorm Child Psychol 43:985–998, 2015

CHAPTER 20

Substance-Related and Addictive Disorders

Kimberly L. Brodsky, Ph.D.
Michael J. Ostacher, M.D., M.P.H., M.M.Sc.

"I don't want to start drinking again, but then I
do and I just can't stop."

"I always think I can stop heroin on my own,
and for a while I can…but soon I'm back to
shooting up and I don't even know how I got
there."

- Alcohol-Related Disorders
- Caffeine-Related Disorders
- Cannabis-Related Disorders
- Hallucinogen-Related Disorders
- Inhalant-Related Disorders
- Opioid-Related Disorders
- Sedative-, Hypnotic-, or Anxiolytic-Related Disorders
- Stimulant-Related Disorders
- Tobacco-Related Disorders
- Other (or Unknown) Substance–Related Disorders
- Non-Substance-Related Disorders

The substance-related and addictive disorders include difficulties associated with 10 classes of drugs—alcohol; caffeine; cannabis; hallucinogens (including phencyclidine); inhalants; opioids; sedatives, hypnotics, and anxiolytics; stimulants; tobacco; and other (or unknown) substances—and gambling. The diagnosis of these disorders is based on a pathological pattern of behaviors in which the essential feature is the continued use of a substance or behavior despite significant problems related to it. This class of disorders, which underwent significant changes in DSM-5 (most notably the elimination of the distinction between substance abuse and dependence) (American Psychiatric Association 2013), is retained in DSM-5-TR (American Psychiatric Association 2022). These changes were made in part because of epidemiological data suggesting overlap between abuse and dependence and lack of clear differences in harm related to each disorder in DSM-IV (American Psychiatric Association 1994). The term *substance use disorder* (SUD) is used to describe all the various presentations of the disorder, from less severe, "mild" substance use to severe, often relapsing, compulsive drug taking that leads to great consequences. The term *drug addiction* is commonly used to describe severe, ongoing drug use and its problems, but it is not applied as a diagnostic classification in DSM-5-TR. The text and diagnostic features of several disorders (notably cannabis and opiate use disorders) have been changed in DSM-5-TR. These changes are summarized in Table 20–1.

The DSM-5-TR criteria for SUDs fit within four overall groupings: impaired control, social impairment, risky use, and pharmacological criteria. Included as a symptom of impaired control is *craving*, which previously was not included in the diagnosis of any SUD. Two symptoms within a 12-month period are required to establish the diagnosis of an SUD, a significant change from the three symptoms required for dependence in DSM-IV. With the abuse/dependence distinction gone, severity (designated as mild, moderate, or severe) is used as a specifier instead.

Common to all substance-related disorders in this diagnostic class is the ability to directly activate the brain reward system via consumption of a substance. The brain reward system involves the reinforcement of behaviors and the establishment of memories; substances with abuse potential short-circuit this system by directly activating the reward system, most often producing feelings of pleasure. This short circuit results in a more intense activation of the reward system than through adaptive behaviors and can result in a lack of attention to and engagement in normal activities. With the exception of hallucinogens, each class of drugs produces behavioral effects that could be described as a "high." With hallucinogens, curiosity is often a motivating factor in their use, rather than a desire for a euphoric experience. Although the term *dependence* has been removed from this category to avoid overlap with pharmacological tolerance and withdrawal, it is important to highlight the physiological aspect of these disorders when they are present. Behaviors associated with SUDs can often be mistakenly viewed as volitional or manipulative; however, it is important to understand these behavioral patterns as a result of alterations in behaviors due to changes in learned reward pathways, which are often tied to physiological dependence and are logical sequelae of the disorders themselves.

Gambling disorder is included in this diagnostic class, given evidence suggesting that gambling behavior activates the brain reward system in a similar way to drugs

TABLE 20–1. Key changes between DSM-5 and DSM-5-TR

Culture-related diagnostic issues have been updated to better address factors such as acculturation, segregation, and westernization and their impact on findings related to substance-related disorders.

Prevalence and gender-related diagnostic issues have been updated for all substance-related disorders in keeping with best evidence.

Poverty, systemic discrimination, and structural inequities have been highlighted as contributing to environmental risk factors for alcohol use disorders.

Diagnostic features, prevalence, and related factors for cannabis use disorders have been updated in keeping with current research and developments in medical and recreational cannabis availability.

Diagnostic features of opiate use disorder have been updated to further clarify the types of opioids and the development of the disorder.

Additional information has been added to address the relationship between each substance-related disorder and suicidal thoughts and behaviors.

of abuse. The addition of gambling disorder is considered controversial by some because it is a *behavior* rather than an exogenous substance; however, the consensus was that the biological evidence merited its inclusion.

The diagnostic class of substance-related and addictive disorders is divided into two subgroups: substance-related disorders and non-substance-related disorders. Each of the substance-related disorders is further separated into SUD (e.g., alcohol use disorder [AUD]); intoxication (e.g., caffeine intoxication); withdrawal (e.g., cannabis withdrawal); other (e.g., other [or unknown] substance use disorder); and unspecified (e.g., unspecified opioid-related disorder). Hallucinogen-related disorders also include phencyclidine-related disorders. In addition, substance-related disorders include tobacco-related disorders (e.g., tobacco use disorder [TUD], tobacco withdrawal) and substance/medication-induced mental disorders. Gambling disorder is the only disorder listed under non-substance-related disorders.

Substance-induced disorders comprise substance intoxication, substance withdrawal, and substance/medication-induced mental disorders included elsewhere in DSM-5-TR (e.g., substance/medication-induced psychotic disorder, substance/medication-induced depressive disorder). Many substances or medications can cause disorders that resemble other diagnoses, with the caveat that typically these symptoms last only temporarily. These disorders are different from substance use syndromes, in which a mix of cognitive, behavioral, and physiological symptoms are identified and contribute to the continued use of the substance, despite significant substance-related problems in functioning. These substance/medication-induced mental disorders are listed in their relevant sections of DSM-5-TR (e.g., depressive disorders, neurocognitive disorders). Symptoms of withdrawal and tolerance can occur during medical treatment involving prescription medications. Tolerance and withdrawal are normal, expected reactions to repeated doses of substances, and when these reactions occur during the course of medical treatment, they should not be counted toward the diagnosis of an SUD. However, tolerance and withdrawal can be important pharmacological signs of the severity of an SUD; furthermore, when prescription medications are used inappropriately or in excess of what is prescribed and other symptoms are present, a diagnosis of a substance-related disorder can be made.

In the clinical approach to an individual who has a substance-related or addictive disorder, it is important to understand that there is often ambivalence about use and its consequences and that this ambivalence can be used to motivate change. Evidence suggests that behavior change is complex and that the locus of change is in the individual with the disorder. This approach is somewhat of a departure from a medicalized approach to care in which the diagnosis is made and then prescriptions for treatment are given. Instead, individuals are led to discuss reasons to change that are within themselves, because most people with substance-related and addictive disorders "know" that they have a "problem"—yet knowing is rarely sufficient to engender change. The shame and stigma of a substance-related or addictive disorder frequently interferes with getting treatment, and although relapses should be an expected part of treatment, individuals (and treatment providers) often view themselves as failures when relapse occurs. Negative views of patients and their behaviors are common in providers and likely interfere with the alliance with the patient—and consequently decrease, rather than increase, the likelihood that the patient will engage in treatment and behavioral change. Consumption of substances, including prescribed medications, may intersect with an individual's cultural background, availability of substances, and local regulatory policies. Intersectionality with culture can have a significant impact on the variability of substance-related disorders.

Many individuals may use substances as an attempt to cope with severe psychosocial stressors or the symptoms of another illness (e.g., major depressive disorder, PTSD, chronic pain). Although this short-term coping mechanism may in fact be quite effective at alleviating distressing feelings of physical or emotional pain, in the long term the sequelae of negative consequences associated with the SUD and the physiological need for the substance take on lives of their own.

IN-DEPTH DIAGNOSIS: ALCOHOL-RELATED DISORDERS

> Mr. James, a 63-year-old man, comes to the clinic requesting services to assist with stopping drinking. He was recently arrested for driving under the influence (DUI) and states that his marriage is "on the rocks." He reports a long-standing history of alcohol use, starting in his teens. He says that he began drinking more frequently in his thirties after his first divorce. He states that he stopped drinking around the time of his second marriage and maintained sobriety for 5 years. However, after his son died in a car crash, Mr. James began drinking again and reports that his use quickly escalated. He states that currently he drinks about 12 beers per day and often will get to sleep with a few additional shots of hard alcohol. He reports frequent blackouts and was told by his doctor that his liver is damaged. He admits that he has had three previous DUIs and is concerned about the possibility of jail time associated with this most recent charge. Mr. James reports that he has worked "on and off" doing landscaping and other odd jobs;

however, he struggles financially. His children will not speak to him any longer, and his wife recently kicked him out of the house when he came home intoxicated. He says that although he knows alcohol has created many problems for him and he cannot really afford the way he drinks, he feels that he cannot stop on his own. He reports that when he tries to stop drinking, he gets the shakes and feels sick to his stomach.

This case highlights the legal and interpersonal ramifications often associated with AUD. It also underscores the tolerance and withdrawal frequently associated with AUD, including physiological symptoms and relapse associated with alleviation of these symptoms. Individuals often will be able to stop using for a period of time; however, once they begin drinking again, their use escalates quickly.

Approach to the Diagnosis

Tolerance and withdrawal are two physiological aspects of alcohol-related disorders to which clinicians often pay special attention. Tolerance develops with continued use of a substance such that greater doses are required to achieve the same effect. Alcohol withdrawal is characterized by symptoms that develop approximately 4–12 hours after the reduction of prolonged heavy alcohol consumption. Withdrawal symptoms are often intensely uncomfortable; therefore, individuals will continue to imbibe alcohol to avoid or reduce these symptoms, despite adverse consequences. In this vicious circle, individuals continue to use alcohol despite psychological and physical consequences (e.g., depression, loss of employment, estrangement from loved ones, liver disease, homelessness). Some withdrawal symptoms (e.g., sleep disturbances) are thought to last up to months and to contribute significantly to relapse. Severe complications of withdrawal, such as delirium and tonic-clonic (grand mal) seizures, affect less than 5% of individuals with AUD.

Individuals may use alcohol in hazardous circumstances (e.g., driving while under the influence of alcohol), and they may continue to use alcohol despite the knowledge that sustained consumption will result in significant psychosocial difficulties. Those who decide to stop drinking often will have successful periods of abstinence; however, once they begin drinking again, their consumption likely will escalate rapidly, and severe difficulties will reemerge. Failed attempts to diminish the amount of alcohol they consume, the need for an alcoholic beverage in the morning to relieve withdrawal symptoms, feelings of guilt or being criticized regarding alcohol consumption, and feelings of needing to cut back on consumption can all indicate an alcohol-related disorder and are important things to inquire about during a diagnostic interview. In addition, major areas of functioning are likely to be affected, resulting in, for example, alcohol-related accidents, school and job problems, interpersonal difficulties, legal problems, and health problems. Unspecified alcohol-related disorder can be diagnosed when a person presents with symptoms characteristic of an alcohol-related disorder that cause significant distress or functional impairment yet do not meet the full criteria for any specific alcohol-related disorder.

The severity of AUD is determined by the number of symptoms endorsed. Having two or three symptoms yields a diagnosis of mild AUD, and having six or more symptoms yields a diagnosis of severe AUD. In general, the more symptoms an individual endorses, the more severe the AUD. Severe AUD, especially in people with antisocial personality disorder, is often associated with criminal acts. For example, more than half of all individuals who commit homicide are believed to have been intoxicated at the time of the event. Severe alcohol use also contributes to feelings of sadness, irritability, and hopelessness, which can contribute to suicidal behaviors.

AUD frequently co-occurs with other SUDs; individuals may use alcohol to alleviate unwanted effects of these substances or to substitute for them when other substances are not as easily available. They may also use alcohol to mask the symptoms of other illnesses (e.g., PTSD, depression) as a way of coping. Symptoms of depression, anxiety, insomnia, and conduct problems frequently co-occur with heavy drinking and can precede it as well.

First alcohol intoxication most often occurs during the mid-teens. Most individuals who develop alcohol-related disorders do so by their late thirties.

Key to the diagnosis of AUD is the use of heavy amounts of alcohol with resulting repeated and significant distress or impairment in functioning. Although many individuals who drink consume enough to become intoxicated, only a minority of them ever develop AUD. This discrepancy is an important part of the assessment in diagnostic interviewing.

As stated in DSM-5-TR, "Alcohol use disorder is an important contributor to suicide risk during severe intoxication and in the context of a temporary alcohol-induced depressive or bipolar disorder. There is an increased rate of suicidal behavior as well as of [completed] suicide among individuals with the disorder" (p. 556). It continues: "Alcohol intoxication is an important contributor to interpersonal violence and suicidal behavior. Among individuals intoxicated by alcohol, there appears to be an increased rate of accidental injury (including death due to behaviors associated with altered judgment, self-harm, and violence), suicidal behavior, and [completed] suicide." (p. 562). Assessment of the risk of suicidal behavior and self-directed violence is a key part of evaluating the person with AUD, and a plan for mitigating risk is an important part of any assessment and treatment approach.

Getting the History

Patient (age 53 years): In my twenties I was drinking about a fifth of vodka a day.
Interviewer: How much and how often do you currently drink?
Patient: I'd say about two fifths per day.
Interviewer: Have you noticed that you need more alcohol to feel the same effects?
Patient: Yes.
Interviewer: How much time do you spend obtaining, using, and recovering from the use of alcohol?
Patient: Basically all of my time. I wake up in the morning and immediately need a drink to feel okay. Then I spend the day drinking and trying to get alcohol.
Interviewer: When you are not drinking, do you have cravings to use alcohol?
Patient: I can't stop thinking about it.
Interviewer: Have you ever used alcohol in a physically dangerous situation?
Patient: Yes, when I'm drunk I've gotten into fights, had my belongings stolen, and gotten arrested for public drunkenness.
Interviewer: Do you feel the need to cut back on your drinking?

Patient: That's why I'm here.
Interviewer: Have you ever tried to cut back, and how did that work?
Patient: A few times, but I always start again.
Interviewer: When you try to stop drinking, what happens?
Patient: I get the shakes, become nauseous, and can't sit still.
Interviewer: Has drinking gotten in the way of work or relationships?
Patient: Definitely. I haven't been able to keep a job, I'm homeless, and my family is fed up with me.
Interviewer: So you feel alcohol has led to some bad things but you still drink?
Patient: Part of me wants to stop so badly, but another part just can't. After all this time, how could I begin to face all of these things?

This interview highlights the key diagnostic criteria for AUD. Initial questions seek to obtain necessary information regarding age at onset, volume of alcohol consumed, and tolerance (determined by inquiring about the need for more alcohol to produce the same effects over time). Symptoms of withdrawal are determined by inquiring about physical signs and symptoms when consumption of alcohol is reduced or the person has tried to stop drinking. Information is also obtained about the amount of time spent consuming, obtaining, and recovering from the effects of alcohol. The interviewer also inquires whether the individual experiences cravings for alcohol and has made unsuccessful attempts to reduce or stop drinking; whether they have used alcohol in hazardous situations (e.g., driving under the influence); and whether they have experienced negative consequences from alcohol consumption and continued drinking despite awareness of these consequences. Ambivalence regarding stopping drinking is a common experience among people who have alcohol-related disorders; the alcohol is often serving some function (e.g., escape from negative emotions, numbing, coping with physical pain), and attempts to stop may have resulted in intense physiological discomfort associated with withdrawal. Clinicians often expect that individuals will present for evaluation certain of their desire to stop drinking; however, ambivalence about change is a natural aspect of modifying any behavior. If this ambivalence is present, recognizing it as a natural aspect of recovery is crucial during an evaluation for both the clinician and the patient. This recognition and acceptance enhance rapport and put in perspective a patient's prior failed attempts at treatment.

Tips for Clarifying the Diagnosis

- Determine answers to the following questions: Is the use of alcohol causing clinically significant impairment in the individual's ability to function? Has it impaired the person's ability to perform at work or school? Has it negatively affected interpersonal relationships?
- Question whether the individual has made unsuccessful attempts to cut back the volume of their drinking.
- Investigate whether there is evidence of a need for increased consumption of alcohol to produce the same effects (tolerance).
- Establish whether physical symptoms of withdrawal have occurred when the individual has reduced or stopped drinking.

- Determine whether the individual has engaged in physically hazardous activities while drinking (e.g., driving under the influence).

Consider the Case

Mr. Kim, a 21-year-old Korean male college student, presents for treatment; he is struggling with his grades and concerned about the possibility of failing out of college. He states that he began drinking alcohol when he and his parents moved to the United States from Korea during his high school years. He found it difficult to fit in and felt that alcohol helped him to make friends and talk to strangers. His drinking escalated during college, partially to cope with the stress associated with classes and the part-time job he works to pay for college and help out his parents at home. Mr. Kim reports that he gets intoxicated easily and that people often tell him that his face becomes flushed when he is drinking. He states that sometimes when he drinks alcohol, his heart will begin to beat rapidly. He states that the first few times he drank, he became so physically ill that he didn't drink again right away, but despite these physical symptoms, he always returned to drinking.

Mr. Kim is somewhat unique in having developed an AUD given that his reports are consistent with those of individuals, often of Asian descent, who have polymorphisms of genes for two alcohol-metabolizing enzymes, alcohol dehydrogenase and aldehyde dehydrogenase, which affect the response to alcohol. Individuals with certain polymorphisms can experience a flushed face and palpitations, which can often be severe enough to prevent further use of alcohol. His treatment is complicated further by the cultural context in which his alcohol use is occurring: he was born in Korea to Korean parents, and he is now immersed in a distinctly U.S. phenomenon of college-age drinking. Clinicians need to be aware of important cultural differences, including the specific meaning of alcohol misuse in Korean culture, and the expectations put on Mr. Kim by his family; these areas need to be explored carefully by treaters and consultation obtained, if necessary.

Differential Diagnosis

The differential diagnosis of alcohol-related disorders includes consideration of the following:

- **Alcohol use disorder:** nonpathological use of alcohol; sedative, hypnotic, or anxiolytic use disorder; conduct disorder in childhood; and adult antisocial personality disorder
- **Alcohol intoxication:** other medical conditions (e.g., diabetic acidosis, cerebellar ataxia, multiple sclerosis); sedative, hypnotic, or anxiolytic intoxication
- **Alcohol withdrawal:** other medical conditions (e.g., hypoglycemia, diabetic ketoacidosis, essential tremor); sedative, hypnotic, or anxiolytic withdrawal
- **Unspecified alcohol-related disorder**

AUD is observed in most individuals with antisocial personality disorder. Because antisocial personality disorder is associated with an early onset of AUD and a worse prognosis, it is important to establish both diagnoses. The signs and symptoms of AUD are similar to those seen in sedative-, hypnotic-, or anxiolytic-related disorders; however, the course is frequently different, particularly concerning associated medical problems. Thus, it is important to distinguish between the two. Individuals with AUD can develop patterns of use that create legal and disciplinary consequences; such patterns should be carefully distinguished from the difficulty with authority and behavioral patterns associated with conduct disorder. Part of the association between depression and AUD may be due to temporary depressive symptoms associated with the acute effects of intoxication or withdrawal; therefore, a diagnosis of major depressive disorder should be made with extreme caution until the person can be assessed outside the context of acute effects of alcohol. Studies have found that, compared with nondrinking individuals, the acute use of alcohol was associated with a significant increase in the risk of suicide attempts, with each drink raising the risk by 30%. Furthermore, heavier alcohol use was a much more potent risk factor for suicide attempts than lower alcohol use. The combination of alcohol and sedatives has been observed to have an even stronger association with suicide attempt. Alcohol use has also been found to be associated with possession of firearms, and people who drink alcohol are more likely to die by suicide with a gun than are those who do not drink.

A key element of AUD involves the large volume of alcohol consumed, which results in repeated and significant distress or impaired functioning. Most individuals who drink alcohol consume enough to feel intoxicated; however, less than one-fifth of them ever develop AUD. Many cultures and age groups encourage drinking at certain events (e.g., college and fraternity events, religious events). Drinking, even daily, and intoxication do not by themselves qualify an individual for diagnosis of AUD. AUD can be diagnosed with or without physiological dependence; however, physiological dependence is not a requirement for the diagnosis. Endorsing two or three symptoms signifies mild AUD, and endorsing six or more symptoms indicates severe AUD. In general, the greater the number of symptoms endorsed and the earlier the age at onset, the more severe the AUD is likely to be.

See DSM-5-TR for additional disorders to consider in the differential diagnosis. Also refer to the discussions of comorbidity and differential diagnosis in their respective sections of DSM-5-TR.

Summary

- Alcohol-related disorders are the most prevalent of the substance-related disorders in the United States.
- First alcohol intoxication most often occurs during the mid-teens. Most individuals who develop alcohol-related disorders do so by their late thirties.
- Suicide risk is elevated with both alcohol use itself and with AUD.
- Polymorphisms of genes for alcohol-metabolizing enzymes are often seen in individuals of Asian descent and can affect their response to alcohol. Individuals with these gene variations experience flushed face and palpitations that may be severe enough to limit the future consumption of alcohol and diminish the risk for the de-

velopment of alcohol-related disorders. However, this protective effect may be modulated by sociocultural factors.

- Alcohol withdrawal is characterized by symptoms that develop approximately 4–12 hours after the reduction of prolonged heavy alcohol consumption. Withdrawal symptoms are often intensely uncomfortable, and individuals may continue to imbibe alcohol to avoid or reduce these withdrawal symptoms, despite adverse consequences.

IN-DEPTH DIAGNOSIS: CANNABIS-RELATED DISORDERS

Mr. Clark, a 27-year-old man, presents with anxiety and insomnia. Questioning reveals that he has been using 1–2 g of cannabis daily for the past 7 or 8 years. He began using cannabis intermittently as a teenager but became a daily user as an undergraduate in college. He denies that his grades were affected by his cannabis use but says he decided not to return to school after his sophomore year because his work in a small café would better help him achieve his goal of running a restaurant. He has been working at several restaurants since, initially as a server, but then he became the assistant manager of a local lunch and dinner restaurant. He decided that "being a waiter is better—I like being in touch with the customers and I get to make my own hours." He often works late, coming home after 2:00 A.M., and he has found that smoking cannabis before going to bed helps him sleep. If he does not use any cannabis, he reports, he generally cannot sleep at all. He smokes on awakening because it helps him relax. He has had periods of trying to stop in the past year because of the cost, but "it's the only thing that helps with my anxiety, and there's no way I can sleep without it." He is not currently in a relationship but lives with three coworkers in a shared apartment.

Cannabis-related disorders are much more likely in adults whose use began in early adolescence. The acceptance of cannabis use is increasing (along with legalized use in some states), and because it is perceived to be less addicting than other substances, even daily use may not be recognized as problematic. School and work performance may be decreased in chronic users, who may achieve less than expected in social and occupational functioning. It is quite difficult for chronic users to stop because of withdrawal effects; people with cannabis-related disorders may believe that withdrawal symptoms such as anxiety, irritability, and insomnia that are relieved by use may represent a benefit of the drug for those symptoms.

Approach to the Diagnosis

As with all substance use (but especially cannabis), the clinician must be aware of either negative or positive feelings about the use of the drug. Cannabis use disorder (CaUD) is difficult to diagnose, in part because of beliefs among both patients and clinicians that the drug is less likely to lead to use disorders than other substances, intoxication is less obvious than for other substances, and the development of dependence is often slower than for other substances. The notion persists that cannabis is less dangerous than alcohol, opiates, stimulants, sedatives, hypnotics, and even nicotine. Although most individuals who use cannabis do not have problems related to its use,

20%–30% of cannabis users do experience symptoms and associated consequences consistent with CaUD; for some people, the drug has a strong negative effect in terms of functioning and ability to control use, and clinicians must be attuned to this. Unspecified cannabis-related disorder can be diagnosed when an individual presents with symptoms characteristic of a cannabis-related disorder that cause significant distress or functional impairment, yet the symptoms do not meet the full criteria for any specific cannabis-related disorder.

Cannabis is used in many forms, most commonly in joints, or cigarette-like forms. It is also smoked in pipes, water pipes, and hollowed out cigars (blunts). Synthetic, oral tetrahydrocannabinol (THC) formulations (pills, capsules, sprays) are also available and can be used for medical purposes. More recent methods of consumption include vaping (vaporizing by heating without combustion to release psychoactive components for inhalation), and dabbing, in which a concentrated butane hash oil is created through butane extraction of THC from the cannabis plant. Cannabis can also be orally ingested in edibles or beverages. Inhalation typically produces more rapid and intense effects than oral administration. Cannabis potency varies greatly across products, ranging from 10%–15% in the plant material to 50%–55% in hash oil. Over the past two decades, the potency of cannabis has steadily increased. Pharmacological and behavioral tolerance to most of the effects of cannabis has been reported in individuals who use it chronically. Generally, tolerance is lost when cannabis use is discontinued for a significant period of time. The abrupt cessation of daily use often results in cannabis withdrawal syndrome, which includes symptoms of irritability, anger, anxiety, depressed mood, restlessness, sleep difficulty, and decreased appetite or weight loss. Although not as severe as opiate or alcohol withdrawal, cannabis withdrawal can cause significant distress and contribute to relapse.

Although medical uses of cannabis remain controversial and equivocal, its use for medical purposes should be considered before making a diagnosis; symptoms of tolerance and withdrawal naturally occur within the context of a prescription for a medical condition and should not be the primary criteria for diagnosis. Increasingly permissive U.S. state medical and recreational cannabis laws have reduced barriers to obtaining cannabis in more than three-quarters of U.S. states. The legal status of cannabis varies by state. Although it currently remains an illegal substance under federal law, cannabis use under state law can involve authorization for medical purposes or a completely legal recreational product. The most common medical purpose for cannabis is chronic pain; however, conditions approved for medicinal purposes vary by state.

Cannabis use may continue despite knowledge of physical or psychological problems associated with it. Individuals with CaUD may use cannabis throughout the day over a period of months or years and may spend many hours each day under the influence. Others may use it less frequently, but their use causes recurrent problems related to family, school, work, or other important activities. Periodic cannabis use and intoxication can negatively affect behavioral and cognitive functioning and thus interfere with optimal performance. Use of cannabis on the job or while working at a place that requires drug testing can also be a sign of CaUD. It is important to query for these signs and symptoms in diagnostic interviews.

Individuals who regularly use cannabis often report that it helps them cope with mood, sleep, pain, and so on. Many people will not report spending an excessive amount of time under the influence, despite being intoxicated most of the day. An important marker supporting a diagnosis is continued use despite clear risk of negative consequences to other valued activities or relationships. It is important to recognize and assess for these common signs and symptoms of cannabis use to better understand the extent of usage. Experienced users of cannabis develop behavioral and pharmacological tolerance. Signs of acute and chronic use include red eyes, yellowing of fingertips (from smoking joints), chronic cough, and exaggerated craving and impulse for specific foods, sometimes at odd times of the day or night.

Cannabis use has been related to a reduction in prosocial, goal-directed activity, which some have labeled amotivational syndrome, manifesting in poor school performance and employment problems. Accidents related to cannabis intoxication can be a concern; studies have shown impaired driving reaction time, diminished spatial perception, and diminished decision-making.

Getting the History

Interviewer: When did you begin smoking cannabis?
Patient (age 32 years): I was 14 years old.
Interviewer: How much were you smoking at that time?
Patient: On the weekends with friends.
Interviewer: When did your smoking increase?
Patient: Around my sophomore year in college, I started smoking during the day before classes.
Interviewer: How much and how often do you currently smoke?
Patient: I'd say about three or four joints per day.
Interviewer: Do you use any other cannabis products?
Patient: Well, I get some gummies sometimes, but I smoke more than use edibles. Sometimes I'll do some dabs if someone has them but mostly I just smoke.
Interviewer: Have you noticed that you need more cannabis in order to feel the same effects?
Patient: Yes.
Interviewer: How much time do you spend getting and smoking cannabis or using other products?
Patient: A lot. I wake and bake in the morning, then I'll use throughout the day; I'm pretty much always high. I get hooked up from my friend who has a prescription, so it doesn't take me too long, but I definitely spend a lot of money on it. When I get edibles, I mostly use them at night. They help with sleep.
Interviewer: When you are not high, do you have cravings to use?
Patient: Totally. Visiting my parents for the holidays is the worst.
Interviewer: Have you ever been high in a physically dangerous situation?
Patient: I guess, but I drive slower when I'm stoned.
Interviewer: Do you feel the need to cut back on your use?
Patient: My girlfriend says I should.
Interviewer: Have you ever tried to cut back, and how did that work?
Patient: A few times, but I always start again.
Interviewer: When you try to stop cannabis, what happens?
Patient: I have trouble sleeping, and my girlfriend says I'm cranky.

Interviewer: Has cannabis gotten in the way of work or relationships?

Patient: Well, it definitely bothers my girlfriend, and sometimes I decide to blow off work and get high. I think my boss suspects something's up. Once I failed a drug test and lost my gig at a video game store. I liked working there too, I used to roll one up and play shooter games—best job I ever had.

Interviewer: So you feel smoking has led to some negative consequences, but you still smoke?

Patient: Part of me wants to stop, but I don't really see too many problems with it.

This interview highlights the key diagnostic criteria for cannabis-related disorders. Initial questions elicit necessary information regarding age at onset, volume of cannabis or THC consumed, and tolerance (determined by inquiring about the need for more cannabis to produce the same effects over time). In individuals with chronic, heavy usage, symptoms of withdrawal are determined by inquiring about signs and symptoms when cannabinoids are no longer used. The interviewer also inquires about whether the patient experiences cravings for cannabis and whether they have made unsuccessful attempts to reduce use or stop using. In addition, the interviewer asks whether the patient has used cannabis products in hazardous situations (e.g., driving while under the influence). Finally, the interviewer inquires about the negative consequences of cannabis consumption and continued use despite awareness of these consequences.

Tips for Clarifying the Diagnosis

- Ask about symptoms of withdrawal during the evaluation of cannabis use.
- Be aware of the cultural context of use, especially the reported medical uses of cannabis.
- Realize that it may be difficult for individuals to identify the social and occupational consequences of cannabis use.
- Carefully evaluate for anxiety and mood symptoms that may have been present before the onset of use or during periods of prolonged abstinence.
- Assess whether the use of cannabis is causing clinically significant impairment in the individual's ability to function, in their ability to perform at work or school, or in their interpersonal relationships.

Consider the Case

Mr. Jackson, a 23-year-old man, presents with severe features of PTSD. Since returning from Iraq, he has been using 1–2 g/day of high-potency cannabis, which he obtains through a cannabis dispensary because he has a prescription to treat his chronic pain. He says smoking helps him cope with his symptoms and relax enough to be around people. He began using cannabis intermittently as a teenager but became a daily user after returning from the war. He works as a security guard at a casino, often for late hours, coming home after 2:00 A.M., and he has found that smoking cannabis or using THC-infused gummies before going to bed "relieves the tension" in his body and allows him to sleep. If he does not use any cannabis, he reports, he generally cannot sleep at all, feels hypervigilant, and is consumed with thoughts about his time in the military.

He smokes on awakening because it helps him get out of bed: "otherwise I'm too stiff." He reports that he has had periods of trying to stop in the past year because of the cost, but "it's the only thing that helps with my pain." He has been planning to apply to the police academy but has not filled out the applications.

The cultural acceptance of cannabis for medical purposes has made its use more acceptable and expanded its availability in certain communities. Currently, cannabis is one of the world's most commonly used psychoactive substances. Cannabis use intersects with ethnicity, religion, and sociocultural practices. This makes teasing out symptoms that may be consequences of use more difficult for clinicians; similarly, individuals have more difficulty defining social or occupational problems resulting from use of the substance. Many people use cannabis in the context of the symptoms of PTSD and anxiety disorders such as generalized anxiety disorder and social anxiety disorder. Evaluation of co-occurring psychiatric disorders is important in providing education, support, and targeted treatment to these individuals. In the case of Mr. Jackson, issues specific to his war-related disorders need to be understood and addressed in the context of his treatment.

Differential Diagnosis

The differential diagnosis of cannabis-related disorders includes consideration of the following:

- **Cannabis use disorder:** nonproblematic use of cannabis; other mental disorders (e.g., anxiety disorders, major depressive disorders)
- **Cannabis intoxication:** other substance intoxication (e.g., phencyclidine intoxication, hallucinogen intoxication); cannabis-induced mental disorders (e.g., cannabis-induced anxiety disorder, with onset during intoxication)
- **Cannabis withdrawal:** withdrawal from other substances; depressive, bipolar, anxiety, or other mental disorders including antisocial personality disorder; another medical condition
- **Unspecified cannabis-related disorder**

Cannabis-related disorders might be characterized by symptoms that resemble those of primary mental disorders. For example, generalized anxiety disorder needs to be distinguished from cannabis-induced anxiety disorder, with onset during intoxication. Chronic cannabis use can result in an amotivational syndrome that resembles chronic depressive disorder. Acute adverse reactions to cannabis need to be distinguished from the symptoms of panic or other anxiety disorders, major depressive disorder, delusional disorder, bipolar disorder, and schizophrenia. Urine screen and physical examination can reveal elevated pulse and red eyes, which can help make the distinction. It is important to query about substance use and determine whether symptoms are present outside the context of recent use and withdrawal. Among adult frequent cannabis users, cannabis withdrawal is associated with comorbid depression, anxiety, and antisocial personality disorder. Reviews of the literature indicate that chronic cannabis use, but not acute use, is associated with suicidal ideation and behavior.

It is essential to the diagnosis to clarify that the cannabis use is problematic and creating impairments in functioning. This assessment can be tricky because social, behavioral, and psychological problems may be difficult to attribute specifically to cannabis use (especially if the individual is also using other substances). Furthermore, denial of heavy use and lack of acknowledgment that cannabis may be related to or causing substantial problems can be common in individuals presenting for treatment at the request or urging of someone else.

See DSM-5-TR for additional disorders to consider in the differential diagnosis. Also refer to the discussions of comorbidity and differential diagnosis in their respective sections of DSM-5-TR.

Summary

- Cannabinoids, especially cannabis, are the most widely used illicit psychoactive substances in the United States.
- Although most users do not have symptoms and consequences related to use, 20%–30% of cannabis users do.
- Compared with males, females report more severe cannabis withdrawal symptoms, especially mood symptoms such as irritability, restlessness, anger, and gastrointestinal symptoms.
- The abrupt cessation of daily use often results in cannabis withdrawal syndrome, which includes symptoms of irritability, anger, anxiety, depressed mood, restlessness, sleep difficulty, and decreased appetite or weight loss.
- Cannabis intoxication does not typically result in the severe behavioral and cognitive dysfunction seen in alcohol intoxication.
- It is essential to the diagnosis to clarify that the cannabis use is problematic and creating impairments in functioning.
- Cannabis-related disorders might be characterized by symptoms that resemble those of primary mental disorders.

IN-DEPTH DIAGNOSIS: OPIOID-RELATED DISORDERS

Emergency physicians treat Mr. Johnson, a 36-year-old man, at the hospital after his girlfriend found him unresponsive on the floor of his apartment and called an ambulance. They revived him by administering intravenous naloxone. Mr. Johnson has a long history of drug and alcohol use, beginning in early adolescence with cannabis and alcohol. In his late teens he began using prescription opiates that he stole from family members; he initially took them orally and later intranasally. This use was followed over the course of several years by the use of intranasal heroin that he bought on the street. By his early twenties, he was using heroin intravenously. He committed petty crimes as a teenager, stealing from neighbors or stealing cars; got into multiple fights with his peers; and was frequently truant from school, ultimately dropping out of high school before obtaining a diploma. He has a history of multiple arrests, with short jail stays but no prison sentences. He was mandated to addiction treatment as a condition of probation, including three episodes of medically supervised withdrawal followed by short-term, abstinence-based residential treatment. During the year of court-mandated methadone maintenance treatment, he successfully remained abstinent from opiates, but he continued to use alcohol and benzodiazepines and left methadone maintenance treatment when his probation ended. He began using intravenous heroin or heroin mixed with fentanyl again, with periods of stopping use by buying buprenorphine/naloxone or methadone on the street. When his girlfriend found him on the floor, he had taken methadone that he had obtained illicitly.

Severe opioid-related disorders are often characterized by physiological dependence and intense cravings that are motivated by both positive rewards (e.g., euphoria) and negative ones (e.g., avoidance of withdrawal symptoms). Users frequently return to use, having limited response to treatment other than maintenance therapy with opioid agonists such as methadone or buprenorphine/naloxone or the long-acting injectable opiate receptor blocker naltrexone. Opioid-related disorders often co-occur with either antisocial personality disorder or antisocial behavior, which is understandable in that people with severe opioid use disorder (OUD) need vast amounts of money to obtain their drugs and may commit crimes as a result.

Approach to the Diagnosis

Opioid-related disorders have traditionally been found primarily in users of illicit opiates, but the rise in nonmedical uses of prescription opiates is striking and of great public health concern. The use of intravenous opiates has shifted somewhat because the purity of heroin sold on the street has increased to the point that intranasal use has become a common entry point for users. The rates of opioid-related disorders from prescription opiates have also shifted, because the prescribing of high-potency opiates such as oxycodone and methadone has increased for noncancer pain, chronic or otherwise. Therefore, young opiate users and older individuals who have been prescribed opiates for pain may develop opioid-related disorders without intravenous use. Fentanyl is typically injected, both medically and nonmedically, and is used medically in transdermal and transmucosal forms. Unspecified opioid-related disorder can be diagnosed when an individual presents with symptoms characteristic of an opioid-related disorder that cause significant distress or functional impairment yet the symptoms do not meet the full criteria for any specific opioid-related disorder.

The approach to different populations must consider at what point the use began (i.e., during adolescence or adulthood), whether users have other substance-related disorders, whether there are comorbid psychiatric illnesses, and whether there are co-occurring medical conditions involving pain. The hallmark of all these opioid-related disorders is the daily use of opiates, with significant periods of withdrawal and cue-conditioned use, often related to reducing symptoms of withdrawal but also related to drug craving.

Although users typically mask or hide their use, if they are not forthcoming it should not be seen as a sign of either severity or lack of willingness to engage in treatment. Questioners should pay close attention to their own responses to patients, maintaining a neutral and nonjudgmental stance. Even doing so may not allow a person to discuss their use freely because they expect a critical response from clinicians.

Clinicians can use the principles of both Screening, Brief Intervention, and Referral to Treatment (SBIRT; Substance Abuse and Mental Health Services Administration 2000) and motivational interviewing (Miller and Rollnick 2013) to allow for more accurate data gathering during initial and subsequent interviews.

As stated in DSM-5-TR,

> opioid use disorder is associated with a heightened risk for suicide attempts and suicide. Some suicide risk factors overlap with risk factors for an opioid use disorder. In addition, repeated opioid intoxication or withdrawal may be associated with severe depressions that although temporary can be intense enough to lead to suicide attempts and suicide. Nonfatal accidental opioid overdose and attempted suicide are distinct phenomena that can be difficult to differentiate but should not be mistaken for each other, if possible. (p. 613)

Opioid overdose is characterized by unconsciousness, respiratory depression, and pinpoint pupils. Overdoses have increased significantly in the United States; since 2010 overdoses due to heroin and since 2015 fatal overdoses due to synthetic opioids other than methadone (generally fentanyl or fentanyl analogues) have become the most prevalent. Studies show that suicide is a common cause of death among regular users of opioids and that they are undercounted and often misclassified. Even after adjusting for psychiatric comorbidity and controlling for demographic factors, OUD elevated the risk for suicide mortality, and among veterans prescribed opioids for pain, suicide mortality increased with higher opioid doses.

Getting the History

Interviewer: When did you begin using opiates?

Patient (age 42 years): Probably when I was 20. I had some friends who got some Oxys [oxycodone tablets], and I started using them.

Interviewer: How much were you using at that time?

Patient: On the weekends with friends.

Interviewer: Were opiates the first drugs you used?

Patient: No, I used to drink in high school, mostly on weekends, and also would smoke pot.

Interviewer: How much oxycodone were you using at that time?

Patient: Just here and there. If I could get a few pills, I would. I wasn't buying them at first, but when I took them I felt like the person I was supposed to be, so I started buying them.

Interviewer: When did your drug use increase?

Patient: Kind of right away. The Oxys were so expensive, but someone I knew had heroin, so I started smoking during the day before classes.

Interviewer: When was the first time you tried to stop?

Patient: Just a few months after I started, but I would get sick—you know, like having the flu, cramps, feeling really like crap—so I would just use.

Interviewer: How much time do you spend getting and using opiates?

Patient: I pretty much plan my day around it, where I'm going to use it.

Interviewer: Have you ever tried to cut back, and how did that work?

Patient: Sometimes I used to slow down by getting some methadone or maybe Suboxone [buprenorphine/naloxone], but I always start again.

Interviewer: Have you been able to stop completely?

Patient: This is really the first time. I was in a methadone clinic once, but I stopped going because the transportation was a hassle, and I couldn't get there every day,
and they wouldn't give me take-home doses, but now that I'm taking Suboxone
I really don't feel like using.

In getting a history of opioid-related disorders, the clinician needs to obtain a history not only of the symptoms associated with use but also of the course of treatment
and attempts to stop using. Individuals who are not presenting for addiction treatment directly are likely to speak about their use in a way that minimizes the negative
reaction they expect from clinicians. It is important to evaluate the symptoms and behaviors associated with use and relapse to use, paying particular attention to the cue-
conditioned behaviors and whether they are hedonically driven or driven by the
avoidance of negative effects common in withdrawal.

Co-occurring psychiatric conditions are common and should be evaluated concurrently. People with opioid-related disorders frequently also have other substance-
related disorders, and these should be evaluated concurrently in any such person.

Tips for Clarifying the Diagnosis

- Determine the answers to the following questions: Is the use of opiates causing
  clinically significant impairment in the individual's ability to function? Has it impaired their ability to perform at work or school? Has it negatively affected interpersonal relationships?
- Question whether the person has made unsuccessful attempts to cut back their use.
- Assess whether there is evidence of a need for increased use of opiates to produce
  the same effects (tolerance).
- Explore whether the person has physical symptoms of withdrawal when reducing
  or stopping the use of opiates.
- Determine whether the symptoms of tolerance or withdrawal are due only to le-
  gitimate medical prescribing of the substance.
- Question whether the individual has persistent craving for opiates after use has
  stopped.
- Determine whether other substance-related disorders are co-occurring.

Consider the Case

Ms. Lark, a 46-year-old woman with no past psychiatric or SUD history other than a tobacco-related disorder, presents on referral from her primary care provider after she ran
out of her opiate pain medication prescription early. She had been well until 1 year
prior, when she fractured her tibia and fibula and required open reduction and internal
fixation. She had a difficult postoperative course and complained of ongoing pain. She
was prescribed opiate pain medication through her recovery. Her doses continued to be
increased after she began ambulating and her casts and splints had been discontinued.
Over months, Ms. Lark continued to complain of worsening pain and went on extended leave from her position in the accounting department of a manufacturing firm.
Her primary care provider continued to increase her dosage of opiates and prescribed
a second course of physical therapy. Several months before, Ms. Lark reported taking

additional opiates after physical therapy "because the pain was so bad" and because she "couldn't function without it." One month she reported that her pills spilled in the bathroom sink, and she lost most of them because they got wet and went down the drain. The primary care provider told her that she could not refill any more prescriptions after that, but this month she called 2 weeks before her refill was due, stating that after a dinner party at her home her prescription bottle was empty. Therefore, the referral was made.

Most of the diversion and nonmedical use of prescription opioids is through opiate pain medication legitimately prescribed to patients, or their relatives or friends, rather than through obtaining the prescriptions from multiple prescribers. In spite of this, many people are able to get more opioids than they were originally prescribed and for longer periods from their prescribers. It is important in the evaluation and treatment of such patients to focus on both their pain (which needs to be adequately addressed) and aspects of their use that are maladaptive. In this case, it is important to be aware of the concerns women have in seeking treatment. Women with OUD appear more likely than men to have initiated use in response to sexual abuse and violence, and they are more likely than men to be introduced to opioids by a partner. There is also evidence of telescoping among women, or progressing to a use disorder more quickly following first use and presenting with more severity when entering treatment facilities in large research samples. Individuals from socially marginalized groups were historically overrepresented among individuals with OUD. However, diagnoses of OUD have become more common among White individuals, and the criteria for OUD perform equally across ethnoracial groups.

Differential Diagnosis

The differential diagnosis of opioid-related disorders includes consideration of the following:

- **Opioid use disorder:** opioid-induced mental disorders (e.g., persistent depressive disorder [dysthymia]); other substance intoxication (e.g., alcohol intoxication; sedative, hypnotic, or anxiolytic intoxication); other withdrawal disorders (e.g., sedative-hypnotic withdrawal)
- **Opioid intoxication:** other substance intoxication (e.g., alcohol intoxication, sedative-hypnotic intoxication); other opioid-induced mental disorders
- **Opioid withdrawal:** other withdrawal disorders (e.g., sedative-hypnotic withdrawal; anxiolytic withdrawal); other substance intoxication (e.g., hallucinogen intoxication, stimulant intoxication); opioid-induced mental disorders (e.g., opioid-induced depressive disorder, with onset during withdrawal)
- **Unspecified opioid-related disorder**

Opioid-induced mental disorders may be characterized by symptoms (e.g., depressed mood) that resemble primary mental disorders (e.g., persistent depressive disorder [dysthymia] vs. opioid-induced depressive disorder, with onset during intoxication). Opioids are less likely to produce symptoms of mental disturbance than are most other substances of abuse. Opioid intoxication and opioid withdrawal are distinguished from the opioid-induced mental disorders (e.g., opioid-induced depressive disorder, with onset during intoxication) because the symptoms in these latter disorders are in excess of those usually associated with opioid intoxication or opioid withdrawal and are severe enough to warrant independent clinical attention.

As stated in DSM-5-TR,

> alcohol intoxication and sedative, hypnotic, or anxiolytic intoxication can cause a clinical picture that resembles that for opioid intoxication. A diagnosis of alcohol or sedative, hypnotic, or anxiolytic intoxication can usually be made based on the absence of pupillary constriction or the lack of a response to naloxone challenge. In some cases, intoxication may be due both to opioids and to alcohol or other sedatives. In these cases, the naloxone challenge will not reverse all of the sedative effects. (p. 614)

Some opioids such as fentanyl and oxycodone are not detected in standard urine tests and need more specialized procedures to be identified. Methadone and buprenorphine also require specialized testing.

According to DSM-5-TR,

> the anxiety and restlessness associated with opioid withdrawal resemble symptoms seen in sedative-hypnotic withdrawal. However, opioid withdrawal is also accompanied by rhinorrhea, lacrimation, and pupillary dilation, which are not seen in sedative-type withdrawal.... Dilated pupils are also seen in hallucinogen intoxication and stimulant intoxication. However, other signs or symptoms of opioid withdrawal, such as nausea, vomiting, diarrhea, abdominal cramps, rhinorrhea, or lacrimation, are not present. (p. 619)

It may be helpful, if opioid withdrawal is a consideration, to use the standard measure of withdrawal, the Clinical Opiate Withdrawal Scale (Wesson and Ling 2003). In recent years, the illicit opioid drug supply, which is primarily fentanyl, has been contaminated with other substances such as xylazine (an anesthetic used in veterinary medicine), so specialized urine drug testing might be warranted in certain patients.

See DSM-5-TR for additional disorders to consider in the differential diagnosis. Also refer to the discussions of comorbidity and differential diagnosis in their respective sections of DSM-5-TR.

Summary

- Opioid-related disorders typically are associated with physiological dependence.
- Co-occurring legal problems and antisocial personality disorder are common among opioid users, especially among intravenous users.
- OUD is often associated with other substance-related disorders, especially those involving alcohol, cannabis, stimulants, and benzodiazepines, which are often taken to reduce symptoms of opioid withdrawal or craving for opioids or to enhance the effects of administered opioids.
- Cue-associated conditioned use is common, is associated with relapse and recurrence, and frequently persists long after cessation of use.

IN-DEPTH DIAGNOSIS: STIMULANT-RELATED DISORDERS

Mr. Wilson, a 36-year-old man, comes to the clinic after getting into an accident during his job as a truck driver. Drug testing revealed he had been using methamphetamine, and his union suggested that he should get treatment. During the course of the interview, he says that he began taking stimulants in his early twenties, when he was driving a beer truck and making deliveries. He states that he was "burning the candle at both ends," trying to party and have fun but also trying to keep his job, which required long hours at times. He states that recently he has occasionally shot up, but typically he just pops pills. Mr. Wilson reports that in between truck routes (and methamphetamine use), he crashes "hard," often feeling down and irritable. He states that he has never really maintained a long-term relationship with anyone but that he likes to engage in sexual activity when using and is concerned that he may have acquired a sexually transmitted infection. He relates that he has always been anxious and describes panic attacks since childhood.

This case highlights the more prolonged course of tolerance and withdrawal associated with oral use of stimulants. Over time, tolerance occurs and use escalates. In addition, Mr. Wilson describes some of the typical patterns of withdrawal, including depressive symptoms and irritability. His use occurs in binges, coinciding with his truck driving. Engaging in unprotected sex and the transmission of infection are frequently associated with use, in particular intravenous use. Frequently, histories associated with panic attacks and anxiety symptoms are reported in individuals with stimulant-related disorders.

Approach to the Diagnosis

Stimulant-related disorders involve the use of psychoactive substances that increase activity in the brain and can temporarily elevate alertness, mood, and awareness. These include amphetamine, prescription stimulants with similar effects (e.g., methylphenidate), and cocaine. Both naturally derived stimulants and synthetic stimulants can produce stimulant-related disorders. This disorder group also covers amphetamine-type stimulants that are structurally different from amphetamines but have similar modes of action, such as methylphenidate, modafinil, armodafinil, and plant-derived stimulants such as *khât*, as well as synthetic chemical *khât* analogues, called cathinones and sometimes known as "bath salts" (e.g., mephedrone and methylone). Unspecified stimulant-related disorder can be diagnosed in cases in which symptoms characteristic of a stimulant-related disorder cause significant distress or functional impairment but do not meet the full criteria for any specific stimulant-related disorder.

Cocaine is derived from the coca plant and is primarily used as cocaine hydrochloride and cocaine alkaloids outside of the indigenous regions where it is grown. Cocaine hydrochloride powder is typically insufflated through the nostrils or dissolved in water and injected intravenously. Crack and other cocaine alkaloids are usually heated and inhaled (smoked), with rapid onset of effects. Given that the effects of amphetamines and amphetamine-like substances are similar to those of cocaine, amphetamine-related disorders and cocaine-related disorders are grouped together in

DSM-5-TR under "stimulant-related disorders," with the particular stimulant being used by the individual being indicated in the diagnostic category (e.g., methylphenidate use disorder).

Stimulant-related disorders can develop over very short periods of time, even in less than a week, because of their strong euphoric effects. Tolerance occurs with repeated use, and withdrawal symptoms include hypersomnia, increased appetite, and dysphoric mood. These symptoms enhance cravings and increase the likelihood of relapse. Use may be chronic or episodic. Aggressive or violent behavior is associated with stimulant use disorder, in particular when high doses are smoked, ingested, or used intravenously. Individuals can present with intense anxiety, resembling panic disorder or generalized anxiety disorder, as well as paranoid ideation and psychotic episodes resembling schizophrenia.

Stimulants can produce rapid and potent effects on the central nervous system, producing instant feelings of well-being, confidence, and euphoria. Individuals may spend large amounts of money and engage in criminal activities to obtain stimulants. Erratic behavior, social isolation, and sexual dysfunction are often long-term sequelae of stimulant-related disorders.

An acute intoxication from high doses of stimulants may manifest in rambling speech, headaches, transient ideas of reference, and tinnitus. Individuals may also present with paranoid ideation, auditory hallucinations, and tactile hallucinations, which they typically recognize as part of the effects of the stimulants. Individuals may present with extreme anger, threats, or acting-out behavior. Mood changes include depression, suicidal ideation, anhedonia, and emotional lability. Disturbances in attention and concentration are also common. These disturbances in mood and cognitive functioning usually resolve within hours to days after cessation of use; however, they can persist for up to a month.

Withdrawal occurs after the cessation or reduction in use of stimulants and may be characterized by fatigue, vivid or unpleasant dreams, insomnia or hypersomnia, increased appetite, and psychomotor agitation or retardation. The substance from which the person is withdrawing should be specified, be it cocaine, amphetamine, or another stimulant.

Individuals with stimulant use disorder often develop conditioned responses to drug-related stimuli (e.g., seeing a pill bottle), which often play a role in relapse and are particularly difficult to extinguish.

As stated in DSM-5-TR, "depressive symptoms with suicidal thoughts or behavior can occur and are generally the most serious problems seen during stimulant withdrawal" (p. 636). Assessment of the risk of suicidal behavior and self-directed violence is a key part of the evaluation of the person with stimulant use disorder, with the risk especially elevated during stimulant withdrawal. A plan for mitigating that risk is an important part of any assessment and treatment approach.

Getting the History

Interviewer: When did you begin using stimulants?
Patient (age 38 years): I was 18.

Interviewer: How much were you using at that time?

Patient: Not much, just for tests and stuff.

Interviewer: When did your stimulant use increase?

Patient: While I was in college. At first I was using just to get my homework done, but then my buddies and I started crushing Adderalls and snorting them, and then I started smoking cocaine, which wasn't hard to find. I dropped out of school and started selling to keep up with my habit, eventually switching to shooting up because it was cheaper and easier to get my hands on.

Interviewer: How much or how often do you currently use?

Patient: Every couple of days or so.

Interviewer: Have you noticed that you need to use more to feel the same effects?

Patient: Yes.

Interviewer: How much time do you spend obtaining, using, and recovering from the use of stimulants?

Patient: I'm mostly always using or recovering; I'll go on a bender every couple of days and then mostly feel miserable the next couple of days.

Interviewer: Have you ever used stimulants in a physically dangerous situation?

Patient: Yes. I'll pick up women when I'm using, and I have had a lot of unprotected sex with people I don't know much about.

Interviewer: Do you feel the need to cut back on your use?

Patient: That's why I'm here.

Interviewer: Have you ever tried to cut back, and how did that work?

Patient: A few times, but I always start again.

Interviewer: When you have tried to stop using, what happened?

Patient: I get really down; I'll even get tearful sometimes. I can't focus on anything. I'm a mess.

Interviewer: Has using gotten in the way of work or relationships?

Patient: Seriously? I dropped out of school, I can't work, I'm homeless; the list goes on.

Interviewer: So you feel stimulants have led to negative consequences, but you still use them?

Patient: I can't stop.

This interview highlights the key diagnostic criteria for stimulant-related disorders. Initial questions elicit the necessary information regarding age at onset, volume consumed, and tolerance (determined by inquiring about the need for more stimulants to produce the same effects over time). Symptoms of withdrawal are determined by inquiring about signs and symptoms when stimulant consumption is reduced or the individual has tried to stop using. Information is also obtained about the amount of time spent consuming, obtaining, and recovering from the effects of stimulants. The interviewer also inquires about whether the patient has cravings for stimulants and has made unsuccessful attempts to reduce or stop use. In addition, the interviewer asks about whether the patient has used stimulants in hazardous situations. Finally, the interviewer inquires about the negative consequences of stimulant consumption and continued use despite awareness of these consequences. Ambivalence regarding stopping use is a common experience of individuals with stimulant-related disorders because the sequelae of tolerance and withdrawal can occur particularly rapidly in those who snort or use intravenously, and attempts to stop may have resulted in intense physiological discomfort associated with withdrawal. The particular stimulant used is noted in the diagnostic category (e.g., "methylphenidate use disorder," "cocaine intoxication," "methamphetamine withdrawal").

Tips for Clarifying the Diagnosis

- Determine answers to the following questions: Is the use of stimulants causing clinically significant impairment in the individual's ability to function? Has it impaired their ability to perform at work or school? Has it negatively affected interpersonal relationships?
- Ask whether the individual has made unsuccessful attempts to cut back the volume of their stimulant use.
- Establish whether the individual requires increased consumption of stimulants to produce the same effects (tolerance).
- Question whether the individual has engaged in physically hazardous activities while using stimulants.
- Consider whether the individual presents with intense anxiety resembling panic disorder or generalized anxiety disorder, or with paranoid ideation and psychotic episodes resembling schizophrenia.

Consider the Case

Mr. Rose, a 31-year-old man, presents to the emergency department with paranoia and reports of hearing voices. He states that he has been walking for several days, trying to get away from the individuals who are after him. He reports that he feels safe in the hospital, although he is fearful that "they" may infiltrate the system. He calms slightly with reassurance that the hospital police force will not allow anyone to interfere with his treatment. He says that he began using drugs, including cannabis and methamphetamine, in junior high school and remembers people being out to get him over the past decade or so; he describes never staying in one place for very long in order to stay safe. He presents as tangential, appearing paranoid and internally preoccupied, telling a rambling narrative interlaced with ideas of reference concerning intricate conspiracies regarding why he was taken to this hospital and devices that are monitoring his movements. At times he becomes agitated and labile during the course of the interview. He describes his belief that thoughts and voices can be inserted into his head through computers and various appliances. His symptoms do not remit over the course of several weeks.

This case may represent stimulant-induced psychotic disorder, one of the most severe instances of stimulant toxicity, although the persistence of Mr. Rose's symptoms makes it difficult to know whether they actually result from a primary psychotic disorder. Individuals with stimulant-induced psychotic disorder may present with delusions and hallucinations that resemble schizophrenia. This patient exhibits paranoia, and he describes fixed beliefs that individuals are funneling thoughts and voices into his head through household items and that others are out to get him and are monitoring him. These symptoms typically remit over time; if they do not, a psychotic disorder diagnosis is warranted. At this point, there is no definitive way to determine whether Mr. Rose's persistent psychotic symptoms are substance induced or due to a primary psychotic disorder.

Although this case may represent the typical presentation of acute intoxication, including rambling speech, emotional lability, agitation, and ideas of reference, the persistence of the psychotic symptoms leads to concerns that Mr. Rose has a psychotic disorder instead. In the case of stimulant intoxication, the severity of the intoxication symptoms exceeds those of stimulant-induced psychotic disorder and indicates separate diagnostic consideration.

Differential Diagnosis

The differential diagnosis of stimulant-related disorders includes consideration of the following:

- **Stimulant use disorder:** primary mental disorders (e.g., schizophrenia, depressive and bipolar disorders, generalized anxiety disorder, panic disorder); phencyclidine intoxication; stimulant intoxication and withdrawal
- **Stimulant intoxication:** stimulant-induced mental disorders (e.g., stimulant-induced depressive disorder, psychotic disorder); other mental disorders
- **Stimulant withdrawal:** stimulant use disorder and stimulant-induced mental disorders (e.g., stimulant-induced intoxication delirium, stimulant-induced depressive disorder, stimulant-induced bipolar disorder, stimulant-induced anxiety disorder)
- **Unspecified stimulant-related disorder**

Patients can present with intense anxiety resembling panic disorder or generalized anxiety disorder, which can be particularly tricky in the context of stimulant-related disorders because individuals who develop these disorders frequently also have histories of repeated panic attacks and generalized anxiety. Getting an accurate timeline can be particularly important, and collateral information may be essential. Urine screening in the context of acute intoxication can also be helpful because individuals may present with paranoid ideation and psychotic episodes resembling schizophrenia.

Furthermore, individuals with stimulant use disorder often have transient depressive symptoms that meet criteria for major depressive disorder. Again, it is important to establish whether these symptoms occur outside the context of use and recovery from stimulants.

There is some association between mortality from suicide and the use of illicit or nonprescription amphetamines and cocaine, and also between suicide deaths and cocaine or amphetamine use disorders, so suicidal ideation and risk must be carefully examined in patients with stimulant use disorders.

In extreme cases, individuals can present with stimulant-induced psychotic disorder, with delusions and hallucinations that resemble the features of schizophrenia. When symptoms persist long after expected from intoxication, a psychotic disorder should be diagnosed.

See DSM-5-TR for additional disorders to consider in the differential diagnosis. Also refer to the discussions of comorbidity and differential diagnosis in their respective sections of DSM-5-TR.

Summary

- Individuals may begin stimulant use to lose weight or to improve performance in school, work, or athletics.

- Stimulant use disorder develops rapidly when the mode of administration involves intravenous use or smoking and progresses over the course of weeks to months. Oral usage typically results in a slower trajectory (months to years).
- The large majority of individuals who present for treatment of stimulant use disorder administer via smoking (66%) rather than injecting (18%) or snorting (10%).
- Individuals tend to stop using stimulants after 8–10 years, which may be associated with the mental and physical sequelae of long-term use.
- Individuals use episodically or daily. *Binges* are a form of use in which high doses are consumed over a period of hours or days. This usage pattern is typically associated with physical dependence. Binges often terminate when the supply of stimulants is depleted.
- Stimulant-related disorders can develop over very short periods of time, even in less than a week, due to their strong euphoric effects. Tolerance occurs with repeated use, and withdrawal symptoms include hypersomnia, increased appetite, and dysphoric mood. These symptoms enhance cravings and increase the likelihood of relapse.
- In the United States, a diagnosis of stimulant use disorder is associated with a 20% increase in 30-day readmission rates following hospitalization, regardless of the cause.

IN-DEPTH DIAGNOSIS: TOBACCO-RELATED DISORDERS

> Mr. Tam, a 46-year-old man, presents with a 33-year history of smoking and is currently smoking one and a half packs of cigarettes per day. He reports beginning smoking at age 13, with daily smoking by age 15. By age 18 he was smoking a pack a day. He has made four or five previous attempts to quit smoking (with abstinence for at least 1 day), with the longest period of abstinence lasting 9 months. He had tried to use a nicotine replacement patch on two of those occasions but had a local reaction to it and stopped each time after 3 or 4 days. He was once prescribed bupropion 300 mg/day, but he took it for only 2 months, stating that he "hates pills" and wanted to quit on his own.
>
> He reports that he currently begins smoking as soon as he wakes up ("even before I go to the bathroom") and that his first cigarette of the day is the most enjoyable. He leaves his building at work to smoke outdoors, and when he cannot smoke for more than an hour or two, he becomes "really irritable—like little things can set me off." He feels that he needs to smoke to "deal with the anxiety" but remains concerned about his health and is interested in cutting down.

Most people who smoke begin before they are age 18, but fewer people who begin smoking after age 21 develop physiological dependence and have difficulty stopping. Many people make multiple attempts to stop smoking, either with or without pharmacological treatment, and recurrence is common. Individuals who report smoking within 30 minutes of awakening are more likely to have a severe disorder and more difficulty stopping. It is important to distinguish between withdrawal symptoms and those of a primary anxiety or mood disorder.

Approach to the Diagnosis

Aside from the overlap of tobacco withdrawal symptoms with other substance withdrawal and psychiatric symptoms, the diagnosis of tobacco-related disorders is rather straightforward. The name of this substance category was changed from "nicotine" in previous editions of DSM to "tobacco" in DSM-5 to reflect that harms from this addiction are largely related to the tobacco and much less to the nicotine. Contrary to general beliefs, adolescents frequently exhibit symptoms of tobacco withdrawal, even without a history of long-term use, so withdrawal is not limited to long-term tobacco users.

TUD can develop with use of all forms of tobacco and with prescription nicotine-containing medications. Individuals who use electronic cigarettes are less likely to develop TUD. The relative ability of these products to produce TUD or to induce withdrawal is associated with the rapidity of the route of administration (smoked over oral over transdermal) and the nicotine content of the product. Nondaily use is infrequently associated with physiological dependence and usually will not be associated with a TUD. One-fourth of people in the United States who currently smoke do so on a nondaily basis. Unspecified tobacco-related disorder can be diagnosed when an individual presents with symptoms characteristic of a tobacco-related disorder that cause significant distress or functional impairment but that do not meet the full criteria for any specific tobacco-related disorder.

The comorbidity of psychiatric conditions in people who smoke is widespread and may mimic the symptoms of withdrawal, so any diagnostic evaluation of tobacco users must include evaluation of past and current psychiatric conditions. Many people, for instance, mistake the symptoms of withdrawal for those of anxiety or depression, but at the same time, symptoms of anxiety and depression may make individuals less likely to attempt to stop smoking or more likely to relapse if they do. Evaluating the temporal relationship between symptoms and cessation of smoking (even if it was only hours before) and the severity of withdrawal is important. The risk of suicide must be carefully evaluated in people who smoke because considerable evidence suggests that, even adjusting for covariates, TUD is associated with an increased risk of suicide.

Getting the History

Interviewer: When did you begin smoking cigarettes?
Patient (age 54 years): When I was 14.
Interviewer: How much were you smoking at that time?
Patient: At first I just started taking cigarettes from my dad, but then I started hanging out and smoking with friends after school. Not every day, anyway.
Interviewer: When did your smoking increase?
Patient: By the time I was in high school, like a junior or something, I was smoking every day. I could buy them myself, so it wasn't a problem.
Interviewer: How much do you currently smoke?
Patient: Less than a pack a day, maybe five packs a week. Last year it was two packs a day, but I have cut down.
Interviewer: Have you tried to completely stop?

Patient: Yes, a few times. Once I made it a week, but the other times I started again in a day or two.

Interviewer: When you try to stop smoking, what happens?

Patient: I have trouble sleeping and am a total bear. In fact, if I have to do something for more than a few hours when I can't smoke, I start to get bad—like anxious and irritable—and my first priority is to get a smoke.

Interviewer: So you feel that smoking has led to negative consequences, but you still smoke?

Patient: Sometimes I want to stop, but at this point I can't see stopping with everything I have going on.

The interviewer should obtain a sense of the longitudinal history of use, including when use started, the pattern of use over time, the involvement of symptoms of craving and withdrawal, and attempts to stop smoking.

Individuals who smoke daily are frequently unable to stop smoking in large part because of persistent withdrawal and craving. Early use in life predicts the severity of use later, and the severity of withdrawal predicts inability to stop. Among adolescents who smoke cigarettes at least monthly, most will become daily tobacco users in the future. Prevalence of tobacco use in the United States varies by age, sex/gender, and ethnoracial background, with lower rates of smoking onset and progression to daily smoking among Black youths, especially young females. Liver enzyme polymorphisms that vary across ethnoracial groups can affect nicotine metabolism and contribute to variation in smoking behavior. Higher TUD prevalence is also associated with exposure to racism and ethnic discrimination. Prevalence of DSM-IV nicotine dependence is higher among adult lesbian, gay, and bisexual individuals than among heterosexuals, possibly due to an association with exposure to sexual orientation discrimination. Lower income and education have both been found to be associated with persistence of DSM-IV nicotine dependence (tobacco use disorder in DSM-5 and DSM-5-TR).

Consider the Case

Ms. Schneider, a 59-year-old woman, reports smoking 10 cigarettes a day, although the number has been increasing over the past year since she began smoking again. She had smoked two packs per day for many years, but 2 years prior she was diagnosed with non–small cell carcinoma of the lung and had a successful resection of her right lower lobe with no mediastinal involvement. She was able to stop smoking after her surgery but eventually began smoking "a few cigarettes a day." She was prescribed varenicline, which she continued for 4 months until her insurance company denied her further treatment, and she decided not to pay for it out of pocket. Two months later she began smoking again and made several attempts to stop, being unable to do so for more than 1 day. She reports that she wants to smoke more than she currently is but knows that it is "bad" for her and is limiting herself to half a pack a day. She is concerned that her smoking will continue to increase in spite of her setting this limit.

Smoking affects males somewhat more than females, but in this case a woman with a severe disorder has relapsed in spite of the past health consequences of her use and her strong desire to not smoke. Research suggests that negative reinforcement (e.g., that smoking relieves negative affect) is a greater motivator in females than in males. It is typical that people who stop smoking continue to have cravings for nicotine long after they are abstinent and may remain at risk of relapse for years.

Differential Diagnosis

The symptoms of tobacco withdrawal overlap with those of other substance withdrawal syndromes (e.g., alcohol withdrawal, caffeine withdrawal); caffeine intoxication; anxiety disorders, such as panic disorder or generalized anxiety disorder; depressive disorders; bipolar disorders; sleep disorders; and medication-induced akathisia. Voluntary smoking cessation or admission to smoke-free inpatient units can induce withdrawal symptoms that mimic, intensify, or disguise other diagnoses or adverse effects of psychiatric medications; for example, irritability thought to be due to alcohol withdrawal could actually be due to tobacco withdrawal.

See DSM-5-TR for additional disorders to consider in the differential diagnosis. Also refer to the discussions of comorbidity and differential diagnosis in their respective sections of DSM-5-TR.

Summary

- Tobacco-related disorders generally begin in adolescence.
- Experiences of racism and discrimination have been found to be associated with the prevalence of TUD.
- TUD is more common in males than in females.
- Suicide risk is elevated in people with TUD, so risk for suicide must be carefully evaluated and managed in these patients.
- An intoxication syndrome does not apply to tobacco; however, withdrawal is common, and its severity is important to assess.
- Many tobacco users have tobacco-related physical symptoms or diseases and continue to smoke.
- Tobacco withdrawal usually has an onset within 24 hours of stopping or cutting down on tobacco use, peaks at 2–3 days after abstinence, and lasts 2–3 weeks.
- Craving persists long after use has ceased and contributes to recurrences.
- Individuals with psychiatric disorders in the United States are three times more likely than others to have TUD.

SUMMARY: SUBSTANCE-RELATED AND ADDICTIVE DISORDERS

The hallmark of substance-related and addictive disorders is that they arise out of a disruption of the normal reward circuitry of the brain. The reward system is usually activated by natural rewards such as food or sex, but addictive substances and behaviors have the ability to produce a more intense activation such that normal activities may be neglected.

The substance-related and addictive disorders include difficulties associated with 10 classes of drugs (alcohol; caffeine; cannabis; hallucinogens [including phencyclidine]; inhalants; opioids; sedatives, hypnotics, and anxiolytics; stimulants; tobacco; and other [or unknown] substances) and gambling. This category of disorders includes both SUDs and substance-induced disorders (intoxication, withdrawal, and substance/ medication-induced mental disorders included elsewhere in DSM-5-TR, such as substance-induced psychotic disorder or substance-induced depressive disorder). Many substances can cause substance-induced mental disorders that resemble other diagnoses, with the caveat that typically substance-induced symptoms last only temporarily.

Consumption of substances, including prescribed medications, may intersect with an individual's cultural background, availability of substances, and local regulatory policies. Intersectionality with culture can have a significant impact on the variability of substance-related disorders.

Alcohol-related disorders are the most prevalent of the substance-related and addictive disorders in the United States. Studies have found that, compared with nondrinking individuals, the acute use of alcohol was associated with a significant increase in the risk of suicide attempts. Cannabinoids, increasingly found in multiple preparations from buds and leaves to tinctures and oils, are the most widely used illicit psychoactive substances in the United States. The abrupt cessation of daily use often results in cannabis withdrawal syndrome, which includes symptoms of irritability, anger, anxiety, depressed mood, restlessness, sleep difficulty, and decreased appetite or weight loss.

Opioid-related disorders typically are associated with physiological dependence. Cue-associated conditioned use is common and associated with relapse and recurrence, and it frequently persists long after cessation of use, suggesting the need for long-term treatment to prevent return to use. Mortality from OUD is high and is increasing. Prevention of overdose, the most serious potential consequence of OUD, must be a part of management.

Stimulant-related disorders develop rapidly when the mode of administration involves intravenous use or inhalation and progresses over the course of weeks to months. Oral usage typically results in a slower trajectory (months to years).

Tobacco-related disorders generally begin in adolescence. An intoxication syndrome is rare among these disorders, but withdrawal is common and its severity is important to assess. Craving persists long after use has ceased and contributes to recurrent use.

Although the term *dependence* has been removed from this diagnostic class to avoid overlap with pharmacological tolerance and withdrawal, it is important to highlight the physiological aspect of these disorders and to understand that the behavioral patterns associated with substance-related and addictive disorders develop as a result of the substance's potential to produce alterations in reward pathways— both negative and positive rewards—and that individuals with these disorders are typically in a cycle of relapse and recovery.

Symptoms of withdrawal and tolerance can occur during medical treatment involving prescription drugs such as opioids, benzodiazepines, and antidepressants. Tolerance and withdrawal are normal physiological responses to repeated doses of substances but do not, in and of themselves, represent a disorder of the brain's reward system. However, tolerance and withdrawal can be important physiological signs of the severity of an SUD; for example, when prescription medications are used in excess of what is prescribed or for nonmedical reasons, and when other symptoms are present, SUD can be diagnosed.

ELEMENTS TO CONSIDER IN THE CULTURAL FORMULATION

- Socioeconomic disparities, access, and availability impact an individual's course of substance-related disorders. These factors as well as cultural context should be considered in diagnosis and treatment of substance-related disorders.
- Research in industrialized countries suggests that exposure to intimate partner violence or childhood mistreatment often co-occurs with stimulant use, especially in women.
- Higher rates of TUD have been found to be associated with exposure to racism and ethnic discrimination.

DIAGNOSTIC PEARLS

- When tolerance and withdrawal occur during the course of medical treatment, they should not be counted toward the diagnosis of a substance-related or addictive disorder; however, when prescriptive medications are used inappropriately or in excess of what is prescribed and other symptoms are present, such a diagnosis can be made.
- Behaviors associated with substance-related and addictive disorders can often be mistakenly viewed as volitional or manipulative; however, these behavioral patterns result from alterations in reward pathways and are often tied to physiological dependence and logical sequelae of the disorders themselves.
- Symptoms associated with substance-related and addictive disorders may meet the criteria for other disorders; however, these symptoms are typically transient (e.g., hallucinations associated with stimulant intoxication or anxiety associated with alcohol withdrawal).
- Many individuals use substances in various contexts; however, it is important to establish the relationship of substance use to functionally significant impairment in order to merit a diagnosis of substance use disorder.
- Consider discrimination, marginalization, histories of interpersonal violence, and exposure to trauma when considering risk factors for substance-related disorders.
- Overarchingly, substance-related disorders correlate with significant increases in suicidal thoughts and suicidal risk behaviors.
- Evaluate for co-occurring psychiatric conditions, which commonly occur.
- Tolerance and withdrawal can be important pharmacological signs of the severity of a substance use disorder.

SELF-ASSESSMENT

Key Concepts: Double-Check Your Knowledge

What is the relevance of the following concepts to the various substance-related and addictive disorders?

- Factors contributing to relapse
- Nonproblematic usage
- Cue association
- Episodic versus chronic use
- Binges
- Tolerance and withdrawal
- Substance use disorders versus substance-induced disorders
- Functional consequences

Questions to Discuss With Colleagues and Mentors

1. How might an individual's cultural background affect the history obtained from them of a substance use disorder?
2. How do gender and cultural factors influence the recognition of symptoms in disorders of addiction?
3. How might cannabis use affect psychosocial functioning?
4. How might the co-occurrence of PTSD affect making a diagnosis of substance-related and addictive disorders?
5. How do the course and associated features of substance use disorders contribute to a cyclical pattern of use and dependence?
6. When symptoms manifest in the context of acute intoxication, what is typically their course?

Case-Based Questions

PART A

Ms. Forsythe is a 43-year-old woman with bipolar I disorder, who is referred for outpatient evaluation and treatment. She was recently hospitalized for 10 days for a manic episode in the context of intermittent adherence to her complex medication regimen. During her hospitalization, she developed increasing agitation and bizarre behavior with unstable vital signs and ultimately was diagnosed with alcohol withdrawal and treated with benzodiazepines. Her mania abated as her medications were reinstituted.

Ms. Forsythe reports that since discharge she has been taking her medications as prescribed, stating, "That last time really scared me, but I still have my glass of Chardonnay every evening. It's really not something I can see giving up." She reports that her mood is "fine" and that she has no thoughts of self-harm or suicidal thoughts.

What are the diagnostic issues in this case? What are the most important principles to consider in evaluation? Ms. Forsythe has a lifelong mood disorder, was admitted to hospital treatment for mania, and was subsequently found to be in alcohol withdrawal. Consideration must be given to the role of alcohol in the development of the mood disorder and a determination made about whether the mood episode was substance induced. It is unlikely in this case, even though Ms. Forsythe's mania was temporally related to her alcohol use, because there is sufficient information to determine that she has bipolar I disorder and that her lack of medication adherence was more likely the proximate cause of her relapse. Further information needs to be gathered—even in the context of what appears to be well-documented alcohol withdrawal—to accurately diagnose the extent of her alcohol use disorder.

PART B

Ms. Forsythe currently smokes between a half and a full pack of cigarettes a day, having started smoking in her teens. She reports making three attempts to stop smoking in the past, with the longest period of abstinence from smoking lasting 7 days. She had been diagnosed with ADHD as a child and was intermittently treated with stimulants. She began using cannabis and drinking alcohol in high school. Her first episode of depression was at age 12, she believes, and she began taking antidepressants and attending psychotherapy at that time. While in her first year of college away from home, she had an episode consistent with mania that required hospitalization, but she finished that year of schooling. She then left college, moved back to her parents' home, and finally got a bachelor's degree at a local college after 6 years.

She reports binge drinking on weekends with friends and some cannabis use in her twenties, but she began drinking regularly during the evenings after she moved out of her family home. She married at age 28 and had two children, but the marriage ended when the children were young, and she shares custody of them with their father. Child protective services had been involved early in the children's lives during a period when Ms. Forsythe was severely depressed, but ultimately she was found fit to parent. She moved back to her parents' house after her divorce but lost her job working at a travel agency and found herself drinking each night, up to two bottles of wine. Because her time was unstructured and her children were at school, she would begin drinking in the late morning. "It's not as if I had the shakes or anything. I just wanted to drink." Her family has made several attempts to get her to stop drinking, including 5 years earlier when she had several days of "bad anxiety," but she went to Alcoholics Anonymous only "a few times." She began drinking again, albeit "only a few glasses a day," after 3 months. She continues to use cannabis, "three joints a week," that she states she buys at a cannabis dispensary "because of my bipolar disorder."

What additional substance use disorders can now be diagnosed? What additional information would be helpful in making these diagnoses? Bipolar disorder often co-occurs with substance use disorders, most commonly with tobacco use disorder but also with alcohol, cannabis, and other substance use disorders. More information is available to more precisely diagnose Ms. Forsythe's alcohol use disorder, which can be done at this time, but further information may be needed to clarify her cannabis use as a disorder. The use of cannabis as medicine is growing because more states and municipalities sanction its use.

Bipolar disorder frequently co-occurs with other psychiatric disorders, including ADHD and anxiety disorders. Further information should be gathered about those disorders because they, in and of themselves, are risk factors for the development of substance use disorders.

Short-Answer Questions

1. What are the 10 classes of drugs in the DSM-5-TR substance-related and addictive disorders diagnostic class?
2. Many substances can cause substance-induced mental disorders that resemble primary mental disorders. What is a distinguishing factor between them in terms of course?
3. What is the typical age at onset of first alcohol intoxication?
4. By what age do most individuals develop alcohol-related disorders?
5. Alcohol withdrawal is characterized by symptoms that develop approximately how long after heavy alcohol consumption?
6. What is the most widely used illicit substance in the United States?
7. How do rates of cannabis use disorder compare in males and females?
8. What are the symptoms of withdrawal associated with cannabis use disorder?
9. How do individuals typically begin using stimulants?
10. How does method of consumption affect the course of stimulant use disorder?
11. What is the typical method of consumption of stimulants with which individuals who have stimulant use disorder present?
12. What is episodic use of stimulants?
13. What are binges?
14. When do tobacco-related disorders typically begin?
15. What is the hallmark of tobacco use disorder?
16. How common are intoxication and withdrawal in tobacco-related disorders?
17. When does tobacco withdrawal typically begin, and how long does it last?
18. How long do tobacco cravings persist?

ANSWERS

1. The 10 classes of drugs are alcohol; caffeine; cannabis; hallucinogens (including phencyclidine); inhalants; opioids; sedatives, hypnotics, and anxiolytics; stimulants; tobacco; and other (or unknown) substances.

2. Typically, the symptoms of substance-induced mental disorders last only temporarily, in keeping with the effects of the substance (e.g., cannabis-induced anxiety disorder, with onset during intoxication vs. generalized anxiety disorder); however, substance use and other mental disorders can be comorbid.

3. First alcohol intoxication most often occurs during the mid-teens.

4. Most individuals who develop alcohol-related disorders do so by their late thirties.

5. Alcohol withdrawal is characterized by symptoms that develop approximately 4–12 hours after the reduction of prolonged heavy alcohol consumption.

6. Cannabinoids are the most widely used illicit psychoactive substance in the United States.

7. Rates of cannabis use disorder are greater among adult males (3.5%) than females (1.7%) and among 12- to 17-year-old males (3.4%) than females (2.8%).

8. The abrupt cessation of daily use often results in cannabis withdrawal syndrome, which includes symptoms of irritability, anger, anxiety, depressed mood, restlessness, sleep difficulty, and decreased appetite or weight loss.

9. Individuals may begin stimulant use in an attempt to lose weight or to improve performance in school, work, or athletics.

10. Stimulant use disorder develops rapidly when the mode of administration involves intravenous use or smoking and progresses over the course of weeks to months. Oral usage typically results in a slower trajectory (months to years).

11. The large majority of individuals who present for treatment of stimulant use disorder administer the stimulant via smoking rather than injecting or snorting.

12. Episodic use of stimulants is separated by 2 or more days of nonuse.

13. Binges are a form of use in which high doses are consumed over a period of hours or days.

14. Tobacco-related disorders generally begin in adolescence.

15. Frequent failed attempts to stop are a hallmark of tobacco use disorder.

16. An intoxication syndrome does not apply to tobacco; however, withdrawal is common and its severity is important to assess.

17. Onset of tobacco withdrawal usually begins within 24 hours of an individual stopping or cutting down on tobacco use, peaks at 2–3 days after abstinence, and lasts 2–3 weeks.

18. Tobacco cravings persist long after use has ceased and contribute to recurrences.

REFERENCES

American Psychiatric Association: Diagnostic and Statistical Manual of Mental Disorders, 4th Edition. Washington, DC, American Psychiatric Association, 1994

American Psychiatric Association: Diagnostic and Statistical Manual of Mental Disorders, 5th Edition. Arlington, VA, American Psychiatric Association, 2013

American Psychiatric Association: Diagnostic and Statistical Manual of Mental Disorders, 5th Edition, Text Revision. Washington, DC, American Psychiatric Association, 2022

Miller WR, Rollnick S: Motivational Interviewing: Helping People Change, 3rd Edition. New York, Guilford, 2013

Substance Abuse and Mental Health Services Administration: Substance Abuse Treatment in Adult and Juvenile Correctional Facilities: Findings from the Uniform Facility Data Set 1997 Survey of Correctional Facilities (Office of Applied Studies, Drug and Alcohol Services Information System Series S-9, DHHS Publ No SMA 00-3380). Rockville, MD, Substance Abuse and Mental Health Services Administration, 2000

Wesson DR, Ling W: The Clinical Opiate Withdrawal Scale (COWS). J Psychoactive Drugs 35:253–259, 2003

CHAPTER 21

Neurocognitive Disorders

Tobin J. Ehrlich, Ph.D.
Brian Yochim, Ph.D., ABPP-CN
Maya Yutsis, Ph.D., ABPP-CN
Jerome Yesavage, M.D.
Allyson C. Rosen, Ph.D., ABPP-CN

"He keeps asking the same thing over and over."

"She left the stove on!"

- Delirium
- Major and Mild Neurocognitive Disorders
  - Major or Mild Neurocognitive Disorder Due to Alzheimer's Disease
  - Major or Mild Frontotemporal Neurocognitive Disorder
  - Major or Mild Neurocognitive Disorder With Lewy Bodies
  - Major or Mild Vascular Neurocognitive Disorder
  - Major or Mild Neurocognitive Disorder Due to Traumatic Brain Injury
  - Substance/Medication-Induced Major or Mild Neurocognitive Disorder
  - Major or Mild Neurocognitive Disorder Due to HIV Infection
  - Major or Mild Neurocognitive Disorder Due to Prion Disease
  - Major or Mild Neurocognitive Disorder Due to Parkinson's Disease
  - Major or Mild Neurocognitive Disorder Due to Huntington's Disease
  - Major or Mild Neurocognitive Disorder Due to Another Medical Condition
  - Major or Mild Neurocognitive Disorder Due to Multiple Etiologies
  - Major or Mild Neurocognitive Disorder Due to Unknown Etiology

The neurocognitive disorders (NCDs) diagnostic class includes disorders of acquired cognitive deficits. Although cognitive deficits may be present in many mental health conditions, only disorders whose *primary* and *core features* are of cognitive decline are included under the NCDs. People will self-report changes in their abilities or, if they lack awareness of them, a caregiver will report them to the clinician. Initial clinical presentation and referral can fall into one of two categories: 1) people who are developing cognitive deficits of unknown cause, for which the clinician must assess the nature, extent, and etiology of these changes; or 2) people who have known neurological injury (e.g., a traumatic brain injury [TBI] or stroke), for whom the clinician must assess the effects of the damage. The individual's experience of the disorder can vary widely from complete awareness of the decline and associated distress to complete lack of awareness and consequent safety concerns (e.g., with regard to driving, cooking, and living alone). In the encounter with the patient, the clinician must take care to express empathy related to this dramatic change in life circumstances, increase insight, and make appropriate referrals as needed.

The NCDs are unique in DSM-5-TR (American Psychiatric Association 2022) because the symptoms are almost entirely cognitive in expression and clearly connected with underlying neurobiological processes. By conducting a thorough evaluation, including input from neurology, psychiatry, and neuropsychology, the clinician can reasonably and confidently establish a neurological etiology. The NCDs involve a decline in cognitive functioning from a previous state, as evidenced by 1) concerns from the individual, an informant, or the clinician; and 2) objective test performance. This evaluation differs from that for intellectual developmental disorders in that intellectual developmental disorders involve a baseline, impaired level of cognitive functioning.

There are three main syndromes of NCDs: delirium, major NCD, and mild NCD. Delirium can be thought of as a behavioral manifestation of an underlying metabolic disturbance that impairs central nervous system functioning to the extent that individuals show reductions in their basic ability to attend to the environment. These individuals show impairment in at least one other cognitive ability, such as memory or language. Delirium differs from major and mild NCDs in that it develops rapidly (i.e., in hours or days) and can be linked to medical conditions, substance intoxication or withdrawal, or other causes. Delirium is also unique in that it can completely resolve if the underlying cause is treated, although residual cognitive deficits can endure. The DSM-5-TR criteria incorporate the reality that delirium can endure for long periods of time, and the clinician can specify whether the disturbance is acute (lasting hours or days) or persistent (lasting weeks or months). Indeed, in medically frail older adults, one condition causing delirium can be ameliorated while another condition surfaces, leading to the net effect of no change in the outward manifestation of delirium. Note that one of the few changes in diagnostic criteria from DSM-5 (American Psychiatric Association 2013) to DSM-5-TR is that, under the category of other specified delirium, attenuated delirium syndrome has been changed to subsyndromal delirium. See Table 21–1 for key changes between DSM-5 and DSM-5-TR.

The term *dementia* has been used previously in DSM editions and is still widely used, including in the ICD-11, so DSM-5-TR allows its use in settings where custom-

TABLE 21–1. Key changes between DSM-5 and DSM-5-TR

Due to increased rates of suicidal behaviors in those diagnosed with a neurocognitive disorder (NCD), added emphasis is made on assessing suicide risk.

Markers of traumatic brain injury (TBI) severity have been expanded.

In cases where there is a likelihood of contributions from both vascular and Alzheimer's etiologies, NCD due to multiple etiologies should be diagnosed.

The table in the section on NCD due to TBI has been slightly modified and is included here.

---

ary; however, NCD extends the domain of acquired brain dysfunction to include people with TBI and other younger-onset acquired disorders. Another advantage of the NCD term is that dementia in DSM-IV (American Psychiatric Association 1994) or in the ICD framework requires more than one domain of dysfunction, but an NCD can refer to a disorder based on a single, disabling deficit, such as aphasia in frontotemporal NCD. Whereas NCDs exist on a continuum of severity, major NCD and dementia both involve functional disability. Mild NCD represents what has been described as preclinical dementia, or mild cognitive impairment, a condition in which the person has cognitive limitations but these are not sufficiently severe to be disabling.

Major NCD typically involves severe impairment in one or more cognitive domains with accompanying impairment in activities of daily living. One exception is in major NCD due to Alzheimer's disease, which requires impairment in two or more domains. The difference between a major and mild NCD is twofold: 1) the cognitive deficits are more severe in major NCD (typically at or below the third percentile) than in mild NCD (typically between the 3rd and 16th percentile); and 2) in major NCD, the deficits must be severe enough to interfere with independence, whereas in mild NCD, the deficits do not interfere with independence, although "greater effort, compensatory strategies, or accommodation" may be needed for the person to remain independent. A key point about the NCDs is that the same etiologies cause the disorder, whether it is a major or a mild NCD.

Once it is established that a person has a major or mild NCD, the next step for the clinician is to determine the most likely etiologies. The etiology can be determined on the basis of a combination of the symptom time course, cognitive domains involved, and associated medical or neurological condition. In some cases, a diagnosis of major or mild NCD depends on the presence of a known medical condition causing cognitive decline, as with the following etiologies: vascular disease, TBI, substance/medication use, HIV infection, prion disease, Parkinson's disease, and Huntington's disease. For other neurodegenerative etiologies, including Alzheimer's disease, frontotemporal lobar degeneration, and Lewy body disease, major or mild NCDs are diagnosed primarily on the basis of the cognitive, behavioral, and functional symptoms present. The term *probable* indicates a higher level of diagnostic certainty, and the term *possible* indicates a lower level of diagnostic certainty. Genetic variants and biomarkers based on diagnostic tests can increase certainty or indicate the level of severity. Some MRI- or CT-based biomarkers, such as stroke for vascular NCD or cerebral contusion for NCD due to TBI, are incorporated in the formal criteria. Other biomarkers, such as those increasingly utilized for NCD due to Alzheimer's disease (e.g., cerebral spinal fluid, positron emission tomography, and blood-based measures of amyloid or tau proteins), are described as used to increase certainty but are not formally part of the diagnostic criteria for discriminating probable or possible diagnoses. Many NCDs have multiple causes, and the diagnostician must undergo a process of ruling out various etiologies. The most common cause of NCD is Alzheimer's disease. This disease most typically causes memory dysfunction in its early stages, although deficits in other areas (e.g., executive functioning) can sometimes manifest as the first symptom. Other categories in this diagnostic class include major or mild NCD due to another medical condition, major or mild NCD due to multiple etiologies, and unspecified NCD. For example, when a comorbid condition contributes to the NCD in an individual with Alzheimer's disease, then NCD due to multiple etiologies should be diagnosed.

IN-DEPTH DIAGNOSIS: DELIRIUM

Mr. Hancock, a 90-year-old man living independently at baseline, was brought by his daughter to the emergency department because he started to "ramble and moan" and could not answer questions or track conversations over the past 2 days. He also started yelling at her about taking his money away but quickly shifted to crying. He started to experience hallucinations of seeing strangers in his room who were "chasing" him. These symptoms fluctuated throughout the day and night.. He was sleeping a lot during the day and was awake much of the night. On admission, he had great difficulty attending to the examiner and answering questions, and he was also disoriented to time, date, and location. He was found to have an acute urinary tract infection. Upon reviewing his medication regimen, the physicians found that he was taking a benzodiazepine for "nerves" and 10 other medications. They decided to taper him off the benzodiazepine and treat the urinary tract infection during a hospital stay. Throughout the hospital stay, Mr. Hancock was provided with a dark and quiet environment at night to aid his sleep and frequent gentle reminders of the date and place, with this information written on a whiteboard next to his bed. His family placed family pictures around the room. After a week of hospitalization, his speech became understandable, he was no longer yelling at his loved ones, and he was able to state the date, his address, and the name of the hospital. Once the urinary tract infection cleared, Mr. Hancock was discharged home.

This case illustrates several key components of delirium. The symptoms developed abruptly and rapidly over a few days, which helped to differentiate delirium from other NCDs. Disorientation and unawareness of surroundings together with a change in sleep-wake cycle further indicated delirium. Mr. Hancock had a rapid change from one emotional state to another—features that are common in delirium. Visual hallucinations are common, and people are often afraid of these experiences; when a person presents with a new onset of visual hallucinations and is older than 40, it is important to consider a delirium process rather than attribute hallucinations to a psychotic disorder. As is common in delirium, Mr. Hancock was found to have more than one contributor to the symptoms: a urinary tract infection and a medication (a benzodiazepine) that is associated with delirium. Polypharmacy is another leading cause of delirium. The urinary tract infection was treated while Mr. Hancock was tapered off the benzodiazepine. (Substance withdrawal, of course, is another cause of delirium, and benzodiazepines must be carefully tapered to prevent delirium.) The medical team made strong efforts to provide a quiet environment for the patient, with frequent reorientation and cues to dates and place to assist in his recovery. It is also helpful for family members or close ones to assist in reorienting patients (e.g., with photographs, as in this case).

Approach to the Diagnosis

Given the complex etiology of delirium, the first line of its assessment is gathering a comprehensive history and establishing a baseline of cognitive functioning. According to DSM-5-TR, the key feature of delirium is a disturbance in attention and awareness that develops rapidly over a few hours to days and represents a change from a typical level of cognitive functioning for the patient. Impaired attention may include difficulty answering questions or repeating words and numbers; difficulty multitasking; becoming distracted by noises, other people, and objects in the room; and difficulty staying on the topic of conversation. Questions often need to be repeated because the person's attention wanders. The individual may provide the same answer to different questions (e.g., answering "35" to both "How old are you?" and "What is your address?"). Lack of awareness of the environment may result in disorientation to date, time, place, and even personal information such as age, marital status, or address. These difficulties may vary throughout the day and even hour to hour, with marked worsening in the evening and at night. The interviewer should assess whether a medical event (e.g., a fall, accident, surgery) may have triggered the aforementioned rapid changes in cognitive status. A physical examination should include a review of current medications, especially those added recently; symptoms of past or current systemic infections; blood work, urine analysis, and imaging to establish whether these changes are due to an underlying medical condition; metabolic issues such as renal or liver dysfunction, hypoxia, hypoglycemia, anemia, or substance intoxication or withdrawal; medication use (e.g., benzodiazepines, anticholinergics, pain narcotics); or a combination of these factors. Because systemic infections, such as urinary tract infections, sepsis, or pneumonia, are a common etiology of delirium, special attention is paid in the history to any symptoms of infection, including changes in urinary symptoms, cough, shortness of breath, and fever.

Given that delirium often occurs in older adults with a preexisting major or mild NCD, which renders them more vulnerable to changes in cognitive status, a cognitive baseline must be established. Because the individual will likely have difficulty answering questions accurately due to impaired attention and disorientation to most personal information, a collateral source or review of outside medical records is needed to establish a cognitive baseline. Data from neuroimaging and other biomarkers can be used to establish whether mild or major NCD of a known etiology, such as Alzheimer's disease, is also present and further renders the person more vulnerable to delirium. In addition to the disturbance in attention and awareness, a change in at least one other cognitive area must occur, such as in recent memory; disorientation to

time and place; language (e.g., rambling speech, mumbling); or perceptual disturbance, including visual hallucinations or misinterpretations. To assess for perceptual
disturbances, the interviewer can ask, "Do you see things other people don't see?" If
the answer is yes, the clinician can follow up with additional questions, such as, "Do
you see animals (people, faces, strangers)? Do these figures appear threatening? What
are they doing?" A collateral source should be asked whether the person has received
a previous diagnosis of mild or major NCD or experienced variability in attention,
alertness, and orientation to date, place, or personal information. The collateral source
should also be asked if the person frequently "stares into space" and appears more
"confused" in the evening. A careful history of the time course of the illness is important to make a separation between delirium and other NCDs.

Getting the History

> Ms. Hart, a 90-year-old man admitted to the emergency department, is unable to an-
> swer questions, appears lethargic most of the day, becomes easily distracted by nursing
> staff walking in and out of the room, and reports "seeing strangers in her room." The
> interviewer first determines the time and course of these symptoms by asking a family
> member who is present in the room a series of questions: "When did you first notice
> that she had difficulty answering questions? Were these issues triggered by a recent
> change in any medications? Has she fallen recently or developed a urinary tract infec-
> tion? Does her alertness vary throughout the day?" If the symptoms vary and devel-
> oped within the past day after she was diagnosed with a urinary tract infection, the
> interviewer may suspect delirium. The interviewer also assesses Ms. Hart's orientation
> to surroundings by asking her, "Can you tell me today's date? What is the name of this
> place? What is your name? How old are you?" If Ms. Hart knows her age and name but
> incorrectly states the date and the name of the place, she is considered disoriented to
> surroundings. Administering a subtest of the Montreal Cognitive Assessment, such as
> digit span, assesses attention. To assess digit span, the interviewer says, "I am going to
> say some numbers, and when I am through, repeat them to me exactly as I said them,"
> and reads a five-number sequence at a rate of one digit per second. If the patient repeats
> fewer than three numbers, her attention is impaired, further indicating delirium. Fi-
> nally, the interviewer assesses perceptual disturbances by asking Ms. Hart, "Do you see
> things that others do not see?" If the answer is yes, the interviewer asks, "What do you
> see? Are these images scary? What are they doing?" The interviewer also asks the pa-
> tient's family member whether Ms. Hart has a history of perceptual disturbances, sub-
> stance use, and other medical problems.

Given that the prevalence of delirium is highest among older adults, the patient's
age of 90 years and the rapid onset of impaired attention are key indicators that a diagnosis of delirium should be high in the diagnostic differential. Ms. Hart experiences
rapid and abrupt onset of impaired attention (repeating fewer than three digits) and
disorientation (not knowing the date and place) over 1 day, triggered by a diagnosis
of urinary tract infection, thus meeting criteria for delirium. Her level of alertness and
inattention varied throughout the day, which further indicates delirium. Ms. Hart
also experienced a new onset of visual hallucinations without a previous history of
psychosis or perceptual disturbances, which usually indicates a neurological problem
or delirium rather than a preexisting mood or psychotic disorder. The interviewer

will want to find out the course and nature of her visual hallucinations because mild or major NCD with Lewy bodies can mimic delirium; it presents with fluctuations in alertness and attention as well as visual hallucinations. However, the short duration and rapid onset of these symptoms support the diagnosis of delirium. A full medical workup and medical chart review would be warranted to rule out other medical problems that may be contributing to the patient's current difficulties.

Tips for Clarifying the Diagnosis

- Evaluate recent lab results.
- Review the person's medical record and current medications, especially ones that were added recently. Assess which over-the-counter medications the person may take that have sedating properties, such as diphenhydramine.
- Assess symptom time and duration and clarify how quickly they developed.
- Explore whether deficits in attention and orientation vary throughout the day.
- Conduct a collateral interview to establish an accurate cognitive baseline for the individual and to verify the medical history and medications. Ask about previously diagnosed major NCDs.
- Evaluate for sensory misperceptions such as visual hallucinations, and question whether the person is frightened by these experiences.

Consider the Case

Mr. Nelson is a 25-year-old man admitted to the hospital following a 10-foot fall from a ladder, resulting in mild TBI and a broken leg. His neighbor found him unconscious on the ground. On admission to the hospital, he was fully oriented to date, time, place, and personal information. He remembered falling off the ladder and "waking up in the emergency room," but he did not know who found him. Duration of posttraumatic amnesia was estimated to last less than 1 hour. On a brief mental status examination, he had difficulty counting backward from 100 in increments of 7 and recalling five newly learned words, indicative of memory impairment. His attention was intact, and he repeated up to five digits forward and three digits backward. He underwent surgery to stabilize his broken leg and was started on morphine postoperatively to aid with pain management. A catheter was also placed. One day following surgery, Mr. Nelson was unable to state the date and the name of the hospital and reported that strangers were "attacking" him. His attention declined significantly; he was unable to answer any questions or repeat three digits forward. The result of a CT scan of his head was negative. His brother informed the staff that Mr. Nelson was allergic to morphine. Upon discontinuation of morphine, Mr. Nelson's attention and orientation returned to his admission level within 3 days. He continued to have difficulty recalling new information, such as a list of five words and the names of new nursing staff or attending physicians.

Delirium often can be triggered by a new medical problem such as TBI, introduction of new medications, or surgery. When multiple risk factors are present, delirium is more likely to develop. In this case, Mr. Nelson experienced a mild TBI, resulting in memory difficulties for recently learned information, which is commonly associated with TBI. However, his attention was initially intact, and he was aware of his surroundings. Following surgery, placement of a catheter, and initiation of an opiate pain narcotic, his attention and awareness of surroundings markedly declined overnight. He was unable to repeat more than three digits forward, to follow conversation, and to answer questions, which indicated impaired attention. (Someone his age should be able to repeat at least five digits forward and three backward.) Visual hallucinations of a frightening nature were also noted. His disorientation to date and place together with impaired attention indicated a major decline in cognitive status compared with his status at admission. Following the introduction of an opiate narcotic, he demonstrated an allergic reaction to morphine, which triggered an acute onset of delirium superimposed onto a recent mild TBI. Once the medication was discontinued, delirium appeared to clear within 3 days. He continued to have memory difficulties, as would be expected with mild TBI 1 week following the injury. Memory impairment due to mild TBI would be expected to resolve completely within 1–3 months.

Differential Diagnosis

The differential diagnosis of delirium is quite broad because the hallmark of delirium is rapid onset of impaired attention, reduced awareness or orientation to the environment, and decline in thinking abilities that includes, but is not limited to, deficits in memory, orientation, language, visuospatial ability, and perception. These difficulties often occur in the context of most major NCDs, medical disorders, and substance/medication-induced side effects, especially postoperatively, with the latter two categories necessitating appropriate medical workup. Similarly, delirium may be seen in many psychiatric disorders (psychotic disorders including, but not limited to, schizophrenia, schizophreniform and brief psychotic disorders; bipolar and depressive disorders with psychotic features; acute stress disorder; malingering; factitious disorder; and substance use disorders). The most common differential diagnosis for delirium includes separating whether a person has major NCD or delirium, both delirium and NCD, or NCD without delirium. Memory problems are common to both delirium and major NCD, such as NCD due to Alzheimer's disease, but the person with only major NCD is typically oriented to personal information, such as their name, age, and children's names, and is aware of surroundings (e.g., hospital vs. home; city and state), and this awareness does not change over the course of the day. Psychotic disorders should also be considered in the differential diagnosis when perceptual changes are present, including visual hallucinations, delusions, or rambled speech. The rapid onset and fluctuation of these perceptual changes would be more consistent with delirium, whereas prolonged onset, chronicity, and stability of these symptoms would suggest the presence of a psychotic disorder. Finally, in the absence of a medical condition or substance that is associated with rapid changes in thinking abilities, malingering and factitious disorder also should be considered.

Two associated features that help with the diagnosis of delirium include change in sleep-wake cycle and rapid changes in emotional states that can vary from hour to hour. Change in sleep-wake cycle may include increased and excessive daytime sleepiness and difficulty falling asleep, and it is often associated with delirium but is not required to make a diagnosis. Rarely, a complete reversal of sleep cycle occurs in which an individual sleeps during the daytime and is awake during nighttime hours. Rapid changes in emotional states include nervousness and anxiety and feeling afraid, depressed, irritable, angry, apathetic, or overly euphoric. Irritability and anger can include behaviors such as screaming, cursing, moaning, rambled speech, and unintelligible sounds. These changes occur rapidly and unpredictably, and they fluctuate from hour to hour. Acute stress disorder and delirium can both be associated with intense feelings of fear, anxiety, and disorientation, but in acute stress disorder these symptoms are precipitated by an easily identifiable traumatic event. Behavioral problems increase in the evening and nighttime with delirium because the environmental cues of light and activity are absent.

See DSM-5-TR for additional disorders to consider in the differential diagnosis, including bipolar disorders, depressive disorders with psychotic features, acute stress disorder, malingering, and factitious disorder. Also refer to the discussions of comorbidity and differential diagnosis in their respective sections of DSM-5-TR.

Summary

- A diagnosis of delirium should be considered when 1) a rapid and abrupt onset of disturbance in attention and disorientation is present, and 2) the alteration represents a change from the individual's cognitive baseline.
- Delirium may be due to substance use intoxication or withdrawal.
- A preexisting history of major NCD highly increases an individual's vulnerability to developing delirium.
- Delirium has diverse causes, including a wide range of general medical disorders (e.g., metabolic issues, hypoxia, hypoglycemia, systemic infections), polypharmacy (e.g., benzodiazepines, opiate narcotics, anticholinergics), recent injury (e.g., TBI, stroke, hypoxia), and psychiatric disorders (e.g., substance use disorders, acute stress disorder, somatic symptom and related disorders, factitious disorder).

IN-DEPTH DIAGNOSIS: MAJOR OR MILD NCD DUE TO ALZHEIMER'S DISEASE

Mr. Green is an 80-year-old man who reports having difficulty finding the right word when speaking, but he attributes this to his age. His wife reports that he increasingly repeats stories to her and asks the same question several times a day. This has progressively worsened over the past year, with no clear precipitating event. His wife also reports that she has taken over managing the finances because he has made a few errors in bill payments in the past year. Upon interview, Mr. Green is unable to describe current events in the news, other than making vague references to wars in parts of the world. On neuropsychological assessment, his performance on measures of memory, naming, and executive ability is at the 1st percentile as compared with adults his age. During the evaluation, he makes several socially inappropriate comments but is friendly and cooperative. Complex attention and visuoperceptual ability are normal for his age and not suggestive of decline. He and his wife report that he has three or four alcoholic drinks per week but has never been a heavy drinker. Each denies that he has any current symptoms of depression. He lost consciousness once for approximately 5 minutes about 20 years ago in a motor vehicle crash, with no other reported brain injuries. MRI reveals cortical atrophy, with pronounced atrophy in the medial temporal lobes shown on a coronal scan and age-appropriate white matter cerebrovascular changes. The result of a recent neurological evaluation was unremarkable except for the presence of observable cognitive difficulties. Mr. Green is physically healthy with no acute infections and has no family history of neurological disease. No genetic testing has occurred.

This vignette highlights several important components of the assessment of major NCD due to Alzheimer's disease. Mr. Green himself does not express concern, whereas a knowledgeable informant, his wife, reports common symptoms relevant to this diagnosis. Clinicians may also see individuals who have concerns, whereas their caregivers lack concerns. Neuropsychological assessment shows impaired performance in two or more domains, with the typical finding of memory impairment associated with Alzheimer's disease. The deficits have interfered with Mr. Green's independence, as indicated by his wife's need to take over financial management. The timeline of progression over the past year and his current health are not suggestive of delirium. Although Mr. Green has a past history of a brain injury, it seems unrelated to his current symptom presentation. MRI findings show atrophy in the areas typically affected by Alzheimer's disease but no evidence of strong cerebrovascular involvement. The unremarkable neurological evaluation result without signs of parkinsonian symptoms or other features of Lewy body disease is also consistent with an Alzheimer's etiology. The deficits in executive ability and mildly socially inappropriate behavior raise concerns about frontotemporal lobar degeneration, but his predominant memory deficits and his age, which is older than that of typical people with frontotemporal lobar degeneration, are less consistent with that diagnosis. It is important to note that complex attention and visuoperceptual ability are normal for his age and not suggestive of decline, although "normal" performance for patients with a high baseline may be indicative of decline.

Approach to the Diagnosis

Assessing a person for the possibility of NCD due to Alzheimer's disease consists of gathering a clear history and obtaining some assessment of cognitive functioning, with an emphasis on memory. The diagnosis of Alzheimer's disease as the cause of NCD can be thought of as a process of ruling out other potential etiologies. Many, if not most, individuals will have more than one suspected etiology (e.g., Alzheimer's disease and vascular disease). These individuals should be diagnosed with major or mild NCD due to multiple etiologies.

Alzheimer's disease involves progressive decline, usually with no precipitating event; but sometimes symptoms, which may simply have not been apparent before, seem to be triggered by a discrete medical event (e.g., surgery, major illness, hospitalization) or a psychosocial event (e.g., major travel, major change in routine). In the interview, it is helpful to gather examples of memory problems, such as forgetting conversations, repeating things, or becoming unable to learn new skills that were previously easy to learn (e.g., how to use the new television remote or the latest type of phone). Other symptoms that individuals or their caregivers may report include word-finding problems in conversation, getting lost, deficits in social functioning, difficulty handling multiple tasks, or other executive deficits described in DSM-5-TR. It is essential to interview not only the individual but also a caregiver, because individuals can under- or overestimate their deficits.

Neuropsychological assessment, if available, is helpful in providing precise measurement of a person's cognitive abilities and comparing them with those of others of a similar age and education level. Neuropsychological testing can also detect mild deficits that screening tools miss. Data from neuroimaging and other biomarkers can be used to establish whether Alzheimer's disease is the underlying cause of deficits found through testing and interview.

Once a clinician suspects Alzheimer's disease as the cause, "probable" or "possible" must be specified. The criteria for probable Alzheimer's disease differ depending on whether the NCD is major or mild. For major NCD, probable Alzheimer's disease requires either 1) evidence of a causative Alzheimer's disease genetic mutation from family history or genetic testing, or 2) a combination of clear decline in memory and one other cognitive domain; progressive, gradual decline in cognition; and absence of other possible etiology. If neither of these criteria are met, possible Alzheimer's disease is diagnosed. Other biomarkers of Alzheimer's disease (e.g., neuroimaging) are not included at this time. For mild NCD, probable Alzheimer's disease is diagnosed only if there is evidence of a causative Alzheimer's genetic mutation. Possible Alzheimer's disease is diagnosed for mild NCD when there is no evidence of a causative Alzheimer's disease genetic mutation, but the other clinical criteria are met.

Lastly, there are two factors to consider in differentiating major and mild NCD related to Alzheimer's disease. Although the general criteria for major NCD involve decline in *one* or more cognitive domains, the criteria for major NCD due to Alzheimer's disease require impairment of *two* domains. This is the only NCD category in which the major specification requires two domains to be impaired. The other key difference between major and mild NCD lies in the impairment in everyday activities involved in major NCD.

Getting the History

Ms. Bell reports that her 77-year-old husband's memory is getting worse. She explains that his long-term memory is normal, but his short-term memory is poor. The interviewer asks, "Can you give me an example?" She reports that he repeats questions throughout the day. When asked about the effects of these memory problems on his everyday living, Ms. Bell is unable to provide a clear answer. The interviewer then asks, "Let's say you had to leave town for a few days. Would you feel comfortable leaving your husband alone at home for a few days?" Ms. Bell then exclaims, "No, I couldn't do that! He would leave on the stove burner and burn down the house! He would also become lost while driving home from the grocery store." After further discussion, the interviewer asks, "Is there some event that seemed to start these problems?" Ms. Bell cannot recall an event that seemed to trigger the problems, but she notes that she knew there was a problem when he had great difficulty learning how to operate the new television they purchased a year ago. She also mentions how their daughter, who lives in another state, came for her yearly visit several months ago and was concerned about how different her father seemed.

Ms. Bell reports difficulties in her husband's "short-term memory." The terms *memory*, *short-term memory*, and *long-term memory* mean different things to different people in the lay public and require clarification when patients or caregivers use them. The examples informants provide may lead the clinician to hypotheses about whether the person is experiencing mild or major NCD, whether the deficits are due to other causes such as a stroke or TBI, how much depression or anxiety symptoms have an impact on functioning, and so on. For instance, if a corporate executive reports difficulty remembering the names of all their employees, this may reflect a mild NCD, whereas if a person is reporting more serious memory problems, such as the ones in this vignette, these may be more symptomatic of major NCD due to Alzheimer's disease. Eliciting examples accomplishes another goal: assessing the effects of the deficits on everyday functioning. Individuals or their caregivers occasionally are unable to provide clear answers about everyday functioning, and the question mentioned in the vignette about leaving town for a few days can help elicit a clear answer. Last, this vignette illustrates how the observation of a new problem often involves the person's being placed in a new situation (e.g., learning how to operate a new appliance) or an infrequent visitor observing the change (e.g., a family member visiting after some time away).

Tips for Clarifying the Diagnosis

- Establish whether the individual shows impairment in one or more cognitive domains, particularly in memory.
- Determine whether this impairment is severe enough to interfere with the person's daily activities.
- Clarify whether the impairment has developed gradually over time or after a particular event (e.g., stroke, brain injury).
- Seek evidence to confirm whether this is a delirium or a chronic disorder.
- Verify whether the person is abusing alcohol or other substances that can cause a reversible memory impairment, or whether they have a history of chronic alcohol abuse that may be the cause of a more permanent impairment.
- Investigate the possibility of parkinsonian motor symptoms or hallucinations related to Lewy body disease, which may suggest a different etiology than Alzheimer's disease.

Consider the Case

Ms. Sato, an 85-year-old woman, reports that her children have requested that she stop driving because she has been involved in three car accidents in the past year. She says that two of the accidents involved other vehicles that "came out of nowhere" and that she hit another car while parking. Her children also note that she sometimes calls them the wrong name when looking at them. When discussing her hobbies, she explains that she used to enjoy reading but has found it more difficult. Ms. Sato lives with her son, and his wife manages her finances and shopping needs. They are of Japanese ethnicity and attribute her symptoms to old age, stating that all older adults eventually must stop driving. Neuropsychological assessment demonstrates performance at the 1st percentile in visual perception, but intact memory, attention, language, and executive ability. She is socially appropriate, quiet, and deferential to medical professionals. She denies any hallucinations, symptoms of rapid eye movement (REM) sleep behavior disorder, or fluctuations in attention. Motor examination results are normal, and she has no parkinsonian symptoms. She denies any history of strokes or TBIs. MRI shows bilateral atrophy in the occipital and posterior parietal lobes. Ms. Sato and her children deny significant history of substance abuse. She denies feeling sad or having physical symptoms of depression, including excessive sleeping and decreased appetite.

This case illustrates atypical mild NCD due to Alzheimer's disease and important components to consider when working with older Japanese Americans. Although Alzheimer's disease typically causes predominant memory deficits early on, occasionally nonamnestic symptoms occur first. This patient is showing some symptoms of the visuospatial variant that results from posterior cortical atrophy, with difficulty perceiving other cars while driving, difficulty reading, and inability to recognize familiar faces. This diagnosis is supported by MRI findings of atrophy in the occipital and parietal lobes. Visual perception deficits can also be caused by Lewy body disease, but Ms. Sato lacks other symptoms of this disease (e.g., visual hallucinations, fluctuating attention, parkinsonian symptoms). Neuropsychological testing found impairment in one area, visual perception, but other areas were intact; thus, mild rather than major NCD would be diagnosed. Ms. Sato and her family are of Japanese ethnicity; individuals from this background are more likely to attribute their symptoms to normal aging and may not seek help when needed. When evaluating for symptoms of depression that may contribute to cognitive presentation, clinicians should keep in mind that people of Japanese ethnicity may be more likely to report physical symptoms (e.g., sleep and appetite disturbances) than depressed mood. It is also important when working with members of this ethnic group to incorporate the closeness of the family unit when planning care.

Differential Diagnosis

Major or mild NCD due to Alzheimer's disease differs from vascular NCD in that most often a discrete cerebrovascular event or a preponderance of vascular damage seen on neuroimaging can be linked with the development of vascular NCD, whereas Alzheimer's disease develops more gradually without a clear precipitant. Other diseases such as Lewy body disease or Parkinson's disease also develop gradually but have symptoms (e.g., visual hallucinations, motor symptoms) that are not characteristic of Alzheimer's disease. Symptoms of executive dysfunction and decline in social cognition can occur in both Alzheimer's disease and the behavioral variant of frontotemporal NCD, and language difficulties (e.g., poor word finding or speech production) can occur in both Alzheimer's disease and the language variant of frontotemporal NCD. However, memory also tends to be impaired in Alzheimer's disease, whereas it is spared in the early stages of frontotemporal degeneration. Frontotemporal NCD occurs most often in patients younger than 65 (although 20%–25% of cases are older than 65), whereas Alzheimer's disease tends to develop later in life, although inherited Alzheimer's disease can have an earlier onset.

Other medical causes of cognitive dysfunction (e.g., vitamin B_{12} deficiency, thyroid disorders) should be ruled out in the assessment through lab work. Symptoms of delirium tend to develop rapidly (e.g., in hours or days), whereas symptoms of Alzheimer's disease typically manifest over the span of months.

Major depressive disorder, generalized anxiety disorder, and PTSD in older adults can often interfere with cognitive functioning. However, these disorders typically do not lead to the cognitive profiles associated with Alzheimer's disease. For example, although individuals with these disorders may have difficulty acquiring new information on memory tasks, they are typically able to retain information over time, whereas people with Alzheimer's disease forget information over time. Likewise, language difficulties occur in Alzheimer's disease but not typically in major depressive disorder, generalized anxiety disorder, or PTSD.

Alzheimer's disease occurs later in life, when persons are more susceptible to a variety of other medical problems. Alzheimer's disease, like other conditions that compromise the brain, increases the risk of delirium, and individuals often are found to be experiencing both conditions. Vascular disease is common in older adults and increases the risk for Alzheimer's disease, in addition to directly causing NCD on its own. Comorbid vascular disease may lead to symptoms of decreased processing speed and executive dysfunction. Depressive symptoms have a strong relationship with Alzheimer's disease; some literature has found that a history of depressive symptoms or recent onset of anxiety may increase the risk of Alzheimer's disease, and newly diagnosed individuals with Alzheimer's disease often develop symptoms of depression or anxiety in response to the diagnosis. Clinicians should be careful to assess suicidal ideation in newly diagnosed patients, particularly those who are demographically at increased risk of suicide (e.g., older White males). Comorbid depressive symptoms also may accelerate cognitive decline in people with Alzheimer's disease. Alcohol abuse in older adults can worsen symptoms of Alzheimer's disease, and individuals should decrease or cease their usage if a history of alcohol abuse is present.

See DSM-5-TR for additional disorders to consider in the differential diagnosis. Also refer to the discussions of comorbidity and differential diagnosis in their respective sections of DSM-5-TR.

Summary

- Alzheimer's disease, the most common cause of NCD, most often involves progressive deterioration in memory and other cognitive abilities.
- Major NCD due to Alzheimer's disease involves impairment in two or more domains and interference with ability to complete everyday activities.
- Mild NCD due to Alzheimer's disease involves decline in one or more cognitive domains, but the deficits do not interfere with independence in everyday activities.
- The criteria for probable versus possible Alzheimer's disease differ depending on whether the NCD is major or mild.

- The main biomarker included in the diagnostic criteria is evidence of a causative Alzheimer's disease genetic mutation from family history or genetic testing.

IN-DEPTH DIAGNOSIS:
MAJOR OR MILD NCD WITH LEWY BODIES

Ms. Farley, a 66-year-old woman, presents with a history of worsening anxiety and depression that began 18 months ago. According to her husband, she had the belief that there was a third person in the house, and she also saw people in the house who were not there. She often slept for several hours during the day and would have periods when she would stare into space. One night she asked her husband what he was doing in her bed, as if she did not recognize him. Her husband had taken over the laundry chores because intermittently Ms. Farley became upset and frustrated that she could not figure out how to use the washing machine, which she had used throughout their marriage. She was hospitalized briefly, during which a full evaluation was conducted with no evidence of a medical contributor to her symptoms. She was given neuroleptic medication, but at the time of her discharge from the hospital, staff noted that she had signs of a movement disorder, and the medication was stopped. Neurological evaluation revealed subtle motor signs consistent with those observed in Parkinson's disease (i.e., bradykinesia and rigidity), which had previously not been noticed by the patient or her husband. Formal neuropsychological evaluation revealed that Ms. Farley has significant executive and visuospatial deficits that could not be accounted for by a movement disorder. She has fears of falling, but her most disabling fear relates to needing to use a bathroom while away from home. Her husband says that she often turns back from leaving the house because she worries that she will need to use the bathroom but not have one available.

Formal neuropsychological assessment documented a significant deficit in executive and visuospatial functioning, so that feature of major NCD is satisfied. Another feature of major NCD—requiring assistance in instrumental activities (i.e., laundry chores)—is also met. Careful interviewing revealed that although the presenting problems are depressed mood and anxiety, they are related to a fixed delusion of a third person in the house and a core symptom of hallucinations. Ms. Farley shows examples of fluctuations in attention and alertness, notably sleeping several hours during the day and displaying episodes of staring into space. The motor signs are subtle and detected only on formal neurological evaluation; these are a core feature. Establishing the timing of onset is problematic with disorders that evolve gradually; however, given that there has not been a formal diagnosis of a movement disorder and the cognitive dysfunction is significant, the diagnosis of NCD with Lewy bodies (NCDLB) would be more appropriate than one of NCD due to Parkinson's disease. Associated features include difficulty with urination and potential susceptibility to falling, of which Ms. Farley appears to be aware. Urinary incontinence or difficulty with urination are not apparent early in Alzheimer's disease but are consistent with NCDLB. In summary, Ms. Farley has more than two core symptoms of functional decline and would thus receive the diagnosis of probable major NCDLB with mild behavioral disturbance.

Approach to the Diagnosis

The three core symptoms of NCDLB are fluctuations in cognition with pronounced variations in attention and alertness, visual hallucinations, and a parkinsonian movement disorder that develops after the cognitive dysfunction. A common reason for which individuals present for clinical evaluation is a late-life, new onset of visual hallucinations, which may be associated with delusions and emotional disturbance. At this point it is crucial to evaluate the other core symptoms of the disorder, because treatment with some neuroleptic medications in patients with NCDLB can lead to enduring disability and be fatal. This adverse response to these medications is described as neuroleptic sensitivity, and symptoms include worsening of movement disorder and impaired consciousness. A previous history of neuroleptic sensitivity is consistent with NCDLB and is a suggestive diagnostic feature. Fluctuations in cognition and attention can be assessed with screening measures (e.g., Ferman et al. 2004; Walker et al. 2000), and it is important to reassure families that the variability in functioning is consistent with the disorder and not intentional. Individuals also may have experienced a REM sleep behavior disorder beginning decades before the illness. REM sleep behavior disorder is a phenomenon in which individuals do not experience the typical paralysis with sleep and may be physically violent during the dream state, which can lead to injuries. This symptom is suggestive; not all persons with REM sleep behavior disorder develop NCDLB. The DLB Consortium consensus statement indicated the symptom was frequent in autopsy-confirmed cases (McKeith et al. 2017).

In DSM-5-TR, the probable versus possible descriptors reflect the level of certainty of the diagnosis: probable NCDLB requires two core features or one core and one suggestive feature, whereas possible NCDLB requires one core feature or one or more suggestive features. The DSM-5-TR criteria agree with the DLB Consortium consensus criteria in designating the cognitive dysfunction as an essential feature and the fluctuating cognition and alertness, visual hallucinations, and parkinsonian features as core features (McKeith et al. 2017); however, the DLB Consortium additionally classifies REM sleep behavior disorder as a core rather than a suggestive feature.

Getting the History

Mr. Greene brings his 68-year-old wife for a diagnostic evaluation. She presents with fluctuations of symptoms, hallucinations, and parkinsonian features. The interviewer asks Mr. Greene about these fluctuations with the following questions: "Do you find that your wife sometimes blanks out, becomes confused, does not know where she is, or can't perform something simple that she should be able to do?" An example is a transient inability to perform an activity, such as brushing teeth without the guidance of a caregiver. Although structured measures of fluctuation can sensitively detect NCDLB (e.g., Ferman et al. 2004; Walker et al. 2000), people using those rating scales often disagree on their ratings if they do not have significant clinical experience with patients who have NCDLB. The interviewer asks, "Is she drowsy during the day, or does she take naps for more than 2 hours?" Content items that differentiate NCDLB from NCD due to Alzheimer's disease include daytime drowsiness, daytime sleep of more than 2 hours, staring into space for long periods, and disorganized flow of ideas. The interviewer asks, "Are there times when she seems disorganized, unclear, or not logical?"

To assess hallucinations, the clinician asks Ms. Greene, "Do you see or hear people or things that others tell you are not there? Describe them." Hallucinations typically are visual, well formed, and commonly of people (less commonly of animals); however, auditory hallucinations or hallucinations of objects do occur. The interviewer asks Ms. Greene, "Does seeing these things make you upset?" It is important to assess whether there is associated emotional distress or delusions. For example, Capgras syndrome, the delusion that an impostor has replaced a family member, can occur. The clinician can inquire into this by asking Ms. Greene's husband, "Does your wife ever treat you as if you were someone else, not her husband?" How a caregiver responds could be important for clinical management, and this information can be elicited by asking, "What do you do when she acts this way?" The interviewer assesses whether particular objects can be important triggers for Ms. Greene by asking her, "Are there places in your house or living space where you are likely to see these people?"

Parkinsonian features are evaluated by asking the patient, "Have you had any falls or difficulty getting around recently?" A neurological examination is required and typically indicates symptoms such as that patients are slow (bradykinesia), are stiff (rigidity), and have tremor. Abnormalities in walking (gait disorder) could also increase risk of falls. Because there may be several contributors to falls in NCDLB (e.g., autonomic dysfunction, gait instability), falls are an early symptom and a risk for further disability. The interviewer asks if the patient has fallen repeatedly. The timing of symptom onset and monitoring of motor symptoms is important over time.

In DSM-5-TR, suggestive diagnostic features include REM sleep behavior disorder and severe neuroleptic drug sensitivity. REM sleep behavior disorder can be assessed by asking Mr. Greene, "Does your wife lie still during sleep or does she behave as if she were acting out a dream, such as talking, yelling, or moving violently?" This symptom is best assessed in a formal sleep clinic. The disorder is important to identify because it is amenable to treatment. Severe neuroleptic drug sensitivity can be evaluated by asking Mr. Greene, "Has anyone ever given your wife medications that changed her ability to move or think clearly? Which medication was given?" Patients who have NCDLB have an extreme sensitivity to anticholinergic and antidopaminergic medications, including typical neuroleptic medications.

This case is an example of an initial interview; however, an evaluation of NCDLB should be multidisciplinary. A basic evaluation ideally includes neurological, medical, and neuropsychological assessments to characterize the motor, autonomic, and cognitive symptoms, respectively. A sleep study would be advisable if symptoms are consistent with REM sleep behavior disorder. Unless otherwise specified, questions are directed to the caregiver, particularly regarding symptoms of which the patient would likely be unaware (e.g., sleep-related behaviors). For clarity, the symptom areas are separated, but it is important to establish roughly when each symptom began in order to differentiate NCDLB from NCD due to Parkinson's disease.

Tips for Clarifying the Diagnosis

- If complex hallucinations first develop in an older adult or marked fluctuations in alertness develop gradually, assess for the other core symptoms of NCDLB.
- Investigate a history of neuroleptic sensitivity, which is suggestive of NCDLB.
- Arrange for a careful medical evaluation, which can assist in discriminating delirium from NCDLB, both of which are characterized by fluctuating cognition, attention, and alertness.

- Question and warn the patient about falls, which are common among people with NCDLB and raise the risk for further disability.
- Differentiate NCDLB from NCD due to Parkinson's disease by establishing the beginning of the major NCD relative to the movement disorder symptoms: major cognitive deficits develop 1 year before symptoms of a movement disorder occur in NCDLB but at least 1 year after such symptoms appear in NCD due to Parkinson's disease.
- Remember that memory is relatively preserved and visuospatial and executive functions are disproportionately impaired early in NCDLB, which distinguishes the cognitive pattern from NCD due to Alzheimer's disease and normal aging.

Consider the Case

Mr. Rodriguez is a 65-year-old retired farm laborer who moved to the United States from Mexico 20 years ago. He presents at the movement disorders clinic for a presurgical evaluation for implantation of a brain stimulation device. Mr. Rodriguez and his wife do not speak English and are interviewed through an interpreter. His wife is eager for the intervention because she believes it will improve her husband's gait and stop him from having falls, symptoms that developed within the past 6 months. When interviewed alone, Mr. Rodriguez describes himself as sad and hopeless because he believes his wife is having an affair. His wife admits that a few times over the past year or two Mr. Rodriguez appeared to be talking to himself and staring off into space. When she asked him if he was hallucinating, he denied it. She is unsure how frequently this occurred because she is often away, assisting other family members. Aside from the stiffness and falls, he appears to be able to care for himself. He has become sedentary over the past year and spends most of his day falling asleep in front of the television. The couple have slept separately for many years because Mr. Rodriguez has dreams in which he thrashes violently, and his wife is worried that she would be injured if she stayed in the same bed. Upon neuropsychological evaluation, the patient demonstrates significant executive dysfunction. He is given a Spanish version of a word list–learning task and displays preserved memory ability.

The evaluation of non-English speakers always has limitations, even with an interpreter. Although Spanish versions of measures are available, educational and cultural differences within subgroups of Spanish speakers must be considered. Relatively strong performance should be trusted more than dysfunction if there is reason to believe language or cultural differences could contribute to poor performance. In this case, neuropsychological testing demonstrated relatively preserved memory as evidence against a diagnosis of NCD due to Alzheimer's disease. Poor performance on measures of executive functioning would support the conclusion of a core feature of major NCDLB, if it can be determined that this performance is not due to the English-based nature of these measures. There is no evidence that the cognitive deficit is associated with functional disability, but this conclusion should have a few caveats.

Another difficulty is the need to rely on an informant when the informant may have limited information. In this case the informant, the patient's wife, is often absent from home, and Mr. Rodriguez leads a largely sedentary life, so that his functional disability may be underrepresented given the minimal demands and his limited activities. In addition, the patient's wife is also expressing a wish that the patient undergo a deep brain stimulation surgery that they believe will improve his physical mobility, so she has an incentive to focus on motor-related symptoms and to minimize other cognitive symptoms. Under this circumstance, clinicians must carefully probe for cognitive dysfunction and hallucinations and explain to patients the limitations and risks of therapeutic interventions. Mr. Rodriguez spends a large portion of his time sleeping, which would be consistent with fluctuations in alertness, a core symptom of NCDLB, and this appears to predate the onset of motor signs. Depression is an associated feature common in NCDLB.

In summary, Mr. Rodriguez has a significant cognitive deficit and at least two core features (i.e., features of parkinsonism, fluctuating alertness) and may experience hallucinations, although limited information is available. In establishing these signs and symptoms, the clinician attempted to select measures appropriate for a non-English speaker to establish the patient's strengths and weaknesses and to consider the entire pattern of symptoms in light of issues related to ethnic diversity and the context of the evaluation. The patient also has evidence of REM sleep behavior disorder, a feature suggestive of NCDLB. The motor symptoms are relatively more recent than the changes in alertness, thus differentiating this disorder from NCD due to Parkinson's disease. He also has other associated features, including a delusion, depressed mood, and falls, that are consistent with the diagnosis. Therefore, the diagnosis is probable major NCDLB without behavioral disturbance.

Differential Diagnosis

The pattern of symptom progression and the relative onset of cognitive and motor dysfunction are important in discriminating NCDLB from other NCDs. When fluctuations are reported, a careful medical evaluation to rule out a delirium is important. Although the patterns of cognitive deficits in NCD due to Parkinson's disease and in NCDLB are similar, major cognitive deficits develop 1 year before symptoms of a movement disorder in NCDLB. In contrast, in NCD due to Parkinson's disease, the stage of major NCD develops at least 1 year after Parkinson's disease has been diagnosed. Assessing whether the patient has suggestive features, REM sleep behavior disorder and a history of an adverse reaction to neuroleptics further supports the diagnosis of NCDLB. Suggestive features such as frequent falls and autonomic dysfunction such as urinary incontinence are important to describe and refer for clinical management (for an extensive review, see Ferman 2013). Once a patient develops motor symptoms and slowing, their depressed scores on speeded measures of executive control will be exaggerated. A comprehensive neuropsychological assessment will help in discriminating mild from major NCDLB and separating the contribution of cognitive dysfunction versus motor dysfunction to functional disability.

Another differential diagnosis to consider with NCDLB is NCD due to Alzheimer's disease; the latter is the most common disorder diagnosed in late life, and both it and NCDLB develop gradually. The cognitive dysfunction in Alzheimer's disease typically involves memory and confrontation naming, domains that are relatively preserved in NCDLB. In contrast, executive and visuospatial dysfunctions are more typical of NCDLB. The three core features of NCDLB (visual hallucinations, motor symptoms, and fluctuating cognition and attention) are not typical of early Alzheimer's disease. NCD due to Alzheimer's disease and NCDLB both develop gradually, unlike vascular NCD, which typically develops in a stepwise pattern and is associated on MRI with strokes and white matter hyperintensities. Fluctuations in alertness and cognition are also not consistent with Alzheimer's disease. Other disorders that lead to hallucinations are peduncular hallucinosis, a rare phenomenon that has MRI findings, and schizophrenia, which has much earlier onset.

See DSM-5-TR for additional disorders to consider in the differential diagnosis. Also refer to the discussions of comorbidity and differential diagnosis in their respective sections of DSM-5-TR.

Summary

- The core diagnostic features of NCDLB are fluctuating cognition, attention, and alertness; visual hallucinations; and movement disorder symptoms.
- Neuroleptic medication can worsen functioning. This associated feature is termed *neuroleptic sensitivity*.
- REM sleep behavior disorder, a condition in which the normal paralysis of movement during sleep is absent, is also a suggestive feature.
- A careful description of the time course of the illness is crucial for discriminating NCDLB from NCD due to Parkinson's disease. In NCDLB, the major cognitive deficits develop before (within 1 year) the onset of motor symptoms, but in NCD due to Parkinson's disease, the major NCD typically evolves long after the movement disorder is established.

IN-DEPTH DIAGNOSIS: MAJOR OR MILD VASCULAR NCD

> Mr. Vicker, a 66-year-old man, and his partner report that he has increasing difficulty concentrating and making decisions. He takes longer to complete projects than he used to. They believe these symptoms began after a day when he experienced left leg numbness and tingling in his left hand. He denied experiencing other neurological symptoms around this time, other than a general, vague sensation of feeling "odd." Neuroimaging shows evidence of small infarctions surrounding the ventricles, predominantly on the right side of his brain. A small degree of atrophy, normal for his age, is also seen on imaging. He has a history of atrial fibrillation, diabetes, cigarette smoking, and hypertension. Neuropsychological assessment finds evidence of mild impairment (15th percentile) in speed of processing, complex attention, and executive functioning, particularly on speeded tasks. Tests of memory show mild difficulty learning new information but minimal forgetting of what he has learned. He is able to continue in his occupation, maintains his level of independence in other areas of functioning, and is aware of his weaknesses.

This case illustrates mild vascular NCD. Mr. Vicker seems to have experienced a mild ischemic event when his left side became numb and tingly. His deficits can be temporally related to this event. Neuroimaging shows evidence of cerebrovascular damage to his brain, which also may be related to the event he described. He shows the typical cognitive profile of impaired information processing, complex attention, and executive functioning. Subcortical vascular damage can result in deficits in these areas. His history of atrial fibrillation, diabetes, smoking, and hypertension provides further evidence supporting a vascular cause. The lack of significant atrophy and his performance on memory testing help to rule out Alzheimer's disease as a cause. Although Mr. Vicker showed impairment in three cognitive domains, the impairments are mild and do not significantly interfere with his independence. Thus, the disorder is mild in severity.

Approach to the Diagnosis

Because of the heterogeneous nature of the presentation of vascular NCD, the approach to the diagnosis also varies considerably depending on the person. Individuals may present with gradually developing cognitive symptoms that can be linked with underlying cerebrovascular disease or with severe cognitive symptoms of a recent stroke. In a general outpatient clinic, a mental health clinician is more likely to encounter individuals whose underlying cerebrovascular disease is less well established. If cognitive decline is suspected by the person, a caregiver, or the clinician, a thorough description of symptoms and a medical history must be gathered. If the symptoms can be linked in time to a discrete vascular event (e.g., "that time when my right hand went numb" or a diagnosed stroke), then a vascular etiology should be suspected. Evidence of stability in symptoms without continual decline is also suggestive of vascular disease as an etiology. However, cerebral autosomal dominant arteriopathy with subcortical infarcts and leukoencephalopathy (CADASIL), which is a rare inherited disorder, typically includes a slow progression of cognitive symptoms. If the symptoms seem more reflective of poor attention, slow processing speed, or executive impairment and less related to memory, a vascular etiology should be suspected. However, individuals occasionally have strokes in the cerebral vasculature feeding the hippocampus, which would lead to memory deficits similar to those seen in Alzheimer's disease. If possible, it is advisable to obtain neuroimaging to assist in the diagnosis. If prominent vascular lesions are seen, with less evidence of atrophy, vascular disease is suspected. The clinician should also always keep in mind that many, if not most, individuals with NCD have more than one etiology and that Alzheimer's disease and vascular disease are very often comorbid, which would result in both atrophy and vascular damage being seen on neuroimaging.

Clinicians also may encounter people who were hospitalized for a stroke but whose cognitive functioning has never been formally evaluated. It is very common for family members to observe significant changes in their loved one after a stroke and to not possess a rudimentary understanding of these deficits. If clinicians uncover a history of a stroke in the recent past that seems linked in time to the onset of a person's deficits, the person should be referred to a neurologist or neuropsychologist for evaluation and diagnosis. Individuals and their caregivers are often very grateful for clarifying information about deficits and remaining strengths that can be used in rehabilitation.

Getting the History

Mr. Lim, a 69-year-old man, presents to the clinic, reporting that his memory seems worse than it used to be. The interviewer asks, "Can you provide examples of what you mean?" and Mr. Lim explains that it is difficult for him to concentrate on driving if the radio is on or if a passenger is speaking to him. He also states that it is difficult for him to keep up in conversations, even though he can understand what people are saying to him. The interviewer asks, "How long have you had these symptoms?" and Mr. Lim answers that it has been almost a year. When asked, "Is there some event that seemed to start these problems?" he states that one day almost a year ago he had difficulty walking and his vision was blurry. When asked if he saw a doctor at that time, he responds that his doctor thought he may have had a "mini-stroke" and prescribed a "water pill" (diuretic). Upon interview, his wife explains that Mr. Lim seems generally slower than he used to be but that he can remember things well if she talks to him in an environment free of distraction (e.g., after turning off the television). The interviewer asks if he has difficulty making decisions (e.g., what to make for dinner or what to order at a restaurant) or if his behavior has changed (e.g., if he says inappropriate things to people), and she answers that he takes longer to make a decision but his social behavior is fine. Last, when asked if his problems have stayed stable or worsened since the "mini-stroke," both Mr. Lim and his wife report that they have stayed the same.

This interview highlights a few important aspects of gathering the history. First, when Mr. Lim was asked to provide examples, he did not endorse memory problems typical of Alzheimer's disease but rather difficulties with complex attention (e.g., difficulty driving with competing stimuli) and slowed processing speed. His difficulty keeping up in conversations seems more to do with slowed processing speed than with symptoms of aphasia. He connects the onset of symptoms with a vascular event described by his physician as a small stroke. His wife reports additional symptoms of executive dysfunction (difficulty making decisions) but also denies memory problems typical of Alzheimer's disease. Lastly, the stable progression of the deficits leads the interviewer toward a diagnosis of vascular NCD rather than a degenerative condition. If possible, the clinician should refer Mr. Lim for neuroimaging and neuropsychological assessment to confirm this diagnosis.

Tips for Clarifying the Diagnosis

- Suspect vascular disease as an etiology when deficits seem to be primarily in attention, processing speed, or executive functioning.
- Use neuroimaging, which is critical in establishing the presence of cerebrovascular damage.
- Take into consideration that when someone has memory deficits suggestive of Alzheimer's disease but also has evidence of extensive cerebrovascular involvement, Alzheimer's disease and vascular disease both may be etiologies. The diagnosis would then be NCD due to multiple etiologies.
- Remember that damage to certain parts of the brain such as the thalamus or angular gyrus can lead to severe deficits that seem out of proportion to the size of the injury. Infarcts in these locations are known as "strategic" infarcts. They can result in symptoms that are more severe than larger infarcts in other parts of the brain.

Consider the Case

Ms. Garcia, a 66-year-old Puerto Rican American woman, sustained a large ischemic stroke 6 months ago; neuroimaging showed a large infarction in the territory of her left middle cerebral artery. Neuroimaging result was otherwise normal, with no significant atrophy suggestive of Alzheimer's disease. She was functioning normally and proficient in English and Spanish before the stroke, but after the stroke she had symptoms of aphasia, with halting, nonfluent speech; difficulty understanding verbal commands; and severe word-finding difficulty. She also showed severe memory impairment. After the event, she was unable to move her right arm. Over the next 6 months, she gained back most of her language abilities with speech therapy, but with lingering word-finding problems and minor memory deficits, scoring at the 15th percentile in auditory memory but with normal memory for visual information. She regained use of her right arm enough to return to work as a graphic designer. Her children are highly involved in her care and report that she does not need assistance with her everyday activities.

Ms. Garcia's case demonstrates that a diagnosis of NCD is not necessarily permanent. With etiologies such as vascular disease (particularly in the form of an acute stroke) and TBI, cognitive functioning may be severely impaired but improve over time to a mild NCD or to the absence of an NCD. Ms. Garcia experienced a major vascular NCD after a large vessel infarction. Her deficits persisted for several weeks, but with the assistance of speech therapy, she was able to regain a large part of her language functioning. It is important to assess and treat language functioning in different languages for a person who is proficient in more than one language, for whom the second language is typically impacted to a greater extent than the first language. Ms. Garcia is left with word-finding deficits and impaired memory for auditory information but is intact in her other abilities and is able to return to her occupation and other activities of daily living. Although she and her family report that she is independent in her daily activities, family members from her culture may provide a great deal of assistance with her daily activities while reporting that she is independent in them. Her work as a graphic designer is less likely than other occupations to require extensive language skills, which facilitates her ability to return to work. Mild vascular NCD thus becomes the diagnosis.

Differential Diagnosis

One key difference between vascular disease and other causes of NCD is that vascular disease, particularly in the form of a large stroke, often can lead to a stepwise pattern of decline, with sudden steep declines followed by periods of stability. In contrast, Alzheimer's disease, Lewy body disease, and frontotemporal degeneration cause a more continual, linear progression of decline. However, vascular disease in the absence of major stroke events can also cause a decline that is continual. In situations such as this, neuroimaging can show cerebrovascular damage significant enough to cause cognitive impairment, and it can be used to assess whether there is significant atrophy suggestive of Alzheimer's disease. Notably, risk factors for vascular NCD (e.g., hypertension, diabetes) are also risk factors for Alzheimer's disease, and patients with evidence of both Alzheimer's disease and cerebrovascular disease meet the criteria for NCD due to multiple etiologies. NCDLB typically involves fluctuating cognition, visual hallucinations, and parkinsonian symptoms, which do not normally occur in vascular NCD. Lastly, frontotemporal degeneration also can cause executive impairment, but in a more gradual fashion than what is seen in vascular NCD and with less involvement of cerebrovascular disease.

Individuals with vascular NCD often have overlapping symptoms of depression related to damage to frontal-subcortical networks. Clinicians must take care to assess whether a person's deficits are caused by a combination of vascular disease and depression or by one factor alone. Concomitant symptoms of depression can worsen the clinical picture and unfortunately may not respond to the same treatments as a nonvascular depression.

Individuals with TBI often experience cerebrovascular damage such as hemorrhages and subdural hematomas. Although these conditions on their own cause deficits that could be considered NCD associated with vascular disease (i.e., strokes), the primary cause is the TBI, and thus the patient would be diagnosed with NCD due to TBI. Strokes in certain locations (e.g., the basal ganglia or the hippocampus) can cause deficits that mimic diseases that are highly associated with these locations (e.g., Parkinson's disease, Alzheimer's disease), but the appropriate diagnosis is vascular NCD. Individuals can also experience delirium when in the acute stages of a stroke. Last, other medical conditions such as brain tumors or multiple sclerosis can also result in cognitive impairment, sometimes with profiles similar to that seen in vascular NCD, and vascular NCD is not diagnosed if these conditions can account for the cognitive deficits.

See DSM-5-TR for additional disorders to consider in the differential diagnosis. Also refer to the discussions of comorbidity and differential diagnosis in their respective sections of DSM-5-TR.

Summary

- Vascular NCD should be suspected if the onset of deficits is temporally linked with a cerebrovascular event or if there is a decline in complex attention (including processing speed) and executive function.
- Probable vascular NCD is diagnosed if there is neuroimaging evidence of cerebrovascular disease, a temporal connection between onset of deficits and a documented cerebrovascular event, or clinical and genetic evidence of cerebrovascular disease.
- Symptoms of depression are particularly common in patients with vascular NCD.
- Patients with vascular NCD can show a stepwise decline, whereas patients with Alzheimer's disease, Lewy body disease, and frontotemporal degeneration will show more gradual decline. However, there are forms of vascular NCD that also have a gradual decline.

IN-DEPTH DIAGNOSIS: MAJOR OR MILD NCD DUE TO TRAUMATIC BRAIN INJURY

Ms. O'Brien, a 60-year-old woman, was involved in a car crash in which her head hit the windshield. She lost consciousness for an estimated 10–15 minutes. She recalls approaching the intersection while driving but cannot remember other details until paramedics arrived on the scene. Her Glasgow Coma Scale score was 14 at the time. She presents in an outpatient primary care clinic 2 weeks later and reports having headaches, concentration difficulties, fatigue, and increased sensitivity to light since the accident. No evidence of seizures, hemiparesis, or visual disturbances is found. A cognitive screen finds deficits in attention and working memory and on speeded tasks. Ms. O'Brien is less productive at work, and she takes twice as long to complete tasks as before the accident. She has to take frequent rest breaks every 2–3 hours and becomes easily fatigued. She left work early several times during the first week after the event but soon resumed her usual work schedule. The findings of her medical workup are otherwise normal, and lab results are in the normal range, ruling out a delirium. An MRI result was unremarkable. Three weeks after the accident, she meets diagnostic criteria for mild NCD due to TBI. Six months after the injury, she completes a neuropsychological assessment. She performs in the normal range on measures of effort, attention, working memory, processing speed, and other domains. She denies experiencing any cognitive difficulties at 6 months postinjury and feels that she is "back to normal."

This case illustrates one important aspect of mild NCD due to TBI that differs from most other NCDs: individuals can experience an NCD at one time point but recover enough that they no longer meet criteria for the NCD (this can also occur with vascular NCD). Ms. O'Brien met diagnostic criteria for mild NCD in the weeks after her injury, which is a common outcome for people who have experienced a mild TBI. It is expected that most such patients completely recover to baseline functioning within 3 months after the injury. Ms. O'Brien showed typical symptoms after the event, including headaches, fatigue, and increased sensitivity to light (i.e., photosensitivity), as well as poor attention, working memory, and processing speed.

Approach to the Diagnosis

The first line of assessment involves a clinical interview and medical chart review to determine the nature and severity of the TBI (mild, moderate, or severe, according to DSM-5-TR severity ratings). Per DSM-5-TR, TBI may include impact to the head or other mechanisms of rapid movement or displacement of the brain within the skull with one or more of the following key features: 1) loss of consciousness, 2) posttraumatic amnesia, 3) disorientation and confusion, or 4) neurological signs (e.g., neuroimaging showing injury, new onset of seizures, a marked worsening of previously diagnosed seizure disorder, visual field cuts, anosmia, hemiparesis) (Table 21–2). Finally, for an NCD to be related to TBI, the cognitive decline must manifest immediately after the TBI or present immediately after recovery of consciousness and persist past the acute postinjury period. A medical chart review should include current medications (e.g., benzodiazepines, anticholinergics, pain narcotics, sedatives, anticonvulsants), history of seizures, lab work examining blood alcohol level, metabolic issues such as renal or liver dysfunction, and substance intoxication or withdrawal.

Cognitive deficits are evaluated in a clinical interview and by a neuropsychological battery of standardized measures focused on attention, memory, executive abilities, and speed of processing information. In an interview, a clinician ascertains whether cognitive difficulties immediately follow the injury by asking about the time of onset and the nature of cognitive difficulties. Although post-TBI cognitive deficits are variable, most involve impaired attention (e.g., difficulty answering questions,

TABLE 21–2. **Classification of traumatic brain injury (TBI) severity**

TBI severity	Mild TBI	Complicated mild TBI	Moderate TBI	Severe TBI
Loss of consciousness duration	≤30 minutes	≤30 minutes	>30 minutes to <24 hours	≥24 hours
Posttraumatic amnesia duration (densely impaired new learning)	≤1 day	≤1 day	>1 day to <7 days	≥7 days
Alteration of consciousness duration (e.g., confusion, disorientation, slowed thinking)	≤1 day	≤1 day	>1 day to <7 days	≥7 days
Glasgow Coma Scale score (30 minutes after the event)	13–15	13–15	9–12	3–8
Computed tomography or magnetic resonance imaging of the brain	Normal	Abnormal	Normal or abnormal	Normal or abnormal

Source.   Reprinted from American Psychiatric Association: *Diagnostic and Statistical Manual of Mental Disorders,* 5th Edition, Text Revision. Washington, DC, American Psychiatric Association, 2022, p. 708. Copyright © 2022, American Psychiatric Association. Used with permission.

completing tasks, or multitasking; losing track in conversations; repeating questions), executive dysfunction (e.g., poor problem-solving and planning, disinhibition, impulsivity, inability to benefit from feedback, inability to create a sequence of steps for complex tasks such as cooking), learning and memory problems for recent information (e.g., interviewer's name and five-word list recall), and slowed processing speed (e.g., longer completion time of tasks, delayed response to questions). Personality changes are also common and include decreased frustration tolerance, irritability, impulsivity, and inappropriate comments in social settings. In severe TBI, the following deficits are commonly seen: aphasia, visual field cuts, hemispatial neglect or inattention, and apraxia (inability to carry out purposeful movement such as brushing one's teeth).

A clinician determines whether the nature and severity of the current cognitive decline meet diagnostic criteria for mild or major NCD. There are two factors to consider when making a diagnosis. First, a diagnosis of major versus mild NCD due to TBI is determined by the extent or severity of cognitive decline from a previous level of functioning rather than the severity of TBI itself. In other words, a mild TBI can result in a major NCD due to TBI if there is evidence of substantial decline on cognitive testing from an estimated previous level of functioning within the first week to months following injury. Second, the course of cognitive decline can vary over time, with major NCD converting to mild NCD, if not completely resolving, because the natural course of cognitive changes involves improvement, if not complete resolution, of symptoms. Except in cases of severe TBI, the typical course of recovery is that of complete or substantial improvement in cognitive, neurological, personality, and mood changes within weeks to 3 months following mild TBI and within 1 year following moderate TBI. For individuals with moderate to severe TBI, cognitive deficits may persist long term and be further exacerbated by neurophysiological, emotional, and behavioral complications. These may include seizures, especially within 1 year after injury, developmental delays in children, PTSD, depression, anxiety, photosensitivity, hyperacusis, irritability, sleep disturbance, fatigue, apathy, and inability to return to work or school. Disruption in social and occupational functioning further negatively affects interpersonal relationships and family or marital functioning. As such, mood assessment should be routinely conducted.

Getting the History

> Mr. Bates is a 25-year-old man who experienced a TBI 3 months ago. He reports increased "concentration" difficulties in college. The interviewer asks, "Can you give me examples of concentration difficulties?" Mr. Bates is unable to provide examples. The interviewer asks follow-up questions: "Do you have to reread the same pages to remember them? Do you lose track of thoughts in conversations? Do you start projects and find it difficult to complete them?" Mr. Bates responds yes to all of these questions, indicating reduced attention. The interviewer then asks, "Does it take you longer to complete tasks?" and the patient nods in agreement and adds that he tends to repeat himself and requires multiple repetitions to learn new information. The interviewer asks, "When did you first notice these difficulties?" Mr. Bates responds that concentration issues started within the week of injury and have improved somewhat over the past 3 months but have not completely resolved. The duration of posttraumatic amnesia and loss of consciousness is determined by asking, "What is the last clear memory you have before your injury? What is the first clear memory following the injury? Did you lose consciousness and for how long?" The patient reports loss of consciousness of 60 minutes, feeling disoriented for 1 day following the injury, no difficulty remembering events immediately preceding the injury, and a first postinjury memory of waking up in a hospital room 2 days later. The interviewer asks, "Have you been feeling unusually blue, tearful, or nervous in the past 3 months?" and the patient denies any signs of emotional distress. Finally, the interviewer asks about difficulty in independent living and self-care (e.g., cooking, driving, managing finances and medications). Mr. Bates denies any changes in independent functioning and is diagnosed with mild NCD due to TBI.

The clinician first establishes the nature of cognitive deficits that the patient experiences. Once reduced attention and processing speed are identified, the time of onset of cognitive deficits is clarified to determine whether the patient meets criteria for mild or major NCD due to TBI, which requires the onset of cognitive difficulties immediately following the injury. Although the severity of initial TBI is not necessarily predictive of mild versus major NCD due to TBI, it is always helpful to assess for the severity of initial injury, which determines prognosis with regard to the timeline of recovery, and to assess whether persisting difficulties are due to other causes (e.g., other medical problems, substance use, anxiety, depression, pain, medication effects). For example, if the patient experienced a mild TBI and continues to experience cognitive deficits 3 months later, other contributing factors should be explored because complete cognitive recovery should occur within weeks to 3 months after a mild TBI. To rule out the presence of emotional distress that can further compound or contribute to ongoing cognitive deficits, the clinician rules out the presence of depression, anxiety, or emotional control issues. Finally, to differentiate between mild and major NCD, the clinician asks about changes in everyday functioning. Compared with those with mild NCD, individuals with major NCD due to TBI have difficulty completing daily activities independently and need assistance.

Tips for Clarifying the Diagnosis

- Determine severity of TBI based on characteristics at the time of injury: loss of consciousness, posttraumatic amnesia, and Glasgow Coma Scale score at the time of injury. Severity of TBI should not be determined by the severity of cognitive decline following injury.
- Establish severity (i.e., mild vs. major) of the resulting NCD due to TBI based on the severity of cognitive decline following the injury and its impact on the patient's ability to perform activities of daily living.
- Clarify the history of the injury and establish the duration of posttraumatic amnesia to better describe the severity of injury:
  - Ask the patient what they remember *last*, *before* the injury, and elicit details.
  - Ask the patient what they remember *first*, *after* the injury. Be sure to differentiate between what the patient has been informed about what happened versus what they remember.
- Assess what characteristics were present before the injury in addition to what has occurred since the injury, because many characteristics associated with TBI (e.g., impulsivity, irritability, depression, anxiety, substance use, high-risk behaviors) may be present before someone experiences a TBI.
- Provide education to patients with mild TBI in regard to recovery trajectory: neurocognitive deficits will likely resolve within the first 3 months postinjury.

Consider the Case

Mr. Daimler is a 24-year-old man who speaks English as his second language. He fell down on the sidewalk while intoxicated, and his forehead struck the concrete. He was unconscious for about 2 hours before paramedics awakened him. His Glasgow Coma Scale score was 10 out of 15 when paramedics arrived. Blood alcohol level was 0.12 at the hospital. He had no memory of the injury or the day before the fall. His first clear memory following the fall was of his sister visiting him at the hospital. He presents to the clinic 1 year after the fall, reporting frequent headaches, shortness of temper, and sensitivity to bright lights. He undergoes a comprehensive neuropsychological assessment and struggles with attention, multitasking, problem-solving, and memory for recently learned information, with these scores ranging from the 5th to the 15th percentiles. He demonstrates adequate effort in the assessment. Since the fall, he has returned to work as a mechanic, although he takes longer to complete tasks (e.g., 90 minutes to perform a standard oil change). He remains independent in his everyday functioning, but his wife has always managed family finances. He reports increased irritability and frequent arguments with his wife. Although he was intoxicated at the time of the fall, he and his wife reported that he typically has no more than three to six alcoholic drinks over the course of a week. He reports some history of depressive symptoms 10 years ago and was treated with an antidepressant medication at that time. He denies feeling depressed or anxious at this time.

Mr. Daimler experienced a TBI of moderate severity, as evidenced by the Glasgow Coma Scale score of 10, loss of consciousness between 30 minutes and 24 hours, and posttraumatic amnesia between 1 and 7 days. Mr. Daimler is within the peak age range for TBI, ages 15–24. Because English is his second language, his neuropsychological test performance should be interpreted with caution because lower scores may underestimate his true abilities. Most cognitive measures were constructed in the English language and with Western notions of cognitive functioning. Research suggests that very few, if any, cognitive tests are immune to these influences; therefore, they may have limited validity in persons who speak English as a second language or who are from different national, ethnic, racial, linguistic, or cultural backgrounds. Although Mr. Daimler's neuropsychological test results indicate at least moderate cognitive deficits, he is independent in daily life and able to return to work, and the tests may underestimate his abilities. Based on this information, he meets diagnostic criteria for mild NCD due to moderate TBI. Alcohol was involved in the fall, which can complicate the assessment of TBI severity, because the sedating properties of severe alcohol intake can depress a Glasgow Coma Scale score, and a clinician may be unable to determine whether the low score is due to the alcohol intake or the brain injury. It is also important for clinicians to determine whether cognitive impairment after a TBI is related to the TBI, whether there is a long history of alcohol abuse that could explain the cognitive deficits, or whether the TBI and alcohol abuse history jointly contribute. Given the family's report of Mr. Daimler's infrequent alcohol use, long-term effects of alcohol on cognitive functioning can be ruled out at this time. Because he denied symptoms of depression and anxiety, it is unlikely that emotional distress is exacerbating, or can explain, his current cognitive difficulties. Last, it is important to assess the effort a person exerts in a cognitive evaluation after a TBI because the possibility of compensation or relief from prior duties may lead a person to perform poorly in an evaluation despite intact cognitive functioning.

Differential Diagnosis

Although the diagnosis of major or mild NCD is not necessarily related to the initial severity of TBI, in some instances the severity of cognitive decline or the lack of expected improvement in symptoms over time may appear inconsistent with the nature and severity of injury. After careful medical record review and ruling out neurological complications (e.g., chronic hematoma, stroke, seizure activity), the clinician should consider the possibility of psychiatric, substance use, and somatic symptom and related disorders. PTSD can frequently co-occur with the NCD and can be the primary diagnosis explaining ongoing cognitive deficits, especially for individuals who experience cognitive deficits that are not necessarily consistent with the severity of the initial TBI. Difficulty concentrating, irritability, sensitivity to noise and light, headaches, depressed or anxious mood, and behavioral disinhibition are common to both PTSD and NCDs due to TBI, but the symptom severity usually improves, if not resolves, in

NCDs due to mild to moderate TBI within 3–6 months, whereas symptoms often persist, if not worsen, when due to PTSD and other psychiatric disorders. When younger adults experience an NCD subsequent to a TBI, a clinician can be confident that the etiology is not a progressive neurodegenerative disorder such as Alzheimer's disease because of the extremely low prevalence of Alzheimer's disease in younger adults. TBI victims often experience vascular damage, such as hemorrhages and subdural hematomas. Although these conditions on their own cause deficits that could be considered NCD associated with vascular disease (i.e., strokes), the primary cause is the TBI; thus, the person would be diagnosed with an NCD due to TBI.

Many symptoms associated with NCDs due to TBI overlap with mood-related disorders, including depressed or anxious mood, headaches, sensitivity to light and noise, and changes in personality (e.g., behavioral disinhibition, irritability, aggressiveness). Substance use (either preexisting or following TBI) is commonly seen in those with NCDs due to TBI and can significantly compound and exacerbate cognitive deficits and functional difficulties in daily life. As noted earlier, many symptoms associated with TBI may overlap with symptoms found in cases of PTSD, and the two disorders can be comorbid, especially in military populations. Additionally, prominent neuromotor features (e.g., ataxia, loss of balance, incoordination, motor slowing) can be present in major NCD due to TBI, but medical and neurological examinations are needed to rule out other neurological causes (e.g., seizures, tumors, movement disorders).

See DSM-5-TR for additional disorders to consider in the differential diagnosis, including factitious disorder and malingering. Also refer to the discussions of comorbidity and differential diagnosis in their respective sections of DSM-5-TR.

Summary

- Mild or major NCD due to TBI is determined by the severity of cognitive decline following injury and its impact on the person's ability to perform activities of daily living. Specification of mild versus major NCD due to TBI is not determined by the severity of injury.
- Severity of injury is determined by characteristics at the time of injury (i.e., loss of consciousness, posttraumatic amnesia, and Glasgow Coma Scale score), not by the severity of cognitive decline following injury.
- A high blood alcohol level at the time of injury can depress the initial Glasgow Coma Scale score and result in an inaccurate measure of injury severity.
- Unlike other NCDs, NCD due to TBI is unique in regard to recovery trajectory: the individual can experience either mild or major NCD immediately after injury, transition from major to mild NCD, and possibly recover enough that they no longer meet criteria for the NCD.
- For NCD due to mild TBI, most patients completely recover to baseline functioning within 3 months after injury.
- The clinician should evaluate the patient's history and current symptoms of mood and substance-related disorders. If neurocognitive deficits worsen or persist longer, it is important to consider other factors (e.g., psychiatric, substance, neurolog-

ical, or somatic symptom and related disorders) that can be contributing to ongoing cognitive difficulties.

SUMMARY: NEUROCOGNITIVE DISORDERS

Table 21–3 summarizes the diagnostic guidelines covered in this chapter for NCDs due to Alzheimer's disease, NCDLB, vascular NCDs, and NCDs due to TBI. Cognitive dysfunction is a common feature of all of these NCDs. Major and mild NCDs are distinguished by the severity of cognitive dysfunction as well as functional impairment. For major NCDs, individuals must have functional impairment, defined as a need for assistance with everyday functioning. Independence in everyday functioning is characterized by the ability to complete instrumental activities of daily living without assistance, such as managing finances and medications, preparing meals, and arranging transportation. In degenerative disorders, in which there is no clear event such as a head injury, the clinician needs to specify probable versus possible, and these criteria vary across the syndromes (as described in Table 21–3). The clinician also needs to indicate whether there is behavioral disturbance. In mild or major NCDs due to TBI, it is important to identify the nature of the injury and the duration of loss of consciousness and posttraumatic amnesia, which occurs immediately after TBI and includes the coma period as well as the time after the recovery of consciousness. It can be assessed by asking a patient what the first thing is that they remember after the event.

ELEMENTS TO CONSIDER IN THE CULTURAL FORMULATION

- In certain cultures, decreased cognitive ability is viewed as a normal part of aging for which the family adjusts to the older adult's abilities.
- Assessing functional decline requires understanding how an individual is able to address the unique demands within their cultural context.
- Individuals from different cultural backgrounds frequently have higher rates of various NCDs.

DIAGNOSTIC PEARLS

- Neurocognitive disorders (NCDs) involve a decline in cognitive functioning from a prior level. These disorders differ from intellectual developmental disorders, which are present from birth or from a very young age.
- It is important to understand an individual's baseline ability to manage instrumental activities of daily living to determine if there has been a decline.
- A decline in functioning needs to be due to a neurocognitive decline and not due to physical, mental health, or other factors.
- Differential diagnosis is informed by considering the typical age at onset.

TABLE 21–3. **Summary of diagnostic guidelines for selected neurocognitive disorders (NCDs)**

Major NCD (all causes)	Mild NCD (all causes)
1. Cognitive deficits interfere with independence in everyday activities.	1. Cognitive deficits do not interfere with independence in everyday activities.
2. Cognition is typically 3rd percentile or less.	2. Cognition is typically between the 3rd and 16th percentile.

Major NCD due to Alzheimer's disease	Mild NCD due to Alzheimer's disease

Symptoms

Insidious onset and gradual progression of impairment in one or more cognitive domains. Disturbance is not better explained by another process.

Probable Alzheimer's disease	*Probable Alzheimer's disease*
Genetic mutation	Genetic mutation
Or all of the following:	*Possible Alzheimer's disease*
1. Decline in memory and learning *and at least one other cognitive domain*	*All of the following:*
2. Progressive and gradual decline	1. Decline in memory and learning
3. No evidence of mixed etiology	2. Progressive, gradual decline
Otherwise, possible Alzheimer's disease	3. No evidence of mixed etiology

Major NCD with Lewy bodies	Mild NCD with Lewy bodies

Symptoms

Insidious onset and gradual progression of impairment in one or more cognitive domains. Disturbance is not better explained by another process.

Probable Lewy bodies: Two core features, or at least one core and one suggestive feature

Possible Lewy bodies: One core feature, or at least one suggestive feature

Major vascular NCD	Mild vascular NCD

Symptoms

Clinical features of vascular etiology, suggested by either

1. Prominent decline in complex attention, processing speed, and executive function; *or*
2. Onset of cognitive deficits is temporally related to one or more cerebrovascular events.

Evidence of cerebrovascular disease.

Disturbance is not better explained by another process.

TABLE 21–3. Summary of diagnostic guidelines for selected neurocognitive disorders (NCDs) *(continued)*

Major vascular NCD	Mild vascular NCD

Probable vascular NCD

 One of the following is present:

 1. Neuroimaging evidence of cerebrovascular disease, *or*

 2. Cognitive deficits with onset temporally due to cerebrovascular event(s), *or*

 3. Genetic and clinical evidence.

Possible vascular NCD

 Clinical criteria are met, but neuroimaging is not available and temporal relationship with one or more cerebrovascular events is not established.

Major NCD due to TBI	Mild NCD due to TBI

Symptoms

Evidence of TBI (at least one of the following):

 1. Loss of consciousness

 2. Posttraumatic amnesia

 3. Disorientation and confusion

 4. Neurological signs

Onset is immediately after TBI or after recovering consciousness and persists past acute postinjury period.

No specification of probable or possible, because the etiology is more clearly established.

TBI=traumatic brain injury.

- Major and mild NCDs both involve impairment in one or more cognitive domains (two or more domains for NCD due to Alzheimer's disease). In major NCD, significant cognitive impairments interfere with independence in everyday activities. In mild NCD, modest cognitive impairments do not interfere with independence in everyday activities.

- Delirium occurs when a medical condition interferes with brain functioning, causing symptoms of disorientation and cognitive impairment.

- The best way to establish the main symptoms of the NCDs (i.e., cognitive deficits) is through cognitive testing. A patient's self-report of cognitive deficits is not sufficient for diagnosis. Moreover, the nature of some NCDs often precludes the patient's own awareness of a disorder being present.

- Unlike other psychiatric disorders, the diagnosis should be thought of as the syndrome (NCD) in addition to the likely neurological cause (e.g., Alzheimer's disease, traumatic brain injury [TBI]).

- Alzheimer's disease is the most common degenerative cause of NCD.

- NCD due to TBI can be acquired at any age, whereas the other NCDs occur most often in older adults.
- To ensure that treatable causes of cognitive dysfunction are considered, cognitive impairment in older adults should be thought of as being due to delirium, unless proven otherwise.
- Hallucinations in delirium as well as in NCD with Lewy bodies are most often visual, whereas hallucinations in schizophrenia are more often auditory, although each disorder can involve hallucinations in other modalities.

SELF-ASSESSMENT

Key Concepts: Double-Check Your Knowledge

What is the relevance of the following concepts to the various neurocognitive disorders?

- Posttraumatic amnesia
- Hallucinations
- Vascular disease
- Learning and memory
- Visuospatial skills
- Stroke or cerebrovascular accident
- Neuroleptic sensitivity
- Loss of consciousness
- Cerebral autosomal dominant arteriopathy with subcortical infarcts and leukoencephalopathy (CADASIL)
- Glasgow Coma Scale

Questions to Discuss With Colleagues and Mentors

1. What tools do you prefer for assessing cognition?
2. Are there certain questions you find helpful for establishing the differential diagnosis?
3. How do you manage patients with neurocognitive disorders who behave inappropriately with you?
4. In your practice, what do you find to be the most common triggers of delirium?
5. Which questions to significant others do you find most helpful for obtaining information to establish a cognitive baseline and decline?

Case-Based Questions

PART A

Ms. Nicolas, a 75-year-old woman, reports that her memory has been declining gradually over the past 2 years. Her partner reports that she frequently repeats questions and occasionally forgets where she set out to go on an errand. Each denies any changes in Ms. Nicolas's personality or behavior.

What disorder might be causing these symptoms? The patient's symptoms sound like those of neurocognitive disorder due to Alzheimer's disease.

PART B

Upon clarification, these symptoms appear to have started abruptly, when Ms. Nicolas presented at the emergency department with complaints of sudden visual disturbance. She believes that the symptoms began then, but her partner believes that some memory deficits were present beforehand.

What can cause a sudden development or worsening of cognitive problems? Sudden onset of memory deficits can be caused by a stroke or other acute medical condition (e.g., encephalitis, expansion of a brain tumor to a critical size). Clinicians often struggle with discrepant reports; in this case, the memory deficits may have started before the event (consistent with Alzheimer's disease), may have been caused by this event (consistent with vascular disease), or may represent precipitant Alzheimer's disease worsened by a stroke.

PART C

Ms. Nicolas undergoes an MRI, which shows evidence of a stroke in the distribution of her hippocampal memory centers and her occipital areas of visual processing. Genetic testing finds that she carries the high-risk polymorphism associated with Alzheimer's disease, apolipoprotein ε4, and she reports that both her parents had been diagnosed with Alzheimer's disease. Neuropsychological testing shows impairments in memory and visual perception but intact functioning in other areas. Review of her medications finds that she recently began taking a benzodiazepine for her "nerves."

What are all the potential etiologies of her deficits, and are any of them reversible? The review of records uncovered three possible causes of Ms. Nicolas's memory deficits: 1) MRI evidence of a stroke in the artery that feeds the hippocampus, which would be expected to lead to memory deficits; 2) genetic testing results consistent with Alzheimer's disease; and 3) recent introduction of a medication (a benzodiazepine) that often interferes with cognition. If she is experiencing symptoms of an anxiety disorder, appropriate treatment must be initiated because anxiety can also interfere with cognition. This case illustrates some of the complexities of assessing and treating cognitive deficits in older adults; many disorders are multifactorial in etiology, with some having reversible causes, some being stable, and some being degenerative.

Short-Answer Questions

1. Which events do patients with Alzheimer's disease have the most trouble remembering: recent events or events from the distant past?

2. True or False: The diagnosis of major neurocognitive disorder (NCD) due to Alzheimer's disease requires evidence of cognitive decline in only learning and memory.

3. Aside from cognitive test performance, what is the key distinguishing feature used to differentiate between mild and major NCD?

4. What is the essential feature of delirium?

5. Visual hallucinations can occur in NCD with Lewy bodies (NCDLB) and what other NCD?

6. What are the three core diagnostic features of major or mild NCDLB?

7. Which cognitive domains are most prominently affected in major or mild vascular NCD?

8. True or False: Probable vascular NCD can be diagnosed if there is neuroimaging-supported evidence of extensive cerebrovascular disease resulting in the neurocognitive deficits.

9. Name five risk factors associated with major or mild vascular NCD.

10. True or False: The diagnosis of mild versus major NCD due to traumatic brain injury is based on the initial severity of brain injury.

Answers

1. Patients with Alzheimer's disease have the most trouble remembering recent events.

2. False. One other cognitive domain must be impaired.

3. Everyday functioning is the key component used to differentiate between mild and major NCD. For mild NCD diagnosis, the patient's ability to function independently is relatively intact, whereas for major NCD diagnosis, the patient depends on others for assistance in instrumental activities of daily living.

4. The essential feature of delirium is a rapid-onset disturbance in attention or awareness.

5. Visual hallucinations can occur in delirium.

6. The three core diagnostic features of major or mild NCDLB are fluctuating cognition (attention and awareness), recurrent visual hallucinations, and spontaneous features of parkinsonism with onset after the development of cognitive decline.

7. Complex attention (including processing speed) and executive function are most prominently affected in major or mild vascular NCD.

8. True. Neuroimaging-supported evidence of extensive cerebrovascular disease resulting in the neurocognitive deficits is sufficient to be diagnosed with probable vascular NCD.

9. Risk factors associated with major or mild vascular NCD include hypertension, diabetes, smoking, obesity, high cholesterol levels, atrial fibrillation, cerebral amyloid angiopathy, and hereditary conditions such as cerebral autosomal dominant arteriopathy with subcortical infarcts and leukoencephalopathy (CADASIL).

10. False. The mild versus major designation is based on the severity of cognitive deficits.

RECOMMENDED READINGS

McKhann GM, Knopman DS, Chertkow H, et al: The diagnosis of dementia due to Alzheimer's disease: recommendations from the National Institute on Aging–Alzheimer's Association workgroups on diagnostic guidelines for Alzheimer's disease. Alzheimers Dement 7(3):263–269, 2011 21514250

Miller BL, Boeve BF (eds): The Behavioral Neurology of Dementia, 2nd Edition. New York, Cambridge University Press, 2017

Smith GE, Bondi MW: Mild Cognitive Impairment and Dementia: Definitions, Diagnosis, and Treatment. New York, Oxford University Press, 2013

REFERENCES

American Psychiatric Association: Diagnostic and Statistical Manual of Mental Disorders, 4th Edition. Washington, DC, American Psychiatric Association, 1994

American Psychiatric Association: Diagnostic and Statistical Manual of Mental Disorders, 5th Edition. Arlington, VA, American Psychiatric Association, 2013

American Psychiatric Association: Diagnostic and Statistical Manual of Mental Disorders, 5th Edition, Text Revision. Washington, DC, American Psychiatric Association, 2022

Ferman TJ: Dementia with Lewy bodies, in Mild Cognitive Impairment and Dementia: Definitions, Diagnosis, and Treatment. Written by Smith GE, Bondi MW. New York, Oxford University Press, 2013, pp 255–301

Ferman TJ, Smith GE, Boeve BF, et al: DLB fluctuations: specific features that reliably differentiate DLB from AD and normal aging. Neurology 62(2):181–187, 2004 14745051

McKeith IG, Boeve BF, Dickson DW, et al: Diagnosis and management of dementia with Lewy bodies: fourth consensus report of the DLB Consortium. Neurology 89(1):88–100, 2017 28592453

Walker MP, Ayre GA, Cummings JL, et al: The Clinician Assessment of Fluctuation and the One Day Fluctuation Assessment Scale: two methods to assess fluctuating confusion in dementia. Br J Psychiatry 177:252–256, 2000 11040887

CHAPTER 22

Personality Disorders

Laura Weiss Roberts, M.D., M.A.

Max Kasun, B.A.

"People always let me down, no matter how hard I try. It's always been this way."

"I can't do anything unless my kitchen is perfectly clean."

- Cluster A Personality Disorders
  - Paranoid Personality Disorder
  - Schizoid Personality Disorder
  - Schizotypal Personality Disorder
- Cluster B Personality Disorders
  - Antisocial Personality Disorder
  - Borderline Personality Disorder
  - Histrionic Personality Disorder
  - Narcissistic Personality Disorder

Adapted from Reicherter D, Roberts LW: "Personality Disorders," in *Study Guide to DSM-5*. Edited by Roberts LW, Louie AK. Washington, DC, American Psychiatric Publishing, 2015, pp 415–440.

- Cluster C Personality Disorders
  - Avoidant Personality Disorder
  - Dependent Personality Disorder
  - Obsessive-Compulsive Personality Disorder
- Other Personality Disorders
  - Personality Change Due to Another Medical Condition
  - Other Specified Personality Disorder
  - Unspecified Personality Disorder

People with personality disorders have enduring maladaptive patterns related to their thoughts, behaviors, reactions, and internal experience that occur across social situations and lead to serious impairment in their lives. Their ability "to love and to work" is diminished, and they often experience distress. The disruptive, negative, or damaging behaviors of people living with personality disorders cause others around them also to have distress. By definition, personality disorders are not episodic; their enduring nature is the key to understanding this diagnostic class.

Personality disorders are not rare, and some are more prevalent in males while others are more prevalent in females. In clinical practice, co-occurring disorders (e.g., disorders of mood or anxiety or substance-related conditions) and significant psychosocial issues are considered the rule rather than the exception. For these reasons, the clinical care of people with personality disorders can be especially challenging, and it requires great conscientiousness, compassion, and tolerance for complexity on the part of health professionals who undertake this work.

In learning about personality disorders, it is helpful to first get a sense of the broad diagnostic class and then to become familiar with the specific criteria for the 10 individual DSM-5-TR personality disorders (American Psychiatric Association 2022). The careful reader will note that the DSM-5 (American Psychiatric Association 2013) criteria for personality disorders have been preserved without changes in DSM-5-TR Section II. Significant scientific work—for example, in the areas of temperament and personality structure—and international comparative studies suggest that future editions of DSM will have new concepts and criteria for personality disorders. The emerging thinking on this domain is detailed in DSM-5-TR Section III, in the chapter "Alternative DSM-5 Model for Personality Disorders." That chapter examines new approaches to consider in personality disorders and provides a more in-depth look at areas of dysfunction often seen in personalities. It also includes a proposed rating scale to calibrate the level of personality functioning. The interested learner is encouraged to review this material in DSM-5-TR.

GENERAL PERSONALITY DISORDER

The criteria for the presence of a personality disorder, in general, must be met before a specific personality disorder diagnosis should be considered. Many negative personality traits may be observed in persons who never meet the general criteria for a personality disorder and who should not be classified with a specific personality disorder (e.g., borderline personality disorder [BPD], dependent personality disorder). Maladaptive personality traits may occur in isolation from other characteristics, or they may occur only in specific situations, in which case they would not constitute a personality disorder diagnosis.

In essence, to meet the criteria for a personality disorder diagnosis, a person's maladaptive patterns of experience and behavior must be essentially fixed in their personality. The traits must in some sense be "calcified" as an aspect of their way of experiencing and behaving across situations. For professionals just entering clinical work, this notion can be hard to understand when, for instance, the trait appears superficially to be dynamic (e.g., because the person is emotionally labile and engages in disruptive behavior) but is actually quite consistent across time and context. This consistency is fundamental to the diagnostic class. The enduring and pervasive nature of personality disorders is why DSM-5-TR specifies that these conditions be apparent across diverse situations and multiple spheres of function, be of long duration, and be traceable to adolescence or early adulthood. Patients can meet the full DSM-5-TR criteria for more than one personality disorder and be correctly diagnosed with each personality disorder when full criteria are met. Moreover, cultural norms and expectations may influence the specific manifestation of personality disorder characteristics. The key to making the diagnosis is the pervasive, maladaptive nature of a trait, rather than the specific ways in which the behavior may present in a clinical situation.

Personality disorder diagnoses are often deferred until the patient is 18 years of age or older because the clinician should identify these experiences and behaviors in an adult personality as opposed to a developing personality. Personality disorders may be accurately diagnosed in patients younger than 18 if symptoms are clearly present for more than 1 year. The one exception is antisocial personality disorder, which cannot be diagnosed in an individual younger than 18. It is also important to note that personality disorders are not necessarily lifelong diagnoses. Patients may develop symptoms meeting criteria for a personality disorder and then no longer meet that diagnostic criteria at another stage of life.

Personality traits are defined in DSM-5-TR as "enduring patterns of perceiving, relating to, and thinking about the environment and oneself that are exhibited in a wide range of social and personal contexts" (p. 735). When personality traits are maladaptive and inflexible, they constitute the patterns associated with personality disorders. Specific constellations of maladaptive personality traits constitute 10 of the 12 personality disorders as defined in DSM-5-TR (p. 733):

- **Paranoid personality disorder** is a pattern of distrust and suspiciousness such that others' motives are interpreted as malevolent.
- **Schizoid personality disorder** is a pattern of detachment from social relationships and a restricted range of emotional expression.
- **Schizotypal personality disorder** is a pattern of acute discomfort in close relationships, cognitive or perceptual distortions, and eccentricities of behavior.

- **Antisocial personality disorder** is a pattern of disregard for, and violation of, the rights of others, criminality, impulsivity, and a failure to learn from experience.
- **Borderline personality disorder** is a pattern of instability in interpersonal relationships, self-image, and affects, and marked impulsivity.
- **Histrionic personality disorder** is a pattern of excessive emotionality and attention seeking.
- **Narcissistic personality disorder** is a pattern of grandiosity, need for admiration, and lack of empathy.
- **Avoidant personality disorder** is a pattern of social inhibition, feelings of inadequacy, and hypersensitivity to negative evaluation.
- **Dependent personality disorder** is a pattern of submissive and clinging behavior related to an excessive need to be taken care of.
- **Obsessive-compulsive personality disorder** is a pattern of preoccupation with orderliness, perfectionism, and control.

Two other conditions are included among the personality disorders: personality change due to another medical condition and other specified personality disorder.

The specific personality disorders are often thought about in three different "clusters" on the basis of similarities between the diagnoses:

- Cluster A personality disorders are those diagnoses characterized by odd beliefs and eccentric behaviors. Cluster A includes paranoid, schizoid, and schizotypal personality disorders.
- Cluster B personality disorders are those diagnoses characterized by erratic and dramatic behaviors and emotional instability. Cluster B includes antisocial, borderline, histrionic, and narcissistic personality disorders.
- Cluster C personality disorders are those diagnoses characterized by fear-based desire for control and by anxiety. Cluster C includes avoidant, dependent, and obsessive-compulsive personality disorders.

It is not uncommon for personality traits to overlap within a cluster. For instance, a person who presents with the full set of signs consistent with BPD may also have some of the traits seen in histrionic personality disorder. The clusters may help clinicians group similar clinical pictures of personality disorders.

A final subgroup, called "other personality disorders," includes personality change due to another medical condition, which is a persistent personality disturbance judged to be caused by a medical condition. This subgroup also includes other specified personality disorder, which describes a condition wherein the definition for personality disorder is met but the full criteria for a specific personality disorder diagnosis have not been met. Last, unspecified personality disorder refers to a presentation that resembles a personality disorder but where there is insufficient information to reach a diagnosis.

Distinguishing personality disorders from other mental health diagnoses, physiological effects of substances, or medical conditions can be difficult but is essential before arriving at the diagnosis of any personality disorder. Discerning whether another

TABLE 22–1. Key changes between DSM-5 and DSM-5-TR

Culture-related diagnostic issues have been updated to better address social determinants of health and sociocultural contexts.

Prevalence and sex- and gender-related diagnostic issues have been updated in keeping with best evidence.

Association with suicidal thoughts or behaviors has been added to all disorders.

The development and course of borderline personality disorder has been updated: The disorder has been found in adolescents as young as 12. Severity does not necessarily lessen with age, as previously thought. Rather, remissions of 1–8 years are very common.

Sex- and gender-related diagnostic issues for borderline personality disorder now note that the disorder is equally prevalent among both sexes according to community samples.

factor or set of factors is shaping the experiences and behaviors that appear to be a personality disorder can be quite difficult, given that patients often present with multiple conditions and states that must be taken into account. Moreover, it is important before making a diagnosis to identify whether seemingly rigid or dysfunctional patterns of behavior are in fact adaptive responses to cultural norms or expectations. Dimensional approaches to diagnosis of personality disorders may help alongside the categorical approach to identify true dysfunction in light of cultural factors. People with personality disorders may elicit strong emotional reactions from others around them—health professionals are not an exception to this pattern. People who have these disorders may not understand their traits to be problematic, even if those traits clearly compromise their well-being and effectiveness in major spheres of life. Paradoxically, people with personality disorders may be successful in some of their activities in society, and in these cases, the diagnosis may be harder to determine. Accurately identifying the presence of a personality disorder diagnosis—and then learning to respond therapeutically rather than to "react" to patients with these conditions—is the mark of a maturing and sound clinician.

This chapter focuses on four personality disorders found in DSM-5-TR: borderline, obsessive-compulsive, schizotypal, and narcissistic. Each of these disorders should be considered in the greater context of the DSM-5-TR criteria for general personality disorder. Key changes between DSM-5 and DSM-5-TR are listed in Table 22–1.

IN-DEPTH DIAGNOSIS: BORDERLINE PERSONALITY DISORDER

Ms. Corrigan is a 26-year-old single woman who presents to the emergency department after consuming 20 tablets of her antidepressant medication. She says she took the pills suddenly after an intense fight and "breakup for the last time" with her boyfriend. Ms. Corrigan called her boyfriend immediately after taking the pills, and he came with her to the emergency department.

Ms. Corrigan reports that she and her boyfriend have had an "on-and-off" relationship—she says she always feels that she "needs" him but they have "lots of fights" and cannot "hold it together" for more than a couple of weeks at a time. Most of her family relationships are strained, but she says her sister is her "best friend" now that they "are on speaking terms with each other again." Ms. Corrigan says that she took the overdose because she "can't stand to be alone." She volunteers that she "sees lots of other guys" and has a pattern of risky sexual behaviors when she and her boyfriend are having problems. She engages in binge drinking ("only when I am really mad") many times each month. Ms. Corrigan reports that she has had "anger issues" and "is always suicidal" since her teenage years. She has been in therapy many times, with many different therapists, because she cannot find one who "understands" her. "At first they seem to 'get me'—understand what I am going through—but then they always pull back at some point."

Throughout the interview, Ms. Corrigan is highly emotional and affectively labile, ranging from intense anger to tearfulness. The interviewer's sense is that the reactions are well out of the appropriate range for the topics discussed. Review of her medical record shows five emergency department visits for "overdose" or "suicidal thoughts" within the past year. Her overdoses have always been with small enough quantities of medication that she only required monitoring without admission to an intensive care unit.

Ms. Corrigan's thoughts, reactions, and behaviors align well with the DSM-5-TR description of BPD as "a pervasive pattern of instability of interpersonal relationships, self-image, and affects, and marked impulsivity, beginning by early adulthood and present in a variety of contexts" (p. 752). Her life story fulfills at least five of the nine criteria for the diagnosis. Ms. Corrigan reports experiences that meet DSM-5-TR criteria for BPD, including efforts to avoid abandonment, intense interpersonal relationships, impulsivity, suicidal gestures, affective instability, and inappropriate anger. The pattern has been pervasive across multiple social spheres and clearly has negatively affected Ms. Corrigan's ability to live a complete, happy, and healthy life.

Ms. Corrigan reports a pattern of self-damaging impulses and recurrent suicidal behaviors. Although she has not yet had a life-threatening overdose, she is at risk for premature death. The fact that she has not yet had a self-harm gesture resulting in serious health impairment or organ damage by no means should reduce the clinician's concern for grave outcomes such as completed suicide. Impulsivity and danger should be evaluated thoroughly when assessing a person with BPD. Although she has demonstrated these symptoms in an enduring and pervasive pattern, the clinician must nevertheless make certain that there is not another mental health condition or substance abuse issue that better accounts for the pattern seen in the case.

Approach to the Diagnosis

BPD often manifests with dramatic flares. Intense relationships, repeated self-harm behaviors, and intense and inappropriate anger can manifest together to create a tempestuous clinical picture. The experience of an unstable and fragmented identity can create additional difficulty for a patient to obtain insight about dysfunctional behavior and can contribute to future patterns of interpersonal hardship. An unstable and fragmented identity can reduce the patient's ability to obtain insight into maladaptive patterns of behavior and can lead to repetitive dysfunction in their interpersonal relationships. Conflicted and emotionally volatile relationships are often impressive with a borderline presentation. The intense emotionality of persons with the diagnosis can sometimes be remarkable—even overwhelming—to the clinician early in assessment; however, more subtle presentations are also possible. Furthermore, the diagnosis of BPD must be arrived at by establishing that the criteria have been present and causing dysfunction over time. Also, before the specific diagnosis of BPD can be given, it must be clarified that the patient's behavior meets the criteria for general personality disorder (see the section "General Personality Disorder" earlier in this chapter and in DSM-5-TR).

As with the other personality disorder diagnoses, the clinician must first clarify that the symptom cluster is not better accounted for by another mental disorder or by the use of substances. This step may be difficult, given the likelihood of comorbidity in BPD. Discerning the diagnosis may also be challenging because the patient's stated reason for seeking care may not immediately line up with the diagnostic criteria for the disorder. A patient with BPD may present with a stated concern of "depression" or "high and low moods," which hints of mood disorder, when in fact the underlying pathology may be the labile mood states seen in BPD. Moreover, people with BPD may develop major mood, anxiety, trauma-related, or substance use disorders. Distinguishing the chronic low mood states seen in persistent depressive disorder (dysthymia) or recurrent major depressive disorder from the chronic feelings of emptiness seen in BPD, for instance, is a challenge that requires attention to the whole clinical picture.

Another potentially confusing issue that may complicate a case is an incorrect diagnosis given in the past or a patient's identification with a different mental health diagnosis. A misdiagnosis may have become the primary issue in the thoughts of the patient. A patient with an earlier diagnosis of bipolar disorder or PTSD but whose condition is more consistent with a personality disorder may focus the clinical attention on the working diagnosis from an earlier time. It is important for the clinician to be aware of these considerations and to place the patient's experiences and behaviors within the greater context.

The transient presence of borderline traits under specific conditions may be another confusing clinical presentation. Some people will use coping strategies consistent with the borderline personality diagnosis but only under specific stresses or in a particular life challenge. This pattern of situational coping does not meet the criteria for a diagnosis of BPD. The pervasive traits of BPD will often be evidenced by a long history of psychosocial complications, such as multiple disruptive and conflicted relationships, employment problems, or legal problems. These impairments in function can be directly linked to behavioral manifestations of the BPD traits.

Problem substance use is a common co-occurring phenomenon in BPD, and patients with BPD should be carefully evaluated for substance-related issues.

It is very useful to try to get a longitudinal history and to obtain collateral information from other people involved with the patient's life (e.g., friends, family). It is often necessary to see a patient on multiple occasions to clarify the pathology's enduring nature. The input from friends and family can clarify the pattern in multiple contexts and help trace the pathology back to adolescence.

Getting the History

Ms. Lane, a 43-year-old woman, describes a history of a pervasive pattern of instability of interpersonal relationships and marked impulsivity beginning by early adulthood and present in a variety of contexts. She reports that she and her family think she is "bipolar" because of her "highs and lows." She says, "I looked up *bipolarism* on the internet, and it is a perfect description of me. I am up and down all of the time! I've been like that since I was a teenager."

To discriminate between affective instability and episodic mania, the interviewer asks, "Can you say more about your 'highs and lows'?" Ms. Lane replies, "I can be fine one minute, and the next minute I am so angry. I get really manic sometimes when I am angry. I will get into an argument, and the mania takes over and I start yelling." The interviewer asks, "How long does that last?" The patient replies, "It can last 20 or 30 minutes. Longer sometimes. I just feel like my emotions are out of control. Sometimes I even throw things. And then I come back down."

The interviewer asks, "When does that happen?" Ms. Lane responds, "When I fight with my ex, but it can also happen out of the blue if I start thinking about all my stress."

When asked when she started noticing this, Ms. Lane responds, "I have been like that since I was little. But it got worse when I moved out of my parents' home—when I got with my first husband." The interviewer asks, "Can you think of times when you weren't like that?" She responds, "Usually when I first start going out with a guy, everything is great, and I am fine. It's when they start turning into jerks that my bipolar gets worse." The interviewer asks, "Do you get angry like that in situations other than with boyfriends?" She says, "Yes, my family says they just can't take it anymore, so I stay away. Also my boss got me all manic a few times by being an idiot, and then he tried to get me fired for it!"

Emotional dysregulation and temper outbursts exemplified in this case are consistent with the affective instability seen in BPD. The mood lability elicited in this history is a long-standing pattern rather than distinct episodes of mania or hypomania. The clinician establishes the pattern of *reactive* mood—different from the pattern present in depression or bipolar disorder, for example. The clinician also clarifies that these mood states are transient and that emotion regulation is a pervasive problem. Ms. Lane has had anger outbursts with many boyfriends throughout her adolescence and early adulthood, as well as with her family and her boss. Because BPD is associated with one of the highest rates of premature mortality among the mental disorders, the clinician should make a diligent effort to identify possible signs of past or intended self-harm or suicidality.

It is confusing that Ms. Lane uses technical terms such as *manic* or *mania* and that she uses the incorrect term *bipolarism*. The clinician must distinguish between DSM-5-TR criteria and what the patient is trying to describe about her life experience.

Tips for Clarifying the Diagnosis

- Establish that the clinical picture is consistent with the definition of general personality disorder.
- Confirm that the DSM-5-TR symptoms of BPD have occurred over a long duration in multiple social settings.

- Explore other diagnoses that may better explain the observed symptoms.
- Consider episodes from mood disorder diagnoses (e.g., major depressive episode or manic/hypomanic episode) and stable mood states as defined by the time span described in DSM-5-TR. In BPD, mood states tend to be unstable and fluctuate rapidly.
- Remember that other mental health diagnoses are commonly associated with the diagnosis.

Consider the Case

Mr. Bush, a 35-year-old single man, presents to a psychiatrist reporting that his girlfriend wants him to "do something for anger management." He reports a history of intense anger and "temper" problems culminating in arguments and, at times, in physical fights with his girlfriend, brothers, and neighbor.

On further interview, Mr. Bush reports that his anger has "always been out of control." He has a long history of temperamental behavior in many different social contexts that has led him to physical fights with family members and "guys at work" and breakups with previous girlfriends. He has been hospitalized three times for suicidal thinking and self-destructive behaviors such as punching himself in the face. Each hospitalization occurred after a breakup with a girlfriend. He is very impulsive, reporting uncontrolled spending and reckless driving as well as binge-drinking episodes. His unstable moods and accompanying behaviors have resulted in a criminal record, including charges for assault, public intoxication, and reckless driving. His conflict-oriented interpersonal style has led to arguments with work superiors and loss of jobs.

When discussing mood, Mr. Bush reports that he has been "depressed since I was a teenager." He endorses chronic feelings of emptiness. Furthermore, he reports reactive "mood swings" that last "a few hours at a time."

On mental status examination, he is hostile and angry for much of the interview. He becomes intensely tearful when discussing his girlfriend. He has surface cuts in different stages of healing on his forearms where he says he has cut himself with razor blades in an effort "to make the pain go away."

The case of Mr. Bush demonstrates many features of BPD. He states that his intense anger is his reason for seeking help, but it is the enduring and pervasive pattern of disruptive, negative, and self-damaging feelings that has caused problems for him in multiple spheres of his life. He meets criteria for general personality disorder and exhibits at least five of the nine criteria for the diagnosis of BPD over a wide range of experiences and in an enduring pattern.

Differential Diagnosis

BPD can manifest with myriad different behaviors or symptoms. These must be distinguished from other mental health issues that can also look similar. For example, the strong emotional content of a borderline presentation can be mistaken for mood disorder episodes. In an effort to describe their affective instability, intense anger, or impulsivity, persons with BPD may endorse symptoms that sound consistent with major depressive episode or manic/hypomanic episode. A diagnosis of bipolar disorder might be incorrectly considered when a patient with BPD describes frequent, intense "highs and lows," when in fact the emotional states are often unstable and more a function of mood lability. Duration of symptoms is a key element in determining episodic, pathological mood states, as in depression and bipolar disorder. BPD tends to be characterized by chronic mood instability, whereas depression and bipolar disorder are characterized by sustained episodes of mood pathology (often with interepisode resolution of symptoms). The differential diagnosis includes, in addition to mood disorders, other personality disorders, personality change due to another medical condition, substance use disorders, and identity problems.

BPD may co-occur with other mental or substance use disorders. Mood, anxiety, and eating disorders are common comorbidities that must be recognized, but each can also become a misdiagnosis when BPD better explains the presentation. The clinician should first establish that the definition for general personality disorder has been met, and then they should systematically explore the specific criteria for BPD while also recognizing that other pathological phenomena, such as eating disorder behaviors or substance abuse, may be present. In this manner, it will be possible to determine whether a patient has additional conditions that fulfill DSM-5-TR diagnoses. These additional diagnoses, when present, should be noted.

Patients may also exhibit maladaptive coping strategies and behaviors that look like BPD only in specific stressful situations, in which case the behaviors are not enduring and do not warrant the diagnosis of BPD.

See DSM-5-TR for additional disorders to consider in the differential diagnosis. Also refer to the discussions of comorbidity and differential diagnosis in their respective sections of DSM-5-TR.

Summary

BPD is characterized by an enduring pattern of emotional instability. Features of the disorder may include any of the following:

- Conflict-oriented, unstable relationships characterized by alternating extremes of devaluation and idealization
- Disproportionate, inappropriate, and intense anger
- Difficulty maintaining a "true sense of self"; identity disturbance
- Impulsive and self-injurious behavior
- Co-occurring mental and substance-related disorders

IN-DEPTH DIAGNOSIS: OBSESSIVE-COMPULSIVE PERSONALITY DISORDER

Mr. Upton, a 37-year-old man, presents with his wife to a mental health clinician for evaluation in the context of having difficulties at work. He says that he believes that he is "fine" but that his boss—and his wife, he adds reluctantly—may have a problem with his "neatness." Mr. Upton has missed opportunities for promotion at work because he has trouble completing tasks, even though he is "the most conscientious worker there." His wife reports that he is a "control freak."

He is puzzled by his boss's attitude toward him. Mr. Upton states, "I'm a real perfectionist. You would think a supervisor would like that!" Mr. Upton is inflexible about matters of morality and ethics. He points out his opinion to coworkers routinely because they are often, he says, so "woolly-headed" about the basics of "right and wrong."

Interviewing the couple reveals that Mr. Upton is very devoted to work activities to the exclusion of leisure activities and family. He is very critical of his wife's inability to maintain his standard of neatness. He will come home from work and redo household cleaning tasks that his wife completed earlier the same day. He scrutinizes their financial budget and has tried to restrict his wife's spending. He says that he wants to make sure they keep some money for "future emergencies."

He reports that he has "always been a stickler for the rules, even as a kid." As a young child he recalls having fits if someone else sat in his assigned seat at the dinner table. He was socially unpopular in high school because he would report schoolmates for "tardiness." His overinvestment in rules has caused conflict in many social spheres from a very young age.

Often people with obsessive-compulsive personality disorder (OCPD) do not see their personality traits as maladaptive. As demonstrated in this case, these individuals see the symptoms as strengths, despite their maladaptive nature and the conflicts and dysfunction that they cause. A clinician needs to assess and interpret the patient's experiences and behaviors carefully when fitting the behavior patterns with the criteria for the disorder. Mr. Upton describes his behaviors as "conscientious," "perfectionistic," and "neat," but he also discloses the problematic nature of them and describes the disability and compromised areas of function that they cause. Mr. Upton's behavior meets criteria for general personality disorder as well as at least four of the eight criteria for OCPD.

Approach to the Diagnosis

DSM-5-TR describes OCPD as "a pervasive pattern of preoccupation with orderliness, perfectionism, and mental and interpersonal control, at the expense of flexibility, openness, and efficiency, beginning by early adulthood and present in a variety of contexts" (p. 771). It is important for the clinician to keep this "big picture" in mind when approaching the patient. To be certain of the diagnosis, a number of factors should be clarified—the first of which is that the patient's behavior meets criteria for a general personality disorder (see the section "General Personality Disorder" earlier in this chapter and in DSM-5-TR)—before refining the diagnosis for a specific personality disorder. A typical presentation of OCPD will capture the essence of the description given earlier, and it must meet four of the eight criteria specified in DSM-5-TR.

Persons with this disorder will have an anxious preoccupation with rules and control to the extent that it causes great interpersonal conflict and dysfunction. Their perfectionism may result in a paralysis rather than excellence. They tend to focus on the trivial details to the extent that their main goals are lost.

Patients may not be aware that their personality traits are pathological. In fact, they may be very invested in their preoccupation with rules or their perfectionism and may believe these traits to be adaptive. This creates a challenge for the clinician to uncover. A patient may present with other complaints, such as interpersonal conflicts or anxiety symptoms. The clinician may have to work to reveal the clinical picture because of the patient's lack of insight.

The transient presence of OCPD traits under specific conditions may create a confusing clinical presentation. Some people might exhibit these traits only under specific stresses, in a particular life challenge, or in a narrow area of their overall social function. Such a pattern does not constitute a diagnosis of OCPD. Moreover, in many instances rigid, rules-oriented traits and excessive attention to detail are adaptive; however, these usually happen in a specific context, such as in a profession that requires great attention to detail, and are not pervasive.

When establishing a diagnosis, it is very useful to try to get a longitudinal history and to obtain collateral information from other people in the patient's life (e.g., friends, family). With OCPD, it is not uncommon for a family member to be able to articulate the clinical picture better than the patient because of the family member's perspective. It is often necessary to see a patient on multiple occasions to clarify the pathology's enduring nature. The input from friends and family can clarify the pattern in multiple contexts and help to trace the pathology back to adolescence.

Getting the History

> Mr. Fox, a 38-year-old man, requested assessment from a psychiatrist because he is having marital difficulties. He tells the clinician that he doesn't think he has a problem, but his wife thinks he has a "control freak personality." Although his wife admits that he has "always been this way," she thinks it is starting to "really bug her." Inviting the patient to explain his concerns in his own words is an important part of getting the history needed to determine the diagnosis. In talking about his orderliness, for example, Mr. Fox mentions that he does not like it when his wife plays his compact discs (CDs) because she "doesn't put them back right." He says, "I like my CDs to be in alphabetical order and on the shelf in a certain way." The interviewer asks, "Can you tell me how you like them to be ordered?" Mr. Fox replies, "I like them to be in order by category and then alphabetically by artist's last name. And my wife doesn't even know that Miles Davis is a jazz musician, let alone how to alphabetize. She usually just leaves them out anyway. She drives me crazy." The interviewer asks, "What do you do when she leaves them out?" Mr. Fox responds, "Well, we argue. And then I put them where they go! In fact, there's no mystery when she's been playing my CDs. She leaves them all over. And out of order." The clinician asks, "What would happen to you if you didn't put them back?" Mr. Fox answers, "I don't know. Nothing. Sometimes I don't, in fact, because I'm too busy picking up some other mess she left." The clinician asks, "Do you ever check the CDs to make sure they're in order?" Mr. Fox responds, "Not really. But that's not a bad idea to check them periodically just to make sure she hasn't messed them up." The clinician asks, "Do you find yourself thinking or worrying about the order of the CDs?" He responds, "Only if I know she was messing them up." The interviewer asks, "Do you spend a lot of time keeping things like the CDs in a particular order?" Mr. Fox replies, "Just when I see she's strewn 'em all over the place. Why do you ask? Don't you think a man's music collection should be respected?"

The clinician, who believes Mr. Fox has an enduring and pervasive pattern of maladaptive personality disorder traits consistent with DSM-5-TR criteria for OCPD, is trying to distinguish Mr. Fox's preoccupation with orderliness around the CDs from an obsessive thought or a compulsion to act, which would indicate possible OCD. In this case, it seems that the patient is describing an example of a preoccupation with order. He has a particular system of rules for his CDs, and he shows annoyance with violations of these rules. However, he does not ruminate and worry excessively about the CD collection. He does not check the CDs spontaneously. Furthermore, he does not experience anxiety when they are out of order. He is just fixated on the orderliness of the collection to the extent that he is willing to let it cause repeated arguments with his wife.

Tips for Clarifying the Diagnosis

- Establish that the clinical picture is consistent with the definition of general personality disorder.
- Confirm that the DSM-5-TR symptoms of OCPD have occurred over a long duration in multiple social settings.
- Explore other diagnoses that may better explain the observed symptoms.
- Look for dysfunction as a result of overvalue of rules and details.
- Remember that other mental health diagnoses are commonly associated with the diagnosis.

Consider the Case

Mr. Singh, a 33-year-old Indian American computer programmer, presents with symptoms of insomnia. In the interview, the psychiatrist uncovers an enduring pattern of preoccupation with orderliness and perfectionism. Further interview reveals some anxiety-based insomnia that bothers Mr. Singh when he works late on projects and then cannot stop thinking about them when he tries to fall asleep.

Mr. Singh goes on to describe a long history of difficulty getting his work done because of his overcommitment to making sure that "everything is perfect" before he logs out. This leads him to work late into the night on projects that colleagues would be able to finish during regular work hours. He reports frustration because his work colleagues are often praised for projects but he is not, even though his projects "have better attention to little details." He will not delegate work to others because, he says, "If you want something done right, you have to do it yourself." He does not engage in many social activities because of his devotion to work and work-related projects. In fact, he does not attend work-related social activities because he doesn't want to "waste company time."

Mr. Singh lives alone and dates rarely, despite pressure from his family to get married. He says that members of his family tell him that he is "not right"—but he feels that "they are the ones who are wrong!" He reports that he cannot stay with a girlfriend because the women he meets are "never just right for me."

He does not have generalized symptoms of anxiety or panic attacks.

He believes that his behaviors make him a better programmer despite feedback that he is struggling at work. He goes on to say that his commitment to orderliness is a culturally appropriate phenomenon and that it is "very Indian." He admits that other Indian Americans in his company "have a more 'American' work ethic."

This case fits with the DSM-5-TR description of OCPD. As frequently occurs in patients with this disorder, Mr. Singh does not see these behaviors as problematic and is stubborn about changing these behaviors. He views them as adaptive in the workplace despite feedback that it is not.

There can be cultural variants that will apply to evaluation of the symptoms of OCPD. In Mr. Singh's case, the behavior pattern is enduring and pervasive and causes dysfunction in multiple spheres, and the symptoms cause significant disability. Mr. Singh does not exhibit thoughts, reactions, or behaviors that align with cultural or social norms, despite the patient's insistence. A patient can normalize something pathological as a cultural nuance when, in fact, it is more of a noncultural, maladaptive trait. Cultural expectations may influence the mindset, interpersonal interactions, and behavioral norms, and individuals may adapt or conform to these cultural expectations. A careful assessment will help determine whether the cultural context of an individual is influencing the clinical presentation of OCPD (p. 774, "Culture-Related Diagnostic Issues," in DSM-5-TR).

Differential Diagnosis

OCPD must be distinguished from other mental disorders (e.g., OCD, hoarding disorder, substance use disorders), other personality disorders and personality traits, and personality change due to another medical condition.

OCD is usually easily distinguished from OCPD by the presence of true obsessions and compulsions in OCD. Descriptively, very often OCD is quite uncomfortable for the individual (ego-dystonic) on an emotional level, whereas OCPD is not necessarily evidently problematic for the person (ego-syntonic). A person with OCPD tends to be less aware of their rigidity and more aware of the conflict that arises from it. When criteria for both disorders are met, both diagnoses should be made.

Other anxiety states may bring out rigid, rules-oriented traits but should not be confused with OCPD.

Other personality disorders may be confused with OCPD because they have traits in common. Therefore, a clinician needs to distinguish among these disorders by the differences in their characteristic features. For example, narcissistic personality disorder (NPD) may also describe perfectionism and a belief that others cannot do things as well; however, narcissism is usually distinguished by inflated self-importance rather than rigid adherence to rules.

Obsessive-compulsive personality traits may be adaptive in certain professional contexts or other situations that reward highly detail-oriented performance. Furthermore, for an individual, the traits may exist only in a context where the trait is adaptive, in which case the diagnosis should not be made.

See DSM-5-TR for additional disorders to consider in the differential diagnosis. Also refer to the discussions of comorbidity and differential diagnosis in their respective sections of DSM-5-TR.

Summary

- Individuals who have OCPD demonstrate an enduring pattern of preoccupation with orderliness, order, and organization.
- OCPD includes an enduring pattern of perfectionism.

- A person with OCPD has an enduring pattern of reluctance to delegate tasks, believing that only they can do such tasks correctly.
- OCPD includes an enduring pattern of rigidity and stubbornness.
- These patterns are pervasive across multiple spheres of social life and create dysfunction.
- Neither obsessions nor compulsions are present in OCPD, which differentiates the disorder from OCD.

IN-DEPTH DIAGNOSIS: SCHIZOTYPAL PERSONALITY DISORDER

Ms. Katz, a 44-year-old single woman, presents with the chief complaint "I am so afraid." She reports anxiety stemming from serious concerns about the world ending with the end of the Mayan calendar in 2012. She believes that the date was actually a miscalculation and that the "true" date is in 2026. She has been interested in the predictions of "end times" from ancient sources such as the myths of the ancient Mayans and the predictions of Nostradamus. She shows the psychiatrist websites that describe the Mayan prediction and possible scenarios for the end of the world. She has "triangulated the data to demonstrate" that the world will end in 2026. "I don't know what is going to happen, but it will be bad," she states.

Ms. Katz says that these fears are "really serious"—she states that she has severe symptoms of anxiety to the extent that she has insomnia and worries about the end of the world. She reports that she has taken precautions for the possibility of catastrophe, like taking self-defense classes and stocking her shelves with water and canned foods. She is involved with a group that takes these predictions seriously. The members of this group are her only major social contacts. Outside this group she has very few social relationships other than first-degree relatives.

Ms. Katz is not shy about sharing her interest in other unusual topics, such as crop circles, UFOs, and her belief that "aliens created many of the natural structures on Earth." She has a pattern of odd beliefs and fascinations with fantasy and science fiction that began in childhood. She was awkward socially and has had a very limited social group since adolescence. She reports that she has never been married and has never had any serious romantic relationships. She is oddly dressed, wearing a pin that says, "The end is near."

Ms. Katz does not have auditory hallucinations. She does not endorse any frankly delusional ideas. She is organized in her behavior. She has never had mood episodes of mania/hypomania or depression.

Ms. Katz's behavior fulfills criteria for general personality disorder, as well as specific diagnostic criteria for schizotypal personality disorder. She has few social relationships. She has very odd beliefs that influence her behavior. These beliefs are odd and eccentric but not clearly of the delusional caliber seen in thought disorders such as schizophrenia. Furthermore, she reports that these patterns have been present for much of her adolescent and adult life. Her interest in and odd ideas around fantasy topics are consistent with the eccentric ideas seen in schizotypal personality disorder. Meanwhile, she does not exhibit the hallmark symptoms of schizophrenia (e.g., she does not have hallucinations or frank delusions, disorganized speech, disorganized behavior, or a flattened affect).

Approach to the Diagnosis

DSM-5-TR describes the essence of schizotypal personality disorder as "a pervasive pattern of social and interpersonal deficits, including reduced capacity for close relationships; cognitive or perceptual distortions; and eccentricities of behavior, usually beginning by early adulthood but in some cases first becoming apparent in childhood and adolescence" (p. 103). A clinician must determine first that a person's behavior fits the definition of general personality disorder (see the section "General Personality Disorder" earlier in this chapter and in DSM-5-TR) and then that they meet five of the nine described criteria for the specific diagnosis. Someone with schizotypal personality disorder typically presents as odd and eccentric and has a limited social network.

Other conditions must be examined when arriving at a personality disorder diagnosis. The prodrome of schizophrenia, for instance, may look very much like schizotypal personality disorder, but the former should be distinguishable because of its timeline as well as its evolution into a primary psychotic disorder.

Individuals may not be aware of their symptoms as pathological. In fact, if they seek mental health treatment at all, they most often present for depression, anxiety, or something other than the personality disorder traits. The clinician must therefore get at the hallmark symptoms through an interview style that uncovers these patterns.

It is useful to try to get a longitudinal history and to obtain collateral information from other people involved in the person's life (e.g., friends, family). Given the individual's lack of insight into symptoms, background history from family members is often helpful. It is often necessary to see a person on multiple occasions to clarify the pathology's enduring nature. Additional information from friends and family can clarify the pattern in multiple contexts and help trace the pathology back to adolescence.

Getting the History

Mr. Willis, a 36-year-old man, reports that he has a background in physical science but dropped out of his doctoral program because of conflicts with his dissertation adviser. Mr. Willis states that the adviser did not understand him because the adviser is not a "time traveler." Mr. Willis then indicates that this is not unusual. "People who don't believe in time travel are just different from me."

His language around the belief is vague and circumstantial, so the interviewer has a hard time distinguishing "odd beliefs or magical thinking" from psychotic delusion.

The clinician asks, "Can you tell me more about the time travel?" Mr. Willis replies, "There are lots of stories about it, but no one really knows if it can work or not, right? With Einstein's relativity, we know that space and time bend." The clinician asks, "But can you tell me about *your* time travel?" Mr. Willis replies, "Different objects vibrate on their own frequencies. And if you get objects from a certain era of time together, they will all vibrate on the frequencies from that time. So I think people can time travel if they have the right objects together around them." The clinician asks, "Have you ever done this time travel?" Mr. Willis replies, "I am still working on getting the right conditions. But I have read about people who have done this. And it's real!" The clinician asks, "Do you mean you've read this in fiction or in real life?" Mr. Willis responds, "It's in science fiction all the time. But I think it's based on things that really happen. And I have read real accounts of this online. The scientific community just ignores it."

The interviewer, who believes that Mr. Willis has an enduring and pervasive pattern of maladaptive personality disorder traits consistent with DSM-5-TR criteria for schizotypal personality disorder, wants to find out if there is a more bizarre idea under the patient's stated belief. The interviewer is seeking to clarify if the unusual belief should be thought of as a psychotic delusion. The clinician asks questions to see how firm the belief is. In this case, the belief is unusual, but Mr. Willis does not hold this belief as absolutely fixed, as he would if it were a psychotic delusion. Furthermore, he is not claiming to have had the experience of time travel, an elaboration that may be present in someone with psychotic symptoms; he simply believes that time travel is possible. It is more along the lines of the odd beliefs seen in schizotypal personality disorder than it is like a psychotic delusion.

Tips for Clarifying the Diagnosis

- Establish that the clinical picture is consistent with the definition of general personality disorder.
- Confirm that the DSM-5-TR symptoms of schizotypal personality disorder have occurred over a long duration in multiple social settings.
- Explore other diagnoses that may better explain the observed symptoms.
- Remember that although they have similarities, people with schizotypal personality disorders should be distinguished from people with primary psychotic disorders.

Consider the Case

Mr. Huffman is a 42-year-old man referred by a physician who performed a necessary work physical examination for evaluation of "possible" depression. The occupational health doctor referred him to a psychiatrist to "rule out a psychotic disorder" because the doctor thinks Mr. Huffman is "very odd."

In his visit with the psychiatrist, Mr. Huffman is dressed oddly, wearing all purple from head to toe. He reports that he likes his work as an information technology technician because he does not have to talk to anyone. He says, "I just fix computers." When asked about depressive symptoms, he says, "I'm okay, I guess. Sometimes I feel discouraged."

He has never been on a date and has never been married. He has few social contacts because he "doesn't trust anyone." He sees his mother every weekend and helps her to "get groceries and pick up the house." His main social network comes from his interaction with people through online video gaming. He is involved in a fantasy-oriented video game that he plays late at night against other fans through the internet. He says that the purple clothes are his "magic colors" from the video game. He wears them every day to bring good fortune and to protect him from "evil." He reports that it has worked for him since he was a child.

Mr. Huffman does not experience auditory hallucinations, and he does not describe frank delusions. He has no history of substance abuse. There is no evidence of autism spectrum disorder. He does not endorse depressive symptoms.

Mr. Huffman's case seems to be consistent with schizotypal personality disorder. The man demonstrates a pervasive pattern of odd and eccentric behaviors within the context of a solitary life with few social relationships. He meets at least five of the nine criteria listed in DSM-5-TR for schizotypal personality disorder. He has eccentric behaviors, odd beliefs, few social relationships, and a generally guarded and suspicious view of other people. The man's belief that the purple colors will protect him is unusual, but it should be viewed as an instance of "magical thinking" rather than as a psychotic delusion. Divergent cultural norms may make magical thinking a difficult phenomenon to categorize, but in this case the belief is inconsistent with any cultural or religious explanation. Cultural variations and beliefs should be considered when determining the traits of schizotypal personality disorder. For instance, a wide range of beliefs might be considered quite ordinary to one culture but as magical thinking in another. Across different cultures and nations, both the actual prevalence of schizotypal traits and the cultural acceptance of schizotypal traits may influence their observed variation in prevalence and expression. The patient's behavior does not meet the diagnosis of schizotypal personality disorder, however, unless there is some disabling impact in his work or life. The presence of odd beliefs and behaviors alone does not make the diagnosis.

Differential Diagnosis

Schizotypal personality disorder must be distinguished from other disorders with psychotic symptoms, neurodevelopmental disorders, personality change due to another medical condition, substance use disorders, and other personality disorders and personality traits.

Schizotypal personality disorder can be distinguished from delusional disorder, schizophrenia, and bipolar or depressive disorder with psychotic features because these other disorders are all characterized by a period of persistent frank psychotic symptoms. Schizotypal personality is characterized by odd and eccentric thoughts and behaviors, including ideas of reference and magical thinking, but it is not characterized by frank psychotic phenomena. It may be challenging to delineate between ideas of reference and delusions and between magical thinking and psychotic delusion, particularly in the context of evaluating a person of a different cultural background. In rare cases, the transient presence of schizotypal traits under specific conditions may be a confusing clinical presentation, but it does not warrant a diagnosis of schizotypal personality disorder.

Special care must be taken to differentiate children with schizotypal personality disorder from those who have autism spectrum disorder.

Substance use disorders can present with similar symptoms as schizotypal personality disorder and must be ruled out. Some psychoactive drugs may mimic symptoms of the disorder.

Other personality disorders may be confused with schizotypal personality disorder because they have common traits. Other Cluster A personality disorders (i.e., paranoid and schizoid personality disorders) may have similar characteristics, such as suspiciousness, lack of close personal relationships, and odd interpersonal dynamics; however, they are usually distinguishable by the broad presentation of trait cluster that defines schizotypal personality disorder. Individuals who have BPD may also have transient, psychotic-like states, but these states tend to be related to intense emotion or dissociation.

See DSM-5-TR for additional disorders to consider in the differential diagnosis. Also refer to the discussions of comorbidity and differential diagnosis in their respective sections of DSM-5-TR.

Summary

- Individuals who have schizotypal personality disorder demonstrate an enduring pattern of reduced interpersonal relationships and suspicious thinking.
- Schizotypal personality disorder includes an enduring pattern of cognitive or perceptual distortions, including magical thinking.
- Schizotypal personality disorder includes an enduring pattern of odd behaviors and eccentricities.
- Patterns are pervasive across multiple spheres of social interaction, and they cause dysfunction.
- Schizotypal personality disorder is not associated with auditory hallucinations or delusions.

IN-DEPTH DIAGNOSIS: NARCISSISTIC PERSONALITY DISORDER

Mr. Klein, a 68-year-old retired businessman, presents with concerns over interpersonal conflicts. He wants to consult with a mental health professional to learn about the pathology of his family and uncover why they are not treating him as he feels he should be treated. He feels that he has been unjustly alienated from his family. He is twice divorced, describing his ex-wives as "girls who were too simple to appreciate what they had in me." He has become estranged from his daughters and grandchildren over time because "they don't give me the respect I deserve in our visits."

Further review of his history reveals a pattern of grandiosity and excessive need for admiration. Mr. Klein tells grand stories of his business endeavors, name-dropping famous businessmen such as Jeff Bezos and Bill Gates as peers. He continuously focuses on his achievements in business and in social interactions. He demonstrates a lack of empathy for those "beneath" him and identifies closely with celebrity businesspeople. From the interview, it is not clear how successful Mr. Klein was in his career. It is clear that he ran into conflicts with superiors, limiting his ability to be promoted. He claims that his bosses "were always jealous" of his talent and never let him "get ahead."

Mr. Klein describes the current problem between him and his family as the source of conflict causing him irritability. He has refused to spend time with his family. He was particularly annoyed that he had to go to the daughters' houses for visits. "They should come see me on my home turf instead." He announced to them that he no longer would travel to anyone's house. For 3 years he has not seen his daughters or his grandchildren. He gets invited to holidays and to the kids' birthdays but refuses to go unless they come to his house first.

Mr. Klein says, "If they want to see me, they know what they need to do."

Mr. Klein meets DSM-5-TR criteria for general personality disorder, as well as specific diagnostic criteria for NPD. A sense of confidence may be useful in the business world, but the pattern of grandiosity seen in this case does not generate success in business or in family life. His rigid rules around expectations for how he is to be treated and respected have been poorly adaptive to achieve his desired goals. Furthermore, there is a sense that other people involved in this patient's life would have very different perspectives on the story.

Approach to the Diagnosis

NPD is described by DSM-5-TR as "a pervasive pattern of grandiosity (in fantasy or behavior), need for admiration, and lack of empathy, beginning by early adulthood and present in a variety of contexts" (p. 760). To make the diagnosis, the person's behavior must meet the definition of general personality disorder (see the section "General Personality Disorder" earlier in this chapter and in DSM-5-TR) as well as at least five of the nine identified criteria for the specific disorder.

The typical presentation of NPD is that of a grandiose individual with an excessive need for admiration. Individuals with this disorder believe that they are superior to others and should be recognized for their superiority. People with NPD tend to lack empathy for others. Some people with NPD intentionally exploit others emotionally, socially, intellectually, or financially.

Other pathology should always be investigated. Often persons with NPD will present for assessment or treatment of symptoms of major mental disorders or because of interpersonal problems. Mood disorders should be considered and ruled out. The grandiosity seen in manic or hypomanic episodes should not be mistaken for NPD because of the episodic nature of grandiosity in bipolar disorders.

Substance abuse should be investigated. Cocaine intoxication, for example, can present as apparent grandiosity.

Individuals who have NPD may not be aware of their symptoms. They do not often present for treatment or evaluation of their personality disorder traits. The diagnosis may be difficult to arrive at initially because of the person's lack of insight.

Adaptive variations of traits must be considered. In limited instances, grandiosity and overconfidence are adaptive traits and promote success. Individuals with NPD may seek to achieve their aims through the exploitation of others emotionally, socially, intellectually, or financially. Usually when these traits are pervasive and enduring, they interfere with optimal function and cause disability. To make the diagnosis of NPD, the clinician must look for the pervasive pattern causing dysfunction.

It is very useful to try to get a longitudinal history and to obtain collateral information from other people involved in the person's life (e.g., friends, family). It is often necessary to see a person on multiple occasions to clarify the pathology's enduring nature. The input from friends and family can clarify the pattern in multiple contexts and help to trace the pathology back to adolescence.

Getting the History

A clinician believes that Mr. Pierce, a 37-year-old man, may meet the DSM-5-TR description of NPD, but the clinician is having trouble fitting Mr. Pierce's presentation to the specific criteria from DSM-5-TR. The patient has described his job as a manager of a paper supply store as a "waste of his talent." The clinician tries to explore this statement as an example of the DSM-5-TR criteria by asking more about it.

The clinician asks, "What do you mean by a 'waste of your talent'?" Mr. Pierce responds, "I mean I am way smarter than anyone in that place. I am the manager of morons. And my boss is a moron. I am the only one in that place with real brains." The clinician asks, "So do you mean you are overqualified to work there?" He responds, "No, I mean I am just way more gifted than anyone else there." The clinician asks, "Do other people see that you are gifted?" He responds, "No, and it drives me crazy." The clinician asks, "How so?" Mr. Pierce responds, "Because no one there appreciates my brains. They can't see that I am smarter. I could snap my fingers and get a better job, but the same thing will probably happen somewhere else!"

NPD may be a tricky diagnosis to make because it is unlikely that a person will answer affirmatively to questions based on the exact criteria from DSM-5-TR. It is doubtful that someone with the disorder would have the insight to say, "Yes, I do require excessive admiration, I have a sense of entitlement, and I am interpersonally exploitative." Therefore, the diagnosis often must be made from inference on the basis of content that comes from the interview.

Tips for Clarifying the Diagnosis

- Establish that the clinical picture is consistent with the definition of general personality disorder.
- Confirm that the DSM-5-TR symptoms of NPD have occurred over a long duration in multiple social settings.
- Explore other diagnoses that may better explain the observed symptoms.
- Remember that other mental health diagnoses are commonly associated with the diagnosis.

Consider the Case

Mr. McCoy, a 22-year-old college sophomore and football player, presents to the student mental health center with irritability after being replaced as quarterback. Despite good athletic performance, he was benched because the coach said that his "attitude stinks." Mr. McCoy says the coach "is blind if he can't see that I'm better than the other players—even the seniors." He quotes his passing and rushing statistics proudly to make the case that he should not have been demoted. Mr. McCoy says, "They call me a prima donna but they need me. Oh yeah. They need me." He is very critical of the other players and will berate them on the field in games. His girlfriend broke up with him recently, saying to him that she could "never love you as much as you love yourself." He laughs at this, saying, "Oh, she'll regret leaving me—she'll never get it so good with somebody else."

Mr. McCoy reports that his "confidence" has always been a "major part of his game." He counts on his abilities to make plays and pick up yards. He says, "I have to be the best to win." He reports that part of his success relates to taking risks—"Going for it, big time!"—and that his coaches have tried to discourage this. "I say to them, 'Hey—no pain, no gain. You gotta take the risk or you won't win.'" He has had excellent performance throughout high school and early college play. He sees this trait as adaptive and productive, despite the feedback he has gotten from the coaches and other players.

This pattern has been present for Mr. McCoy throughout his adolescence and young adult life. It has caused him problems in family and intimate relationships.

Confidence can be adaptive, especially in sports, and some of the traits associated with NPD can be helpful and positive in very specific contexts. However, these traits tend to be maladaptive when inflexibly applied across multiple settings and when they are unchanging over time. Mr. McCoy has applied extreme confidence and risk-taking to be competitive in games, and the strategy has worked to a great enough extent that he has had success and earned the role of starting quarterback. However, his interpersonal relationships are hindered to the point that he has lost his spot on the team. Furthermore, he is failing in other areas of functioning as a result of his rigid patterns.

Differential Diagnosis

NPD must be distinguished from mania or hypomania, substance use disorders, and other personality disorders and personality traits. Grandiosity often manifests as part of manic or hypomanic episodes. The inflated sense of self that relates to bipolar disorder should be present only in the context of a mood episode, whereas it is an enduring trait of the personality disorder. Manic or hypomanic states would not necessarily mimic other traits of NPD.

NPD also must be distinguished from symptoms that may develop in association with persistent or intermittent substance use.

Other personality disorders may be confused with NPD because they have certain features in common. Other Cluster B personality disorders (i.e., antisocial, borderline, and histrionic personality disorders) may share the most overlap with NPD traits. Antisocial personality disorder shares the characteristic lack of empathy and manipulation of others. The two disorders are usually easily distinguished by the other symptoms in the DSM-5-TR description. Antisocial personality disorder is usually characterized by lack of regard and violation of the rights of others as evidenced by aggressiveness, deceit, and lack of remorse, whereas the lack of empathy seen in NPD is usually a result of an inflated sense of self.

Many highly successful individuals display personality traits that might be considered narcissistic. Only when these traits are inflexible, maladaptive, persisting, and causing significant functional impairment or subjective distress do they warrant a diagnosis of NPD.

See DSM-5-TR for additional disorders to consider in the differential diagnosis. Also refer to the discussions of comorbidity and differential diagnosis in their respective sections of DSM-5-TR.

Summary

- Individuals with NPD may demonstrate an enduring pattern of grandiose sense of self-importance.
- People with NPD may have an enduring pattern of lack of empathy.
- People with NPD may have an enduring pattern of excessive need for admiration.
- These patterns are pervasive across multiple spheres of experience, and they cause dysfunction.

SUMMARY: PERSONALITY DISORDERS

To be diagnosed with any personality disorder, the person must first meet the threshold criteria that define the presence of a general personality disorder. Personality disorders are defined as enduring patterns of experience and behavior that are pervasive across social situations and lead to serious impairment in important areas of life function. The enduring quality is a key to understanding the concept of the diagnosis because these phenomena are related to personality traits that are generally consistent throughout adulthood and are nonepisodic.

If the clinical case meets the description of general personality disorder, a specific personality disorder diagnosis may be considered. Many maladaptive personality traits may be observed in persons who never meet general criteria for personality disorder and should not be classified with a specific personality disorder. Maladaptive personality traits may occur in isolation or only in specific situations, in which case they would not be associated with a personality disorder diagnosis.

The concept of general personality disorder suggests that the maladaptive patterns of experience and behavior are fixed into an individual's personality. This is why DSM-5-TR specifies that personality disorders must be of long duration and traceable to adolescence or early adulthood. Although it is possible to give a personality disorder diagnosis in a person younger than 18, personality disorder diagnoses are often deferred until the person is older than 18 because the clinician should identify these experiences and behaviors in an already firmly established personality rather than a developing personality.

Distinguishing personality disorders from other mental health diagnoses, physiological effects of substances, or medical conditions is a challenging necessity for any personality disorder diagnosis. This can be a difficult step given that individuals often present with multiple conditions and states that must be taken into account.

ELEMENTS TO CONSIDER IN THE CULTURAL FORMULATION

- Culturally determined characteristics, such as those regarding religious beliefs and practices, may appear dysfunctional to outsiders.
- Behaviors are influenced by sociocultural contexts and life circumstances.
- Social demands may evoke certain behaviors.

DIAGNOSTIC PEARLS

- Personality disorders are associated with maladaptive personality traits.
- In personality disorder, the maladaptive traits must be enduring over a long period of time (i.e., fixed in the personality) and pervasive across many social situations; they are not episodic.

- The enduring and pervasive pattern of maladaptive experience and behavior must lead to impaired function to be classified as a personality disorder.
- Personality disorder traits can be traced to the development of adult personality (adolescence or early adulthood).
- Specific personality disorder diagnoses can be made only if the criteria for general personality disorder have been met.
- Personality disorders may be confused with other mental disorders, substance abuse, or medical conditions. Understanding the long-lasting patterns of behavior is essential to making a correct diagnosis. This understanding usually involves knowing a person long term or having a very extensive and complete history.
- Individuals should be evaluated in the context of their cultural milieu.

SELF-ASSESSMENT

Key Concepts: Double-Check Your Knowledge

What is the relevance of the following concepts to the various personality disorders?

- General personality disorder
- Pervasive and inflexible pattern
- Onset in adolescence or early adulthood
- Stability of pattern over time
- Ten specific personality disorder diagnoses
- Cluster A: odd or eccentric profiles
- Cluster B: dramatic, emotional, or erratic profiles
- Cluster C: anxious or fearful profiles

Questions to Discuss With Colleagues and Mentors

1. If a patient exhibits six of the nine symptoms listed in the DSM-5-TR criteria for borderline personality disorder only when they are under a particular stressor, is the diagnosis of borderline personality disorder appropriate?
2. A person develops personality disorder traits after the onset of a medical condition in the fifth decade of life. Their symptom profile meets six of the seven criteria for paranoid personality disorder. What is the most appropriate way to apply DSM-5-TR diagnoses to this case?
3. If all of the diagnostic criteria are met for more than one personality disorder in two separate clusters, can one patient be given two diagnoses?
4. How are personality disorders different from episodic mood disorders?
5. Personality disorder traits can work to an individual's benefit in certain situations. Why is it important to examine the pervasiveness of patterns to make the diagnosis of a personality disorder?
6. How is a diagnosis of other specified personality disorder or unspecified personality disorder useful in practice?

Case-Based Questions

PART A

Ms. Bailey, a 26-year-old single woman, presents to the clinic with a pervasive pattern of instability of interpersonal relationships, self-image, and affects and marked impulsivity, beginning by early adulthood and present in a variety of contexts. She has a prior diagnosis of unspecified bipolar disorder. She does not report a history consistent with manic or hypomanic episodes; however, she does report a mood history consistent with depressive episodes. She also reports some very unusual and eccentric beliefs, but no frank delusions and no auditory hallucinations.

Ms. Bailey's presentation reveals anger outbursts and constant irritability. Identity disturbance also seems to be a serious issue. She identifies closely with a small group of friends in a club that plays a fantasy game. The few romantic relationships she has had have been with members of this group and have been unstable and intense. She claims that her identity is closely related to her character in the game (and to the fantasy club in general).

Ms. Bailey does not drink alcohol, but she does use hallucinogenic drugs fairly regularly (once every few weeks). She says she does these drugs with her friends from the fantasy club. She is odd in her dress.

What diagnosis can be made?   With the information provided, it seems clear that the criteria for general personality disorder are met. Ms. Bailey appears to have traits from the DSM-5-TR criteria for borderline personality disorder, but the clinical picture is complicated by her odd beliefs and eccentricities. She does not seem to meet symptom criteria for bipolar disorder.

PART B

When exploring Ms. Bailey's fantasy interests more closely, the concept of schizotypal personality disorder enters the thoughts of the clinician. The patient speaks of the fantasy club in very vague terms, and she does not distinguish the members of the club from their characters in the game. In fact, she refers to herself by the name of her character about half the time. When asked about her unusual dress, she reports that this is typical dress "for an elf." When specifically asked, she reports that she does not think she is an elf, but her character in the club is. She says that, like her character, she has "special gifts for reading people." When asked in more detail, she reports that her character is clairvoyant and "to some extent, so am I."

She reports that she believes that people outside of her fantasy club are untrustworthy.

When she uses hallucinogenic drugs, she reports that she "enters the real kingdom" (referring to her fantasy game). But she goes on to say, "That only happens when I trip."

Can one individual be diagnosed with more than one personality disorder?   Yes. In the second part of this case, the clinician uncovers traits consistent with schizotypal personality disorder in addition to the borderline personality disorder traits. Two specific personality disorder diagnoses can be made if the person fulfills the criteria for both. This case is complicated further by the use of hallucinogenic drugs, which may cause odd ideas or magical thinking.

Short-Answer Questions

1. If a person meets seven of the nine criteria for borderline personality disorder (BPD), but only in the context of a hypomanic episode, is the diagnosis of BPD appropriate?
2. A senator has an "overly inflated ego" and enjoys the admiration she gets from others. She is in a successful marriage and is high-functioning without the perception of distress in her life. Should the diagnosis of narcissistic personality disorder be considered?
3. Which personality disorder is most associated with self-harm behaviors?
4. Which two symptom criteria does OCD have that obsessive-compulsive personality disorder lacks?
5. Can a 17-year-old be correctly given a personality disorder diagnosis?
6. Is a personality disorder necessarily a lifelong or permanent diagnosis?
7. Can personality disorders be diagnosed cross-culturally?
8. Which sex has a higher prevalence of BPD?
9. What diagnoses are in the differential for schizotypal personality disorder?

ANSWERS

1. No. BPD is not diagnosed when the criteria that are met occur in the context of a hypomanic episode.

2. No. The features of a personality disorder must cause distress or dysfunction.

3. BPD is the personality disorder most associated with self-harm behaviors.

4. Obsessions and compulsions occur in OCD but do not occur in obsessive-compulsive personality disorder.

5. Yes. A 17-year-old can be diagnosed with a personality disorder if the features have been present for at least 1 year—with the exception of antisocial personality disorder, for which an individual must be 18 years of age or older to receive the diagnosis.

6. No. A personality disorder is not necessarily a lifelong or permanent condition, although when a personality disorder is present, it must have emerged early in life.

7. Yes. Personality disorders can be diagnosed cross-culturally.

8. Females have a higher prevalence of BPD.

9. In the differential diagnosis for schizotypal personality disorder are other mental disorders with psychotic symptoms, neurodevelopmental disorders, personality change due to another medical condition, substance use disorders, and other personality disorders and personality traits.

REFERENCES

American Psychiatric Association: Diagnostic and Statistical Manual of Mental Disorders, 5th Edition. Arlington, VA, American Psychiatric Association, 2013

American Psychiatric Association: Diagnostic and Statistical Manual of Mental Disorders, 5th Edition, Text Revision. Washington, DC, American Psychiatric Association, 2022

CHAPTER 23

Paraphilic Disorders

Richard Balon, M.D.

"I have this urge to show my genitals."

"I have recurring sexual fantasies of being beaten by my partner."

- Voyeuristic Disorder
- Exhibitionistic Disorder
- Frotteuristic Disorder
- Sexual Masochism Disorder
- Sexual Sadism Disorder
- Pedophilic Disorder
- Fetishistic Disorder
- Transvestic Disorder
- Other Specified Paraphilic Disorder
- Unspecified Paraphilic Disorder

The diagnostic class of paraphilic disorders includes disorders of sexual interest and behavior that are characterized by intense and persistent fantasies, interests, or behaviors far beyond what is considered a normative sexual interest or behavior and that cause significant distress or impairment. As noted in DSM-5-TR, "the term *paraphilia* denotes any intense and persistent sexual interest other than sexual interest in genital stimulation or preparatory fondling with phenotypically normal, physically mature, consenting human partners" (American Psychiatric Association 2022, p. 779).

The term *paraphilia* literally means love (*philia*) beyond the usual (*para*). The focus of paraphilic behavior could be either the target of sexual activity or fantasy (e.g., nonhuman objects, children or nonconsenting adults, animals) or the sexual activity itself (e.g., spanking or whipping a sexual partner or oneself to cause pain or humiliation). It is important to note that this interest or behavior should exceed interest in what is considered regular sexual intercourse and relationship with a consenting sexual partner, because some elements of this behavior may occur during what is considered normal sexual activity.

The crucial distinction made in DSM-5 (American Psychiatric Association 2013) and DSM-5-TR as compared with DSM-IV (American Psychiatric Association 1994) is between paraphilic disorder and paraphilia. *Paraphilia* is the description of specific sexual arousal and behavior (Criterion A of each paraphilic disorder, which requires a duration of at least 6 months), whereas *paraphilic disorder* is the paraphilia plus its consequences (e.g., acting on the sexual urges or fantasies with a nonconsenting person, the paraphilia causing clinically significant distress or impairment in social, occupational, or other important areas of functioning—Criterion B of each paraphilic disorder). This distinction advanced by DSM-5 and consequently DSM-5-TR avoids labeling every nonnormative sexual behavior as psychopathological and also provides more specific guidance for clinical intervention. Examples in which this distinction is important include fetishism or transvestism: if the person using a fetish or engaging in cross-dressing during sexual activity is not distressed or impaired by this behavior, the diagnosis of fetishistic or transvestic disorder should not be entertained. In the absence of a disorder, clinical intervention is not indicated.

Paraphilic interest and behavior occur along a spectrum from occasional nondistressing behavior during normative copulatory behavior (e.g., mildly spanking a sexual partner); to intense urges, fantasies, and behaviors that are still not distressing and not causing any impairment; to intense or persistent urges, fantasies, or behaviors that also cause distress or impairment in various areas of functioning; to intense or persistent urges, fantasies, or behaviors that the individual acts on with a nonconsenting partner or that cause distress or impairment in various areas of functioning. The careful use of both Criterion A and Criterion B (and, possibly, specifiers, severity ratings, and patient self-measures) allows for clearer distinction and delineation of occasional nonconsequential behavior, paraphilia, and paraphilic disorder.

One individual may be diagnosed with more than one paraphilic disorder (e.g., pedophilic disorder and voyeuristic disorder) or co-occurring paraphilia and paraphilic disorder (e.g., fetishism and sexual sadism disorder). Paraphilic disorders can also be comorbid with other mental disorders (e.g., personality disorders, substance use disorders).

Interviewing individuals with suspected or diagnosed paraphilic disorder(s) or paraphilia(s) may be a challenging task. These disorders may have far-reaching medicolegal impact and consequences; thus, the individual may not be willing or eager to discuss their innermost fantasies, urges, and behaviors in the paraphilia realm. Thus, the interview must be conducted in an atmosphere of respect, rapport, and confidentiality (with understandable limitations). The interviewer should be aware of their countertransferential feelings, which could be fairly strong in this area, especially in cases of paraphilic disorders involving children or violence. When legal issues are relevant, the limits on confidentiality should be explained. The interviewer should attempt to obtain insight into the feelings and possible distress of the individual with paraphilic disorder. Some individuals not only recognize the problems, unacceptability, and consequences of their urges, fantasies, and behaviors toward others (victims, families) and themselves, but they also agonize over them despite being unable to resist them.

DSM-5-TR delineates eight paraphilic disorders:

- **Voyeuristic disorder**: becoming sexually aroused by observing an unsuspecting person being naked, disrobing, or engaging in sexual activity.
- **Exhibitionistic disorder**: becoming sexually aroused by exposing one's genitals to nonconsenting person(s).
- **Frotteuristic disorder**: becoming sexually aroused by touching or rubbing against a nonconsenting person.
- **Sexual masochism disorder**: becoming sexually aroused from being humiliated, beaten, bound, or otherwise made to feel pain during sexual activity.
- **Sexual sadism disorder**: becoming sexually aroused by the physical or psychological distress of another individual.
- **Pedophilic disorder**: becoming sexually aroused by fantasies, urges, or behavior involving sexual activity with prepubescent children (generally those age 13 or younger).
- **Fetishistic disorder**: becoming sexually aroused from using nonliving objects (e.g., clothing) or highly focusing on nongenital body parts of a sexual partner.
- **Transvestic disorder**: becoming sexually aroused from cross-dressing as a member of the opposite sex.

These eight paraphilic disorders do not encompass all possible paraphilias or paraphilic behaviors. They have been traditionally selected in the DSM diagnostic system because they are relatively common in relationship to other paraphilias and paraphilic disorders, and because some of them entail actions that, because of their noxiousness or potential harm to others, are classified as criminal offenses. Numerous paraphilias have been described, such as acrotomophilia (erotic focus: amputation in partner), necrophilia (erotic focus: corpses), telephone scatologia (erotic focus: obscene phone calls), and zoophilia (erotic focus: animals). In cases of clearly distinctive paraphilic behavior that is not included in the eight delineated disorders, has been present for at least 6 months, and is causing distress or impairment, the diagnosis of other specified paraphilic disorder should be used, specifying the specific reason or paraphilia. When paraphilic behavior causes significant distress or impairment in social, functional, occupational, or other areas but does not meet the full criteria for any disorder in this diagnostic class (or insufficient information is available to make a more specific diagnosis), clinicians should use the diagnosis of unspecified paraphilic disorder. Key changes between DSM-5 and DSM-5-TR diagnostic criteria are summarized in Table 23–1.

TABLE 23–1. Key changes between DSM-5 and DSM-5-TR

General description has been updated; the word *normophilic* has been replaced by either *nonparaphilic* or by the descriptive sentence "sexual interest in genital stimulation or preparatory fondling with phenotypically normal, physically mature, consenting human partners."

Diagnostic features have been updated for paraphilic disorders, emphasizing the importance of the number of victims in strength of clinical inference of the disorder (e.g., for voyeuristic disorder, exhibitionistic disorder, frotteuristic disorder, sexual sadism disorder).

Association with suicidal thoughts or behaviors was added for sexual masochism disorder and sexual sadism disorder.

Prevalence has been updated for most paraphilic disorders.

Culture-related diagnostic issues were added for sexual masochism and sexual sadism disorders.

Some language has been changed; for example, under transvestic disorder, wording for autogynephilia was updated from "self as female" to "self as woman," and in fetishistic disorder "fetishistic behavior without fetishistic disorder" is replaced by "fetishism."

IN-DEPTH DIAGNOSIS: EXHIBITIONISTIC DISORDER

Mr. Ward, a 25-year-old male, was referred for an evaluation by the court. He was arrested by the police after he exposed himself to a female fast-food restaurant worker. While the woman was handing him his order in his car at the drive-through window, he exposed his genitalia. After the woman began to scream, he drove away. The woman was able to get his license plate number and contacted police immediately. He was arrested about a mile away while still masturbating in the car. During the interview he reveals that he has been exposing his genitalia to unsuspecting women for several years. Mr. Ward likes to expose himself to women with "big breasts, if possible." He has exposed himself several times to women at drive-through restaurants or to women passing by his car in parking lots. Exposing himself to unsuspecting women and subsequently masturbating has been his preferred sexual activity, although he had a girlfriend with whom he was sexually active. Mr. Ward occasionally masturbates while imagining exposing himself to female movie stars. At times, he cannot control his urge to expose himself and drives "around to see where I can do it." He has been very nervous lately because "I have almost been caught by police several times, but I cannot stop myself. It is hopeless." He denies any other unusual sexual behavior. He works part-time and lives by himself. He occasionally has contact with his parents and rarely with coworkers.

This heterosexual man was referred for psychiatric evaluation by the criminal justice system. Individuals with exhibitionistic disorder do not usually seek help themselves. Mr. Ward presents a typical case of exhibitionism because he is a male deriving sexual arousal from exposing his genitals to multiple unsuspecting females on separate occasions. This behavior has been ongoing for several years, with onset around age 20. Furthermore, he was not seeking treatment himself, although he has been distressed by possible consequences of his behavior and the inability to stop his urges.

Approach to the Diagnosis

A substantial number of individuals who expose themselves or who have a strong impulse to expose themselves may never be referred and diagnosed with exhibitionistic disorder. If these individuals are not distressed by their fantasies and urges, are not impaired by this sexual interest in other important areas of functioning, and have self-reported, psychiatric, or legal histories indicating that they do not act on their interest, they could be, according to DSM-5-TR, ascertained as having a paraphilia (i.e., exhibitionism) but are not diagnosed with exhibitionistic disorder. Those individuals who are distressed by their behavior or are impaired in some area(s) of their functioning (e.g., relationship, occupation due to legal issues) should be diagnosed with exhibitionistic disorder. The urges, interests, fantasies, and behaviors must be intense and recurrent over at least 6 months to meet the diagnostic criteria for this disorder.

Although the paraphilic behavior or the distress or impairment from the behavior is the key feature, the duration of the recurrent and intense sexual arousal is necessary for making the diagnosis. These features help to determine whether the general criteria are fulfilled for the disorder.

The intensity or severity of the disorder may vary during its course. DSM-5-TR provides specifiers regarding the preference of the person to whom the individual likes to expose themselves (i.e., prepubertal children, physically mature individuals, or both) and in what environment. The "in a controlled environment" specifier was added as an acknowledgment that behavior such as exhibitionism may be difficult to assess in individuals who have limited opportunity to expose themselves because they are in a controlled environment (e.g., such exposure may not be possible in prison or during military service). The exhibitionistic disorder could also be specified as being in full remission, meaning that the individual has no distress or impairment in functioning and has not acted on exhibitionistic urges for at least 5 years while in an uncontrolled environment.

DSM-5-TR notes that the disorder is highly unusual in females and that it tends to emerge in males in adolescence or early adulthood. Little is known about its persistence over time. No specific tests are useful for making this diagnosis. Thus, the approach to this diagnosis is clinical and descriptive.

Getting the History

A 35-year-old man reports having problems being sexually aroused unless he is "in some special situations." The interviewer, even if they know (from the referral) or suspect that the individual exposes his genitals to unsuspecting strangers, should ask for a better description of the situation in which arousal occurs and accept the individual's description as a starting point, no matter how evasive or minimalizing the description is.

Once the occurrence of exhibitionism is established, the interviewer should ask how the individual feels during the exposure, immediately after it, and later on, and investigate whether he masturbates during or after the exposure: "Do you get really aroused when you show your genitals to some unknown woman? Do you masturbate when she is surprised or shocked?" The following questions should focus on how long, how often, and in what situations the behavior occurs: "When did you first expose yourself? How often do you expose yourself and where do you usually expose yourself?" Finally, the interviewer should ask whether the individual is disturbed by the behavior: "Does the exposing to people bother you? Do you feel upset about it? Have you had any legal or other problems related to exposing yourself?"

The interview should establish an atmosphere of trust, good rapport, and confidentiality (with understandable limits)—without confronting the individual about their behavior and its legal consequences—to elicit all symptoms of exhibitionism. The description of the behavior—exposure of genitals to unsuspecting strangers—and the fact that the behavior arouses the individual are crucial for recognizing *exhibitionistic disorder*. The questions about being distressed or impaired in some area of functioning are helpful for making the diagnosis. The individual may be evasive about their arousal or behavior, its frequency, and associated problems (e.g., legal trouble). The clinical interview is the cornerstone for making the diagnosis. Previous records of exhibitionistic behavior (e.g., police reports, victim statement, prior evaluations) or a corroborating interview (e.g., with parents in the case of a juvenile offender or with the individual's partner) also may be helpful. Evaluations conducted for forensic purposes have different confidentiality requirements that should be reviewed with the person being interviewed.

Tips for Clarifying the Diagnosis

- Determine whether the exposure of genitals happens in the presence of unsuspecting strangers.
- Explore whether the person is unable to control their urges to expose themself.
- Establish whether the exposure is accompanied or followed by masturbation.
- Evaluate whether the person is apprehensive about or distressed by their behavior.
- Investigate whether the individual has the opportunity to go out and expose themselves.

Consider the Case

Mr. Carson, a 50-year-old man, seeks help for "sexual deviation." He states, "My wife caught me making calls to some pay-for-sex phone numbers and talking about sex while touching myself." Mr. Carson admits during the interview that what he calls "phone sex" is just a substitution for what he really likes: "getting out of the car in some unknown neighborhood, watching some people in their bedrooms, and then, when I get excited, finding an unknown woman to whom I show my penis. That really makes my day, when she screams, and I come. But, you know, this has been a very tough winter. I cannot get out because it is really cold outside, so I tried those phone numbers." He says that he has never gotten caught over the 15 years he has been exposing himself; however, he has been a bit nervous since he read in the newspaper that police were looking for an older man who likes to expose himself. His wife, with whom he has a "regular but boring sex life," had not known about his behavior until recently. "She did not push me to seek help, but she told me I was nuts, deviant, someone with whom she does not want to have sex. That made me think."

The onset of Mr. Carson's exhibitionistic behavior developed relatively late in his life, which is unusual but possible. Although he reports himself for help and treatment, his self-referral is not totally voluntary; he has been forced by some circumstances, such as by reading about police looking for someone who is exposing himself and by his wife's comments. He is heterosexual, married, and engaged in regular sexual activity with his wife. However, he has been deriving more satisfying arousal and sexual satisfaction from paraphilic behaviors, such as watching people in their bedrooms (voyeurism), exposing himself, and talking about sex over the phone (telephone scatologia). His preferred source of paraphilic arousal is exposing himself to unsuspecting females. It is important to realize that paraphilic disorders can overlap or coexist. Exhibitionism also can occur in an individual who is involved in regular sexual activity with a partner. Organic brain changes may be considered in older individuals in which paraphilia or paraphilic disorder develops de novo. However, Mr. Carson has shown no signs of cognitive impairment and has no history of brain injury. A further neurological workup may be needed to anchor the diagnosis.

Differential Diagnosis

The differential diagnosis of exhibitionistic disorder is relatively narrow because the description of the paraphilic behavior is specific—exposing one's genitalia to unsuspecting strangers. This behavior may occur strictly within exhibitionistic behavior or within the frame of several co-occurring paraphilic disorders (e.g., voyeuristic behavior or disorder, fetishistic disorder). The exposure of genitals may also occur in a psychotic disorder such as schizophrenia (where the exposure would probably be more nondiscriminatory), manic episode, major neurocognitive disorder, intellectual developmental disorder, personality change due to another medical condition, conduct disorder, antisocial personality disorder, and substance use disorders (especially during intoxication). Unless the exhibitionistic behavior occurs at times other than in the context of these disorders or conditions, the diagnosis of exhibitionistic disorder should not be made. The exhibitionistic disorder should also be distinguished from nudism—individuals with exhibitionistic disorder usually do not expose themselves at nudist places. The diagnosis of exhibitionistic disorder should not be made if the person has not acted on intense urges by exposing themselves to unsuspecting individual(s), or if distress or impairment in various areas is not present.

The course of the disorder likely varies with age, and little is known about persistence over time when it emerges in adolescence or early adulthood. Advancing age may be associated with decreasing exhibitionistic sexual preferences and behavior. Depression and substance use may develop as a consequence of exhibitionistic disorder and then affect the clinical presentation. Denial or minimization of the behavior could hinder the differential diagnosis.

See DSM-5-TR for additional disorders to consider in the differential diagnosis. Also refer to the discussions of comorbidity and differential diagnosis in their respective sections of DSM-5-TR.

Summary

- Exhibitionistic disorder involves recurrent and intense sexual arousal from the fantasies, urges, or behavior of exposing one's genitalia to nonconsenting, unsuspecting strangers.

- In the context of an intense exhibitionistic sexual interest, the diagnosis of exhibitionistic disorder can be made if the individual has exposed their genitalia to a nonconsenting person or when the individual has distress or impairment in various areas of functioning because of the exhibitionistic urges or fantasies.
- A careful history should help rule out other mental disorders (e.g., psychotic disorder, manic episode, major neurocognitive disorder, intellectual developmental disorder, substance use disorder, personality disorder) and other paraphilic disorders.

IN-DEPTH DIAGNOSIS: PEDOPHILIC DISORDER

Mr. Flynn, a 50-year-old businessman, reports being attracted to "little girls, when they barely have any breasts and have no body hair. Their bodies enormously arouse me." He says that he has always been sexually attracted to female children. His first sexual encounter around age 16 was with a "neighbor's girl. She was about 9. She excited me, unlike my classmates." He started to touch her and then undressed them both and fondled her genitalia, although "she was pushing me away." He then masturbated in front of her. He adds that when both their parents found out, his parents punished him, but the "whole thing was swept under the rug. Everybody said that kids are curious and like to play." He states that although he has had sexual intercourse with adult women and is married, he has always been much more excited by "those little girls." He regularly masturbates while viewing child pornography. He has had sexual interactions with female children around the country. "You know, in some cities, you can get a little girl easily." He has also traveled to other countries to have sexual interactions with young females because "it is quite easy to get girls in some countries. Their families offer them for almost nothing." He has spent all his money on travel to "get girls" and on child pornography. His wife divorced him when she found him masturbating using child pornography. He has no friends because "nobody would understand me." He has the urge to look at "pictures" at work and is afraid that he will be fired, should he follow the impulse and be discovered.

Mr. Flynn has always been aroused by prepubescent females. His parents and others considered his first sexual encounter with a 9-year-old female to be child's play or an act of curiosity. It is difficult to establish a firm sexual interest during adolescence because many children and young adolescents are curious about seeing other children naked, but they lose their curiosity during puberty. This patient has remained sexually aroused by prepubescent females as an adult and clearly prefers sexual interactions with prepubescent females over sex with adult females. He has acted on his fantasies and urges, either by masturbating while watching sexually explicit content depicting children or by having sexual interactions with prepubescent females. He does not seem to be distressed by his attraction (some individuals with pedophilic disorder are not distressed by and do not feel guilty about what they consider to be a sexual "preference"). Mr. Flynn's pedophilia (sexual attraction to prepubescent females, acting out on his fantasies and preferences) has caused significant impairment in his social functioning (divorce, no friends), in his work setting, and probably in his personal finances (spending substantial money on pornography involving children and travel for sexual interactions). As sexual arousal decreases with age, it is possible that his pedophilic activities and their frequency may decrease.

Approach to the Diagnosis

Most individuals with pedophilic disorder are evaluated after being caught or reported for having sexual interactions with children (prepubescent or pubescent), soliciting sexual activity with children, trading sexually explicit content involving children, or being caught watching such content. Individuals with pedophilia or pedophilic disorder frequently may deny sexual attraction to children because they are aware of the legal ramifications of their attraction. It is important to note that pedophilia is not synonymous with sexual offending against children. Some individuals may report sexual attraction to children (prepubescent males or females), yet they do not feel guilty, ashamed, or distressed about it, and they have never acted on their fantasies or urges. Thus, the interviewer may ascertain that these individuals have pedophilia but not pedophilic disorder.

Pedophilic disorder occurs mostly in males. It also occurs in females, but the prevalence of this disorder in females is likely a small fraction of that in males. Pedophilia or pedophilic disorder develops around the time of puberty and is usually stable across the life span. Pedophilic disorder should be suspected in any adult individual whose behavior suggests sexual interest in or preference for children.

Some individuals with pedophilic disorder are not distressed by and do not feel guilty or ashamed about their sexual attraction and behavior. However, they should be diagnosed with pedophilic disorder if they have acted on their fantasies or urges with a prepubescent child or children or if they have been socially, economically, or otherwise impaired because of their sexual preferences (e.g., divorce, job loss).

As DSM-5-TR Criterion C specifies, the person must be age 16 or older and at least 5 years older than the child or children they are attracted to or involved with. The age difference of 5 years between the individual acting on pedophilic urges and fantasies and the child is an important issue and an area where medicine and law may differ. An 18-year-old male who has been having sex with a fully sexually developed 14- to 15-year-old female is not considered to have pedophilia or pedophilic disorder in medical terms; however, he may be labeled as a sexual offender in many jurisdictions, which may have lifelong consequences. These individuals should not be diagnosed with pedophilic disorder.

The diagnosis of pedophilic disorder should specify whether it is *exclusive type* (attracted only to children) or *nonexclusive type* (attracted to children as well as sexually mature adults), as well as whether the individual is sexually attracted to men, women, or both (gender specifier). Finally, it should be specified whether the pedophilic disorder is limited to incest.

Assessment tools that may help in diagnosing pedophilic disorder in special settings include penile plethysmography (sensitivity and specificity may vary from place to place), viewing time (using photographs of nude children may be difficult because possessing such photographs may violate American law, and that would leave the clinician susceptible to criminal prosecution), and self-report measures. Clinicians must be careful in interpreting the results of these diagnostic markers because they indicate relative sexual response to stimuli depicting children compared with stimuli depicting adults, rather than absolute response to child stimuli.

Getting the History

The individual evaluated for possible pedophilic disorder has usually been suspected of, if not clearly "caught," being involved in pedophilic behavior. To the extent possible, the interviewer should establish an atmosphere of trust, because many individuals deny their pedophilic urges, fantasies, and behavior. The discussion of the limits of confidentiality should be also included. The interviewer should ask first about the individual's understanding of the reasons for the evaluation and clarify what happened. Then the interviewer should move to more specific questions, such as determining the sexual attraction: "Do you get sexually aroused by fantasizing about sexual activity with adults, young adults, kids? Have you ever masturbated while thinking about sex with younger persons? How old were they? Does watching pornography arouse you sexually? What kind of pornography? How frequently do you do this?" The interviewer should determine whether the individual acted on their urges, which may be difficult information to obtain. They may start by asking the patient about touching children, spending time with them, and the activities the individual did with children.

Once the existence and nature of the pedophilic disorder is established, the individual should be asked about the distress and possible consequences: "How have you been feeling about being sexually aroused by children? Have you ever had any problems because of watching child pornography? What about your relationships with others—have they said anything about your sexual interests? Have you been in any legal troubles because of your sexual urges and acting on them?" It may be useful to watch the reactions to such questions, such as hesitation to answer, pauses, vehement denial, and refusal to answer, and then to modify subsequent questions on the basis of these reactions.

Tips for Clarifying the Diagnosis

- Investigate whether the person becomes sexually aroused by fantasizing about having sexual interactions with children.
- Explore whether the individual has acted on these fantasies or urges.
- Verify whether the individual is age 16 or older.
- Confirm the person is at least 5 years older than the child or children of interest.
- Clarify whether the individual is attracted only to children.
- Assess the sexual preferences in terms of gender (boys, girls, both).
- Determine whether the individual's urges, fantasies, or sexual behaviors are limited to children in their nuclear family only (i.e., biological or stepchildren).

Consider the Case

Ms. Dixon is a 25-year-old nanny. She and a 12-year-old boy were found naked by his parents when the parents came home unexpectedly. She admitted that she has been "playing with him for a few months." She says that she has been sexually aroused by looking at him since she started to work for his family a year ago. She used to bathe him and his sister and enjoyed playing with his genitals when drying him off. She fantasized about having oral sex with him. When he started to get erections while she was playing with his genitals, she finally performed fellatio on him. They have been engaged in regular sexual activities since then, whenever his parents were not at home. Ms. Dixon usually performs oral sex on him and masturbates during it. She admits feeling guilty and anxious and worried about being caught all the time. She says, "I know it's illegal, but I could not help it. I love him and love his young body." She had an older boyfriend when she was 18 years old but did not like having sex with him. "He had too much body hair and was a bit rough." She has not had a boyfriend since she ended that relationship and has not been sexually attracted to adult males. However, she has been fantasizing about sexual interactions with young males, "just as they stop being little." She was dismissed from her previous job as a nanny because her employers became suspicious when she was rubbing their son for a long time after he took a bath.

Pedophilic disorder occurs mostly in males, but rare cases of female pedophilia or pedophilic disorder have been reported. Ms. Dixon began fantasizing about having sexual interactions with pubescent males shortly after ending an adult sexual relationship with an older man, when she realized she was not sexually attracted to adult men. She gradually started to act on her fantasies, fondling the young male's genitals and finally performing oral sex and masturbating while doing so. She clearly prefers sexual interactions with pubescent males, has been intensely aroused by pubescent males, and has acted on her fantasies and urges. At age 25, she is more than 5 years older than these pubescent males. She has been feeling guilty, knows it is illegal, and is worried about her behavior. She has been dismissed from one job. She clearly meets the criteria for pedophilic disorder in that she has pedophilic fantasies and urges, acts on them, and is distressed about her behavior and losing her job because of it.

Differential Diagnosis

The differential diagnosis of pedophilic disorder includes other paraphilic disorders (e.g., exhibitionistic disorder, voyeuristic disorder), antisocial personality disorder, and substance use disorders. The distinction between pedophilic disorder and other paraphilic disorders should focus on the object of arousal (children) and the character of sexual behavior (sexual intercourse, masturbation). Individuals with pedophilic disorder may also be diagnosed with antisocial personality disorder; however, antisocial personality disorder does not explain pedophilic disorder and should not supplant it. Individuals with substance use disorders may get involved in sexual activity with children while intoxicated, but their pedophilic activity usually occurs during intoxication only and does not have a chronic character. Individuals with neurocognitive disorders may fondle children, but this behavior develops uncharacteristically in older age and within the context of neurocognitive impairment. OCD may include obsessions involving sexual activity with children, but individuals with OCD do not act on those urges; their thoughts or urges are ego-dystonic, and they worry about them.

Individuals with pedophilic disorder may have comorbid anxiety, depression, bipolar disorder, substance use disorder, antisocial personality disorder, and other paraphilias or paraphilic disorders. These disorders may affect the presentation of pedophilic disorder—for example, depression may be associated with profound feelings of guilt, but not necessarily about the pedophilic disorder. Pedophilic behavior may become more disinhibited in individuals with substance use disorders, especially during intoxication. The comorbid antisocial personality disorder psychopathology may also affect the presentation of pedophilic disorder, in terms of a lack of distress or impairment in various areas of functioning.

See DSM-5-TR for additional disorders to consider in the differential diagnosis. Also refer to the discussions of comorbidity and differential diagnosis in their respective sections of DSM-5-TR.

Summary

- The defining feature of pedophilic disorder is intense sexual arousal from fantasies, urges, and behaviors involving sexual activity with prepubescent children.
- To meet the criteria of pedophilic disorder, the person must act on the sexual urges or the urges or fantasies must cause marked distress or interpersonal difficulty.
- The individual with pedophilic disorder should be age 16 or older and at least 5 years older than the child or children by whom they feel sexually aroused.
- Pedophilic disorder occurs predominantly in males, but the disorder has been reported in females.
- Pedophilic preference, age difference between the individual and child, and acting on the preference—or experiencing distress or interpersonal difficulty resulting from the sexual urges and fantasies—all must be present to make the diagnosis of pedophilic disorder.
- Careful history should help to differentiate pedophilic disorder from other mental disorders and other paraphilic disorders.

IN-DEPTH DIAGNOSIS: FETISHISTIC DISORDER

> Mr. Griffith, a 30-year-old man, reports being ashamed and stressed out about "my sexual practices." Since he became sexually active more than 10 years ago, he has been extremely aroused by holding his partners' "used panties and smelling them while having sex or while masturbating." He also asks his partners to cut a substantial piece of their hair, which he uses to play with while masturbating or puts over his partner's face during sex. Mr. Griffith says that he has had sex or masturbated without these objects, but "it is not the same, and I am not even able to come without them at times." He adds that, alternatively, when he has everything "together," "the sex could be pretty amazing, I get very aroused." He was not originally distressed by using fetishes. However, because several of his girlfriends were turned off by his practices and called him "a pervert," he started to wonder whether he "was normal." He began to feel more guilty that "I am not able to have sex without bothering my girlfriend with those panties and hair." His current girlfriend has flatly refused to let him cut her hair and use her panties during sex. She has threatened to leave him unless he stops this behavior.

Mr. Griffith's use of fetishes during sexual intercourse and masturbation developed in his late teens and was not originally associated with distress, so at first, he had a fetishism. However, over the years, his sexual partners have been complaining about his use of fetishes, and he has gradually become distressed. He has started to doubt himself and feels a lot of shame. His relationships with several girlfriends have been impaired due to his adamant requirement for fetishes during intercourse. Thus, he now meets the criteria for fetishistic disorder. He has been using more than one fetish, and his behaviors have included holding and smelling worn underwear and requiring his partner to have pieces of her hair on her face during intercourse. Interestingly, he reports lesser arousal during intercourse when not using any fetish—impaired sexual functioning may occur when a preferred fetish is not available during intercourse or masturbation.

Approach to the Diagnosis

Most individuals with fetishism (use of fetishes during sexual intercourse or mastur-bation or fantasizing about using them) do not seek help or get diagnosed. Their sex-ual partners may tolerate their behavior. The diagnosis of fetishistic disorder is made only when the individual has significant distress or impairment in important areas of functioning due to their fetishism. Individuals with either distress or impairment due to using fetishes—thus meeting the diagnostic criteria for fetishistic disorder—are more likely to be diagnosed because their distress or impairment may bring them to clinicians. Fetishistic disorder is usually considered harmless unless it leads to crimi-nal activity, such as stealing items for a specific fetish or collection of fetishes (some could be quite special or expensive). Fetishes involve not only nonliving objects but also may include very specific nongenital parts of the body, such as feet, toes, and hair.

Individuals (mostly male) with fetishistic disorder may use one specific fetish, more than one fetish, or a specific combination of fetishes. Behaviors involving fetishes may include holding them, rubbing them, smelling them, touching them, inserting them, asking a sexual partner to wear them, and kissing or sucking them (e.g., nongen-ital body parts), all during sexual intercourse with a partner, masturbation, or intense sexual fantasies. The fetishistic behavior should not be limited to cross-dressing or to use of devices designed to increase sexual stimulation, such as vibrators. It is import-ant to note that the diagnosis of fetishistic disorder does not require the use of fetishes during sexual intercourse. The condition could involve using fetishes during mastur-bation or fantasies only.

Impairment of sexual functioning may occur when a preferred fetish is not avail-able during sexual intercourse. Sexual dysfunction due to the lack of a fetish should be distinguished from sexual dysfunction due to other reasons, such as physical ill-ness, depression (even due to fetishistic disorder), or medication use.

The diagnosis should specify whether nonliving objects or specific body parts are the focus of fantasies, urges, or behaviors. The diagnosis should also specify whether the behavior is in full remission (i.e., no distress or impairment for at least 5 years in an uncontrolled environment) and whether it occurs in a controlled environment (i.e., setting where opportunities to engage in fetishistic behaviors are restricted).

Fetishes can develop before adolescence or, more commonly, during puberty. Fe-tishistic disorder tends to be a chronic condition that fluctuates in intensity and frequency of urges or behavior. In clinical samples, it is nearly exclusively reported in males. No specific tests are useful for making this diagnosis. Thus, the approach to this diagnosis is clinical and descriptive and relies on clinician judgment.

Getting the History

Individuals will usually present to the clinician their focus on a fetish in sexual fantasies, urges, and behaviors (e.g., intercourse, masturbation). The interviewer should further explore whether the individual derives intense arousal from using fetishes and what kind of fetishes by asking, "Do you get aroused using some objects—for instance, panties, bras, or your girlfriend's shoes? Does kissing or sucking your girlfriend's feet or toes excite you during sex? Does any other part of her body, besides her breasts and private parts, arouse you sexually?" Once the interviewer establishes that the individual becomes aroused by using a fetish or fetishes, further clarification should focus on duration and intensity: "How long have you been using these [e.g., panties, bras, socks, toes] to get aroused during intercourse, masturbation, or fantasizing about sex? Are you able to have sex (or masturbate) without using them?" The interviewer should also rule out other paraphilic disorders by asking, for example, "Do you wear women's clothes during sex? Does it excite you? Do you use your fetish to slap or beat your partner during sex?"

Finally, the interviewer should establish whether the use of a fetish is causing any distress or impairment by asking, "What does your partner think about using your fetish during sex? How do you feel about using the fetish or fetishes? Do you feel guilty or ashamed that you have to use it? Have you had any problems related to your use of fetishes, such as being chastised or being apprehended obtaining a fetish that did not belong to you?"

The description of the behavior—using various fetishes such as undergarments or a partner's foot or toe—and the fact that the behavior arouses the individual are crucial for recognizing *fetishistic behavior* or *fetishism*. The questions about being distressed or impaired in some area of functioning are crucial for making the diagnosis of *fetishistic disorder*. Obtaining a detailed description of the objects, behaviors involved (e.g., touching, smelling), and their frequency may be straightforward; however, the individual may be evasive about some associated problems, such as a partner's tolerance, associated sexual dysfunction when a fetish is not used, or associated criminal activity. It is important to establish a trusting atmosphere to elicit all symptoms of fetishism. The clinical interview is the cornerstone for making the diagnosis.

Tips for Clarifying the Diagnosis

- Explore whether the individual becomes sexually aroused by the use of nonliving objects or a focus on nongenital body parts.
- Question whether the individual uses fetishes during sexual intercourse or masturbation or whether they fantasize about using them during sexual activities.
- Determine if this behavior has been ongoing or is an occasional experimentation.

- Consider whether this behavior is limited to the use of a vibrator.
- Investigate whether the individual derives sexual arousal from cross-dressing.
- Evaluate whether the individual is apprehensive or distressed by their behavior.

Consider the Case

Mr. Owen, a 45-year-old man, was arrested for breaking a fashion clothing store window and stealing a couple of female mannequins but no clothing. This was his third arrest for the same offense. During the interrogation by police, he admitted, "I needed them for sex. I cannot help it." He was referred for an evaluation by the court. He reports, "These slender mannequins really excite me when I hold them while I masturbate or when I look at them while having sex with my wife." He prefers mannequins without any clothing. He says he does not know why he likes to use them, but "I really like them." He has not tried to have sex with mannequins; he just touches them or looks at them during intercourse or masturbation. He describes that his attraction to mannequins developed over the past 5 years, after he and his wife moved from a small town to a big city where he started frequenting shopping malls with stores that have mannequins in their windows. Mr. Owen says that his wife tolerates him having the mannequins at home but threw the previous ones out "when the kids started to ask why we have them in our bedroom. She tolerated me having them because our sex has become better since I got my first mannequin, and I do not chase other women."

Mr. Owen developed the attraction and use of a fetish—slender female mannequins—at a relatively late age of 40. Most paraphilic disorders, including fetishistic disorder, develop during puberty or adolescence. He has been touching or looking at the fetish (mannequin) during sexual intercourse or masturbation. The presence of the mannequin enhances his sexual arousal. The use of fetishes is frequently accepted or tolerated by sexual partners. This patient's wife tolerates his attraction to mannequins because their sex life has improved since he has been using them. He has not used mannequins as sexual surrogates. He could not explain his attraction to mannequins, and most individuals with fetishistic behavior are unable to explain their attraction to fetishes. He has displayed serious functional impairment because he has been arrested for burglary (stealing mannequins) and destroying property several times. He has not been able to control his illegal behavior.

Differential Diagnosis

The differential diagnosis of fetishistic disorder is relatively narrow. The disorder should be distinguished from other paraphilias, namely transvestic disorder (sexual arousal derived from using a fetish vs. sexual arousal derived from cross-dressing—in both cases, female undergarments may be used) and sexual masochism disorder (sexual arousal derived from using fetishes to touch, smell, or hold oneself vs. sexual arousal derived from the sexual partner using a variety of objects to slap, hit, or bind the individual). Fetishistic disorder may co-occur with other paraphilic disorders. The distinction between fetishistic disorder and transvestic disorder could be difficult to make at times because their phenomenology is similar; however, this differential diagnosis is fairly straightforward—in transvestic disorder, the articles of clothing are worn exclusively during cross-dressing. Fetishistic disorder is not diagnosed when the object used is genitally stimulating because it was designed for that purpose (e.g., a vibrator).

Some individuals may use fetishes (e.g., licking partner's toes, wearing leather boots) during foreplay or sexual activity and not be distressed about it—this behavior should be categorized as fetishism. Fetishistic disorder may also occur in individuals with other mental disorders, such as personality disorders, mood disorders, and im-pulse-control disorders.

Fetishistic disorder occurs mostly in males, and the course of the disorder is chronic. Depression and substance use may develop as a consequence of fetishistic disorder and then affect the clinical presentation. Sexual dysfunction may develop during the times when fetishes are not available. Denial or minimization of the behavior could hinder the differential diagnosis. Occasionally, an injury may occur when a fetish is inserted or when fetishistic behavior such as sucking gets extreme or switches to more harmful behavior such as biting.

See DSM-5-TR for additional disorders to consider in the differential diagnosis. Also refer to the discussions of comorbidity and differential diagnosis in their respec-tive sections of DSM-5-TR.

Summary

- The hallmark of fetishistic disorder is the use of nonliving objects (e.g., undergar-ments) or nongenital body parts (e.g., partner's feet, toe, hair) to become sexually aroused.
- Establishing the use of fetishes for sexual arousal confirms the presence of fetish-ism, not fetishistic disorder.
- Distress over fantasies, urges, or behavior—or impairment in various areas of functioning—is necessary for establishing the diagnosis of fetishistic disorder.
- Taking a careful history should help rule out other mental disorders (e.g., psy-chotic disorder, substance use disorder, personality disorder, impulse-control dis-order) and other paraphilic disorders, such as transvestic disorder and sexual masochism disorder.

SUMMARY: PARAPHILIC DISORDERS

Paraphilic disorders are rarely observed in routine practice. The diagnostic class in-cludes disorders with sexual interest and behavior characterized by intense and per-sistent sexual fantasies, interests, or behaviors other than sexual interest in genital stimulation or preparatory fondling with phenotypically normal, physically mature, consenting human partners. Examples of paraphilic behaviors include being sexu-ally aroused by any of the following: watching a nonconsenting person who is naked, disrobing, or having sex; exposing one's genitals to nonconsenting strangers; rub-bing or touching a nonconsenting person; being humiliated, beaten, or otherwise made to feel pain; causing the physical or psychological distress of another person; having sexual activity with prepubescent or pubescent children; using a nonliving object or nongenital body part during sexual intercourse or masturbation; and cross-dressing. Some sexual interests and behaviors may be relatively harmless (e.g., fetishism, transvestism), and at times they do not distress the individuals; in those cases, only paraphilia is identified, and paraphilic disorder is not diagnosed. The origin or basis of paraphilic behavior or disorder is unknown. There are many paraphilias beyond those discussed in depth in DSM-5-TR. These are usually very rare and thus have not been included in the DSM system. Almost any of them could, by virtue of negative consequences for the individual or for others, rise to the level of a paraphilic disorder.

Paraphilic disorders occur almost exclusively in males (with the exception of sexual masochism disorder), for unclear reasons. Paraphilic disorders usually develop during late childhood or during puberty or adolescence and have a chronic, lifelong course.

ELEMENTS TO CONSIDER IN THE CULTURAL FORMULATION

- Knowledge of and appropriate consideration for normative aspects of sexual behavior are important factors to explore to establish a clinical diagnosis and to distinguish clinical diagnosis from a socially acceptable sexual behavior, such as in the case of fetishism.
- Cultural acceptance of some paraphilic disorders varies across countries.
- Paraphilias and paraphilic disorders are more prevalent among males than among females, with the exception of sexual masochism disorder.
- It is important to distinguish self-harming behaviors that occur during collective accepted religious and spiritual practices (e.g., self-flagellation and other painful ordeals) from sadomasochistic behavior conducted for sexual arousal.
- The legal status of sexually sadistic behavior ranges across countries and societies, suggesting potential for variation in distress and functional impairment.

DIAGNOSTIC PEARLS

- The diagnostic class of paraphilic disorders includes intense or persistent sexual interest or behavior that is not conventionally considered normal sexual interest or behavior.
- The diagnosis of paraphilic disorder is made if the individual with the non-normative sexual behavior (e.g., fetishism, cross-dressing) describes being distressed by their behavior or having impairment in various areas of functioning due to the behavior.
- In the absence of distress or impairment regarding the paraphilia, if the individual has acted on the sexual urges with children (pedophilic disorder) or nonconsenting persons (exhibitionistic disorder, frotteuristic disorder, or sexual sadism disorder), the diagnosis of paraphilic disorder applies.

- The delineation of the paraphilic urges, fantasies, and behaviors as "intense" and "persistent" may be difficult in some cases and should then be defined as paraphilic only if clearly greater or equal to intense and persistent sexual interest in genital stimulation or preparatory fondling with phenotypically normal, physically mature, consenting human partners.

- The urges, fantasies, or behaviors should occur for at least 6 months.

- Most paraphilic disorders occur almost exclusively in males, with sexual masochism disorder being an exception.

- Although paraphilic preferences may persist to the end of an individual's life, it is believed that paraphilic expressions or performances of paraphilic behavior decrease with age.

- Paraphilic disorders may overlap with other disorders within the diagnostic class (e.g., fetishistic disorder and sexual masochism disorder) or may be comorbid with other mental disorders (e.g., depressive disorders, substance use disorders, personality disorders).

- Evaluation of paraphilic disorders should be done in an atmosphere of respect and confidentiality. Medicolegal aspects should be considered.

- Paraphilic disorders are usually considered pervasive and enduring traits; however, the behaviors may decline with age.

- Paraphilic disorders frequently coexist with other paraphilic disorders.

SELF-ASSESSMENT

Key Concepts: Double-Check Your Knowledge

What is the relevance of the following concepts to the various paraphilic disorders?

- Intense and persistent sexual interest other than sexual interest in genital stimulation or preparatory fondling with phenotypically normal, physically mature, consenting human partners
- Sexual fantasies, urges, and behaviors
- Sexual preferences for an object of behavior (fetish, nonconsenting stranger)
- Marked distress over sexual preferences or behavior
- Recurrence of fantasies, urges, and behaviors
- Exposure of genitals
- Fetish—nonliving object, nongenital body part
- Age difference between perpetrator and child in pedophilic disorder
- Role of a controlled environment

Questions to Discuss With Colleagues and Mentors

1. Do you routinely discuss sexual functioning, preferences, and behaviors with your patients?

2. If you suspect a patient has paraphilic behavior or preferences, what specific questions do you ask?

3. Do you have difficulties asking your patients about their sexual practices? Do you avoid certain questions about their preferences and practices? Why?

Case-Based Questions

PART A

Mr. Foster, a 20-year-old man, reports that he is a bit uneasy about being fixated on his need to have his sexual partners (of both sexes) wear a special tight leather garter belt, "otherwise I don't really get excited. But some of my previous partners got really upset with me and refused to wear it."

What diagnosis would you consider for Mr. Foster's behavior at this point? He seems to have fetishism because he becomes really aroused only when his partner wears a specific piece of clothing. He requires both males and females to wear the clothing, but because Mr. Foster does not wear it himself, his behavior is not related to cross-dressing. He seems to be uneasy about his demand. The existence of distress and the duration of 6 months need to be explored to establish the diagnosis of fetishistic disorder.

PART B

Upon further questioning, Mr. Foster also states that he is sexually attracted to young males and females, and he does not get excited thinking about having sex with adults. He says that he prefers sexual interactions with both male and female adolescents "a few years younger than I am, when they have some pubic hair, but no body hair, their skin is soft, girls' breasts are just budding." He has had sexual interactions with several male and female adolescents looking like that. "They really arouse me."

Does the additional information change your diagnostic consideration? Would you change Mr. Foster's diagnosis or add another one? In addition to his fetishism, Mr. Foster has pedophilic disorder and is sexually attracted to both males and females. It would be important to establish how old his sexual partners are and what the age difference is, but he clearly prefers early pubescent males and females, has acted on this interest by having sexual interactions with several male and female adolescents, and thus meets the diagnostic criteria for pedophilic disorder. Various paraphilic disorders may co-occur.

SHORT-ANSWER QUESTIONS

1. How long must any paraphilic fantasies, urges, or behaviors last to meet the diagnostic criteria for paraphilic disorder?
2. What is the difference between paraphilia and paraphilic disorder?
3. What is the usual age or time period at onset of paraphilic disorders?
4. What are the usual fetishes?

5. In which sex does paraphilia almost exclusively occur?
6. What are some examples of paraphilias and their other specified paraphilic disorders?
7. What personality disorder must be considered in the differential diagnosis of pedophilic disorder?
8. What is the minimum age difference between the individual with pedophilic disorder and their victim?
9. Why was the specifier "in a controlled environment" included in the diagnostic criteria of most paraphilic disorders?
10. Can substance use modify paraphilic behavior? Can paraphilic behavior appear during substance use and during intoxication?

ANSWERS

1. **Any paraphilic fantasies, urges, or behaviors must last at least 6 months to meet the diagnostic criteria for paraphilic disorder.**

2. **The diagnosis of paraphilic disorder includes the paraphilia and the distress or impairment caused by the paraphilia. In the absence of distress or impairment regarding the paraphilia, if the individual has acted on the sexual urges with children (pedophilic disorder) or nonconsenting persons (exhibitionistic disorder, frotteuristic disorder, or sexual sadism disorder), the diagnosis of the paraphilic disorder applies.**

3. **Childhood through puberty or adolescence is the usual age at or period of onset of paraphilic disorders.**

4. **The usual fetishes are nonliving objects (e.g., undergarments) and nongenital body parts (e.g., feet).**

5. **Paraphilia almost exclusively occurs in males.**

6. **Some examples of paraphilias with their other specified paraphilic disorders include acrotomophilia and acrotomophilic disorder, necrophilia and necrophilic disorder, telephone scatologia and telephone scatophilic disorder, and zoophilia and zoophilic disorder.**

7. **Antisocial personality disorder must be considered in the differential diagnosis of pedophilic disorder.**

8. **Five years is the minimum age difference between the individual with pedophilic disorder and their victim.**

9. **It may be more difficult to objectively assess an individual's propensity to act on paraphilic urges when the individual has no opportunity to act on those urges (e.g., because of being in a controlled environment, such as prison).**

10. Yes. Substance use can modify paraphilic behavior, and paraphilic behavior can appear during substance use and during intoxication.

REFERENCES

American Psychiatric Association: Diagnostic and Statistical Manual of Mental Disorders, 4th Edition. Washington, DC, American Psychiatric Association, 1994

American Psychiatric Association: Diagnostic and Statistical Manual of Mental Disorders, 5th Edition. Arlington, VA, American Psychiatric Association, 2013

American Psychiatric Association: Diagnostic and Statistical Manual of Mental Disorders, 5th Edition, Text Revision. Washington, DC, American Psychiatric Association, 2022

PART 3

Q&A

CHAPTER 24

Questions and Answers

Max Kasun, B.A.

Willa Roberts, B.A.

Jodi Paik, M.F.A.

In this section, we provide a series of questions to help learners apply and consolidate their knowledge of the concepts presented in this *Study Guide to DSM-5-TR*. Many of the questions are embedded in a series of fictional cases that exemplify "classic" diagnoses from DSM-5-TR or highlight phenomena that relate to key diagnostic features. Other questions test terms that are important for accurate understanding and communication of diagnoses in DSM-5-TR. Many of the questions are very straightforward and underscore basic diagnostic concepts, whereas other questions present atypical situations that will, we hope, be a bit more challenging.

Adapted from Roberts LW, Bajestan SN, Balon R, et al: "Questions and Answers," in *Study Guide to DSM-5*. Edited by Roberts LW, Louie AK. Washington, DC, American Psychiatric Publishing, 2015, pp. 461–506, with additional questions by chapter authors.

1. A 10-year-old boy who has severe developmental delay exhibits immediate and involuntary repetition of ambient sounds and vocalizations made by other people. What is the term for this phenomenon?

    A. Dysarthria.
    B. Echolalia.
    C. Echopraxia.
    D. Word salad.

    Answer: B

2. Match each description with the personality disorder for which it is most highly characteristic (you may use each disorder once, more than once, or not at all):
    _____ Chronic feelings of emptiness or boredom.
    _____ Consistently uses physical appearance to draw attention to oneself.
    _____ Failure to conform to social norms and without remorse.
    _____ Frantic efforts to avoid real or imagined abandonment.
    _____ Grandiose sense of self-importance.
    _____ Self-dramatization, theatricality, and exaggerated expression of emotion.

    A. Antisocial personality disorder.
    B. Borderline personality disorder.
    C. Histrionic personality disorder.
    D. Narcissistic personality disorder.

    Answers: B, C, A, B, D, C

3. A 45-year-old Latino man presents to his primary care doctor, complaining of chronic chest pain for the past year. He has seen multiple specialists, who tell him the pain is from uncomplicated acid reflux; however, he thinks he must have serious heart disease. He continues to worry about his heart despite reassurance from multiple cardiologists; he acknowledges that it is possible the cardiologists are correct. He denies hallucinations, and there is no evidence of delusional content in his thought process. His concern about his heart has prevented him from vacationing with his family. He denies feeling depressed or anxious or having any problems with sleep or appetite and continues to enjoy hobbies at home. What is the likely diagnosis?

    A. Generalized anxiety disorder.
    B. Illness anxiety disorder.
    C. Major depressive disorder.
    D. Panic disorder.

    Answer: B

4. A 33-year-old Indian man presents to a psychiatrist with concern of excessive handwashing. He reports that he has a ritualistic washing routine that takes at least 20 minutes, which he performs multiple times per day for fear of contamination with infectious disease. When interviewed further, he states that he has recurrent and persistent thoughts about handwashing and risk of contamination, which he tries unsuccessfully to suppress. He reports an overwhelming sense of anxiety if he does not wash his hands or if he does not complete the "ritual." He says the behavior is "out of control." He recognizes these thoughts as functions of his own mind. He has no symptoms of psychotic disorders. What is the likely diagnosis?

A. Obsessive-compulsive disorder.
B. Obsessive-compulsive personality disorder.
C. Schizophrenia.
D. Specific phobia.

Answer: A

5. Which of the following symptoms or experiences is more characteristic of major depressive disorder secondary to bereavement than to prolonged grief disorder?

A. Feelings of longing, yearning for the deceased.
B. Experienced in relation to loss of a specific person.
C. Pervasive low mood, sadness.
D. Bittersweet or pleasant emotions evoked by memories of the deceased.

Answer: C

6. A man brings his 35-year-old wife, who has a history of previous psychiatric hospitalizations, to the emergency department because of her unusual behavior. He states that she just spent $3,000 on a shopping spree. She speaks animatedly and loudly: "I just remembered all these things I wanted to buy!" She looks down at her hand and said, "I need this ring on my finger for good luck." She has been sleeping 5 hours per night, and her days are "packed with events, booked from morning to evening!" She describes her mood as "stressed," and her affect is labile. Her mental status examination is notable for a slender, well-groomed woman with meticulous makeup and good eye contact. She is cooperative on interview, but at times she is verbose and difficult to redirect. Her thought process is occasionally tangential, and her speech is fluent, with rapid rate. She denies any hallucinations. There is no evidence of psychomotor abnormalities. Her urine toxicology screen result is negative for illicit substances. What is the likely diagnosis?

A. Bipolar I disorder.
B. Borderline personality disorder.

    C. Obsessive-compulsive disorder.

    D. Schizophrenia.

Answer: A

7. A chronically ill man with schizophrenia tells his psychiatrist that the ideas in his head are not his own. The Central Intelligence Agency (CIA) transmits the thoughts into his brain through a microchip planted in his spinal column. What sort of delusion is described here?

    A. Grandiose delusion.

    B. Somatic delusion.

    C. Referential delusion.

    D. Nihilistic delusion.

Answer: B

8. Brain regions involved in the pathology of dissociative identity disorder include which of the following:

    A. Orbitofrontal cortex.

    B. Hippocampus.

    C. Parahippocampal gyrus.

    D. All of the above.

Answer: D

9. A 25-year-old man with no other medical or psychiatric history than anemia travels frequently for his job. He has trouble on long flights because he feels the need to move his legs about and unfasten his seat belt to do so. When he is not permitted to get up, especially on red-eye flights, he feels symmetrical burning and tingling in his legs. He is also very exhausted and notes that his sleep is not restful. He takes no medications except a daily multivitamin. What is the likely diagnosis?

    A. Adjustment disorder.

    B. Akathisia.

    C. Parkinson's disease.

    D. Restless legs syndrome.

Answer: D

10. A 26-year-old man seen in the emergency department acknowledges persistent substance use until about the past 2 days, when he was evicted from his apartment. Which cluster of symptoms is typical of stimulant withdrawal?

A. Depression, fatigue, insomnia.
B. Diarrhea, nausea, anxiety.
C. Hypertension, tachycardia, seizures.
D. Vivid dreaming, nightmares, confusion.

Answer: A

11. Twelve-year-old Donny feels tired of standing out so much at school. Several times a day he feels an uncomfortable sensation in his throat and then feels he "has to" cough or grunt, which temporarily makes the uncomfortable sensation go away. He also repeatedly shrugs his shoulders and stomps his feet at what appear to be random moments throughout the day. The other students no longer make fun of him the way they did when they were younger. However, he still feels demoralized because he just wants to fit in with them. What is the likely diagnosis?

A. Obsessive-compulsive disorder.
B. Obsessive-compulsive personality disorder.
C. Persistent motor or vocal tic disorder.
D. Tourette's disorder.

Answer: D

12. Police bring a 30-year-old man experiencing homelessness to the psychiatric emergency department after he called 911, concerned that people were controlling his mind through "microwaves." He has no previous psychiatric or medical history, and his urine toxicology screen result is negative for any substances. On interview, he appears very guarded, repeating that he does not belong on a psychiatric unit. "I am not the problem," he says. "These microwaves are all around us, even if you can't feel them." He denies any mood symptoms. Until a few years ago, he was working full-time, but he is unwilling to divulge his occupation "because I don't trust anyone." On examination, his speech is fluent with normal volume and rate, but his thought process is disorganized when discussing the "microwaves." His affect is blunted, and no psychomotor abnormalities are noted. He denies seeing or hearing anything that others do not, but during the interview he occasionally stares behind the interviewer intently. What is the likely diagnosis?

A. Bipolar disorder.
B. Delusional disorder.
C. No psychiatric diagnosis.
D. Schizophrenia.

Answer: D

13. In the previous example (question 12), which term best describes the patient's experience of "microwaves"?

    A. Ideas of reference.
    B. Hallucination.
    C. Delusion.
    D. Illusion.

    Answer: C

14. Which of the following physical signs does not suggest intoxication with cannabis?

    A. Decreased heart rate.
    B. Difficulty with motor tasks.
    C. Impaired short-term memory.
    D. Reddening of eye membranes and dry mouth.

    Answer: A

15. A 29-year-old woman and her boyfriend had an unplanned pregnancy culminating in a first trimester miscarriage last year. She has always considered herself an anxious person, but she felt even more anxious after the miscarriage. She became pregnant a second time, again unplanned, and she gave birth to a healthy boy after an emergency cesarean-section delivery. Their son is now 4 months old. Her boyfriend has become increasingly distant and unavailable. He moved out of their apartment 2 weeks after the birth, stating, "I am not ready for this life." Beginning around the same time, she has experienced escalating low mood, irritability, tearfulness, poor sleep, and constant fatigue. She is most anxious about the thoughts she has been having that "sometimes I feel I could not care less about taking care of my son or, even worse, that I want to just physically push him away. It is really scary. How can I ever be a good mother to him? I am miserable. I do not know if I can take it anymore." Her first psychiatric contact was at age 22, when she was treated with citalopram for a depressive episode precipitated by being laid off from her first postcollege job. She says, "I have never quite been happy again since then. Life has been hard." What is the likely diagnosis?

    A. Bipolar II disorder, current episode depressed, with peripartum onset.
    B. Brief psychotic disorder, with peripartum onset.
    C. Major depressive disorder, with peripartum onset.
    D. Persistent depressive disorder.

    Answer: C

16. Which statement is correct regarding the domains DSM-5-TR evaluates in the Clinician-Rated Dimensions of Psychosis Symptom Severity Scale?

    A. The scale assesses only the three most important domains of hallucinations, delusions, and disorganized speech.
    B. The scale is based on symptoms experienced by the patient in the previous 7 days.
    C. The scale is most accurate if patients, rather than clinicians, provide the responses.
    D. The scale should only be completed if the clinician is certain of the symptom severity.

    Answer: B

17. A diagnosis of conduct disorder with onset prior to age 15 precedes which of the following disorders?

    A. Antisocial personality disorder.
    B. Attention-deficit/hyperactivity disorder.
    C. Narcissistic personality disorder.
    D. Oppositional defiant disorder.

    Answer: A

18. A woman brings her 32-year-old husband to a psychiatrist for "unusual behavior." She says that for the past 5 days he has been cleaning the house extensively, often late into the night. He wakes up 2 hours earlier than usual the next morning but does not appear tired. He feels "very happy and productive—the best I have ever been!" His wife denies any dangerous behaviors at home and reports he is able to continue working at his current job, albeit more productively than before. She recalls that 6 months earlier, he seemed very depressed, with loss of interest, poor sleep, low energy, and impaired concentration that lasted 1 month. She denies he has history of any previous psychiatric hospitalizations. On interview, he is pleasant and cooperative. His speech is pressured but redirectable. His thought process is linear, and he denies any hallucinations. His urine toxicology screen result is negative. What is the likely diagnosis?

    A. Bipolar I disorder.
    B. Bipolar II disorder.
    C. Schizophrenia.
    D. Substance-induced mood disorder.

    Answer: B

19. A 32-year-old Latina woman presents to the emergency department, requesting help for back pain. She says that she has wrestled with this pain for 2 years, after a minor skiing accident, and no medications or interventions have helped. No physical evidence explains the degree of pain she reports. The pain prevents her from working as a ballerina. She loves her job but says that for the past few years, budget cuts have stressed the entire ballet company. She denies any problems with sleep, anxiety, or mood. Her body weight is 90% of expected, and she denies any problems with her weight or diet. She is cooperative, and her thought process is linear. What is the likely diagnosis?

    A. Adjustment disorder.
    B. Anorexia nervosa.
    C. Major depressive disorder.
    D. Somatic symptom disorder with predominant pain.

    Answer: D

20. A 21-year-old college student complains he has developed "an uncomfortable relationship with food." His current symptoms seem to be consistent with an eating disorder. Which of the following pieces of information would help distinguish between a diagnosis of anorexia nervosa and of bulimia nervosa?

    A. He has lost significant weight and appears emaciated.
    B. He is highly critical of his body.
    C. He regularly binges on high-calorie, high-fat foods.
    D. He uses large quantities of laxative tablets each day.

    Answer: A

21. A 3-year-old girl in a park attempts to sit on the lap of a person experiencing homelessness. She is pulled away by her mother, a 32-year-old woman who was recently out of town. In that time period the child had been under the care of a grandmother who did not have time to engage with her. The child is noted to not respond to affection from her mother or grandmother but is indiscriminately affectionate with strangers. She has no evidence of motor abnormalities, and she has met all developmental milestones appropriately. What is the likely diagnosis?

    A. Autism spectrum disorder.
    B. Borderline personality disorder.
    C. Reactive attachment disorder.
    D. Rett syndrome.

    Answer: C

22. A 30-year-old retail manager at a cosmetics store with no previous psychiatric history finds herself feeling distinct periods of intense anxiety two to three times a day. She is concerned because she has never experienced anything like this in the past. She describes the episodes as feeling tremulous, hot, and faint, with palpitations and fear of loss of control. She denies any drug use and any recent stressors. This problem has been getting worse over the past few months and has affected her ability to function at work. She also has been losing weight and eating more. She is worried that her health has affected her appearance because her skin looks different, her hair is thinning, and she has swelling in her neck. What is the likely diagnosis?

    A. Agoraphobia.
    B. Anxiety disorder due to another medical condition.
    C. Generalized anxiety disorder.
    D. Social anxiety disorder.

    Answer: B

23. Joey, a 34-month-old boy, rarely initiates eye contact with his mother and does not seem to engage in play with other children in his peer group at day care. At times, he behaves aggressively toward the other children. He is only minimally communicative with speech but, when vocal, is prone to repetitively use only single words. He gets very upset when his mother varies his morning clothing routine, always insisting, for example, that she put on his right sock first, before any other piece of clothing. What is the likely diagnosis?

    A. Autism spectrum disorder.
    B. Global developmental delay.
    C. Major depressive disorder.
    D. Intellectual developmental disorder.

    Answer: A

24. A 24-year-old woman complains of mood dysphoria and anhedonia affecting her ability to perform well at her job. Which of the following additional pieces of information would be more consistent with a diagnosis of major depressive disorder than with premenstrual dysphoric disorder?

    A. The patient has been feeling cognitively hazy, confused, and forgetful.
    B. The patient has had suicidal thoughts every day for the past 3 weeks.
    C. The patient was very irritable and rejection sensitive for 4 days last week, followed by rapid resolution.
    D. The patient's symptoms have caused strain on her relationship with her boyfriend.

    Answer: B

25. Match each description with the sexual dysfunctions diagnosis for which it is most highly characteristic (you may use each disorder once, more than once, or not at all):

    _____ Involves inability to attain and maintain arousal.
    _____ Involves inability to have vaginal intercourse or penetration.
    _____ Involves anorgasmia or delayed orgasm.
    _____ Involves orgasm before the person desires.

    A. Erectile disorder.
    B. Female orgasmic disorder.
    C. Genito-pelvic pain/penetration disorder.
    D. Premature ejaculation.

    Answers: A, C, B, D

26. A 56-year-old biologist has had a very successful career publishing extensive research on the aging process. Now he believes he has found the key to eternal life. For the past several months, he has been quite secretive and refuses to come to work group meetings regarding upcoming projects. He has installed a dead bolt on his office at home and insists that extra security personnel be hired to guard his research lab. He refuses to present his material or discuss it with his colleagues or family, claiming the knowledge is too powerful to be made public. He is not having any visual or auditory hallucinations, and he is able to support his statements with logical arguments. He has a history of depression. What is the likely diagnosis?

    A. Schizophrenia.
    B. Major depressive disorder with psychotic features.
    C. Delusional disorder, grandiose type.
    D. Stimulant intoxication, cocaine, without perceptual disturbances.

    Answer: C

27. A 33-year-old man arrives at the hospital by ambulance after his girlfriend called the police during a dispute. While arguing with his girlfriend, the patient had locked himself in a bathroom and swallowed 40 tablets of clonazepam. On evaluation, the patient is drowsy but responsive to voice. He has thin, linear, parallel scars on the extensor surface of his left wrist. He states that he wanted to show his girlfriend how much she was hurting him and then says, "She is probably going to leave me, just like everyone else has." What is the likely diagnosis?

    A. Adjustment disorder.
    B. Borderline personality disorder.
    C. Histrionic personality disorder.
    D. Dependent personality disorder.

    Answer: B

28. Evie is a 9-year-old third grader. Although she started grade school 1 year behind in reading, she quickly caught up in proficiency and has since become an avid reader and writer. She has been described as a "social butterfly" and has a range of interests similar to those of her classmates. Evie frequently mimics the mannerisms and phrases of certain adults, including her teacher and the lead character in her favorite popular television show. She insists on wearing clothing that matches theirs, and she turns down new clothing selected by her parents that does not show a clear resemblance. When asked to speak in her "Evie voice," she becomes unusually frustrated and unable to communicate the source of her distress, behaviors that her parents "thought she grew out of" in first grade. What is the likely diagnosis?

    A. Obsessive-compulsive disorder.
    B. Language disorder.
    C. Autism spectrum disorder.
    D. Echolalia.
    E. Dissociative identity disorder.

    Answer: C

29. A 35-year-old man tells his therapist that he is having marital problems because the object of his sexual arousal is his wife's underwear. He reports that he and his wife have sexual intercourse in a limited fashion, much less than she prefers. He does not wear women's clothing, but he fulfills his sexual desires through masturbation while holding his wife's underwear or other women's undergarments that he has purchased. This activity is his longstanding pattern of sexual behavior and has been problematic in the relationship with his wife from early in their relationship. He reports that his wife has "caught" him masturbating with women's undergarments on multiple occasions and she thinks he is "weird."What is the likely diagnosis?

    A. Erectile disorder.
    B. Fetishistic disorder.
    C. Gender dysphoria in adolescents and adults.
    D. Transvestic disorder.

    Answer: B

30. Fellow Theravada Buddhist monks living at a temple bring a 27-year-old Laotian man to the hospital 17 days into a fast. The man is acutely dehydrated and is admitted to the medicine service. He is delirious at first, but when he improves, the psychiatric consult service is called because of his "odd manner." He is unkempt and unshaven, which is in sharp contrast to the two other members of his order. He appears withdrawn and responds very briefly to the other monks, at times laughing inappropriately. The monks say that the patient's family, who had recently emigrated from Laos, brought him to the order nearly 1 year ago. Although he has been with-

drawn since they have known him, the monks say that this is the first time he has embarked on such a fast. He told them that he was instructed to do so by "spirits" who watch his daily activities and comment on whether he is being appropriately observant. The members of his order are familiar with the names of the spirits from Laotian religious traditions, but they are not familiar with this particular tradition of fasting. They acknowledge that the patient is from a remote part of Laos which may have different customs, but this behavior is new in him. What is the likely diagnosis?

A. Culturally appropriate behavior.
B. Major depressive disorder.
C. Psychotic disorder due to another medical condition.
D. Schizophrenia.

Answer: D

31. A woman brings her 73-year-old father to the hospital because she is extremely concerned that he has virtually no memory of the day's events. He cannot recall where he has been or what he has done. Which additional piece of information would be more consistent with a diagnosis of dissociative amnesia than with neurocognitive disorders?

A. He cannot name the current president.
B. He has a hand tremor and slowing on rapid alternating movements testing.
C. He has extensive history of chronic alcohol use.
D. He was the victim of a mugging that morning.

Answer: D

32. A primary care doctor refers a 46-year-old Russian woman for psychological assessment after she receives a negative workup result for several medical conditions. The psychologist learns that the patient has an extensive history of physical complaints without medical basis. Her physical symptoms have been multisystemic and unlike the constellation of symptoms associated with specific medical illnesses. The referring doctor also reports that the patient has frustrated many primary care doctors in the past and has transitioned from one to another. When the psychologist talks to the patient, she is also frustrated. She says, "None of this is in my head. It is real. Those doctors just cannot figure it out." She describes a long history of multiple physical symptoms that are not explained by medical diagnosis even after multiple, long workups. What is the likely diagnosis?

A. Body dysmorphic disorder.
B. Somatic symptom disorder.
C. Factitious disorder.
D. Functional neurological symptom disorder (conversion disorder).

Answer: B

33. A 40-year-old woman says she is "very anxious about public speaking," to the point of having episodes that resemble panic attacks when she faces speaking before even small audiences. Her division chief expects employees to present at conferences before he will promote them. She is not only unable to give large presentations but also avoids most social events related to her work. She feels as if she is "acting like an idiot" when she is with colleagues, especially her work superiors. The anticipation of a meeting with her boss can cause severe anxiety. She does not have anxiety in other contexts, and she is aware of the dysfunction her anxiety causes and wants to make changes. What is the likely diagnosis?

    A. Generalized anxiety disorder.
    B. Major depressive disorder.
    C. Obsessive-compulsive personality disorder.
    D. Social anxiety disorder.

    Answer: D

34. What is a hallmark feature of the symptoms of oppositional defiant disorder?

    A. They exceed what is normative for that particular age group.
    B. They fall short of what is normative for that particular age group.
    C. They occur exclusively when the individual is in a certain setting.
    D. The disruptive behaviors are targeted only toward authority figures.

    Answer: A

35. A gynecologist refers a 32-year-old pharmaceutical employee to a psychiatry clinic, noting that the patient requested a prescription for testosterone and also a surgical referral for double mastectomy. On review of the patient's previous physical examination, the gynecologist notes that the patient has normal female development and anatomy with no clinically concerning findings. What is the likely diagnosis?

    A. Autism spectrum disorder.
    B. Schizophrenia.
    C. Depersonalization/derealization disorder.
    D. Gender dysphoria in adolescents and adults.

    Answer: D

36. A 5-year-old child believes that their thoughts, words, and actions cause specific outcomes in nature, and these outcomes defy the commonly understood laws of cause and effect. What is this phenomenon called?

    A. Magical thinking.
    B. Hallucination.

C. Illusion.

D. Grandiosity.

Answer: A

37. A man brings his 36-year-old wife to a new primary care doctor because she has lost patches of her hair recently. He notes that her previous doctor sent her to a dermatologist, who felt an underlying skin condition was unlikely. In a private exam room without her husband present, she says that she secretly pulls out her hair in clumps to relieve tension. The act of pulling her hair brings her relief. She denies changes in mood, sleep, concentration, or energy level. What is the likely diagnosis?

    A. Generalized anxiety disorder.
    B. Major depressive disorder.
    C. Tic disorder.
    D. Trichotillomania.

Answer: D

38. A 50-year-old woman presents to the community hospital complaining of "a drug problem." She says that for the past 3 years her use of cocaine has been uncontrollable, to the point that she has lost her housing and her job. She reports using increasing amounts of cocaine over the past year to "reach the same high." When she stops using cocaine, she experiences intense symptoms of anxiety, depression, fatigue, and nausea. She has tried multiple times to quit using cocaine altogether, but her efforts have been unsuccessful. She experienced a transient stroke once during a cocaine binge. She denies any mood problems or hallucinations prior to using substances. What is the likely diagnosis?

    A. Bipolar I disorder.
    B. Stimulant intoxication, cocaine, without perceptual disturbances.
    C. Stimulant use disorder, moderate, cocaine.
    D. Stimulant withdrawal, cocaine.

Answer: C

39. Which movement disorder has a symptom pattern that antipsychotics can cause by blockade of dopamine receptors within the striatum?

    A. Huntington's disease.
    B. Parkinson's disease.
    C. Sydenham's chorea.
    D. Tourette's disorder.

Answer: B

40. Mary, a 55-year-old woman, has a history of HIV. She has been prescribed antiretroviral therapy but for years has been only intermittently adherent. Currently, her CD_4 count is 200 and her HIV viral load has been escalating. She complains that over the past several months she has been less mentally agile than she used to be. It takes her significantly longer to read the newspaper each morning. When she wants to communicate with her daughter, concentrating on writing a text message is difficult, and she even finds "my fingers do not cooperate with me when I try to type." Her fine motor skills appear to be worsening. Mary denies any other physical symptoms, such as fever or headache. There are no focal findings on neurological exam. Head CT, MRI, electroencephalogram, lumbar puncture, non-HIV viral PCR testing, antibody screens, metabolic parameters including hepatic and renal function, and urine toxicology results are all negative. Neuropsychological testing shows impairment in information processing speeds, motor skills, and attention. What is the likely diagnosis?

    A. Cryptococcal meningitis.
    B. Major depressive disorder.
    C. Mild neurocognitive disorder due to HIV infection.
    D. Vitamin B_{12} deficiency.

    Answer: C

41. A 53-year-old woman presents for a psychiatric evaluation for her long-standing depression. She has had several bouts of depressive episodes and was hospitalized once for a suicide attempt. She describes childhood sexual abuse from her father and neglect by her mother. During the interview, while talking about her childhood, she suddenly switches to talking in a childlike, high-pitched voice, while pulling her legs under her in a chair and starting to rock backward and forward. While rocking, she says, "Don't hurt me, don't hurt me." Later during the interview, when she is talking and behaving in her original manner, she endorses having multiple episodes of lost time and not being able to recount her activities during several hours per day. What is the likely diagnosis?

    A. Major depressive disorder and dissociative identity disorder.
    B. Major depressive disorder and schizoaffective disorder.
    C. Major depressive disorder and schizophrenia.
    D. Major depressive disorder and somatic symptom disorder.

    Answer: A

42. Match each term with the correct definition (you may use each term once, more than once, or not at all):
    _____ Loss of appetite.
    _____ Loss of control over speech such that socially unacceptable or obscene words are uttered.
    _____ Loss of interest or pleasure.

_____ Loss of muscle tone, with weakness.
_____ Loss of response to outside stimuli and muscular rigidity.

A. Anhedonia.
B. Anorexia.
C. Cataplexy.
D. Catatonia.
E. Coprolalia.

Answers: B, E, A, C, D

43. DSM-5 and DSM-5-TR assigned to new categories some diagnoses that DSM-IV included in the section on diagnoses in infancy, childhood, and adolescence. Which of the following statements is correct regarding these changes?

A. Selective mutism was added to anxiety disorders.
B. Selective mutism was added to depressive disorders.
C. Separation anxiety disorder was added to dissociative disorders.
D. Separation anxiety disorder was added to schizophrenia and other psychotic disorders.

Answer: A

44. Jolene, age 12, is getting along poorly with her parents and teachers. She is highly argumentative and defiant at home. She has attempted to humiliate her teacher in front of the other students and uses profane language. She never seems to take responsibility for the hostility that seems to be present in many of her social interactions. Because of her uncompromising negativity with her teachers, other students have begun to keep their distance from her. In the past 5 years, Jolene's parents have gotten divorced. Her mother then remarried, but that marriage subsequently ended in a rapid divorce. Jolene is not particularly unpleasant during the psychiatric assessment but only moderately cooperates in responding to questions. What is the likely diagnosis?

A. Antisocial personality disorder.
B. Conduct disorder.
C. Major depressive disorder.
D. Oppositional defiant disorder.

Answer: D

45. A primary care physician refers a 60-year-old Cambodian man to a psychiatrist to rule out a psychotic disorder. The patient was previously given a diagnosis of schizophrenia because he "hears voices." He has been prescribed a large dosage of an antipsychotic medication, which he takes daily,

with very little symptom relief. He states that the medicine helps him sleep. The psychiatrist learns that the patient is a survivor of the Cambodian genocide of the 1970s who survived torture under the Khmer Rouge regime, witnessed executions, and endured forced labor in Communist Cambodia. He reports that subsequent to the extremes of traumatic experience he sustained, he has had chronic symptoms of anxiety with panic attacks. He also reports concern of "thinking too much." When asked to clarify what he means, he describes ruminating worried thoughts about his past traumas. He reports severe insomnia and nightmares about Cambodia at night. He describes hearing voices other people do not hear. Further questioning reveals that the voices he hears are of Khmer Rouge officers, and he "hears" them when he is remembering his experiences of violence. When the psychiatrist asks him to clarify this, he says the "voices" are more like memories than hallucinations. What is the likely diagnosis?

A. Bipolar I disorder, current episode manic.
B. Panic disorder.
C. Posttraumatic stress disorder.
D. Schizophrenia.

Answer: C

46. In the previous example (question 45), the "voices" are likely an example of what?

A. Auditory hallucinations.
B. Intrusive memories.
C. Nightmares.
D. Panic attacks.

Answer: B

47. Match each description with the diagnosis for which it is most highly characteristic (you may use each disorder once, more than once, or not at all):
_____ Memories of deceased provoke fear and horror.
_____ Unremitting symptoms experienced in relation to the loss of a
    specific person.
_____ Hypervigilance.
_____ Pervasive low mood, sadness.
_____ Yearning, longing for the deceased person.

A. Major depressive disorder secondary to bereavement.
B. Prolonged grief disorder.
C. Posttraumatic stress disorder secondary to bereavement.

Answers: C, B, C, A, B

48. A 62-year-old veteran underwent lung transplantation for idiopathic pulmonary fibrosis 6 months ago. His postoperative course has been complicated by prolonged intensive care unit stay, renal insufficiency dependent on dialysis, atrial fibrillation, pneumonia, and severe deconditioning. He has difficulty working with physical therapy on his strengthening because he becomes anxious and worries about his perceived shortness of breath. He frequently asks to avoid or postpone these sessions and has been described as noncooperative with his treatment. This behavior, in turn, impedes his recovery. On evaluation by psychiatry, the patient denies depressed mood, reports enjoying visits from his family and watching the news, and is hopeful about his recovery. What is the likely diagnosis?

    A. Adjustment disorder.
    B. Generalized anxiety disorder.
    C. Posttraumatic stress disorder.
    D. Psychological factors affecting medical condition.

    Answer: D

49. A 67-year-old man has been living by himself for decades in an apartment, but his daughter is concerned about his safety there. His rooms are stacked to the ceilings with multiple items such as books and souvenirs, to the point that he cannot move around without shifting items. She worries he may trip himself in the apartment and has offered to help discard items; however, he finds it distressing to remove anything because he thinks everything will be of use to him someday. He denies any anxiety with his current living situation and prefers it to remain this way. What is the likely diagnosis?

    A. Delusional disorder.
    B. Hoarding disorder.
    C. Generalized anxiety disorder.
    D. Obsessive-compulsive personality disorder.

    Answer: B

50. A 76-year-old widowed, retired history professor comes to the clinic with his daughter for memory difficulties, which started about 3 years ago and have progressed gradually. He stopped driving after being involved in a car accident. He recently moved in with his daughter, and she has been taking him to appointments, managing his finances, and attending to his care. A recent brain CT scan shows cortical atrophy and ventricular enlargement. His thyroid stimulating hormone and vitamin B$_{12}$ levels are within normal limits. His daughter starts crying while reporting that he has had many fights with her and has been accusing her of controlling him. What is the likely diagnosis?

    A. Delirium.
    B. Intermittent explosive disorder.

C. Major neurocognitive disorder due to Alzheimer's disease.

D. Major neurocognitive disorder with Lewy bodies.

Answer: C

51. A 40-year-old woman sees a psychiatrist for the first time. She complains of low energy and fatigue for the past year and endorses additional symptoms of depressed mood, poor sleep, and decreased concentration. She exhibits significant psychomotor retardation on examination. She denies any suicidal ideation or hallucinations. She takes medication for hypothyroidism but has not seen a primary care doctor in more than 10 years. Her thyroid stimulating hormone level is 7.6, and her urine toxicology screen result is negative. What is the likely diagnosis?

A. Primary insomnia.

B. Bipolar II disorder.

C. Major depressive disorder.

D. Major depressive disorder due to another medical condition.

Answer: D

52. A woman brings her 45-year-old husband to a neurologist for "memory and behavior" problems. She states that for the past several years, he has been alternately dependent or hostile toward her, as if he were two distinct individuals. When he is dependent, he follows her around everywhere, like a child. When he is hostile, he ignores her and will curse at her if she asks him to do household chores. He also tells her to call him by a different name. Each of these phases lasts for months at a time. He has forgotten important details of his childhood, such as the names of his parents and the town where he grew up. His wife denies that he uses any alcohol or other substances and denies that he has a history of seizures or sleep disturbances. She has not noticed any impulsive or unsafe behaviors. On examination, the patient is silent and stares blankly at the wall, without evidence of psychomotor abnormalities. He responds very briefly to questions but denies any hallucinations, changes in mood, or elevated anxiety. What is the likely diagnosis?

A. Bipolar I disorder.

B. Dissociative identity disorder.

C. Major depressive disorder with psychotic features.

D. Schizophrenia.

Answer: B

53. A doctor sees a middle-aged man experiencing homelessness who was admitted to the medical unit 24 hours earlier for a workup of heart failure. The patient has received appropriate medication for his heart but reports puzzling symptoms unrelated to his cardiac condition, such as feeling very

dysphoric, with nausea and vomiting, muscle aches, and insomnia over-night. On physical examination, the patient is sweating profusely, and his pupils are dilated. He keeps asking the nurse for "morphine for pain." At admission he tested positive for opioids. What is the likely diagnosis?

A. Alcohol withdrawal.
B. Factitious disorder.
C. Opioid intoxication.
D. Opioid withdrawal.

Answer: D

54. A husband brings his 35-year-old wife to a psychiatrist because he thinks she has been buying a lot of jewelry over the past few years. In private, she admits that she stole all the jewelry from department stores. She describes feeling aroused by the prospect of stealing and then gratified after each theft. She denies hallucinations or mood disturbances or any other motives for acquiring the jewelry. She denies any distress associated with the desire to steal or the act of theft. On examination, her thought process is linear with fluent, normal speech, and she presents with no evidence of psychomotor agitation. She denies any problems with sleep. What is the likely diagnosis?

A. Bipolar I disorder.
B. Delusional disorder.
C. Kleptomania.
D. Obsessive-compulsive disorder.

Answer: C

55. A 22-year-old woman is brought to the hospital after being found wandering in a school playground. She is not able to read or fill out basic paperwork. On examination, she is noted to be perusing the picture books in the pediatric waiting area and laughing in a childlike manner. She is wearing a T-shirt, sweatpants, and shoes with hook-and-loop fasteners and has a wristband with her identification and her mother's contact information. She can say her name and address and answer simple yes/no questions but cannot answer compound or complicated questions. She begins to cry after not being able to answer many questions. On review of her records, she has no psychiatric history but is noted to still see her pediatrician and her mother accompanies her to all appointments. There is a recent record of IQ testing that places her at an IQ of 50. She has no basic laboratory abnormalities and a negative urine toxicology screen. What is the likely diagnosis?

A. Conduct disorder.
B. Dissociative disorder.
C. Intellectual developmental disorder.
D. Selective mutism.

Answer: C

56. A man with schizophrenia manifests a failure to express feelings either verbally or nonverbally, even when talking about issues that one would expect to engage emotions. His expressive gestures are very limited, and there is little animation in his facial expression or vocal inflections. Which term best describes the patient's affect?

    A. Blunt.
    B. Depressed.
    C. Inappropriate.
    D. Labile.

    Answer: A

57. A mother brings her 6-year-old son to the pediatrician because of difficulty at school. His mathematical abilities are below his grade level, but he is otherwise an average student in all his other classes. His mother denies any problems with hyperactivity or impulsivity, and he is social with peers at school. His teachers also deny any behavioral problems at school and say he is an attentive student. He met all his developmental milestones appropriately. What is the likely diagnosis?

    A. Attention-deficit/hyperactivity disorder.
    B. Autism spectrum disorder.
    C. Global developmental delay.
    D. Specific learning disorder.

    Answer: D

58. Which developmental stage represents the usual age at onset of pedophilic disorder?

    A. Childhood.
    B. Puberty.
    C. Middle age.
    D. Late life.

    Answer: B

59. A mother who recently moved to a new area brings her 6-year-old son for evaluation by a pediatrician. She worries that he is having diarrhea because she finds stool stains on his underwear. She is not sure how often he goes to the bathroom or the nature of his stools because for many years she has worked two to three jobs and has left him in day cares. On examination, he is shy and avoidant of social interaction but appears to have no developmental delay with respect to cognition and language. The pediatrician notes a hard golf ball–sized structure on the patient's left abdomen on deep palpation. What is the likely diagnosis?

    A. Conduct disorder.

    B. Encopresis.

    C. Enuresis.

    D. Intellectual developmental disorder.

Answer: B

60. For which DSM-5-TR diagnosis is there a greater prevalence in females than males?

    A. Alcohol dependence.

    B. Bipolar I disorder.

    C. Major depressive disorder.

    D. Schizophrenia.

Answer: C

61. A Native American mother brings her 15-year-old daughter to a psychiatrist's office. She says that for the past year, her daughter has not said a word to her teachers. With her family members or friends, however, she is very talkative and engaging, without any speech impairments or language abnormalities. The mother notes that her daughter met all developmental milestones appropriately and reached puberty at age 14. She never had to repeat a grade in school, although her grades this year are faltering because she does not speak in class. She is otherwise attentive and does well on homework. The mother denies any impulsive behavior. The patient does not speak to the psychiatrist when addressed, but shakes her head no when asked if she experienced any hallucinations, mood disturbances, or traumatic episodes in her past. She sits patiently in her chair, without any fidgeting or unusual movements. What is the likely diagnosis?

    A. Attention-deficit/hyperactivity disorder.

    B. Autism spectrum disorder.

    C. Schizophrenia.

    D. Selective mutism.

Answer: D

62. A plastic surgeon refers a 22-year-old hairdresser with no previous psychiatric history to a psychiatrist. The patient had undergone facial reconstruction and other surgeries after a disfiguring fire at her salon. When she was seen at a 1-year follow-up appointment, her reflection in the examination room mirror alarmed her. She said that she "felt apart from" her body and was markedly distressed. She described the sensation as disabling because it occurs often at work. However, she is not able to clearly characterize her symptoms, aside from feeling "outside" herself. Aside from emotional distress from her symptoms, she has intact reality testing ability. What is the likely diagnosis?

A. Acute stress disorder.

B. Conversion disorder.

C. Depersonalization/derealization disorder.

D. Dissociative amnesia with dissociative fugue.

Answer: C

63. Which statement is correct regarding the neurodevelopmental disorders category of DSM-5-TR and DSM-5 in comparison with earlier versions of DSM?

A. Consolidated social cognitive disorders under autism spectrum disorder.

B. Eliminated diagnoses such as global developmental delay and social communication disorder.

C. Reduced the use of adaptive functioning as a criterion for neurodevelopmental disorders.

D. Tightened age criteria for childhood-onset fluency disorder.

Answer: A

64. A primary care physician refers a 45-year-old Japanese man to a psychiatrist for evaluation of his anxiety. The patient explains that he worries that there is something seriously wrong within his abdomen but that his primary care doctor has not been able to identify it. He shares that he has had intermittent pain in his abdominal area, and although physical examination, laboratory work, endoscopy, imaging, and expert consultation have not revealed abnormalities, he is worried that his pain is a sign of cancer that is being missed. He relays lifelong concerns about his health. His wife shares that he is always hypervigilant about any signs of illness, and she embarrassingly chuckles that their primary care doctor "must be a very patient man" because her husband constantly emails and calls him with various concerns. She describes her husband as an overall healthy man. The patient denies feeling depressed but again states how anxious he is that something serious is being missed. What is the likely diagnosis?

A. Body dysmorphic disorder.

B. Illness anxiety disorder.

C. Generalized anxiety disorder.

D. Somatic symptom disorder.

Answer: B

65. Age at onset for anorexia nervosa is typically

A. Infancy or toddler.

B. Early childhood before puberty.

C. Adolescence.

D. Older than age 40.

Answer: C

66. A 35-year-old man gets into an altercation with his neighbors, whom he believes to be spying on him and his wife. His wife and others do not believe this to be plausible, and he is ultimately referred to a psychiatrist to evaluate for delusional disorder. Which of the following symptoms would most suggest that other diagnoses should be considered?

    A. A belief that the neighbors are being controlled by Martian scientists.
    B. A belief that his wife is conspiring with neighbors against him.
    C. Auditory hallucination of his neighbors putting listening devices in his walls.
    D. Significant distress about the situation, including that others do not believe him.

    Answer: A

67. What term best describes a person's mental status when they are responsive to external stimuli but unable to stay awake?

    A. Agitated.
    B. Comatose.
    C. Delirious.
    D. Lethargic.

    Answer: D

68. A woman takes her 32-year-old roommate, who has a history of migraines, to the hospital after her roommate experienced sudden-onset blindness in both eyes. Her most recent migraine was 1 month ago, and she is currently not experiencing any headache symptoms. The preliminary visual examination reveals no blink to threat in either eye. The patient is unable to describe colors or identify people standing near her bed. Her CT and MRI results are normal, and stroke is ruled out. Ophthalmological examination reveals no abnormal findings. The blindness persists for 3 days, during which time she is hospitalized. Further discussion with medical providers reveals that her boyfriend broke up with her the night before admission. What is the likely diagnosis?

    A. Functional neurological symptom disorder (conversion disorder).
    B. Dissociative identity disorder.
    C. Major depressive disorder.
    D. Somatic symptom disorder.

    Answer: A

69. Bryan is a pleasant 12-year-old student who has developed difficulty staying awake in class for the past 6 months. He is very upset that no matter how much he tries, he suddenly becomes very sleepy, even during his fa-

vorite classes, and then falls asleep and naps. He feels refreshed after these naps but feels embarrassed when other students laugh at him or when teachers notice these episodes, which happen at least three times per week. His parents ensure that he goes to sleep at a regular time and sleeps for at least 8 hours, but this regularity has not helped with his lapses into sleep during the day. Recently, he started having episodes where he suddenly loses muscle tone and falls but remains conscious. These falls usually happen when he is excited or laughs. He has had a few such falls over the past month. The previous time, it happened when he got very excited because his school's basketball team won the state championship, and he felt very embarrassed in front of his classmates. He has begun avoiding social events at school because he is worried he may have one of these falls. The extensive neurological and cardiac workup results were unrevealing. The nocturnal sleep polysomnography shows rapid eye movement sleep latency less than 15 minutes. What is the likely diagnosis?

A. Circadian rhythm sleep-wake disorder.
B. Narcolepsy.
C. Non–rapid eye movement sleep arousal disorder.
D. Rapid eye movement sleep behavior disorder.

Answer: B

70. Police arrest a 21-year-old man for arson, and a psychiatrist evaluates him in jail. On interview, the patient describes an intense fascination with fire since his teenage years. He feels excited whenever he lights matches and enjoys watching the flames "dance" before him. He denies a history of unstable relationships, getting into fights, or deceiving others. He denies any suicidal or homicidal ideation, attempts, or gestures. His record shows no other legal charges besides arson. He denies hallucinations or unstable mood, and his thought process is linear. What is the likely diagnosis?

A. Borderline personality disorder.
B. Conduct disorder.
C. Delusional disorder.
D. Pyromania.

Answer: D

71. For which DSM-5-TR diagnosis is there a far greater prevalence in males than females?

A. Depersonalization/derealization disorder.
B. Exhibitionistic disorder.
C. Major depressive disorder.
D. Narcolepsy.

Answer: B

72. Beth is a talented sophomore at a prestigious college, where she lives in a dorm. She describes herself as "shy" and "slow to warm up" in social situations. She used to drink one or two cans of beer on social occasions. She found that drinking alcohol reduced her anxiety, so she started taking her "social lubricant" before most social events. After a difficult breakup with her boyfriend about 15 months ago, she began drinking larger amounts of alcohol to "forget him." She has become irritable and impatient with friends and has lost many of them. Her mother found empty bottles of hard liquor in her room during a visit and confronted her. Beth exploded and yelled at her mother, but she finally admitted that alcohol was contributing to her erratic behavior and promised to cut back. Despite her efforts, Beth has found it difficult to reduce her drinking. Every night, she decides to drink only one beer but craves more and eventually ends up drinking a few shots as well and fails to do her schoolwork. She has been skipping her morning classes because she feels sick and has to have a drink to prevent shaking, sweating, and anxiety. Beth has also stopped hiking with friends on the weekends because she worries that she may start shaking in the middle of a hike. Once, she fell off her bike while she was drunk and broke her wrist. Her grades have started to deteriorate. An instructor asked her to see a doctor after he became aware of her drinking behavior. What is the likely diagnosis?

    A. Adjustment disorder.
    B. Alcohol intoxication.
    C. Alcohol use disorder.
    D. Alcohol withdrawal.

    Answer: C

73. A 56-year-old patient who is 14 days out of surgery has just begun to consume solids in part because of antiemetics. He begins to stick out his tongue at the staff and wink at them. He also makes gestures with his lips to kiss them and smiles much more. He is not sure why he is doing this and appears fully alert with intact cognition when these movements occur. He has no psychiatric history. What is the likely diagnosis?

    A. Adjustment disorder.
    B. Delirium due to multiple etiologies, hypoactive.
    C. Schizophrenia.
    D. Tardive dyskinesia.

    Answer: D

74. Concerned parents bring a 33-year-old man to the psychiatrist. He appears to be his stated age, with erythematous face and holding his reddened and chapped hands away from his body. He takes a few minutes to adjust into the seat. He appears to be very embarrassed during the evaluation as he shares his story. He describes being very concerned about getting sick from

the germs in the environment. This concern translates into frequent hand-washing and showering. He explains that he has a particular ritual for these grooming procedures and that if he feels that he made a mistake, he has to repeat the whole procedure from the start. He spends approximately 5 hours per day on his grooming rituals. He also shares that things in his room have to be in a particular order; otherwise, he feels very uncomfortable and spends significant time readjusting these items. Moreover, when driving, he frequently worries that he ran over someone, and he has to go back to make sure that no body is lying on the ground. This worry has led him to avoid driving. He realizes that his concerns are irrational but cannot stop his rituals because they help with the significant anxiety that accompanies his troubling thoughts. He has not worked for the past 5 years because his rituals and worries caused him to be late and inefficient at his job. He currently lives with and is supported by his parents. He finally agreed to come in for an evaluation at their urging. What is the likely diagnosis?

A. Generalized anxiety disorder.
B. Obsessive-compulsive disorder.
C. Obsessive-compulsive personality disorder.
D. Panic disorder.

Answer: B

75. Men account for less than 10% of the diagnoses for which of the following disorders?

A. Bulimia nervosa.
B. Major depressive disorder.
C. Obsessive-compulsive disorder.
D. Schizophrenia.

Answer: A

76. Daisy is an 11-year-old girl who enjoys doing math problems and is always enthusiastic when doing experiments in the science lab. However, in English and history class, she sits in the back of the classroom and avoids reading out loud when asked. Her reading comprehension test results show that she is well below grade-level expectation. She does not make spelling mistakes in her homework assignments. What is the likely diagnosis?

A. Specific learning disorder.
B. Specific learning disorder, with impairment in mathematics.
C. Specific learning disorder, with impairment in reading.
D. Specific learning disorder, with impairment in written expression.

Answer: C

77. A 55-year-old woman presents to the hospital for treatment of acute my-
    eloid leukemia, which was diagnosed 1 month ago. Her husband passed
    away 1 year ago from a cancer that he had battled for 2 years. She reports
    seeing a therapist for the past 2 years while dealing with her husband's ill-
    ness and death. Her primary care team noted that she is frequently tearful
    in the hospital and asked for a psychiatric evaluation. On interview, she re-
    ports feeling sad much of the day but that she is trying to stay upbeat about
    her treatment. She also reports feelings of guilt and hopelessness. Her ap-
    petite and sleep have been poor, and she has lost 50 pounds since the death
    of her husband. She reports feeling isolated from friends and family as well.
    She makes a vague complaint of anxiety, which "comes and goes" through-
    out the day and is being treated with a round-the-clock schedule of benzo-
    diazepines. She says that she "does not care if cancer kills her too."What is
    the likely diagnosis?

    A. Major depressive disorder.
    B. Adjustment disorder.
    C. Generalized anxiety disorder.
    D. Uncomplicated bereavement.

    Answer: A

78. Each week a 52-year-old woman bakes bread using the recipe and tech-
    niques taught to her by her grandmother. She describes this behavior as an
    important "ritual" in her life. When does this behavior become a symptom
    that would appropriately be considered a part of a diagnostic assessment?

    A. At all times this behavior should be considered a symptom.
    B. At no time should this behavior be considered a symptom.
    C. When engaging in this behavior is no longer of interest or becomes distress-
       ing to her.
    D. When engaging in this behavior is very time consuming for her.

    Answer: C

79. Hallucinations and delusions feature prominently in schizophrenia. In
    their absence, it is still possible to meet diagnostic criteria for schizophre-
    nia, but this would require the presence of which of the following symp-
    toms?

    A. Agitated behavior.
    B. Catatonia.
    C. Disorganized speech.
    D. Negative symptoms.

    Answer: C

80. Which statement is correct regarding the World Health Organization Disability Assessment Schedule 2.0 included in DSM-5-TR?

    A. The scale assesses only the three most important domains of hallucinations, delusions, and disorganized speech.
    B. The scale is based on symptoms experienced by the patient in the previous 7 days.
    C. The scale is most accurate if patients, rather than clinicians, provide the responses.
    D. The scale should only be completed if the clinician is certain of the symptom severity.

    Answer: B

81. Eddy is in first grade. Since kindergarten, his mother reports, Eddy has not seemed to fit in with his classmates. He has a difficult time fully engaging in conversations with them. Instead, he seems to talk "at" them. For example, in a monotone voice he persistently shares elaborate and detailed information about his favorite subject, classic cars, even when the other kids are very disinterested. Although Eddy met all motor milestones appropriately, he often exhibits a repetitive behavior of stacking his cars in a line. What is the likely diagnosis?

    A. Global developmental delay.
    B. Language disorder.
    C. Autism spectrum disorder.
    D. Social phobia.

    Answer: C

82. Eight-year-old Liam wets the bed approximately 2 nights a week. He has been invited to a weeklong summer sleep-away camp but feels afraid to go because of the bedwetting. He is particularly upset because he did not have this problem the previous year. He feels a little less embarrassed when he finds out that his dad had the same problem when he was a boy. His father moved out of the home the previous year after marital separation. Liam does not take any medications, nor does he have any known medical problems. What is the likely diagnosis?

    A. Enuresis, diurnal only.
    B. Enuresis, nocturnal only.
    C. Enuresis, nocturnal and diurnal.
    D. Encopresis.

    Answer: B

83. Police arrest a 26-year-old man for smashing the windows of a coworker's car after an argument at work. The man's wife says that he has a history of destroying property or items of value when provoked, in a manner that is "extreme"as compared with the magnitude of the inciting trigger or event. He denies any history of head trauma, difficulty with attention, depressed or labile mood, restlessness, or any problems with sleep or appetite. When he is not provoked, he is calm and pleasant. He denies any alcohol or substance use, and his wife corroborates this information. There is no evidence of fidgeting or psychomotor agitation on examination. What is the likely diagnosis?

    A. Attention-deficit/hyperactivity disorder.
    B. Bipolar I disorder.
    C. Intermittent explosive disorder.
    D. Panic disorder.

    Answer: C

84. James is a 66-year-old moderately obese man with a long history of hypertension. He is seen for a follow-up appointment after his second stroke, which happened about 2 months ago. He reports that the weakness in his right leg is improving with physical therapy, but he has had difficulty finding his way back from the rehabilitation center, which is only a few blocks away from his home. His wife reports that after James's first stroke, which happened about 2 years ago, he started having memory difficulties. James used to enjoy playing chess with his grandchildren, but his memory deteriorated so significantly after his second stroke that he is unable to play and even forgets their names frequently. James is pleasant and well-articulated but shows significant difficulty finding words. He is not oriented to time, performs poorly in calculation, and is unable to name familiar objects such as a pen or watch. While reviewing his medications, James shows significant difficulty remembering the medications' names and instructions. He appears frustrated and asks for a pen to write down the instructions. What is the likely diagnosis?

    A. Delirium.
    B. Major neurocognitive disorder due to Alzheimer's disease.
    C. Major neurocognitive disorder due to another medical condition.
    D. Major vascular neurocognitive disorder.

    Answer: D

85. Match each description with the paraphilia diagnosis for which it is most highly characteristic (you may use each disorder once, more than once, or not at all):
    _____ Involves exposing one's genitalia to unsuspecting people.
    _____ Involves intense sexual arousal from observing an unsuspecting person disrobing or being naked.

_____ Involves intense sexual arousal from prepubescent or early pubescent children.

_____ Involves intense sexual arousal from the significant physical or psychological distress of another person.

A. Exhibitionistic disorder.
B. Fetishistic disorder.
C. Pedophilic disorder.
D. Sexual sadism disorder.
E. Voyeuristic disorder.

Answers: A, E, C, D

86. A 20-year-old college freshman is brought to the attention of her resident assistant for not attending meals in the dining hall. The student says she feels anxious about being in the crowded kitchen and dining hall. Similarly, she has ordered all of her schoolbooks online to avoid being in the bookstore because of her anxiety and discomfort. She also has not attended some of her crowded lectures. The student is able to have a good conversation in the hall of the dorm with the resident assistant and denies fearing scrutiny by others. She explains that she avoids some places because she found that in malls or other crowded areas, she feels very worried, faint, diaphoretic, and dizzy, as though she is losing control, and she fears she cannot escape. What is the likely diagnosis?

A. Acute stress disorder.
B. Agoraphobia.
C. Posttraumatic stress disorder.
D. Social anxiety disorder.

Answer: B

87. Using the DSM-5-TR criteria to "diagnose" celebrities is not considered ethically acceptable in the professions for many reasons, but especially for which reason?

A. Celebrities do not like to be diagnosed.
B. Media do not accurately portray celebrities.
C. The DSM-5-TR diagnostic criteria do not apply to celebrities.
D. The DSM-5-TR diagnostic criteria rely on information gathered through a comprehensive evaluation.

Answer: D

88. A mother learns during a conference with her 6-year-old son's schoolteacher that her son tends to blurt out answers when students are asked to raise their hands. Also, he often intrudes on other children's activities during

playtime, which has caused some disputes with his classmates. The mother notes that he often forgets to bring home his schoolwork. In addition, he will often willingly start a chore around the house, such as cleaning his room, but then switch to another activity and fail to finish the original task. What is the likely diagnosis?

A. Attention-deficit/hyperactivity disorder.
B. Obsessive-compulsive disorder.
C. Oppositional defiant disorder.
D. Tourette's disorder.

Answer: A

89. Marcus is a 45-year-old high-powered businessman. His employees often commiserate about their difficulties working with him. They say he seems arrogant and self-obsessed. He was overheard stating, "With my leadership track record, I should be running the whole country!" He is prone to retaliate and humiliate others when he receives even gentle constructive criticism. His employees feel used and manipulated by him. They feel he has no empathy for them, yet he seems to desire their reassurance much of the time. In his personal life, Marcus has been divorced three times "because my wives were way too jealous of me." What is the likely diagnosis?

A. Antisocial personality disorder.
B. Borderline personality disorder.
C. Histrionic personality disorder.
D. Narcissistic personality disorder.

Answer: D

90. Match each description with the personality disorder for which it is most highly characteristic (you may use each disorder once, more than once, or not at all):
_____ Behavior that is odd, eccentric, or peculiar, with odd beliefs or magical thinking that influence behavior and are inconsistent with cultural norms.
_____ Neither desires nor enjoys close relationships, with emotional coldness, detachment, or flattened affective responses to others.
_____ Suspects that others are exploiting or deceiving them, and persistently bears a grudge against others for perceived insults or slights.

A. Avoidant personality disorder.
B. Paranoid personality disorder.
C. Schizoid personality disorder.
D. Schizotypal personality disorder.

Answers: D, C, B

91. Match each term with the correct definition (you may use each term once, more than once, or not at all):

    _____ Inability to comprehend language despite intact sensory function.
    _____ Inability to perform motor activities despite intact motor function.
    _____ Inability to produce language despite intact motor function.
    _____ Inability to recognize objects despite intact sensory function.

    A. Agnosia.
    B. Anhedonia.
    C. Aphasia.
    D. Apraxia.

    Answers: C, D, C, A

92. Myra is a 29-year-old graduate student. Her boyfriend broke up with her 2 months ago, and she continues to feel devastated. She immediately moved back into her parents' home for support. Her parents are used to this, she says, because "this happens all the time." Her parents help her with everything, including choosing her clothes each morning, washing her laundry, and making all of her meals. They recall, "Her boyfriends would always pay her bills and even choose her friends for her. She has never made it on her own." Despite their concerns, in many ways her parents like having her at home because she is always agreeable and respectful. She even volunteers to scrub all the bathrooms from top to bottom, "whatever I have to do so you will let me stay here until I find a new boyfriend." What is the likely diagnosis?

    A. Avoidant personality disorder.
    B. Borderline personality disorder.
    C. Dependent personality disorder.
    D. Generalized anxiety disorder.

    Answer: C

93. Nia is in second grade. Last year her paternal grandfather died from cancer. Since then, her parents have become increasingly concerned about her. Last week a babysitter said that Nia sat staring at the front door almost the entire night, waiting for her parents to return from their date night. Nia keeps asking to stay home from school. She pleads for her mother to stay home with her, stating, "I do not want you to drive to work. What if you get in an accident? Just stay home with me." Before she goes to bed at night, she complains of headaches, which only seem to subside if she sleeps in her parents' room. They have stopped allowing her to sleep there, but some mornings they find her sleeping in the hallway right outside their bedroom door. She refuses to attend sleepovers with friends because she always feels "sick" while she is there. What is the likely diagnosis?

A. Major depressive disorder.
B. Panic disorder and agoraphobia.
C. Separation anxiety disorder.
D. Social anxiety disorder.

Answer: C

94. What is the time criterion for oppositional defiant disorder symptom manifestation for patients age 5 or older?

A. Must occur once per week for at least 3 months.
B. Must occur most days for at least 3 months.
C. Must occur once per week for at least 6 months.
D. Must occur twice per week for at least 6 months.

Answer: C

95. To receive a diagnosis of bipolar I disorder, an individual must have experienced in the past which of the following events, even if the event was not formally diagnosed and did not lead to an episode of clinical care?

A. Manic episode.
B. Depressive episode.
C. Head injury.
D. Psychological trauma.

Answer: A

96. Police bring a 34-year-old woman to the hospital after neighbors called them to her apartment to investigate a burning smell. They found her naked, with excoriations all over her body, which she claims are caused by "worms and lice" that have infested her skin. In her stove, the police found masses of burnt clothing, which the patient says she was "disinfecting." During the interview, the patient keeps turning her head, as if responding to a sound, and demands, "Turn down that horrible music," before she begins to laugh because she sees "like, Disney characters, like, Barbara Bush, coming 'poof' out of your head." She denies any recent substance use and becomes verbally abusive when her urine toxicology result comes back positive for methamphetamines. She accuses a nurse of "pissing into my cup" and has to be restrained when she attempts to strike the nurse. She does not have a history of mental illness. What is the likely diagnosis?

A. Borderline personality disorder.
B. Schizoaffective disorder, bipolar type.
C. Schizophrenia.
D. Substance/medication-induced psychotic disorder.

Answer: D

97. Police bring a woman to the hospital after they find her in an alley behind a restaurant. She appears to be in her late twenties. She cannot say who she is or where she lives and is considered gravely disabled. When asked what she was doing earlier, she recounts a reasonable story about having dinner at a restaurant and then having a few drinks. However, she looks worn, as though she has been exposed to the elements for hours or days. Her results are negative for alcohol and drugs on laboratory testing. Aside from mild dehydration, she is medically stable. Physical examination shows no neurological abnormalities. Finally, staff members find in her belongings an employee identification card from a mall where a shooting occurred 2 days earlier. When asked about that event, she has no recollection of it and seems unbothered. Her speech is clear and fluent, and she denies any perceptual changes. Police match her to a missing person report that her mother placed the previous day. What is the likely diagnosis?

    A. Bipolar I disorder.
    B. Depersonalization/derealization disorder.
    C. Dissociative amnesia with dissociative fugue.
    D. Schizophrenia.

    Answer: C

98. Police arrest a 26-year-old man who got into a fight at a bar after he was discovered in the act of stealing the wallet of another customer. He defended his behavior to the police, stating that the other man had provoked him earlier in the evening by calling him a profane name. Review of his criminal record reveals charges, including some as a minor, for credit card fraud and selling cocaine. He lives alone and is currently unemployed. He has no psychiatric history and does not report any recent hallucinations or changes in his mood or sleep. What is the likely diagnosis?

    A. Antisocial personality disorder.
    B. Conduct disorder.
    C. Narcissistic personality disorder.
    D. Stimulant use disorder, moderate, cocaine.

    Answer: A

99. Rachel is a 37-year-old single mother. She divorced her husband about 8 months ago and has custody of their two daughters. She went back to work full-time to make ends meet. About 2 months ago, while at work, she began to feel extremely anxious. Within a few minutes, she developed heart palpitations and difficulty breathing and almost fainted. Her coworkers rushed her to the hospital; however, the thorough medical workup was unrevealing. Within 1 week, she had another attack at the local grocery store and felt embarrassed because she had to lay down on the floor for about 10 minutes while she was surrounded by the store's concerned customers until the symptoms subsided. She has had two other attacks in different sit-

uations. She has constant concern that another panic attack may happen. She has been skipping meetings at work to avoid embarrassment in front of her coworkers in case she "goes crazy" again. What is the likely diagnosis?

A. Panic disorder.
B. Generalized anxiety disorder.
C. Social anxiety disorder.
D. Specific phobia.

Answer: A

100. Tara is struggling in second grade. Her teacher called her parents for a conference because of concerns that she is forgetful in class, is often daydreaming, and has difficulty following multistep directions. Her mother noted that "in second grade there is some real homework, and she cannot sit down and focus on doing it. Half the time she even forgets it at home in the morning." Her teacher recalls careless errors Tara made on simple mathematics assignments. Her father reminds them, "She has been this way for years! You cannot get her to focus, even if it is on making her bed or brushing her teeth." What is the likely diagnosis?

A. Conduct disorder.
B. Major depressive disorder.
C. Attention-deficit/hyperactivity disorder, predominantly hyperactive/impulsive presentation.
D. Attention-deficit/hyperactivity disorder, predominantly inattentive presentation.

Answer: D

101. Which diagnosis was added to the depressive disorders category of DSM-5 and DSM-5-TR that did not appear in earlier versions of DSM?

A. Prolonged grief disorder.
B. Premenstrual dysphoric disorder.
C. Persistent depressive disorder.
D. Disruptive mood dysregulation disorder.

Answer: B

102. The hematology service requests that a 45-year-old nurse receive a psychiatric consult because they cannot find a cause for her generalized bruising, for which she has been on their service three times in the past 5 months. She is not taking any medications. On interview, she is very tearful. Bruising is predominantly circumferential on her arms and legs, with none on her face or torso. She does have some venipuncture marks on her abdomen, however, as well as a wristband from another hospital. She appreciates the con-

sult but asks the psychiatrist to leave when her ex-husband comes for his daily visit to watch videos of their daughter. She explains that they lost their daughter to a chronic illness at age 8. What is the likely diagnosis?

A. Conversion disorder.
B. Factitious disorder.
C. Malingering.
D. Somatic symptom disorder.

Answer: B

103. Xavier is a 16-year-old high school student. He reports trying to intentionally lose weight over the past year. At this time, Xavier started counting calories and continues to set strict calorie limits each day. He also stopped eating foods high in sugars and fats that he previously enjoyed, including all desserts. He currently only eats fruits, vegetables, and lean proteins. Xavier plays on his school's soccer team and practices three times a week. On days that Xavier does not have soccer practice, he reports spending at least 2 hours at the gym. Over the past 6 months, he has lost 20 pounds. His weight is currently 125% of expected BMI for his age. Xavier reports that he plans to lose more weight and expresses a definite fear of becoming fat. He denies intentional vomiting or using laxatives, diuretics, or diet pills. He also denies binge eating. He reports experiencing dizziness, syncope, and constipation. His parents noticed that Xavier is less social, more irritable, and has trouble sleeping. Xavier continues to succeed academically, and his parents deny any additional concerns beyond his eating and health. Based on this information, what is the most likely diagnosis?

A. Avoidant/restrictive food intake disorder.
B. Bulimia nervosa.
C. Binge-eating disorder.
D. Other specified feeding or eating disorder (atypical anorexia nervosa).

Answer: D

104. To diagnose paraphilia, a behavior must manifest for which of the following durations?

A. 1 week.
B. 1 month.
C. 6 months.
D. 12 months.

Answer: C

105. A 22-year-old college student presents to a mental health clinic for an initial visit. She has not turned in any of her papers on time this term because she

worries about getting poor grades, and this worry has affected her ability to concentrate. She is also very concerned about getting a job after she graduates, despite multiple meetings with a career counselor. She says that she is concerned with the sanitation at the local gym and prefers not to play recreational sports because she might be injured. She does not have any rituals or checking behaviors. She describes her mood as "irritable" and says that she feels "tense all the time." Her appetite has not changed, and she continues to enjoy watching movies. She denies low energy and has not had any thoughts of harming herself. She tried cocaine last year but has not used any illicit substances or alcohol recently. What is the likely diagnosis?

A. Adjustment disorder.
B. Generalized anxiety disorder.
C. Major depressive disorder.
D. Obsessive-compulsive disorder.

Answer: B

106. John is a 24-year-old veteran who was involved in combat in the Middle East, where he was exposed to a few explosions. Since he returned about 4 months ago, he has had difficulty sleeping and has experienced frequent nightmares. He has avoided going out because any loud noise startles him, disturbs him significantly, and brings back memories of the explosions. He sees himself as a failure and believes that he was not strong enough to tolerate combat. When his friends approached him, their comments and jokes irritated him, and he isolated himself more. He has not been able to concentrate well and failed to pass the online courses he had been taking for his college degree. His mother has become increasingly concerned and encouraged him to come to the clinic. What is the likely diagnosis?

A. Acute stress disorder.
B. Adjustment disorder.
C. Posttraumatic stress disorder.
D. Social anxiety disorder.

Answer: C

107. Which statement is correct regarding the schizophrenia spectrum and other psychotic disorders category of DSM-5 and DSM-5-TR in comparison with earlier versions of DSM?

A. Elimination of duration criteria for the diagnosis of schizophrenia.
B. Elimination of the negative symptom criteria.
C. Elimination of the requirement for a delusion, hallucination, or disorganized speech for the diagnosis of schizophrenia.
D. Elimination of the subtypes of schizophrenia, except the catatonia specifier.

Answer: D

108. A 16-year-old presents to his high school counselor after running out of his programming class because he was asked to explain a piece of code. He had trouble answering and had felt this sort of difficulty in the past, but today it was worse. He is not able to explain clearly to the counselor what happened because he was still having the same speaking problems as he had in class. He has broken words, keeps getting stuck on sounds like "aye" and "ah." He seems to spit out words. He writes down on a piece of paper that he has been thinking about dropping out of school because of his difficulty speaking; his older brother dropped out of school for similar problems. The counselor later observes him working in the computer lab and notices no abnormal behavior. What is the likely diagnosis?

    A. Autism spectrum disorder.
    B. Childhood-onset fluency disorder.
    C. Social anxiety disorder.
    D. Tourette's disorder.

    Answer: B

109. An 18-year-old presents to the clinic after 6 weeks of low mood and trouble sleeping. At first, she attributed her poor sleep to getting up every 2 hours to feed her 8-week-old daughter, but more recently, her mother has been caring for the baby at night. Despite this, the patient reports continuing poor sleep, with low energy and poor concentration. She is less interested in leaving the house and seeing others and less excited about playing with her daughter. She is not very interested in eating but pushes herself to eat, "because I want to make good milk for the baby." She denies wanting to harm herself or others and feels that, with her mother's help, she is able to care for the baby well. What is the likely diagnosis?

    A. Bipolar I disorder, current episode depressed, with peripartum onset.
    B. Major depressive disorder, unspecified.
    C. Major depressive disorder, with peripartum onset.
    D. Persistent depressive disorder.

    Answer: C

110. Which of the following symptom profiles most likely indicates the diagnosis of delirium?

    A. Disorientation, fluctuating attention and awareness, hallucinations.
    B. Anhedonia, hopelessness, fatigue.
    C. Defensiveness, inability to compromise.
    D. Euphoria, risky behavior, disrupted sleep.
    E. Disorganized speech, blunted affect, hallucinations.

    Answer: A

111. Which statement is correct regarding how DSM-5-TR diagnoses and documents personality disorders?

    A. DSM-5-TR has eliminated personality disorder diagnoses.
    B. DSM-5-TR has introduced new personality disorder subtypes.
    C. DSM-5-TR has maintained the use of the Axis II system for documenting personality disorders.
    D. DSM-5-TR has preserved the same diagnostic criteria as in DSM-IV-TR for personality disorders.

    Answer: D

112. A 32-year-old woman is brought to the emergency department by her daughter, who witnessed the patient having a "shaking spell" after learning that the patient's husband had an extramarital affair. In the emergency department, the patient has an event characterized by shaking movements that progress into wildly thrashing movements. The patient calls out her husband's name several times during the spell. The event lasts approximately 1 minute. Following the event, the patient resumes a conversation with her daughter, who is at bedside. Which is the most appropriate next step in the evaluation?

    A. Obtain an electroencephalogram.
    B. Discharge with reassurance.
    C. Initiate an anticonvulsant.
    D. Referral to psychodynamic psychotherapy.
    E. Admit to inpatient psychiatry.

    Answer: A

113. A 26-year-old woman is admitted to the hospital for a workup of hypoglycemia after she fainted at work. The patient states that she enjoys her position and finds her work rewarding. She is looking forward to coworkers visiting her while hospitalized. Prior to her scheduled discharge, the nurse noticed an empty insulin vial in her bed; however, the patient does not have a diagnosis of diabetes. What is the most likely diagnosis?

    A. Malingering.
    B. Factitious disorder.
    C. Somatic symptom disorder.
    D. Functional neurological symptom disorder.
    E. Borderline personality disorder.

    Answer: B

114. True or False: Suicidality is a common problem among those with a dissociative disorder.

A. True.
B. False.

Answer: A

115. Which of the following is required to make a diagnosis of schizoaffective disorder?

   A. The presence of psychosis during a mood episode.
   B. The presence of psychosis outside of a mood episode.
   C. Mood symptoms are present any time there is psychosis.
   D. Criteria for either psychosis or a mood episode are met at all times.

Answer: B

116. Match each term with the correct definition (you may use each term once, more than once, or not at all):
   _____ Repeated behavior that a person feels driven to perform.
   _____ Repeated expression of psychological issues through physical symptoms, concerns, or complaints.
   _____ Repeated, irrational, and enduring fear of an object or situation.
   _____ Repeated thought or image that provokes anxiety.

   A. Compulsion.
   B. Obsession.
   C. Phobia.
   D. Somatization.

Answers: A, D, C, B

117. A 21-year-old college student is preoccupied with the appearance of her nose. She has a small, 0.2-cm soft tissue nodule from a biking accident many years ago, but the area is well healed. She feels it is a serious flaw on her face, however, and is thinking about plastic surgery to correct the defect. She is concerned about dating anyone as long as she has this nodule on her nose, although she continues to enjoy spending time with friends. She denies any pain or discomfort, and she has no concerns about her body weight, which is average for her height. She continues to bike the same route daily at school. What is the likely diagnosis?

   A. Anorexia.
   B. Posttraumatic stress disorder.
   C. Body dysmorphic disorder.
   D. Somatic symptom disorder.

Answer: C

118. A mother brings her 3-year-old daughter to the pediatrician because she "does not talk very much." Her vocabulary consists of only 10 words, and she speaks only 1 word at a time. Her past medical history is notable for delays in developmental milestones: she walked independently by age 2, developed a pincer grasp at age 15 months, and continues to have stranger anxiety. The result of a hearing test completed in the clinic was normal. What is the likely diagnosis?

    A. Autism spectrum disorder.
    B. Global developmental delay.
    C. Selective mutism.
    D. Tic disorder.

    Answer: B

119. A 28-year-old woman seeks psychiatric consultation. She says that 10 years ago, she had a panic attack while presenting her project at the high school science fair. Since then, she has developed an intense fear of being embarrassed or humiliated in a public venue. She is constantly worried that others are scrutinizing her. She is very self-conscious and afraid that she will have heart palpitations, trembling, or stuttering or that her mind will go blank. She refuses to go on dates and is not being considered for a new job because she declined the interview. She is tired of living such an isolated life. What is the likely diagnosis?

    A. Avoidant personality disorder.
    B. Obsessive-compulsive disorder.
    C. Panic disorder.
    D. Social anxiety disorder.

    Answer: D

120. A 12-year-old girl persistently misbehaves at home. She called 911, reporting that her parents were forcing her to go to school and claiming they were hitting her. She also locked her younger siblings out of the house in cold weather. Although her parents attempt to set limits, she frequently responds with prolonged tantrums and attempts to get revenge. After one serious tantrum, her parents took her to the emergency department. She was hospitalized and viewed as quite charming by several members of the staff, whereas others thought she was "a very, very difficult patient."What is the likely diagnosis?

    A. Attention-deficit/hyperactivity disorder.
    B. Conduct disorder.
    C. Intermittent explosive disorder.
    D. Oppositional defiant disorder.

    Answer: D

121. The emergency department calls a psychiatrist to evaluate a 35-year-old man who was brought in by police after he was found in a park yelling at passers-by. The patient explains that he has been experiencing homelessness for the past 8 years, since emigrating from a small island nation. He describes having a special relationship with animals, with whom he can communicate telepathically. He reports that this communication with nature is a common belief in his culture and that he has this special "gift." He says that he receives "special signals" from birds that influence his behavior, and he can "hear them talking to him." He is notably emaciated and malodorous, with poor hygiene. He acknowledges that his eating schedule may seem unusual to others, but that he eats when instructed to do so by the animals. He has been itinerant, so has few social connections, but has recently received some support through a church attended by people from his country of origin. Nothing is found on urine drug toxicology. What is the likely diagnosis?

    A. Delusional disorder.
    B. Culturally appropriate behavior.
    C. Major depressive disorder with psychotic features.
    D. Schizophrenia.

    Answer: D

122. In the previous example (question 121), the patient's belief that he receives special messages from animals dictating his eating schedule is most likely an example of which of the following?

    A. Culturally appropriate belief.
    B. Delusion of reference.
    C. Idea of reference.
    D. Magical thinking.

    Answer: B

123. In the previous example (question 121), which of the following information would support a diagnosis of schizophrenia?

    A. The patient's disturbance has been present for 8 months.
    B. The patient reports that he feels so depressed he no longer enjoys books that used to fascinate him.
    C. The patient has been using psychoactive substances for religious purposes.
    D. The patient's parents report developmental delays and that he was always "quirkier" than his siblings.

    Answer: A

124. A 34-year-old woman presents to the emergency department for new suicidal thoughts. She describes worsening depression and isolation from her

friends and family over the past month. She feels tired all day but still has difficulty falling asleep at night. Her self-care has markedly declined, and she has not showered in 5 days. When asked about symptoms of psychosis, she endorses concerns about being watched by her neighbors, as well as hearing voices that make derogatory statements about her. She had several previous depressive episodes and two psychiatric hospitalizations with similar presentations. What additional information would most support a diagnosis of schizoaffective disorder?

A. Her auditory hallucinations are present only in the context of her mood symptoms.
B. She has had at least one manic episode.
C. She has periods of hearing voices for weeks without depressed or elevated mood.
D. She has heard similar voices before when she was depressed.
E. She is experiencing both hallucinations and delusions.

Answer: C

125. Which disorder involves both a loss of control over eating and performance of compensatory behaviors, such as self-induced vomiting or laxative use?

A. Binge-eating disorder.
B. Rumination disorder.
C. Bulimia nervosa.
D. Pica.

Answer: C

126. A wife brings her husband, a 55-year-old with chronic conditions of diabetes, obesity, and hypercholesteremia, to his primary care doctor. She is upset that her husband has no energy to go on outings with her, that he is always tired—even though he would like to do things with the family, he consistently declines to do so. She gave him her own prescription for sleeping medication ("I know I should not do that! I was just hoping it would help us!"), but all that she noticed is that he snored "more than usual." She is worried about the well-being of their marriage, given her husband's changes. The husband notes that he is interested in life, their marriage, going out to dinner, and so on, but he does not know why he feels so exhausted. What is the likely diagnosis?

A. Adjustment disorder.
B. Anorexia.
C. Major depressive disorder.
D. Obstructive sleep apnea hypopnea.

Answer: D

127. The neurology department refers a 39-year-old Latina woman to psychiatry because she has been experiencing tonic-clonic movements of extremities without loss of consciousness for the past 2 months. The extensive neurological workup was unrevealing. The patient is cooperative throughout the session but shows restricted range of affect. Her husband says that she has been under treatment for infertility for many years and miscarried a very expected pregnancy approximately 3 months ago. She does not show significant changes in her affect in reaction to this information from her husband. What is the likely diagnosis?

    A. Depressive disorder due to another medical condition.
    B. Factitious disorder.
    C. Functional neurological symptom disorder (conversion disorder).
    D. Somatic symptom disorder.

    Answer: C

128. Which statement is correct regarding the bipolar disorders category of DSM-5 and DSM-5-TR in comparison with earlier versions of DSM?

    A. Addition of increased activity or energy as a new core mood elevation symptom.
    B. Consolidation of bipolar disorder under the category of depressive disorders.
    C. Elimination of anxious distress as a feature of bipolar disorder.
    D. Elimination of cyclothymia.

    Answer: A

129. What is the time criterion for intermittent explosive disorder symptom manifestation?

    A. Once weekly for the past 3 months.
    B. Twice weekly for the past 3 months.
    C. Once weekly for 6 months.
    D. Twice weekly for 6 months.

    Answer: B

130. Partners in a long-term affectionate and intimate relationship have recently begun to "experiment" with wearing costumes with especially soft fabrics and engaging in role-play during their sexual encounters. They are enjoying this practice and find that it enriches their sexual life together. Does this pattern meet criteria for fetishistic disorder?

    A. No, because neither partner is experiencing distress.
    B. No, because soft fabrics do not represent a fetishistic object.

C. Yes, because role-playing represents a fetish.

D. Yes, because this "experimentation" is new.

Answer: A

131. A diagnosis of depersonalization/derealization disorder cannot be made if the symptoms are occurring exclusively in the context of

A. A major depressive episode.

B. Current panic disorder.

C. Posttraumatic stress disorder.

D. Dissociative identity disorder.

E. All of the above.

Answer: E

132. A 41-year-old man reports to the psychiatrist that he is afraid of dentists. He has a history of extreme anxiety on entering a dental office, to the point that he feels dizzy and nauseated. He becomes excessively anxious in the waiting room and has a very difficult time completing visits. He is so fearful about dentists that he reports he cannot take his own children to their dentist because he has "anxiety attacks" in the office. Rather, he insists that his wife take the children. His aversion of dentists has led to his missing regular appointments for more than 6 years. He plans to go soon, only because he has severe tooth pain and believes he may need a root canal. He does not have anxiety in other contexts. What is the likely diagnosis?

A. Adjustment disorder with anxiety.

B. Generalized anxiety disorder.

C. Posttraumatic stress disorder.

D. Specific phobia.

Answer: D

133. A 35-year-old man with a history of migraine headaches and hypertension presents for a routine follow-up appointment with his primary care physician. According to the patient's electronic medical record, the patient has had more than 10 emergency department visits for headaches and dizziness in the past 8 months. At those visits, he requests head imaging as he believes a brain tumor is causing his symptoms. Head imaging to date has not revealed any abnormalities. The patient feels like the physicians are being dismissive of his concerns. He has joined online support groups for individuals with brain cancer so he "can learn what to anticipate after the diagnosis." What is the most likely diagnosis?

A. Illness anxiety disorder.

B. Adjustment disorder.

C. Somatic symptom disorder.
D. Generalized anxiety disorder.
E. Obsessive-compulsive disorder.

Answer: A

Index

Page numbers printed in **boldface** *type refer to tables or figures.*